Biocultural Aspects of Disease

Contributors

William B. Bean

William E. Bertrand

Wilma B. Bias

Denis P. Burkitt

Horacio Fabrega, Jr.

Jeffrey R. Fisher

Robert R. Franklin

Ralph M. Garruto

Leonard Hayflick

Claude F. Jacobs

B. Krompholz

Reijo Norio

Koji Ohkura

D. F. Roberts

Robert S. Robins

Henry Rothschild

Maurice L. Sievers

V. Simko

Rosalind Y. Ting

Elizabeth S. Watts

Anthony B. Way

Biocultural Aspects of Disease

Edited by
Henry Rothschild

Department of Medicine and Anatomy
Louisiana State University Medical Center
New Orleans, Louisiana

Coordinating Editor
Charles F. Chapman

Editorial Office
Louisiana State University Medical Center
New Orleans, Louisiana

1981

ACADEMIC PRESS
A Subsidiary of Harcourt Brace Jovanovich, Publishers
New York   London
Paris   San Diego   San Francisco   São Paulo   Sydney   Tokyo   Toronto

ACADEMIC PRESS, INC.
111 Fifth Avenue, New York, New York 10003

United Kingdom Edition published by
ACADEMIC PRESS, INC. (LONDON) LTD.
24/28 Oval Road, London NW1 7DX

Library of Congress Cataloging in Publication Data
Main entry under title:

Biocultural aspects of disease.

Includes bibliographies and index.
1. Epidemiology. 2. Health and race. 3. Medical
anthropology. 4. Medical geography. I. Rothschild,
Henry, Date. [DNLM: 1. Anthropology, Physical.
2. Ethnology. 3. Disease. WA 300 B615]
RA651.B53   616.07'1   81-12714
ISBN 0-12-598720-X   AACR2

PRINTED IN THE UNITED STATES OF AMERICA

81 82 83 84   9 8 7 6 5 4 3 2 1

To Tanea, Shoshana, and Jamin

Contents

I Conceptual

1 The Biological Race Concept and Diseases of Modern Man

ELIZABETH S. WATTS

2 Changing Patterns of Ideas about Disease

WILLIAM B. BEAN

3 Culture, Biology, and the Study of Disease

HORACIO FABREGA, JR.

4 Genetic Polymorphisms and Human Disease

WILMA B. BIAS

5 Geography of Disease: Purpose of and Possibilities from Geographical Medicine

DENIS P. BURKITT

6 Disease, Political Events, and Populations

ROBERT S. ROBINS

7 Ethnic Groups: A Paradigm

HENRY ROTHSCHILD

II Populations and Disease

8 Diseases of North American Indians

MAURICE L. SIEVERS AND JEFFREY R. FISHER

13 Culture and Disease in Britain and Western Europe

D. F. ROBERTS

14 Diseases of Eastern Europeans

V. SIMKO AND B. KROMPHOLZ

15 Illness in Black Africans

ROBERT R. FRANKLIN, CLAUDE F. JACOBS, AND WILLIAM E.
BERTRAND

16 Diseases of Jews

HENRY ROTHSCHILD

17 Disease Patterns of Isolated Groups

RALPH M. GARRUTO

18 Genetic Disparities of Senescence

LEONARD HAYFLICK

List of Contributors

Numbers in parentheses indicate the pages on which the authors' contributions begin.

William B. Bean * (25), Institute for the Medical Humanities, University of Texas Medical Branch, Galveston, Texas 77550

William E. Bertrand (483), Department of Epidemiology and Biostatistics, Tulane University, Tulane School of Public Health and Tropical Medicine, New Orleans, Louisiana 70112

Wilma B. Bias (95), Department of Medicine, The Johns Hopkins University School of Medicine, and Department of Epidemiology, The School of Hygiene and Public Health, Baltimore, Maryland 21205

Denis P. Burkitt (133), Unit of Geographical Pathology, St. Thomas Hospital, London, England

Horacio Fabrega, Jr. (53), Departments of Psychiatry and Anthropology, University of Pittsburgh, Western Psychiatric Institute and Clinic, Pittsburgh, Pennsylvania 15261

Jeffrey R. Fisher (191), Department of Internal Medicine, Indian Health Service, Phoenix Indian Medical Center, Phoenix, Arizona 85016

Robert R. Franklin (483), Department of Epidemiology and Biostatistics, Tulane University, Tulane School of Public Health and Tropical Medicine, New Orleans, Louisiana 70112

Ralph M. Garruto (557), Laboratory of Central Nervous System Studies, National Institutes of Health, Bethesda, Maryland 20205, and Department of Medical Genetics, University of South Alabama Medical School, Mobile, Alabama 36688

Leonard Hayflick (599), Center for Gerontological Studies, University of Florida, Gainesville, Florida 32611

*Present address: Department of Internal Medicine, University of Iowa College of Medicine, Iowa City, Iowa 52242.

Claude F. Jacobs (483), Department of Epidemiology and Biostatistics, Tulane University, Tulane School of Public Health and Tropical Medicine, New Orleans, Louisiana 70112

Brigita Krompholz (459), Department of Epidemiology and Preventive Medicine, University of Maryland School of Medicine, Baltimore, Maryland 21201

Reijo Norio (359), Department of Medical Genetics, Väestöliitto (The Finnish Population and Family Welfare Federation), SF-00100 Helsinki, Finland

*Koji Ohkura** (293), Department of Human Genetics, Medical Research Institute, Tokyo Medical and Dental University, Tokyo, Japan

D. F. Roberts (417), Department of Human Genetics, University of Newcastle-Upon-Tyne, Newcastle-Upon-Tyne, NE24AA, England

Robert S. Robins (153), Department of Political Science, College of Arts and Sciences, Tulane University, New Orleans, Louisiana 70118

Henry Rothschild (177, 531), Department of Medicine and Anatomy, Louisiana State University Medical Center, New Orleans, Louisiana 70112

Maurice L. Sievers (191), Department of Internal Medicine, Indian Health Service, Phoenix Indian Medical Center, Phoenix, Arizona 85016

V. Simko (459), Department of Internal Medicine, College of Medicine, University of Cincinnati, Cincinnati, Ohio 45267

Rosalind Y. Ting (327), Department of Pediatrics, University of Pennsylvania School of Medicine, and The Children's Hospital of Philadelphia, Philadelphia, Pennsylvania 19104

Elizabeth S. Watts (3), Department of Anthropology, Tulane University, College of Arts and Sciences, New Orleans, Louisiana 70118

Anthony B. Way (253), Department of Preventive Medicine and Community Health, Texas Tech University Health Sciences Center, Lubbock, Texas 79430

*Present address: Yushima 1-5, Bunkyo-ku, Tokyo, Japan 113.

Preface

The ancient Greeks had no difficulty accounting for the differences in, and the existence of, things and beings, surrendering graciously to artful myth where reason was limited or inelastic. Brought to observe that some men are dark-skinned and others light-skinned, they attributed the variation in skin color to sun and climate by this fable: Sun god Helios let his son, Phaethon, drive the golden sun chariot across the sky, and, in the pattern of wayward youth, the lad-god drove too close to some parts of the earth, burning black the skin of the people there, and too far from the other parts, causing the people of those regions to pale from the cold.

Since that time, observable differences among peoples have led scientists to consider race as an aid in classification in defining normal health and in diagnosis and treatment of disease. Unfortunately, stereotyping people by highly visible characteristics has often led to a sociological definition of race and to rationalizing racism and preconceptions. The enslavement of blacks in America and the Nazi atrocities in Europe were "justified" by a doctrine of racial supremacy. Even with the advance of science during the nineteenth and twentieth centuries, including the Darwin-stimulated studies of Galton, Pearson, Spearman, and others, objectivity often was buried by intent, as has recently been shown of British psychologist Sir Cyril Burt's designs for education in England. These historical examples of the destructiveness of superficial racial classification aside, knowledge of culture, genetic traits, and diseases among specific ethnic groups is potentially useful.

This book attempts to explore the relationship of disease to ethnicity. Such knowledge may not only enable physicians to better understand the pathogenesis of diseases and thus improve treatment of individual patients, but it may also provide an economically feasible basis for screening populations for disease detection. Comparative ethnogenetics, a fresh field in which questions may be cultivated anew and unexpected insights harvested, may delineate some of the

xvii

factors of evolutionary change. Most importantly, however, knowledge of disease distribution may provide a model for studying the mechanisms underlying complex diseases and thereby help to distinguish between the roles of exogenous and endogenous factors in the causes and pathogenesis of these diseases.

Here we explore the role of genetics and culture in relation to disease, defining culture in terms of environmental, nutritional, or exogenous factors. The text is divided in two parts: a forepart that is conceptual and general, and an aftpart that is applicable and specific, providing in its major portion information on the demography of diseases in various ethnic groups and also attempting to systemize knowledge about the diseases of such groups.

Our choice of ethnic groups is selective rather than comprehensive and is focused on populations that have been influential in shaping the American culture. Because of the vastness of the theme, not all significant ethnic groups are included; many were excluded because information is scant, others merely because we could not include all such groups in one volume. The omission of any group in no way detracts from its significance. Contrariwise, some groups were included because information on them is extensive but has never been presented as a cohesive unit. To our knowledge, the information on such groups as the American Indians and the Chinese has not been organized previously into a comprehensive unit. Some chapters are mere surveys because the areas they cover are too immense or the pertinent data are not available in current medical literature, but each is a start at systematizing the data.

This book is interdisciplinary, with contributors representing a diversity of approaches and areas of expertise. Some of the authors are geneticists, others epidemiologists; some are clinicians, others basic scientists. Whereas some authors emphasized the practical, others focused on the philosophical aspects of their respective topics. Some chapters emphasize ethnogenetic diseases, but in others, especially those covering topics for which genetic data are scarce, other aspects are emphasized. The contributors were given carte blanche to pursue the question of biocultural aspects of diseases pertinent to their specific interests. Our guiding principle has been to retain the writing style of each contributor in his work while shaping the whole to conform to a consistent and readable text. Treatment of the subject matter differs in each chapter, and we did not attempt arbitrarily to produce uniformity of viewpoint or style.

The mass of knowledge cataloged is small in proportion to the vastness of the accumulated data. This book, structured to be both interesting and informative, is a beginning toward fulfilling the need for such a collection. Although the concept is not original, we are unaware of any comparable work. Several excellent books have been written on diseases affecting individual groups, such as Jews and Blacks, but none has comprehensively collected multiethnic information.

Knowledge of group variation in disease is important to many disciplines related to human biology and human health, most especially demography and public health. Sociologists and physical anthropologists must be aware of group differences when studying the interactions among persons. Geneticists, epidemiologists, and behavioral scientists, too, must consider these in their studies.

If this book whets the reader's appetite, stimulates interest, and highlights the need for gathering more data on biocultural interactions, it will have served well.

Henry Rothschild

I
Conceptual

1

The Biological Race Concept and Diseases of Modern Man

ELIZABETH S. WATTS

I. INTRODUCTION

Few subjects have been more controversial than the race concept in anthropology. Despite the assumption that they are the most knowledgeable about the evolutionary biology of the human species, contemporary physical anthropologists hold radically differing views of race. At one extreme is the position that human races are clear-cut biological entities deeply rooted in man's evolutionary past (Coon, 1962, 1965). At the other is the view that the concept of race is biologically invalid and totally inapplicable to *Homo sapiens* (Brace, 1964; Livingstone, 1964; Montagu, 1964a). Between these extreme positions lies the view that the race concept, though it has strong limitations and cannot be used uncritically, has some utility in teaching, research, and other activities that involve generalizing and communicating about genetically differing groups of mankind (Garn, 1961; Baker, 1967; Brues, 1977). Even those who agree that races can be delineated in man often differ about the number of racial categories to be defined and on the placement of various populations within them.

Given the lack of consensus among specialists, the nonanthropologist can

3

BIOCULTURAL ASPECTS OF DISEASE
Copyright © 1981 by Academic Press, Inc.
All rights of reproduction in any form reserved.
ISBN 0-12-598720-X

scarcely be blamed for understanding little of what race means biologically and what its legitimate uses might be with reference to the human species. This chapter presents some of the factors responsible for the confusion and controversy surrounding the racial classification of man, explains as clearly as possible what the race concept means in contemporary physical anthropology, and, finally, discusses briefly the utility of race for the understanding, prevention, and cure of human diseases.

II. PROBLEMS WITH THE CONCEPT OF RACE

Most of the problems pertaining to race in man relate to four main sets of causes: semantic, sociopolitical, historical, and evolutionary. Problems in each of these areas will be considered separately, for clarity, but the reader will come to realize that their occurrence is due to a set of interrelated causes that accompany the growth of scientific knowledge in many fields.

A. Semantic Ambiguities

The difficulty with the scientific utility of the race concept is partly semantic. The word "race" has many meanings and the physical anthropologist and the nonscientist use it differently. Compounding the problem of ambiguity is the word's frequent use in emotionally charged situations and contexts. Both the differences in meaning and the attached emotionalism have been cited as reasons for abandoning the use of "race" altogether in biological discourse.

Semantic difficulties with the word race stem from its many general meanings and, in particular, from the difference between its use in biological taxonomy and public parlance. Popular usage of the word reflects an underlying confusion about the nature of cultural and biological phenomena and the way they act and interact in human groups. The mixture of cultural behavior and biology in connection with race can be seen in older classifications that included both behavioral and somatic traits as racial characteristics, and in contemporary confusion between biological and sociological usage of the term.

One naive concept of race, which undoubtedly grew out of folk belief, was perpetuated in some of the earlier racial classifications of the eighteenth century, and still survives today among the scientifically ignorant and racially prejudiced. The belief is that biological attributes such as skin color, hair form, or facial features are somehow inextricably linked with emotional, mental, and behavioral characteristics in human racial groups. Figure 1 shows an example of such thinking—the 1758 racial classification of Linnaeus. Although this idea of linkage between physical features and behavior is totally unsupported by research in cultural anthropology or human behavioral genetics (Brace *et al.*, 1971), its

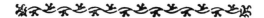

MAMMALIA.

ORDER I. PRIMATES.

Fore-teeth cutting; upper 4, parallel; teats 2 pectoral.

1. HOMO.

Sapiens. Diurnal; varying by education and fituation.
2. Four-footed, mute, hairy. *Wild Man.*
3. Copper-coloured, choleric, erect. *American.*
   Hair black, ftraight, thick; *noftrils* wide, *face* harfh; *beard*
   fcanty; *obftinate*, content free. *Paints* himfelf with fine red
   lines. *Regulated* by cuftoms.
4. Fair, fanguine, brawny. *European.*
   Hair yellow, brown, flowing; *eyes* blue; *gentle*, acute, inventive.
   Covered with clofe veftments. *Governed* by laws.
5. Sooty, melancholy, rigid. *Afiatic.*
   Hair black; *eyes* dark; *fevere*, haughty, covetous. *Covered*
   with loofe garments. *Governed* by opinions.
6. Black, phlegmatic, relaxed. *African.*
   Hair black, frizzled; *fkin* filky; *nofe* flat; *lips* tumid; *crafty,*
   indolent, negligent. *Anoints* himfelf with greafe. *Governed*
   by caprice.

Monftrofus Varying by climate or art.
1. Small, active, timid. *Mountaineer.*
2. Large, indolent. *Patagonian.*
3. Lefs fertile. *Hottentot.*
4. Beardlefs. *American.*
5. Head conic. *Chinefe.*
6. Head flattened. *Canadian.*

The anatomical, phyfiological, natural, moral, civil and focial
hiftories of man, are beft defcribed by their refpective writers.

Vol. I —C   2. SIMIA.

Fig. 1.   Racial classification of man published by Linnaeus. [From Sir Charles Linne, "A General System of Nature" (William Turton, transl.). Lackington, Allen, London, 1806. Courtesy of Rare Book Room, Perkins Library, Duke University.]

persistence is not difficult to understand. Cultural and genetic distinctiveness do tend to go together in human populations. The casual observer of human populations quickly notes the association between physical attributes and behaviors and, unfortunately, just as quickly draws erroneous conclusions about the nature of the relationship between the two.

In contemporary speech ''race'' more often refers to a person's membership in a socially defined group than in a biologically defined one. The term race is applied to culturally defined entities such as national, linguistic, or religious groups, as well as to genetically defined population groups. Because the public uses race most often in its sociological sense, Montagu (1964a), Alland (1971), and others have suggested that the word be omitted from biological discourse and ''ethnic group'' be substituted for its sociological meaning. This restricted usage would solve the problem of the lack of fit between genetic and social classifications in contemporary American society. Here, for example, many people of substantial European genetic background are socially classified as ''black'' or ''Afro-American,'' whereas others with even more African genetic ancestry than the former may be called ''Puerto Rican'' or ''Hispanic.'' Ethnic group, implying membership in a socially defined population, is appropriate in such situations. However, rather than drop the word race entirely, restricting its use to the biological meaning would be preferable. Coining substitute terms, such as genogroup, as suggested by Montagu (1964a), for race in the biological sense simply skirts the issue and perpetuates confusion. The best solution for the biologist is to define race as clearly as possible and continue to use the term in its appropriate biological sense.

I shall discuss the meaning of race in physical anthropology more thoroughly later in this chapter. For the moment, however, let race refer to a unit of biological taxonomy (i.e., a system of classification). Populations are classified into races on the basis of similarities and differences in the frequencies of their genes. These gene frequencies, and hence the classification based on them, should reflect the evolutionary relationships among the populations classified.

B. Sociopolitical Uses and Abuses

Homo sapiens has often been claimed to be the only species that contemplates itself. One source of constant challenge, but of real constraint, to the study of human evolutionary biology is humankind's pervading interest in itself. Statements about the evolution of fruit flies or bats may interest a handful of specialists, but when one speaks of man virtually everyone listens. In the study of man the potential impact of theories, facts, and discoveries on public life and thinking is indeed great. As will be evident below, public attitudes have also had a great deal of influence on scientific thinking about race. So when one deals with the human species, more than with any other, science is not separable from the rest of human existence.

Racial classifications, when the biologist uses them properly, are a way of characterizing the evolution of human populations below the species level, reflecting their time separation, degree of genetic divergence, and adaptation to the environments in which they live. For various reasons, notions of a qualitative dimension to racial categories, a ranking according to supposed superior or inferior characters, are sometimes implied or read into them. When this happens, racial classifications become tools to be used in promoting social and political oppression of groups of human beings. In these instances neither the classification itself, nor the act of classifying, need be questioned, but rather the supposed superior or inferior characters attributed to the peoples classified. In nearly all cases of the misuse of racial classifications to promote racism, the groups involved have been defined more socially than biologically. So-called racial prejudice is actually social prejudice, though it cannot be denied that genetically based phenotypic characteristics may trigger such prejudice and biological reasons given to justify it. To condemn all racial classifications on the grounds that they might be used to further social injustice would probably accomplish nothing. Any method for classifying human beings is potentially subject to that abuse, whether it be based on biological characteristics, such as sex, stature, and fatness, or cultural ones like religion, ethnic origin, or language. In fact, racial classifications are actually being used in the United States in attempts to enforce equal opportunity legislation and school desegregation; here again, however, the concept of race being used is more sociological than biological.

C. Historical Perspectives

Part of the problem with modern racial classification stems from its origins in the pre-evolutionary thought of the eighteenth century. The theoretical framework and purpose of biological taxonomy in general have undergone profound changes following the discoveries in evolution and genetics made during the past two centuries. However, despite these changes, several archaic ideas continued to be associated with the race concept as it was applied to man, long after major advances in biology, particularly evolutionary gentics, showed them to be untenable. Retention of such ideas is but one example of the conservatism often seen in the application of new biological theories and discoveries to the human species.

Race, like all units of biological taxonomy used today, grew out of early attempts by European naturalists to bring the variety of living organisms into an orderly classification. The culmination of these attempts is presented in the famous work of Carolus Linnaeus (Carl von Linné), "Systema Naturae," originally published in 1735 (Linnaeus, 1758). This work, which went through many editions during the author's lifetime, put forth a hierarchical, binomial system of classification of plants and animals that formed the basis of modern taxonomy. The classification itself was based on careful observations of resemblances and differences among living organisms. The largest units were the kingdoms, plant and animal, which were subdivided into smaller and smaller categories including organisms with increasing numbers of similarities. Though Linnaeus' system predates Darwin's theory of evolution by a century, it provided an important basis for the discovery of evolution by arranging organisms in a way that reveals their descent from common ancestry. This basis explains why the system is still used today, though its scientific meaning has changed.

Although the meaning of biological taxonomy in general has altered with each new discovery, the approach to human variation below the species level continued to embody some outdated notions right up to the mid-twentieth century. In the view of the eighteenth and early nineteenth century naturalists, the world was to be studied for revelation of the Divine Plan. According to Biblical dogma, plant and animal species were believed to be products of Divine Creation that had been brought into being at a single point in time and did not change thereafter. The overriding assumptions were that the natural world had a permanent order, and the purpose of science was to discover, describe, and classify it. Foremost among the elements of pre-evolutionary thought that clung to the concept of race were (1) a preoccupation with classification; (2) the assumption that races actually existed as biological units in nature; (3) the belief that races could be distinguished by a set of more or less permanent criteria; and (4) the view that each race could be characterized by setting forth the attributes of an ideal physical type that best represented the race itself (Garn, 1957; Montagu, 1963; Washburn, 1951).

Anthropologists working during the last half of the nineteenth century and the first half of the twentieth century gathered much data on human biological variation throughout the world. However, they continued to use their observations primarily to construct racial types and classify races. In pursuing these goals, they constantly searched for stable characters that were not subject to change by natural selection. The unchanging nature of racial differences was stressed, and variation within racial groups, or deviation from the average type, was de-emphasized. These ideas about the static nature of races and the concept of the racial type were not only pre-evolutionary they were antievolutionary. According to evolutionary theory, most racial differences originate because of adaptive changes. The process of natural selection that is responsible for these changes works on individual variations, not types. A large number of racial classifications of man were generated during that period. They were based on more complete and more objective data than previous classifications and had finer subdivisions, but there was little agreement among classifiers. This lack of agreement is not surprising since, given the independent assortment of genes and the discordant nature of geographical variation in the human species, the more traits one uses the more difficult it becomes to arrive at a neat classification, with each population clearly distinguished from all others.

Beginning about 1930, the synthesis of Mendelian genetics and evolutionary theory gave biologists a new perspective on diversity in the natural world. This outlook has been called the populational approach because it stresses genetic variability in populations, through space and time, as the key to understanding the evolutionary process. Populational thinking, which emphasized individual genetic variability and its evolutionary role, eventually won out over the older Platonic notion of the ideal type. Variation within the species, and more importantly within the breeding population, became the focus of evolutionary study. Individual differences were no longer viewed as fortuitous deviations from the true type of the species.

The conflict between the older typological thinking and the newer populational approach affected the entire field of biology during the rise of population genetics and the formation of the modern synthetic theory of evolution that took place during the 1930s and 1940s (Mayr, 1963). It is, therefore, not surprising that his controversy eventually reached the study of human races. However, it did so after a considerable time-lag and in conjunction with a particular set of sociopolitical events. Neither nineteenth century Darwinian evolution nor the rise of the modern genetical theory of evolution in the 1930s had any immediate impact on thinking about human racial variation. It was not until the 1950s, some 20 years after the development of population genetics in biology, that those studying human subspecific variation questioned the use of types. This aspect of the race concept was fairly thoroughly demolished by various writers during the 1960s.

The older typological approach in biology is compatible with the racial stereotyping racists use to justify their prejudices. Both tend to ignore individuality and treat individuals as mere manifestations of a type. Likewise, Dobzhansky (1967) points out the philosophical compatibility between populational thinking and racial liberalism when he states:

> The populational approach is simply that an individual is himself, not a pale reflection of some archetype. Every person has a genotype and a life history different from any other person, be that person a member of his family, clan, race, or mankind. Beyond the universal rights of all human beings (which may be a typological notion!), a person ought to be evaluated on his own merits.*

It is probably no coincidence that physical anthropologists were debating and rethinking the biological meaning of the race concept during the same decades that saw the rise of the civil rights movement in the United States.

In any case, 1950 saw the introduction of the populational approach to human variability. Two other trends also began to make headway about that time and continued to gain impetus during the decade that followed, so that they eventually supplanted concern about classification altogether. These were the interests in evolutionary dynamics and in biological adaptation of human populations. Change and adaptation are both integral parts of evolutionary theory. However, in actual practice, workers interested in evolutionary dynamics have generally emphasized only simply inherited traits, such as the blood group antigens and serum proteins. Those interested in adaptation have concentrated on physiologi-

*Quoted with permission from ''Genetic Diversity and Human Behavior'' (J. N. Spuhler, ed.), Viking Fund Publications in Anthropology, No. 45. Copyright 1967 by the Wenner-Gren Foundation for Anthropological Research, Incorporated, New York.

cal and morphological characteristics of multifactorial inheritance and have studied the relationship of those characteristics to geography and climate. Although tracing a detailed history would not be appropriate here, several publications stand out as symbolic of, if not actually responsible for, the beginnings of this newer and more dynamic approach to studying living human populations. On a theoretical level, the writings of Washburn (1951, 1953) clearly showed the applicability of the new biological theory of evolution to the study of man. Boyd's (1950) "Genetics and the Races of Man" showed that blood group antigens could be used in applying the genetic theory of evolution to human populations. Because of their relatively simple mode of inheritance, blood groups are useful for characterizing populations in terms of actual gene frequencies and for investigating evolutionary dynamics by looking at changes in these frequencies. "Races" by Coon et al. (1950) re-emphasized the geographical nature of human racial variation and the need to account for population differences in terms of natural selection and adaptation to environmental features.

The new outlook was not completely accepted by all anthropologists. The most notable exception is represented by the works of Coon (1962, 1965), who put forth a concept of race and a theory of racial origins that were strongly typological and that largely ignored genetic theory. Briefly, Coon argued that there are five races of modern man and that these races actually predate the existence of *Homo sapiens*. These races evolved into the modern species independently and at different times. Although Coon's hypothesis can be reconciled somewhat with modern evolutionary theory (Johnston, 1964), it was widely attacked as antiquated and racist (Birdsell, 1963; Dobzhansky, 1963; Montagu, 1964b). As with much of the writing about race in the 1960s, the criticism of Coon's work was leveled against both race and racism. The feeling of the time, that the very concept itself was racist and should be abandoned, was partly an overreaction attributable to the same sociopolitical climate that favored the civil rights movement.

Of course, in the light of evolutionary theory sound reasons existed for abandoning the older typological notion of race and the assumptions that were carried over with it from the pre-evolutionary era. From the re-evaluation of the race concept in the 1960s a new outlook emerged. It contrasts with the older view presented at the beginning of Section II,C in the following ways. Today the major aim in studying human population differences is *understanding* the process of human evolution. Classification is useful only insofar as it contributes to that aim. Races, like all units of taxonomic classification, are arbitrary categories that exist only in the minds of classifiers, not in nature itself. Races, and the genetic characteristics that distinguish them, are, and have been, constantly subject to evolutionary change. Human populations are genetically variable and are best characterized and compared, where possible, using frequencies of genes.

As might be expected, given the change in emphasis stated above, concern with racial classification per se in the last decade has been slight. Some anthropologists continue to use various existing classifications of man as suits their needs in teaching and research. But attempts at making new classifications have virtually ceased, as has discussion of the subject in general. After some 200 years of effort and debate, an ideal racial classification of man was never developed. For reasons that will become evident in Section II,D, most workers have come to realize that such a classification is not achievable and that there are more important things to do. Meanwhile, the investigation of human population differences and their evolutionary implications is more vigorous and productive than ever (Roberts, 1975; Salzano, 1975).

Thus, during the 1960s the concept of race was widely and severely criticized on the grounds discussed above, mainly, that it was ambiguous, promoted racism, and was scientifically outmoded. All of these criticisms are justified to some extent. But the major question for the physical anthropologist concerns the relationship of racial categories to human genetic variation in time and space, and ultimately to the processes of evolution.

D. Biological Taxonomy, Human Variation, and Evolution

As stated earlier, race refers to a system of classification, not a biological entity. Much of the confusion surrounding the race concept comes from a general misunderstanding of zoological taxonomy, its principles, its purpose, and, in particular, its limitations. Some of the difficulties with race are common to all taxonomic levels, while others are peculiar to the subspecies. Some problems occur in other animal groups whereas a few are unique to man.

Zoological classification is not absolute. There are many possible ways of classifying human or animal populations and many potential classifications depending on one's purposes. However, the classification that is most widely useful and meaningful to the modern zoologist is the one based on the Linnaean system. Initially it arranged animals according to morphological resemblances, but in post-Darwinian times it classifies them according to genetic similarities and presumed evolutionary relationships. Each grouping implies common ancestry. Therefore, the primary standard by which one judges whether a particular arrangement of organisms is "better" than another is how well it reflects their evolutionary relationships (Simpson, 1961). Because biologists may hold differing opinions about the evolutionary relationships of animal groups, they may use different classificatory schemes to express those opinions. Zoological classifications, therefore, represent broad statements about evolution.

Simpson (1961) pointed out, however, that taxonomy cannot be expected to express fully evolutionary relationships among organisms, even though it should be consistent with these relationships as discerned from the evidence available.

From the evolutionary point of view, the Linnaean hierarchical system's major limitations are that it is static and arbitrary. Forcing the results of the dynamic and multiplex process of evolution into a simple two-dimensional static set of pigeonholes cannot be done without losing information. Phylogenetic information, where known to the classifier, is not really lost, of course; it is simply not expressable within the framework of the classification. Classifications may change with expanding knowledge of the evolutionary histories of animal groups, but even were such histories completely known it might be possible to construct different and equally valid classifications of the groups involved. With all zoological taxonomy, one can reach a point where science leaves off and art begins. At that point, in Simpson's (1961) words, "A basic principle of taxonomic art is that its results should be useful."

Obviously, then, racial classifications, like all taxonomic classifications, cannot fully express evolutionary relationships among human populations. At best they provide useful rough approximations of relationships. Yet much of the anthropologists' dissatisfaction with the biological validity of racial classifications lies in the inability of a set of racial categories to express adequately the complicated historical and evolutionary processes that lead to the present-day patterns of human genetic variability. Human populations can be classified in ways that are broadly consistent with their genetic affinities, just as they can be characterized by lists of "typical" traits and genes. However, they cannot be understood in those terms. Races as genetic groups can only really be understood in terms of the process by which they originated (Brace, 1964; Livingstone, 1964).

Exactly what taxonomic level the term race refers to has sometimes been uncertain. Although I have stressed that all taxonomic categories are arbitrary, the one that most nearly represents an actual grouping in nature is the species. The species is usually (though not always) most easily definable because it has rather clear-cut genetic boundaries. By applying the time-honored criterion of interbreeding, Mayr (1963) defined species as, "groups of actually or potentially interbreeding natural populations that are reproductively isolated from other such groups." From the viewpoint of genetic exchange a species is usually a closed system. Genes may be exchanged among populations within the system but not outside of it. Though smaller entities are biologically meaningful, the smallest unit of taxonomy recognized by biologists is the subspecies (Simpson, 1961). The individual organism is not considered classifiable in a taxonomic system. The breeding population (Mendelian population, or deme) is a local group definable by frequency of mating, i.e., a group of organisms that mate with each other more frequently than with members of other populations. The breeding population, with its genetic structure, is considered the most important unit for the study of evolutionary change, but it is not a taxonomic unit. Therefore, races are subdivisions of species that are composed of groups of breeding populations.

Yet within this area, below the species and above the breeding population, more than one level of population group is possible. During the past two centuries, classifiers have enumerated from 2 to 200 races of modern *Homo sapiens*. The numbers of races proposed often differ because authors work at different levels (Garn and Coon, 1955). The term race has been applied both to large continental population groups and to smaller regional or local assemblages. Naturally the latter practice will yield a larger number of races than the former. The problems caused by the use of different levels below the species are not restricted to human biology but occur also with other animal groups (Simpson, 1961). Most often the discrepancy of number can be resolved by considering the smaller groupings as subdivisions of the broader ones. However, in man such consideration will sometimes not work because some local population groups do not fit genetically with the remainder of the populations inhabiting their continental area. These groups exist because of some rather special circumstances of human prehistory that will be explained below.

Garn and Coon (1955) propose the terms "geographical race" for the larger groupings, "local race" and "microgeographical race" for the smaller ones, to eliminate confusion and apparent conflict caused by using different levels. However, several arguments favor restricting the biological usage of the term race to the larger geographical groups of man, which older writers called "stocks" or "divisions" and more recent writers call "geographical races" or "continental races." First, these geographical subdivisions correspond most closely to the only legitimate taxonomic unit below the species level, the subspecies of the biologist. Mayr (1963) defined a subspecies as "an aggregate of local populations of a species, inhabiting a geographical subdivision of the range of the species, and differing taxonomically from other populations of the species."

Second, for more than 200 years attempts at classifying human populations have consistently resulted in a relatively small number (usually between five and ten) of geographically delimited groups, no matter what combination of characteristics was used (Linnaeus, 1758; Blumenbach, 1781; Huxley, 1870; Boyd, 1950; Garn, 1961; Coon, 1962, 1965; Brues, 1977). This scheme is the most workable because it shows the best fit to many kinds of genetic variation seen in the largest number of living populations, and the number of racial categories is small enough to keep it from being overly cumbersome. Table I shows a comparison of several racial classifications of man dating from the eighteenth century to the present.

Finally, these broad subdivisions correspond to genetic differences that reflect evolutionary differences, that is, they reflect the isolation, differential adaptation, and time separation among the populations being classified (Baker, 1967). For these reasons, the term race as applied to man is considered here to be the equivalent of the biologist's subspecies. For some purposes it may be desirable and necessary to define smaller population groupings, but one should not call them races or attempt to give them taxonomic status. Many human populations, usually

TABLE I

Some Racial Classifications of Man from the Eighteenth Century to the Present

Blumenbach (1781)	Huxley (1870)	Boyd (1950)	Garn (1961)	Coon (1962)	Brues (1977)
Caucasian	Xanthocroid	Caucasoid (Early European)	European	Caucasoid	Caucasoid
	Melanocroid		Indian		
Ethiopian	Negroid	Negroid	African	Congoid	Negroid
				Capoid	
Mongolian	Mongoloid	Mongoloid	Asiatic	Mongoloid	Mongoloid
American		American Indian	Amerindian		
			Polynesian		
			Micronesian		
Malay			Melanesian		
	Australoid	Australoid	Australian	Australoid	Australoid

called "breeding isolates" or "religious isolates" manifest some degree of genetic distinctiveness due to restrictive mating practices. The genetic isolation of such groups may be due to cultural or religious rules barring mating outside the group, or to geographical barriers, as in the case of remote island populations. In these usually small and isolated groups, inbreeding and genetic drift have produced somewhat distinctive gene frequencies and phenotypic appearances. Though peculiar in genetic makeup, these groups are not true races, as defined above, because most are of comparatively recent origin and some show evidence of considerable admixture with other populations, despite religious prohibitions. The castes of India and the Jews, Amish, and Dunkers are familiar examples of such isolates.

Racial differences exist because they have evolved. Thus they are of interest to the contemporary physical anthropologist, who is concerned with ongoing evolution in the human species. The evolution of races is due to the same processes responsible for the evolution of species—geographical isolation and genetic differentiation. Genetic divergence results from adaptation of populations to differing environments by the process of natural selection acting on random mutations, and from chance effects such as genetic drift. However, because the isolation between races is neither complete nor longstanding, the process does not result in reproductively isolated species. What emerges are population groups that differ in the frequencies of certain genes but are still able to interbreed. Though the factors that produce them are the same, races should not be viewed as incipient species. They are only temporary "evolutionary episodes" that emerge and disappear along with the conditions that favor their formation (Hulse, 1962). Many human genes show strong geographical patterning, whether they be genes for morphological features such as pigmentation, dental traits, and body build, or biochemical ones such as the blood groups and serum proteins. In most cases these geographical patternings reflect long-term adaptations of the gene pools of human populations to their environments.

If racial classifications are to have evolutionary meaning, genetic similarities among populations of the same race should be due to common ancestry. A "racial" characteristic is one that is shared by a particular group of populations because of their common evolutionary heritage. Skin color, often regarded as a racial characteristic in man, is actually a poor indicator of evolutionary affinities. Like all pigmentation, skin color is clinally distributed on a geographical gradient (Gloger, 1833). Dark skin is found in several Old World population groups living in humid zones near the equator in subsaharan Africa and southern India as well as Australia and the Western Pacific. Older racial classifiers (see, e.g., Deniker, 1900; Haddon, 1924), sometimes grouped these dark-skinned populations together and tried to account for their far-flung geographical distribution by supposed migrations. However, the evidence of many other genetic systems indicates that these populations are not particularly closely related (Boyd, 1963). The most probable explanation is that they developed dark skin color independently as an adaptation to high levels of ultraviolet solar radiation (Loomis, 1967). Thus, the most valid racial classifications are those based on evidence from several different genetic systems. Similarities in one or a few traits do not necessarily indicate common ancestry.

Most of the world's human populations can be successfully classified into a series of major groups. Ideally, such a set of racial categories implies a series of population groups with clear-cut boundaries, each separated from the others by about equal amounts of genetic distance and containing populations that are genetically homogeneous. However, the fit of such classifications to genetic and evolutionary reality is far from perfect. None of the implications stated above is true of human and racial groups, which are genetically heterogeneous, have indistinct boundaries, and are not all related in the same way. Knowledge of the nature of evolution below the species level, of the geography of human variation, and of certain events in human prehistory helps to explain why these difficulties exist.

To appreciate why human populations defy precise classification one must understand the geographical patterning of human genetic variation. Maps depicting the distribution of genes and characters, such as those provided by Biasutti (1959) for pigmentation and morphology, or by Mourant et al. (1976) for the blood group alleles, are useful for this purpose. Racial boundaries are not discrete from either the genetic or the geographical point of view. Genetic differences among races involve only the proportions of genes they possess. Few genes are found only in a particular race and not in any other. No given gene is universal in a particular race that is not found in another. Interbreeding of contiguous populations is possible below the species level, and it usually occurs. Therefore, zones of intergradation between races nearly always exist, where populations showing intermediate characteristics may be found. The sharpness of the genetic boundaries separating races depends on the degree to which mating, and gene exchange, between adjacent populations has been reduced by geographical features such as oceans, deserts, or major mountain chains. For example, striking genetic differences exist between peoples living on either side of the Himalayas, but to the north, across the Eurasian plain, European gene frequencies simply grade into Asian ones, with no perceptible break.

Most human genetic variation is clinal in nature. Clines are geographical gradients where the frequency of a gene or morphological character changes gradually throughout its distribution. The presence of clines, whether due to a gradual change in selective factors or to interbreeding of contiguous populations, or to both, makes it difficult to define racial boundaries except arbitrarily. That presence also means that populations are not genetically homogeneous within a large geographical area. These problems are compounded by the fact that clines for different traits or genes are frequently discordant and crosscut each other. In Europe, for example, the clines for pigmentation and body size are distributed on a generally north-to-south gradient, with body size decreasing and pigmentation increasing in a southerly direction. The clines for blood group antigens, however, generally run from east to west, with the frequencies of A and r decreasing in an easterly direction. Although some clusters of traits are typical of certain areas of the world, existing human variation does not conform to the neat packages that racial classifications imply.

Though they may cause problems for classification, clines are interesting with regard to natural selection. Because different genetic loci respond to different selective factors, it is not surprising that clines may run in different directions. Often the study of the geographical distribution of genes provides important clues to the evolutionary forces operating on them. Some well-known examples are the geographical correlations between climate and body build, ultraviolet radiation and skin color, or malaria and the abnormal hemoglobins. Thus, for understanding evolution, studying clines rather than races or populations is sometimes more profitable (Livingstone, 1964).

Most existing racial classifications are based on the distribution of human populations as they existed in the fifteenth century and ignore the widespread migration, displacement, and hybridization of peoples that has occurred more recently. This practice may be justifiable in terms of ease of understanding adaptive and evolutionary relationships. However, the evidence is ample that such phenomena are not limited to recent centuries but occurred on a wide scale in prehistoric times as well (Hulse, 1957; Menozzi et al., 1978). As noted earlier, racial classifications are necessarily time bound because evolutionary processes are constantly operating to change the characteristics of existing populations. Also, largely because of cultural factors, some groups are disappearing, others expanding, and new ones emerging. The relative sizes of human racial groups today differ from what they were in the past (Hulse, 1957), and they can be expected to change in the future. Hulse (1955) has pointed out that, in the past, all other things being equal, the groups with better technologies were those that left more offspring. At present we may be witnessing a reversal of this trend with the effects of industrialization and improved technological means of birth control on lowering reproductive rates. Now, and possibly in the future, groups with better technologies may be those that leave fewer offspring. In any case, the present numerical predominance of certain groups does reflect historic and prehistoric changes in technology.

On the continents of Europe, Africa, and Asia the human populations that are most numerous and best conform to the description of the continental race are descendants of populations that were the earliest and most successful agriculturalists. On all three continents are smaller, genetically distinctive groups representing descendants of nonagricultural populations that were gradually absorbed, displaced, and outnumbered by the expanding agriculturalists. These populations, although living within the geographical boundaries of the larger continental races and showing some resemblances to them, are too distinctive to be considered as subdivisions of the larger race. The best known groups of this kind are the Pygmies, Bushman, and Hottentots of Africa, the Ainu and Negritos of Asia, and the Basques and Lapps of Europe. All differ somewhat from surrounding populations in gene frequencies and physical appearance and most speak languages that appear to be distantly related to those around them, thus reinforcing the idea of their long separation. These groups have always presented problems for racial classifiers, who have devised various means of dealing with them. In Table I one sees that Coon (1962) gives the Bushman-Hottentot groups the status of a major race, designated Capoid. Boyd (1950) names a hypothetical Early European race, of which the Basques represent the only descendants. Garn (1961) and Brues (1977) omit these groups from their classification of principal races but discuss them as distinct local races. The location of some of these groups may be seen in Fig. 2. Though most workers agree that these represent remnant groups of past races, they often decline to give them racial status because of their reduced numbers.

Another phenomenon of racial history that leads to complication in classification is past expansion and colonization of new territories. American Indians and populations of Micronesia and Polynesia all descended from migrants who came at various times from Asia. They show a number of genetic differences from present-day Asians, and from each other, which can be attributed to genetic change; yet all show some resemblances to Asians as well. Table I shows that some classifiers include these populations in a single race along with Asiatic Mongoloids, whereas others give them separate racial status. Here the disagree-

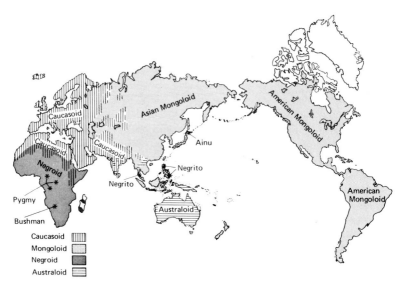

Fig. 2. Geographical distribution of principal human races and some minor ones, as of 1500 A.D. (From Alice M. Brues, "People and Races." Macmillan, New York, 1977.)

ment results from differing opinions about the degree of genetic distinctiveness a population group must show to be counted a major race. Even those who give American Indians separate racial status admit American Indians are closer to Asians genetically than to any other racial group.

From the global view, existing genetic variation in human populations can be explained by a combination of evolutionary processes and historic events. Overlying the patterning and clustering of genes produced by geographical barriers, proximity and distance, and adaptation is a second set of patternings resulting from three major kinds of historic (and prehistoric) events. These were the settling of the Americas and the Pacific Islands from Asia, the invention and spread of agriculture on three continents, and, finally, the voyages of exploration of the fifteenth century that led to the dispersal of Europeans and a smaller number of Africans to many parts of the globe. Undoubtedly many more small-scale events account for the distribution of genes on a local or regional level (see, e.g., Livingstone, 1958). The distribution of population groups and genes resulting from the factors mentioned above is complex and unclassifiable by any scheme that is both accurate and simple enough to be useful. Today we know at least the broad outlines of prehistoric population relationships from the genetic, archaeological, and linguistic data available. We are beginning to understand the evolutionary mechanisms and forces that lie behind genetic variation within and between population groups. Though much progress has been made on both of these fronts since the eighteenth century, it has not simplified the task of classification. If anything, this knowledge has complicated the task.

III. RACIAL VARIATION, HEALTH, AND DISEASE

Having stated that improved understanding of human variation has not greatly aided classification, I believe it is appropriate to inquire whether classification can lead to improved understanding. That racial classifications by themselves have little explanatory value should now be evident. They are merely modes of roughly codifying and expressing existing knowledge about population relationships. Physical anthropologists have abandoned race as a subject of research but continue to use the biological race concept, either explicitly or implicitly in teaching, research, and communication to generalize about genetic variation in the human species when necessary. Most realize that racial classifications cannot be taken too literally for the reasons discussed above. Race is no longer either a starting point for research on human evolution or an end. However, as Baker (1967) has pointed out, it can be a useful tool in some kinds of research. He argues that racial taxonomies based on the evidence of multiple genetic systems represent the best available estimates of genetic distance among human populations. Therefore, race is a useful concept to apply in many types of research where the investigator wants to compare either genetically similar or genetically different populations. Herein lies its value to those interested in causes, diagnoses, and treatments of human diseases. When diseases are being related to genetic factors, or when such relationships are being ruled out, biological race is an easily applied general indicator of the genetic makeup of populations and individuals.

Later chapters will show that many diseases are either population specific or show decidedly different incidence in various human groups. In many cases these associations may be at least partially the consequence of genetic factors. However, I must stress that not all genetic diseases are racial, nor do all racial differences in disease patterns have genetic causes. Many relatively rare disorders are due to recurrent mutations at single genetic loci. Because most of these disorders are caused by recessive alleles, their incidence in human populations may vary, depending on the culturally determined mating patterns of the groups. Their incidence will usually increase with inbreeding. However, the mutation rates for these alleles do not seem to vary among racial groups (McKusick, 1967). Disorders such as albinism or hemophilia occur in all of the major racial groups and may vary among populations within a race but would not be expected to vary between races.

After their existence has been demonstrated, associations between race and disease have two interesting aspects that can and should be pursued. One is the role of diseases as selective mechanisms in maintaining genetic polymorphisms and producing evolutionary change. The other is the role of the genotypes of individuals in either predisposing them to, or protecting them from, diseases. Racial variation in the frequency of the allele for hemoglobin S provides a striking example of both aspects of the problem. Here is a gene that causes a severely debilitating genetic disease (sickle cell anemia) but is polymorphic because it lends resistance to an infectious disease (falciparum malaria). In passing, I should point out that, although sickle cell hemoglobin is considered a racial trait in the United States, it is not found in all African Negroid populations and it does occur in other racial groups (Mourant *et al.*, 1976).

In discussions of diseases of genetic origin, single gene disorders usually predominate because they represent cases where the genetic component is most obvious. As mentioned above, most are relatively rare diseases that may show elevated frequencies in certain ethnic groups, but have little to do with race in the sense used here. However, few such diseases are due to polymorphic genes that vary among races. The best known examples are some of the hemoglobin variants that produce severe anemia in the homozygotic state and the Rh fetal-maternal incompatibility that may result in hemolytic disease of the newborn. The latter disease can occur only in populations that are polymorphic for the *r(cde)* allele. Hence, it is found primarily in Europeans, is rare in Africans, and is virtually unknown in other racial groups. Diseases produced by genetically mediated reactions to particular substances should also be mentioned here. Examples are lactose intolerance and glucose-6-phosphatedehydrogenase (G6PD) deficiency (producing favism and primaquine sensitivity), which show racial variation in their frequency (Omenn and Motulsky, 1978).

In addition, a fairly large number of diseases of uncertain etiology show differing frequencies in various races and may have a genetic component. Damon (1969) tabulated these diseases, which include diabetes mellitus, pernicious anemia, certain cancers, and birth defects. If a genetic component exists, multiple genetic loci are probably involved and a strong environmental contribution as well. Numerous racial differences in morphology, physiology, and biochemistry may account for the differential incidence and severity of these diseases across racial groups. A better understanding of them can only come from research utilizing complicated and carefully controlled designs. However, the race concept is a useful device, at least in the initial stages of this research, where one may want to compare disease rates of genetically similar populations living in different environments and genetically differing populations living in similar environments. When this approach is applied, race can be used as a general measure of genetic similarity and difference. With large samples, it has a practical utility that more valid, but necessarily more complicated, biological classifications do not possess. I should caution, however, that this kind of comparative approach must be carefully applied and controlled if one is to avoid the common pitfalls that have led to erroneous conclusions in the past. Genetic and environmental "similarity" cannot be assumed in a naive way but must be demonstrated. The groups to be compared must be carefully chosen and every effort made to eliminate confounding variables.

Once statistical relationships between a particular race and a specific disease are demonstrated, further work must be done to establish a functional relationship between the biological attributes of the individuals of that race and the disease. And, finally, a causal relationship must be proved. However, the existence of strong statistical associations between race and disease is an aid to the clinician in identifying populations and persons at risk for certain diseases. Damon (1969) has pointed out that the same symptoms may have different implications, depending on the race of the person manifesting them.

Race is a useful concept for health as well as disease. Because of racial differences in body size, shape and composition, growth and maturation, and many physiological and biochemical variables, the use of race-specific standards for assessing normality is necessary (Damon, 1969; Garn and Clark, 1976). Whether one is interested in assessing nutritional adequacy, obesity, child development, or bone loss during aging, or in evaluating the results of specific clinical tests, the race of the individual or population makes a difference.

Though race may be an obsolete concept in the evolutionary biology of the human species, it still has practical value in several areas. Its main value in relation to health and disease lies in its use as a general system for assessing the genetic makeup of populations and individuals. The race concept continues to be a useful tool in some areas of clinical medicine, epidemiology, and public health. For those interested in the causes as well as those concerned with diagnosis and treatment of human diseases, an important first step is discovering patterns of association between particular diseases and other biological attributes of the persons they strike. When these associations are sought, race provides an important means, but certainly not the only means, of subdividing the human species along biological or genetic lines.

REFERENCES

Alland, A., Jr. (1971). "Human Diversity." Columbia Univ. Press, New York.
Baker, P. T. (1967). The biological race concept as a research tool. *Am. J. Phys. Anthropol.* **27**, 21–25.
Biasutti, R. (1959). "Le Razze i Popoli Della Terra," 3rd ed. Unione Tipografico-Editrice Torinese, Torin.
Birdsell, J. B. (1963). The origin of human races. *Q. Rev. Biol.* **38**, 178–185.
Blumenbach, J. F. (1781). "De generis humani varietate nativa," 2nd ed. Cited *in* "The Anthropological Treatises of Johann Friedrich Blumenbach" (T. Bendyshe, ed.). Longmans, Green, London, 1865.

Boyd, W. C. (1950). "Genetics and the Races of Man." Little, Brown, Boston, Massachusetts.

Boyd, W. C. (1963). Four achievements of the genetical method in physical anthropology. *Am. Anthropol.* **65**, 243-252.

Brace, C. L. (1964). A nonracial approach to the understanding of human diversity. *In* "The Concept of Race" (A. Montagu, ed.), pp. 103-152. Free Press of Glencoe, New York.

Brace, C. L., Gamble, G. R., and Bond, J. T. (1971). "Race and Intelligence." Am. Anthropol. Assoc., Washington, D.C.

Brues, A. M. (1977). "People and Races." Macmillan, New York.

Coon, C. S. (1962). "The Origin of Races." Knopf, New York.

Coon, C. S. (1965). "The Living Races of Man." Knopf, New York.

Coon, C. S., Garn, S. M., and Birdsell, J. B. (1950). "Races." Thomas, Springfield, Illinois.

Damon, A. (1969). Race, ethnic group and disease. *Soc. Biol.* **16**, 69-80.

Deniker, J. (1900). "The Races of Man." Scribner's, New York.

Dobzhansky, T. (1963). A debatable account of the origin of races. *Sci. Am.* **208**, 169-172.

Dobzhansky, T. (1967). On types, genotypes, and the genetic diversity in populations. *In* "Genetic Diversity and Human Behavior" (J. N. Spuhler, ed.), pp. 1-18. Aldine, Chicago, Illinois.

Garn, S. M. (1957). Race and evolution. *Am. Anthropol.* **59**, 218-224.

Garn, S. M. (1961). "Human Races." Thomas, Springfield, Illinois.

Garn, S. M., and Clark, D. C. (1976). Problems in the nutritional assessment of black individuals. *Am. J. Public Health* **66**, 262-267.

Garn, S. M., and Coon, C. S. (1955). On the number of races of mankind. *Am. Anthropol.* **57**, 996-1001.

Gloger, C. L. (1833). "Das Abandern der Vogel durch Einfluss des Klimas." Breslau.

Haddon, A. C. (1924). "The Races of Man and their Distribution." Cambridge Univ. Press, London.

Hulse, F. S. (1955). Technological advance and major racial stocks. *Hum. Biol.* **27**, 184-192.

Hulse, F. S. (1957). Some factors influencing the relative proportions of human racial stocks. *Cold Spring Harbor Symp. Quant. Biol.* **22**, 33-45.

Hulse, F. S. (1962). Race as an evolutionary episode. *Am. Anthropol.* **64**, 929-945.

Huxley, T. H. (1870). The geographical distribution of mankind. *J. Ethnol. Soc. London.* **2**, 404.

Johnston, F. E. (1964). Racial taxonomies from an evolutionary perspective. *Am. Anthropol.* **66**, 822-827.

Linnaeus, C. (1758). "Systema Naturae," Vol. I, 10th ed. (1956 facsimile ed., Br. Mus. Nat. Hist., London).

Livingstone, F. B. (1958). Anthropological implications of sickle cell gene distribution in West Africa. *Am. Anthropol.* **60**, 533-562.

Livingstone, F. B. (1964). On the nonexistence of human races. *In* "The Concept of Race" (A. Montagu, ed.), pp. 46-60. Free Press of Glencoe, New York.

Loomis, W. F. (1967). Skin pigment regulation of vitamin D biosynthesis in man. *Science* **157**, 501-506.

McKusick, V. A. (1967). The ethnic distribution of disease in the United States. *J. Chronic Dis.* **20**, 115-118.

Mayr, E. (1963). "Animal Species and Evolution." Belknap Press, Cambridge, Massachusetts.

Menozzi, P., Piazza, A., and Cavalli-Sforza, L. (1978). Synthetic maps of human gene frequencies in Europeans. *Science* **201**, 786-792.

Montagu, A. (1963). The concept of race in the human species in the light of genetics. *In* "Race, Science and Humanity" (A. Montagu, ed.), pp. 1-10. Van Nostrand, Princeton, New Jersey.

Montagu, A. (1964a). The concept of race. *In* "The Concept of Race" (A. Montagu, ed.), pp. 128-128. Free Press of Glencoe, New York.

Montagu, A. (1964b). On Coon's *The Origin of Races. In* "The Concept of Race" (A. Montagu, ed.), pp. 228–242. Free Press of Glencoe, New York.

Mourant, A. E., Kopec, A. C., and Domaniewska-Sobczak, K. (1976). "The Distribution of Human Blood Groups and Other Polymorphisms." Oxford Univ. Press, London and New York.

Omenn, G. S., and Motulsky, A. G. (1978). "Eco-genetics": Genetic variation in susceptibility to environmental agents. *In* "Genetic Issues in Public Health and Medicine" (B. H. Cohen, A. M. Lilienfeld, and P. C. Huang, eds.), pp. 83–111. Thomas, Springfield, Illinois.

Roberts, D. F., ed. (1975). "Human Variation and Natural Selection." Taylor & Francis, London.

Salzano, F. M., ed. (1975). "The Role of Natural Selection in Human Evolution." Am. Elsevier, New York.

Simpson, G. G. (1961). "Principles of Animal Taxonomy." Columbia Univ. Press, New York.

Washburn, S. L. (1951). The new physical anthropology. *Trans. N.Y. Acad. Sci.* **13**, 298–304.

Washburn, S. L. (1953). The strategy of physical anthropology. *In* "Anthropology Today" (A. L. Kroeber, ed.), pp. 714–727. Univ. of Chicago Press, Chicago, Illinois.

2
Changing Patterns of Ideas about Disease

WILLIAM B. BEAN

I. INTRODUCTION

Here I can do no more than reflect on a few ideas about the long partnership of people and illness and how their intimate interrelationships have changed. We cannot reconstruct the prehistory of ideas. Archeologists of thought gain insight

BIOCULTURAL ASPECTS OF DISEASE
Copyright © 1981 by Academic Press, Inc.
All rights of reproduction in any form reserved.
ISBN 0-12-598720-X

of unmeasurable accuracy by observing today, as unobtrusively as possible various primitive peoples *in situ* whose customs and beliefs are our best clues about what could have been the early stages of societies that now, however naively, look on themselves as civilized.

My comments are provisional and best seen as a partial—though perhaps tolerably correct and coherent—account of how things might have been. The first five ideas are painted with broad strokes, about like whitewashing a board fence. The remainder, which might be reckoned easier because we come within the realm of history, is unhappily no more secure. The elusiveness of beliefs and ideas, central though they may be, still leaves much obscurity and uncertainty. But such is the nature of the subjective, the realm of feeling, notions, and mind for which matters crudely referred to in current jargon as "hard data" are so regularly rejected by the intellect as indigestible and no suitable pabulum for the mind.

The thoughtful person comes to realize that each family, group, tribe, society, or civilization not only develops its own concept of disease or illness but also produces them. Sometimes this development arises out of sheer ignorance or confusion. Today—with a world of information available—part of our dilemma resides in a strong residual belief in magic that few would admit to and the almost universal feeling that the laws of cause and effect will extract their troublesome or fatal toll from everybody else but not from me. Indeed, with all its fine qualities the capacity of the human mind to deceive itself has no apparent limit. Each person with an illness gives that illness meaning in light of the state of general knowledge and the time and the place in the world's history. Naming an illness, giving it a label, though it conveys confidence, unhappily does not introduce an explanatory principle, nor does it guarantee an easily understood or correct interpretation. Even a person ignorant of the history of medicine may realize that the structure of medical ideas and medical practices changed profoundly during the prehistoric, the historic, and even the recent past. Those familiar with history also realize that many persons living in various epochs or periods have thought that the rate of medical advance in their own particular time was greater than had ever occurred before. No one can deny that the rate of development of the understanding of lesions and pathophysiology and, to some extent, vital and basic mechanisms is changing at an increasing rate. Rarely, change correlates with advance. Real progress may come unexpectedly with a sharp reorientation of our intellectual emphasis or emotional attitude toward disease.

The natural history of health and disease is full of obscurities and puzzles. For example, for more than 150 years there has been a slow secular trend in the decline of the incidence, frequency, and severity of tuberculosis. This decline has been influenced little by ideas of pathogenesis or forms of therapy. Surely environmental causes and perhaps changes in the characteristics in the infecting tubercle bacillus as well as the host are important. Manifestations of psychological pressures in combat soldiers in World War I often were classified as hysteria and neurocirculatory asthenia. In World War II, stress reactions involving the alimentary canal and other systems predominated, at least in the frequency of diagnosis. One is almost tempted to say that a change in concept produces a vacuum into which diseases flow.

Because the concepts of disease change and the mental image of diseases shifts rather than stays fixed, traditional views are not always reliable or satisfactory. Fortunately, new and more vigorous ideas or concepts do not eliminate older ones. Rather, they extend them. Quantum physics and relativity did not repeal the Newtonian laws, which are still a splendid guide for our ordinary confrontation with the force of gravity. In distant but still historic times, medicine was often a matter of opinion supported by other opinions. Self-appointed or otherwise recognized authorities reigned supreme. Insofar as physicians had any effective function, it was in exemplifying and practicing medical arts. Galen inadvertently fastened an intellectual straitjacket on medicine that bound it for more than a 1000 years, right up into the Renaissance. Although rules of logic and argument governed the speculative debates of the ethereal dialectics of the Middle Ages, the Renaissance found bold men ready to question nature instead of trying to deal with the racy quiddities of abstract thought uncontaminated by the crudities of reality. Opinion and speculation have a disproportionate role in the dominant themes of treatment, even today.

Until the dissection of the human body became not only possible but a fairly common practice, medical science could not exist; indeed, it could not be conceived. Anatomy had to come first. The fabric of the human body must be understood. Within the fabric, that is, in the organs and systems of the dead body, are found clues of physiology, since structure in large degree modulates function. Thus, common sense recognized the complimentarity of structure and function. But before physiology gained any headway, pathology emerged from the study of anatomy. Not only did war and accident influence it but practicing barbers gave it strong impetus. Those journeymen with their scalpels and bandages, kept the spark of practical medicine alive while the dialecticians—the professors of the long robe—took centuries to creep out from under the dark cloak of necromancy, astrology, alchemy, and magic. Their posture was epitomized in the old wood cuts showing a formidable ancient professor inspecting a flask of urine held up to the light, pompously prescribing and prognosticating. Up to that time, pathology had been mostly recognition of combat wounds and other massive injuries causing death. Men saw and wondered about exsanguinating hemorrhages that had no external or other apparent cause. Often enough were seen the destructive ruin of various tissues by fatal neoplasm, the mechanical obstruction of a person's various tubes and conduits, and the anomalies and congenital deformities. The most perplexing were likely ill-developed, misshapen, or ambiguous and ambivalent sex organs.

After the Dark Ages, physicians and scholars began to regain and extend insights that had been smothered by the long period of intellectual surmise and scientific inactivity after the decline of Alexandria and the Roman Empire. Dramatic advances came after the primitive probings gave rise to more sophisticated study, such as Harvey's illuminating demonstration of the hydraulics of circulation. This discovery was not just a great discovery but the birth of physiology.

The long inertia of the human intellect is evident when we recall that Harvey had the same technical equipment as was available to Aristotle and his predecessors: scalpel, tweezers, needles, scissors, thread, and rather weak magnifying glasses. The body's function could not be understood until the circulation was comprehended. The ebb and flow of mystical humors, coction, and concoction began to be blown away with the mists of mysticism as the clarifying concepts of physiology emerged. Breathing and the interchange of gasses in the lungs could be understood only when the curious nature of the air around us was investigated and the laws regulating the way a special gas is dissolved and distributed in the other gasses and fluids became known. Only then did the dynamics of respiration and energy exchange begin to make sense.

Then the development of the microscope carried anatomy into a whole new order of things, particularly as the knowledge of optics led to achromatic lenses and corrected for other aberrations. Tissue- and cell-staining brought a further advance. Then formed elements in the circulating blood could be removed and even counted. Microorganisms were tackled, and with the development of solid media for cultures a single organism could be isolated in pure culture. As the forces of electricity became better known, electrophysiology and neurophysiology advanced greatly, particularly with techniques for amplifying tiny electric currents of heart and brain and other organs. Whole new worlds have been explored in more recent times with the electron microscope. Molecular biology has brought us close of the dwelling place of the molecule and atom, although many secrets remain veiled.

As science brought the laboratory closer to the sick patient, more and more was learned about the mechanisms of metabolic disorders, genetics, microbiology, enzyme chemistry, and immunology. A clinical puzzle led to tests. If its essence could be abstracted, its nature might be explored and explained. Then the ideas were referred back to the patient to see whether the information fit the real life of a sick person or whether further modification was required. It was also essential for the answer to be exact and to lead to clearer diagnosis and management.

Diseases have not been invented or discovered in the laboratory and then brought to be recognized in a sick person. Linus Pauling could never have been concerned with the nature of the physical flaw in the hemoglobin of sickle cell anemia if Castle or someone else had not given him the crucial hint. Castle, in turn, knew about it because James Herrick had described the trouble in a sick person decades earlier.

The history of ideas in medicine depends to a surprising degree on the quality of nosography, the formulated constitution and bylaws of illness. Any history of ideas reminds us that our present place is along a continuum and not on a magnificent isolated pinnacle, detached from the past and unmindful of the future. Those who practiced medicine began as observers and collected data. Generalizers then extracted principles from phenomena, concentrating on progressively narrower fields. The description of disease varies with the conception of disease. Ideas have always run ahead of observation. In ancient times, and recently in primitive peoples disease meant the invasion by magic from outside, whether a spirit, a demon, a wizard, or a substance—or the loss of the soul, or the power of gods or ghosts to wreak vengeance for disobedience or breaking laws.

The person familiar with medicine only as seen today fails to get historic insights and thus loses the opportunity to develop wisdom that comes from the firm realization of the changing, sometimes ephemeral, nature of so many concepts of illness, disease, or health. Many ideas about disease have become coherent and usable. They not only affect but also determine the conditions for the practice of medicine.

Our view of the early stages of any society indicates that its attitudes include sacrifice and propitiation, the exploitation of unknown natural powers, spirits, and deities, always in uneasy symbiosis with a society's slowly developing effort to control the environment and manage sources of energy. Nomadic hunters encountered a different life from tribes that domesticated plants and animals. By providing for a more or less steady source of food for energy, human beings found leisure for thinking, observing accurately, and speculating. From earliest time, magic and experience have gone along together, sometimes hand in hand and separable only with difficulty, sometimes in conflict. Their uncertain and often paradoxical balance set up whatever tentative and often flimsy barrier human beings could erect against the surrounding and encroaching chaos. With work to control environment, the rise of civilized society consolidated its victories, large and small. Magic and divine powers shrank and lost prerogative. The gods of the storm and weather shrivel when meteorology becomes sophisticated, but each tornado tells us it is hardly yet a science. Rationalization and rationalism become habit forming, suggesting that knowing is control. A side effect is inevitable hubris, the pride that is prelude to peril.

As any society develops and tends toward rational and logical understanding of the environment, terror and confusion continue because current events have not yet led to a new understanding to free us from the old myths, demons, horned and beaked griffins, sphinxes and unicorns. Ultimately they lose force as they become tamed and rationalized. The unknown outer world remains strange, unpredictable, and baffling. The gods, prompted by self-interest even as man was, were conceived as having enormous power. Thoughtful persons must have stood in danger of being crushed by the unknown, by native ignorance, by the insecurity of daily existence, and by the frightening and fantastic dread of divine jealousy, divine poisons, or divine miasms. Burdens from such pressures would have been unendurable without some sense of purpose, such as the oracle at Delphi gave to the Greek nation, indicating that a pattern of knowledge and purpose must exist behind the all-pervading chaos. Here now are the ancient ideas.

II. EARLY GENERALIZATIONS

A. Magic and Sorcery

Whether one looks at disease as error, as magic, as inadequacy, or as pain, clearly culture, the general state of ideas, and the stage and kind of civilization are all important in coloring our notions. Probably many intelligent persons have wondered what would happen if a newborn babe, kidnapped from some advanced society, were transplanted to a primitive clan or family. Clearly the results would be determined to an unusually large degree by the altered environment. A slightly older child, lost in the wilds, who managed to survive alone, growing up in the environment without people would be like a wild animal. Thus, a person in the most primitive state would, perhaps without articulation or with little help from words, exist as does the growing person in primitive societies who knows the difference between injury and noninjury. The primitive would recognize pain, disablement, and malfunction whether from injury, accident, or warfare.

Problems arose about the significance and management of pain or bleeding or breathlessness or bloating or diarrheas or great thirst and excretion of urine, as primitive societies advanced. These problems occurred without any noticed change in the external environment and thus required an interpretation that gave names and identified mysterious forces. The problems were not susceptible to any validation beyond that of experience. If nothing like a spear or an arrow or a sword entered the body but stabbing pain were felt, something magical must be at work. Probably no primitive people looked on such symptoms as being natural or in the ordinary way of things but as extra- or supernatural. Thus, from earliest times, an illness or a disease that came without an evident external cause, such as a fall, a bite, or a wound, would be interpreted as coming from mystical but hostile forces in the totally personified environment, where every tree or object had a spirit or a hidden essence influencing those around it. The sting of serpents, poisonous plants or berries, the bites of insects, the fickle toadstool—that is so like a mushroom—bees, wasps, electric eels: by millenia of hard won and slowly accumulated knowledge from trial and error, human beings from many a thousand unplanned or planned events learned by improvement how to survive in a hostile environment.

In addition to natural accidents or injuries, troubles caused by the human agency—a lash, beating, strangling, stabbing, killing—were recognized and avoided as far as possible. When things became more organized, struggles were called battles or wars. Thus, the human agency in disease and disability was added to what nature could do by accident or error. In addition to the constant presence of environmental hazards or perils and those troubles that man's inhumanity to man inflicted, there were forces thought to involve spirits or essences and to be under the control of magical or supernatural forces that might or might not be controlled by man's sorcery and incantations. These forces were as real to primitive folk as a knife, rock, or claw.

Probably no people or tribe is so primitive that belief in sorcery as a cause of illness and disease does not exist and often flourish. Most primitive Australian aborigines or the Fuegians accept a well-organized pattern of sorcery by which a person or a spirit may invade or shoot into a victim something that ruins his relationship to his environment or disturbs his own spirit. Sorcery as a cause of disease is so universally distributed that it occurs everywhere primitive peoples live. Indeed, the culture of western Europe and those derived from it still have vestiges not only among the ignorant but among those supposed to be sophisticated. Thus, the idea of sorcery comes close to being instinctive in primitive persons and lingers on today. Whether sorcery arose independently among many peoples, as seems probable, or whether it had one origin and diffused with their migrations, we do not know. Possibly one type gave rise to another or perhaps various types of sorcery had single foci or origin and spread, adding new layers to primitive concepts.

Sorcery and witchcraft encompass all those hypotheses that ascribe illness in a gently or cruelly paranoid way to the manipulation of others, through their control of magic or their ability to make others work for them, to exercise their will against another person by supernatural means. The sorcerer can gain control in two ways, mastering the name of a person or making a model, a small image of the body. Thus, he may say things with a formula, a ritual, or customary incantation and, by naming that person, cause illness and perhaps even death. Or he may take his homemade image or model, pierce it will pins or needles or thorns, burn it, or otherwise damage it. Whether he damages the model or the name, he has demoralized or destroyed the essence, spirit, or health of the victim.

If one cannot get the victim's name, or if the image of the person is inadequate, another way to gain control is to get a small part of the person, a bit of his or her jacket, hair from his or her head, nail clippings, menstrual blood or whatever, any part of or from a person can personify the person. By what is called contagious magic, the victim can be controlled. An advance of this idea is the firm conviction that a person with such skills can project, hurl, spit, or send by gun or arrow a plague or poison into a person. Boning—pointing with the bone—casts a spell and gains desired control.

In general, these are the means and methods of sorcery and magic. In the long prehistory of man the local village bully or wise man might gain or claim control of an entire group by demonstrating to one and all incredible power of mysterious force that could be deployed to produce all manner of harm, evil, or (sometimes) even good. As time moved on, a medicine man or shaman might be able to protect his people from external magic and sorcery by countervailing power. The evil-eye (perhaps Etruscan, certainly older than Rome), spells, hexes, looking, and pointing appear in many primitive groups. Darkness was especially feared. What person cannot recall the experience in a strange town, a strange house, of awakening in the dark with an eerie feeling of being lost and fearful, that the very walls were peopled by unknown forces or spirits of harm or evil? One does not have to project far into the past to perceive the uneasy influences that our not-so-ancient ancestors grew up with and felt around them, not just at times but constantly. We do not have to go with Fraser into the woods of Nemi to witness, not the change of the guard, but the changing of a king, slain by a shrewder, younger, wilier seeker for power under the sway of the mystic mistletoe, The Golden Bough. The new king who took the place of the old eventually was in turn hunted down and replaced.

B. Soul Loss

The enormous difference between a living person and that person's body after death, so apparent even to a child, exemplifies a great mystery of existence. Sleep, resembling but still a counterfeit of death, has observable but nonetheless mystifying analogies. Dreams that occur during sleep naturally might be interpreted by primitive peoples as a temporary departure of the soul. The soul, or the essence of a person, detached from the physical body, may be off visiting other places, having other experiences, doing other things, pleasant or terrifying. There are certain related bits of deeply embedded lore, such as the notion that during dreams or during sleep the soul enters a mouse or small animal and scurries away. Sickness may result if the spirit does not return before the sleeper awakens. Therefore, many primitive peoples have a strong feeling that a person must never be disturbed during sleep for fear that the soul will not be able to return to the body in time.

One entertaining and interesting notion, traces of which still exist in today's customs, is that a sneeze signifies the soul's departure. Here, of course, it is departing at the time of a spasmodic, partially uncontrollable event, during the time when a person is awake. Various salutations and magic words, urging it to come back, are altogether natural. Although the notion that soul loss as the cause of disease has disappeared from most contemporary Western cultures, "Gesundheit" and "Bless you" and various other folk expressions survive long after their original purpose has been forgotten. Perhaps because sneezing was usually harmless and did not occur when the person was asleep, some believed it signified the re-entry and not the exit of the soul.

The belief that dreams are the experience of a wandering soul is closely linked with the conception of disease as soul loss. Ghosts can steal up on a sleeping person and crush him or stop his heart or breathing. Related to the phenomenon of the soul departing during sleep is the feeling of many primitive people that an absent person must never be mentioned by name. Thus, in some respects one's name is like the soul. Control of it gives an ill-wisher certain powers. Although the belief in soul loss is widespread in certain areas, the continuity of spread cannot be demonstrated, suggesting that it either originated spontaneously in several regions or that the belief was lost from many areas.

Since the concept of soul or spirit is difficult for the clearest thinkers and the wisest persons to comprehend, it is not surprising that primitive peoples have had a great variety of beliefs. Most seem to look on the soul or spirit as a kind of double, an image or ethereal part that resembles the body but has no tangible embodiment. Certainly the soul would seem to be much more than nothing and to have substance but not be subject to the ordinary controls. In more sophisticated terms, it might be called a Vital Principle. A dreamer may dream of dead or distant persons. On awakening he is convinced he has been with them. But because his body has not moved, those in his dream could not have been the actual people, particularly when the dream was about the dead. Some such sources must have given rise to a belief in spirits as bodily images.

The essential life force or factor appears to be inseparable from the body during coma or sleep and disappears only with death. The ethereal image, though, can escape at any time, wander about, appear to persons at a distance and, at length, return. These two notions combine in the belief of a ghost soul that for health and comfort must reside steadily in the body. It is essential for health and for life. Illness, temporary or protracted, represents the absence or malfunction of this essence.

Because the notion of the soul or spirit is almost universal, we must assume that it results from a fundamental psychological and mental similarity of the human brain among diverse races of peoples. For practical purposes it does not really matter whether such ideas originated once and spread erratically, leaving a patchy trail or whether the notions originated altogether independently at different times and places. The fact is that, given the appropriate circumstances, the concepts did develop somewhere, indicating that they might develop in other places.

Among some peoples certain spirit losses were thought to have particular avenues of departure. The newborn, the infant whose fontanel has not yet closed, was assumed to have a special portal of entry or exit for the spirit. Having learned how to get in or out, the spirit managed to use the same portal even after the bone had fused and become solid, forever able to enter or escape from the top of the head by remembering the old, secret way.

Other primitive peoples thought that the heart, with its mysterious beating, was the home of the spirit, which it could enter or leave at will. Others believed the soul loss could occur only when the soul was dislodged by fright. It then might be eaten or destroyed by its captor. Further notion of the hearth and home of the soul held that it might reside in the liver, in the fat around the kidney, or even in the gall bladder. Nobody has ever calculated why the Ojibway Indians of the Great Lakes put the soul in the gall bladder, but there it was.

Another widespread belief was that children, because they are clearly fragile and subject to injury and illness in their precarious existence, are more easily separated from their souls than are adults. This belief, again, might relate to the soft fontanel, though such ideas have not been codified.

Very primitive peoples have believed that one person's soul can kidnap and cannibalize the souls of others by trapping and capturing them and savoring them at will. Thus, some believe that illness is characterized by the capture of the soul and that death follows when the soul has been eaten by the captor.

Burials of late Paleolithic times give evidence of truly elaborate ceremonies including all sorts of gear and provisions for a journey, implying a belief that something or some spirit or ghost or soul survives after death and goes on a long journey. If the concept of the soul arose in the Paleolithic period, it is not unreasonable to suppose that the notion of soul loss as a cause of sickness came not very long afterward. Why the idea of soul loss as a cause of disease remained most highly developed in Siberia—even into recent times—is not clear.

C. Breaking Taboos

Taboo as related to disease is a sophisticated idea. It requires an established belief in gods or spirits more complicated than household dieties or ancestral shades. The rudiments of law and order derive from it. For taboo to be an effective force, belief that spirits or gods are directly concerned with and intervene in human affairs must be universal. Their goodwill must be earned or regained by expiation or placation of some sort. The idea of divine punishment for transgression and expiation by confession seems perfectly logical. Apparently it arose independently in different parts of the world. Most highly developed in Polynesia, the idea seems to have been extremely important in ancient Palestine, Babylonia, and Assyria. A parallel belief is that illness may result from failure to do one's recognized duty or from committing a forbidden deed. Curiously, in Mesopotamia, where breach of taboo was accepted as a cause of illness, confession did not find any effective place in therapy. On the other hand, confession as a part of organized Christianity has suggested to some that its role in Polynesia and in other places has been a fairly recent acquisition from missionaries, though we do not have detailed information to verify that idea.

It is easy to believe that faith in penitence, often with something like a sacrament or offering, which made a tremendous impression on the natives, explains the atonement or confession as treatment. The evidence strongly indicates that, at least in the Americas, these ideas were well established in pre-Columbian times. Thus, breach of taboo encompasses all hypotheses that contain explanations of illness as punishment sent by gods for breach of prohibitions that might be religious or legal in a social structure that gave them divine sanction.

Breach of taboo might occur from error or ignorance of a taboo and thus be completely unrecognized by a person who broke the rule. Whether accidental, unintentional, or willful seemed to make no difference in its capacity to be a real cause of illness. Likewise, whatever might have been the reason for breaking taboo, confession—arbitrary and automatic—was the sovereign remedy (except in Mesopotamia, the exception that proved the rule).

Every family or group—even two people, a man and wife, parent and child, any small group living and working together—has customs that should not be breached, well-recognized rules that must be obeyed. Rules that cannot be broken without bad consequences can be as simple as the law of gravity or acting on the belief that running a car at full speed into a wall is likely to cause trouble. If rules as simple as these or much more subtle are broken and the gods are in control, punishment must ensue. Whether illness results basically from error, ignorance, or willful disobedience of a recognized rule matters little. Stupidity, perversity, or bravado may lead to the same unhappy result.

Taboos, as far as we can trace their mysterious origins, seem to have grown up as appropriate reactions to something that was dangerous to an individual, represented peril to the family or clan, or was just plain useless or frivolous. They may represent folk comprehension of public health, as in the Hebrew practices described in Leviticus. Residues of simple taboos are preserved and observed when children in their hopscotch jumps and dances have certain rules that must be followed with the utmost care or bad things will happen. We all know the childish chant, "If you step on a crack you will break your mother's back." Possibly this arose from ancient and insecure bridges over roaring cataracts, but perhaps not. Such codes or practices may have evolved from many different reasons, not all of which are clear, but they had in common the fact that they were considered to have community value. If a single person or a small group defied them, challenging the rules and regulations of the clan, a local taboo was breached and serious consequences followed. Disease in the form of a deity's retribution or revenge was the meting out of judgment to those who did not obey the law or did not follow the taboo. Living with taboos, to some extent prepared our way for obeying law and abiding by custom. The more intelligent among human beings have recognized that manners, thoughtfulness, and the obedience of regulations provide the lubricant that makes the often groaning and grinding wheels of daily life move more quietly and smoothly. If everyone could re-member this, at least some of our all-prevailing social malaise might be reduced or mitigated.

D. Object Invasion of the Body

Object invasion is one of the most natural and simplest of all supposed or postulated causes of illness and disease. Something gets into a person that should not be there. That something may be either a normal, natural thing or something intrinsically harmful, poisonous, or lethal. The concept seems to have been more prevalent in the western hemisphere than in other parts of the world, but its worldwide though scattered existence gives evidence of its importance. Certainly there was a rational basis for object intrustions, since arrowheads, spears, snake bites, splinters, thorns, pebbles, and so forth might enter and sometimes become embedded in the flesh. The object itself, when a natural one, produced injury that could be understood as rational and logical. This cause was of a different order from a more mysterious cause that could be known only from the results it produced, such as pain, when its nature was neither seen nor understood. As an example, among some primitive peoples disease of the teeth was thought to result from worms in the teeth. That idea might have arisen from the observation of worms in the jaws of dead persons or dead animals. One might expect that the therapy of object intrusion would be more rational than therapy of other sorts, but that is not necessarily true. The intruding arrow or an impaling sword might be removable, might be pulled out. Clearly, a large splinter might require either massage or the use of the thumb and fingernail as tweezers, but the major means of extraction was suction, though certainly it was not organically necessary to deal with the object intrusion concept. Such treatment embodies a whole battery of ideas.

In some instances, removing a disease object is not practical, and removal is simulated by trickery. The shaman or priest–physician may carry, secreted about his person, all sorts of objects that might cause disease. Called in to treat a patient, he may, while sucking over an affected spot, produce, by legerdemain, an object he had put into his mouth or had palmed at the appropriate time. The object is exhibited to the patient, his family, and his friends. One and all are relieved. Variations on the method may include manipulation and massage of some unaffected surface of the body or the extraction of an artifact manually from one of the body's orifices. Because of its stylized and formal complexity, this phenomenon probably had a single focus of origin, despite its being widespread.

Object intrusion is probably of extreme antiquity. Its greatest residual importance has been among primitive peoples in North America and Australia.

E. Spirit Invasion of the Body

With the development of the belief in a spirit or soul as an essential element of the human condition also grew the idea that a person's disease might result from invasion by a foreign and hostile spirit. Rarely did it seem to come as a friend or helper, though a shaman might overcome the effect of an invading force by producing a stronger opposing one. The differences between the western hemisphere and Old World forms of spirit invasion are extensive enough that one may reasonably suppose the idea arose independently in the two regions. Though plausible, this development cannot be proved.

Spirit intrusion has many ramifications involving religion, magic, medicine, and related aspects of life. When belief in spirits is universal, it is not surprising that they might be looked on as beneficient or destructive. Anamism is consistent with uniform credence in spiritual beings. How the idea of the intrusion of a harmful spirit could have arisen, even when no other reason to explain illness or sickness was obvious, is a little difficult to see, nor does ordinary experience have much to suggest or make reasonable such an intrusion. Perhaps we cannot recapture the ancient past.

If spirit intrusion is accepted as a cause of disease and even of death, then the casting out of the spirit, exorcism, becomes a required form of therapy. Practiced widely in North, South, and Central America, the Caribbean, Asia, Indonesia, Polynesia, and Africa, exorcism is, indeed, not unknown in Europe. Not just in the Bible is the transference of spirits in persons to animals recognized. Such transference has been recorded in India, Africa, and ancient Rome and other parts of Europe. Even more widespread, particularly in North and South America, is the transference to plants or objects of an invading spirit. The identification of spirit intrusion with insanity or odd behavior has many parallels. As with the mechanical extractions, the casting of spells, the saying of magic words, and the exhibition of amulets seem to be essential as therapy. Obviously, if a demon can cast itself in or be cast into a person, it can be cast out. The question is how to get it out and where to have it land or what to do with it. Exorcism seems to be especially developed among the higher cultures of the Old World. Organized religions surely had as an important part of their beginnings the elaboration of the concept of spirit intrusion and the development of exorcism by expert priests and shamans as treatment. Spirit intrusion seems to have occurred rather late among ideas about disease.

Spirit intrusion and its implications influenced the Egyptians in their ideas about life after death and the preservation of bodies by embalming, particularly of the rich and powerful. No one seems to have believed that disease and death were natural. Rather, the invasion of man by invisible malignant spirits caused him to weaken and sicken. By such means the soul of a dead man could assail the living, either by some cunningly contrived means of entry into his body or by attacking him with overwhelming violence from the outside. Once the evil spirit had established a foothold, it might scour the skin, addle the wits, suck the blood, crush the windpipe, suck the marrow, drink the blood, strangle the lungs, break the bones, gnaw the intestines, or devour victims in a wasting disease. The priest, physician, or exorcist must discover the nature and quality of the spirit in possession. Discovery was easy if the spirit's name could be learned, and thus power over it could be obtained. By direct attacks a shaman could destroy the spirit or remove it, but only by exhibiting a more powerful magic. The skill in making amulets and in saying incantations was highly developed. Ultimately the lore of astrology, mathematical arts, and religious ceremonies all had an important place during the time when we see the rise of Imhotep, whom Osler described as ''the first figure of a physician to stand out clearly from the mists of antiquity.'' By now we find the magical approach involving animals in therapy; saliva, urine, bile, blood, feces, and various parts of animal bodies boiled, dried, or powered. Those materials make up a remarkable and mystical pharmacopea, including unicorn's horns and such. Indeed, desiccated thyroid and pituitary extract survive even into the modern period. Just think what solace an eager patient must have found when he knew that he was to be subjected to the properties resident in elephant, lion, rhinoceros, crocodile, or the 79 Egyptian preparations made from the hyena.

Some argue that when one of the five major ideas of the cause of disease has dominated, it has eroded or displaced other ideas. We may never know with gratifying assurance whether multifocal origin or single origin with diffusion accounts for similar beliefs the world over. One would suggest a powerful similarity of peoples long separated so that certain ideas recurred at different times and places. Multifocal origins suggest that the nature of people and their mental functions cause beliefs to form at a certain stage, when the time is ripe, and that these beliefs will be closely similar if not identical, though they arose independently. The idea of diffusion would suggest tenacious and powerful cultural transfer and continuity, with the dispersal of peoples and races. Object intrusion to explain disease rarely exists along with any of the other concepts except magic and sorcery. Generally, the older the concept the more likely it is to have eroded in certain areas and to have disappeared. A belief that is almost universal among primitive peoples suggests strongly that it is of relatively recent origin.

III. CONCEPTS OF ILLNESS AND DISEASE

Though the terms are often used interchangeably and loosely, illness focuses attention on the person and disease focuses the attention on the lesion and process. Much overlapping of the various concepts occurs, and, though they are presented separately, they are rarely found in absolutely pure culture.

A. Ontologic Concept

Ontology is the branch of knowledge that studies the nature, essential properties, and relations of being as such. It is distinct from such concepts as spiritual existence. An early notion of disease that survives in many traces is the ontologic concept. Illness was represented as something foreign or alien to the healthy person, a literal invasion of the victim's body by a thing, a spirit, a magic spell, a curse, a glamor, a devil, or a witch. As a thing identifiable and separate from the person who harbored it, disease had its own identity, ran its own course, had its own prognosis, and had its own specific therapy. To some extent, this concept encouraged the search for specific and external causes of disease. What was not clear in the early phases of this belief was why, in different victims, the harm seemed able to go in so many different directions and involve so many functions and such a large array of organs or organ systems. Treatment, often in the hands of a shaman or priest–physician, involved countermagic, spells, amulets, witchcraft, or incantation to exorcise or drive out the invading evil. Prognosis often dealt with the telling of magic days, the reading of horoscopes, the study of the influence of the moon and stars. Disease was a thing, tangible, palpable, sometimes even personifying an attacking enemy. Medicine has not been able to expunge the traces of ontology from its system of beliefs. Symbolically, it has some use. We hear the expressions "He caught a cold," "The flu hit him," "He had an attack of pneumonia," "She had a seizure," and many other expressions that are almost instinctive and have universal currency. The shortcomings of the idea are that the disease is seen as a thing and not a process, that a label gives a static picture of disease, and that emphasis on the changing reactions of a specific, genetically and historically unique person is missing. The ontologic concept ignores the fact that the patient is, at any moment, the sum of bodily characteristics, genetic traits and experiences, reacting to the stimuli that evoke illness.

Much of the ontologic concept remains today, as seen in folk speech and in the talk of well-trained physicians. As such, it remains a strong but inexact force in our current ideas about health, illness, and disease.

B. Platonic Concept

The rise of the Platonic concept of illness illustrates the great power of ideas. It was dreamed up, invented, made up out of other ideas and thoughts, rather than arrived at by a study of objective findings in sick persons. Disease was viewed as an unnatural state of excess, deficiency, or imbalance of one or more of the four mystical elements of existence: earth, air, fire, and water. In essence it was subjective, mysterious, almost religious. Where belief in the imbalance of nonexisting entities is a conviction, confusion must prevail. The ancient idea of balance—with moderate proportions producing health, and imbalance producing disease—was rooted in aesthetics. Like the graphic arts, painting and sculpture, its end result was inherently static. Its nature was intrinsically artificial and kept losing vitality when it was bruised or abraded by the data of clinical reality. Because it was not easy to destroy, this concept has to its credit a long catalogue of human misery. It found expression in the Brunonian system and, in a negative way, in homeopathy. The Platonic concept accounted for the blood baths of the heroic but misguided Benjamin Rush, advocate of the bleeding system, in efforts to rid the body of unknown bad humors. Vapors, migrims, disposition, resistance, and temperament connoted much, but denoted little, and failed to explain as they missed the nature of living and the essence of reality.

Perhaps a Platonic view of systems, forces and balance survives in the negative form of denial. This is also true of the Stoic Concept. Szasz claims mental illness is largely a figment. Illich can find no progress or any good in physicians or medicine and so encourages paranoia. McKeown can find no progress or advance in medicine, seeing errors in statistical and semantic interpretation. Whenever ideas depart far from the bedrock of data, error follows. The resulting mischief will be great or small, depending on the skill of the prophet and the intellectual strength of the audience.

C. Biographic or Anthropologic Concept

The Hippocratic canon, the codification of the Hippocratic school, had a strong influence, introducing into medicine the most intense reality imaginable. Rather than generalize, it looked at each person and the illness in terms of the kind of person who had the illness and that person's environment. It did not retreat into abstraction and generalization. It rejected sacred diseases and magic. It was environmental, descriptive, and, in its best aspects, approached a broad ecologic view. The concept was based on understanding places, seasons, diets, rhythms, and disposition. Detailed and complicated history taking and the actual inspection and touching of the sick person made it practical and workmanlike. At its best it used a string of consecutive anecdotes to arrive at an understanding of disease or illness in terms of the person's story. It proponents tried to understand the person and to avoid abstract labels.

The biographic approach traces symptoms back to their origins, establishes stages of illness, and develops prognostic signs in emphasizing the explicit historical view. Emphasized too are premonitory signs, early stages, rhythm, the day-to-day variations in disease with focus on precise duration and outcome. Prevention is implied, although it may not be expressed in any formal way. Prognosis developed in terms of critical, crucial, or mysterious days, related to Pythagorean concepts of the sacredness of numbers, to be corrected by observation. This departure from the reality of clinical experience was dangerous. It was not entirely mystical, though, as malaria, pneumonia, typhoid, typhus, and the plague all had a pattern of regularity with many variations on a central theme. Empirical wisdom prevails in observation of some courses of disease. Being sequences of events, diseases do unfold as dramas, tragedies, or comedies, or often as rather drab and undramatic stories. Illness may advance in a crescendo to a crisis that may be surmounted or—as in Greek tragedy—may end in death. In prying into the future by judging the past, but without controls or statistics, the biographic concept often ran aground on post hoc reasoning. Its virtues were its practical observations, still too rough for adequate generalizations. The great advance was the practical reality of observations, its earthiness, and the physical contact of patient and physician.

The biographic concept is essential in modern understanding of disease and in evaluating disease and illness. It is essential but not complete and sufficient. It can be flawed by willful deceit, forgetfulness, or a mind deficient or obtunded. When the story is accurate, obtained by openminded and open-ended questioning, and not obscured by proliferation of the irrelevant, good physicians get the understanding essential for diagnosis and treatment. Examination of the person, physically and by the necessary technical methods, must be added.

D. Stoic Concept

The Stoic concept is the most elegantly simple of all. It confronts the reality of illness by rejecting it. Thus, to treat disease, one denies it exists. The Stoics simply renounced the reality of the external world. Their medical philosophy was a sort of miscegenation of schizophrenia and Christian Science. For the Stoic, the subjective reality of his inner world was the decisive one. The past forgotten, the future unseen, he lived in the present. Intellectually rejecting disease by saying it did not exist, he set a concept that eliminated time and gave a static view. A paradoxical upshot of the Stoical idea was that life, based on the bland tranquility of peace of mind, ceases to exist as an actively moving enterprise. Here would be no substance to pain, no basis for disease, no hope of treatment, and no fear of death—only the glacial calm of a spirit in intellectual and emotional deep freeze. The concept was heroic enough but unreal. It did not help with the doubts, worries, and fear that come with pain or injury to the strong and weak alike.

E. Moral or Metaphysical Concept

The moral or metaphysical concept views disease as retribution and punishment. Greedy man, ever seeking new gratification and continuing to try to satisfy fancies and fanciful needs at the expense of his fellow human beings, brings revenge on himself. He has broken custom or taboo. We see sin and repentance, error and correction, good and evil as polarities. In the moral concept, disease arises from a never-ending struggle for new satisfactions, giving rise to pain, suffering, and death. With Rousseau the concept held that increasing civilization leads to increasing discontent and unhappiness. Origins of the moral concept of disease are lost in the dim mists of antiquity. Traces are common in most systems of medicine, including the ontological. The concept lives today. The notion that disease results from sin has remained frustrating and futile, because, by its neglect of the physical, it limits investigation of mechanisms and appropriate therapy. It also led to ecclesiastical extravagances, such as inquisitions and torture, and saw witches everywhere. Organized misconstruction, when it institutionalizes morality, increases human woes and sorrows wherever pain is conceived as punishment and psychosis is considered as witchhood. The difference between ignorance and innocence is essential. Millions of lives have been sacrificed because a man's symptoms do not reveal their origin. The causes of health are not self-evident. The conflict between good and evil, which Freud says is indispensable in the production of neurosis, suggests that man, freed from conflict, would be protected from disease. But such a state, by definition, is mythological. A person cannot avoid conflict any more than he can live without stimulus or stress. Properly reacted to and properly surmounted, conflicts lead to development and growth, not to disease.

A sense of guilt may be veiled by the usual "Why me?" that affects most families and many friends of an ill person. The idea of retribution and punishment runs deep in human beings. Even if separated from formal religion, guilt remains part of the human condition. Particularly traumatic in dying persons and those close to them, it is also part of the hurt and grief of bereavement. Thus, as moral creatures, we carry a burden of guilt as all encompassing as it is unreasonable.

F. Anatomic Concept

The anatomic concept had a slow start. Accidents and wars gave some early glimpses of the fabric of the body. Despite the need for detailed anatomical knowledge for embalming, the study of anatomy never reached sophistication in ancient Egypt. It advanced under Galen in Rome, but there the focus of study was on animal rather than human anatomy, and was misleading when extrapolated in identity. With the decay of the Roman Empire, the church's prohibition of dissection made all study of anatomy languish. With Vesalius and other early anatomists, a powerful revival occurred. Morgagni, adding to his own large experience by gathering together that of others, both predecessors and contemporaries, systematically tried to link the facts of clinical history and observation with the lesions found on examining the body after death, combining Hippocratic and Galenic elements. He related symptoms to lesions as effect and cause. His classic book was arranged according to regional anatomy, but the subdivisions were clinical. The materials in each book were grouped around symptoms—pain, cough, palpitation, syncope, hiccough, vomiting, stammering, aphonia, aphasia, epilepsy, gout, arthritis, apoplexy, dropsy, breathlessness, jaundice, edema. Here disease was related to organs. Then Bichat tried to establish a connection between texture and disease, believing that structure had inherent disease-shaping propensities, as developed in his "Treatise on the Membranes." Bichat retained the physiological and clinical approach, discussing disease in terms of symptoms, sites, signs, and clinical events. Virchow originally made a total transfer to anatomy; for him, the cell was the seat of disease. Later he became deeply interested in man and the social problems of existence. He said:

> Should Medicine ever fulfill its great ends, it must enter into the larger political and social life of our time; it must indicate the barriers which obstruct the normal completion of the life-cycle and remove them. Should this ever come to pass, Medicine, whatever it may then be, will become the common good of all. It will cease to be medicine and will be absorbed into that general body of knowledge which is identifiable with power. Then will Bacon's prediction be accomplished fact: what seemed causal in theory will become established rule in practice.

Some conflicts in his views remain unresolved. The problem of local and generalized disease was misinterpreted, for it was all forced into too artificial a system. The shortcoming of the strictly anatomical approach was its failure to comprehend the patient as a human being in distress or to think of relief by rational therapy. Claude Bernard, who was not a clinician, was mainly concerned with all the new things about mechanisms he could find in his laboratory. But he conceived of disease in terms of humors, a somewhat physiological approach, although his emphasis was still anatomic. The disasterous emphasis of the anatomic view was that its advocates were content with predicting from exact clinical studies, careful history, careful examination, what would be found when the body was examined after death. The concept was inherently pessimistic, therapeutically inert, and, after initially advancing the arts and science of medicine, slowed down their progress. Nevertheless, it still has essential contributions to make despite the decline in autopsies in the recent past. Autopsies must be revived if clinical medicine is to have its own necessary diagnostic correctives.

The anatomic concept provides an essential basis for conceptualizing disease, but structure without function falls short. Structure determines function and provides the physical machinery, but human life exists in structure functioning in an environment. Disease and illness occur whenever there is significant failure of fabric, function, or any of the forces and facts of our environment.

G. Physiologic Concept

It was natural that out of the anatomic notion of structure the physiologic idea of function should arise. They are, indeed, hand and glove. Galen, using motion and locomotion as models, conceived of disease as malfunction, albeit rather obscurely, but he was shrewd enough to hold on to empirical ideas. He distinguished primary from secondary lesions and, following Hippocrates, differentiated between diathesis and disease. Most subsequent ideas of disease have derived from or been influenced by the physiologic or functional concept of disease.

Our increasing technical virtuosity has not brought new principles in but has rather developed older principles to a high degree of specification and precision. Thus, a physiological or function element was suspected before the rise of the anatomical concept of disease during the Renaissance gave it the basis of form that made it real. With the flowering of pathology in the eighteenth century, lesions and malfunction were studied as cause and effect. The development of bacteriology as a major contribution of the nineteenth century continued such combinations.

Sir Francis Walshe emphasized for us the difficulty physiologists encounter. The problem, one of abstraction, is exemplified by the neuropathologist as he surveys the neurophysiologic scene. The more exclusively electronic his methods are, the greater the danger is that his ideas become rigid and fixed, losing touch with the realities of true structure and function. We cannot conceive of a neuron exercising its natural function in a biologic vacuum, valuable as such Platonic divineness may be in other circumstances. An understanding of normal and altered function undergirds all modern understanding of illness and disease.

The physiologic concept is central to any comprehension of illness and disease. But it must add anatomic and environmental aspects, for function cannot occur detached from the substance of structure and living organisms must exist and act somewhere, in some environment.

H. Aristotelian Concept

An etiologic concept of disease depends on the Aristotelian hierarchy of causes, logic, and rational thought. It makes the sensible, though not always realistic, assumption that man can understand himself and perhaps even govern the course of his own life and the direction society may take. The Aristotelian texture of causality dominates this view. It runs aground because we do not necessarily understand the disease more deeply or more truly by knowing the nature of the soil in which it flourishes.

Though Pasteur himself was aware of the importance of both host and invading organism, he was enshrined as the high priest of the etiologic concept. Later Freud was to have disciples distort some of his ideas, too. The new emphasis of bacteriologic cause of disease was opposed by more than the inevitable resistance to change. Pidoux was aroused to criticize Pasteur's advocacy of the etiologic concept at the time Pasteur was initiated into the French Academy, as follows:

> Disease is the common result of a variety of external and internal causes (that) bring about the destruction of an organ by a number of roads which the hygienist and physician must endeavor to close.

The fading out of a purely etiologic concept of medicine has come partly from medicine's tendency to be dominated by machines and technology and partly because causality was conceived in too narrow and rigid a framework. Failure to realize the multiplicity of causes in the genesis of illness, their sometimes simultaneous, sometimes sequential timing, as well as the individuality of each patient, limited this concept's value. It really ran aground in seeking a single cause. When only a few of the necessary facts or bits of information are at hand, failure is inevitable. The concept's doom was sealed by failure to look for multiple causes operating in a flux.

The science of causes still influences concepts of illness but can be helpful only if the strict rules of logic and causality operate using the data of medical arts and medical science. If one sets forth using wrong data or wrong premises, the most perfect logic will not lead him to understand the ill, the ailing, and the sick nor to understand their illnesses or diseases.

I. Psychologic Concept

Another idea of disease is the psychologic concept, with borrowings from the moral or metaphysical concepts. Man turned to the stars, spirits, demons, witches, and to the heavens, and the gods, which he saw everywhere in the world about him. Renaissance man experienced himself as a world unto itself, looking back a little to the Stoic view. He was a lesser world in a macrocosm, receiving his power from a greater force. The cosmic yielded to the psychic. Ultimately this concept had man looking to himself as the cause of his own misery. This self-analysis has led perceptive men to put the blame on themselves, as Cassius so nobly did in "Julius Caesar" when he said, "The fault, dear Brutus, is not in our stars, but in ourselves, that we are underlings."

Man saw disease as resulting from his own shortsightedness. Indeed, man was breaking his own visualized and understood taboos and thus—in varying degrees—producing his own illness. The questions in psychoanalytical terms is, does moving man's destiny from the stage of objective events to conflicts and matters of conscience bring relief and liberation? Is man's own shortsightedness or are external events mainly responsible? Does facing the inevitability of aging, infirmity, incurable disease, or death carry consolation? Because they are inevitable and unexplainable, man is left with only a reduced sphere for action. Limitations of the psychologic concept of disease are seen in its efforts to revise or prevent disease. The psychologic approach is not necessarily more successful than other methods.

J. Socioeconomic Concept

With the social or economic concept, disease is conceived as maladaptation to bad or changing environments. The concept makes difficult the evaluation of social and economic effects that are neither constant nor predictable. It risks being forced onto shoals by the fact that, stated simply, what is one man's meat is another man's poison. Can we root out disease by changing the social context of its origin? According to my view, we simply substitute one form of disease for another. No great wisdom is needed to realize that nothing in life, no event or modification of life or nature, exists that cannot cause disease. Remember that under certain circumstances eating, drinking, walking, running, or breathing may be not only dangerous but fatal.

Other forms of illness seem to fill any vacuum produced by corrections in harmful environments. The socioeconomic view combines certain elements of the anatomic and physiological concepts of disease, selecting what it needs from the etiologic and rejecting the ontologic, Platonic, and moral and metaphysical concepts.

Many students of health and illness emphasize the strong socioeconomic forces that may contribute to ill health and disease. Crowding, slums, poor water and hygiene, bad nutrition, inadequate heating, cooling, or clothing, or unsatisfactory education and work certainly undermine the body's proper function and structure. Though most agree that these are harmful circumstances, no one seems able to break the spinning cycle and change the direction.

K. Nosographic Concept

Another and partially composite view of disease is the nosographic concept. Medicine's greatest step forward came when the physician and his forerunners turned to the sick persons to observe disease, to examine and treat those patients. The sick person became the source of the therapeutic endeavors, guided by what had happened to him in the past and what he could reveal to the observer who actually examined him and who then could introduce the approriate treatment. As we work with a sick person, moving from the inspection and examination, we reach a working diagnosis in progressing from biography to nosography. This approach is precarious business because the tendency is strong to consider disease as a state, as fixed, and existing at a certain instant, rather than as the constantly changing evolution of a process, a reaction to stimuli with a sequential unrolling of successive processes.

In a formal sense, nosography, as it survives in medicine, is important for what it has assimilated from other concepts. Little is left of any independent concept as such.

L. Concept of Social Pathology

Suicide, singly or of masses in cults, fictitious disease in all forms but notably in the Munchausen syndrome, a patient's willful sabotage by lying or failure to follow directions, self-abuse by narcotics and alcohol, the following of pipers of strange and dangerous fads that have neither carefully observed experience nor prospective studies to support their seductive promises of the unreal or the impossible—all these are real enough. So are the innocent ignorant whose gullibility has provided untold wealth for an army of alert quacks. Though many of these aberrations cause illness and death, we do not know enough about human nature to have clear ideas of prevention. Treatment is difficult and cure is rare without something like a religious conversion taking place.

Social pathology is a pessimistic subject and so is the ruin of many a sociopath. We are not even sure which is more sick, society or some of its members.

M. Ecologic Concept

The ecologic concept is a composite, a mosaic of portions of other notions. It conceives of man and existence as comprising many parts and many forces, mutually interacting but in complicated ways. Internal and external forces act and interact, change and grow. When an infinite number of forces gets out of balance, when the homeokinetic flux becomes homeostatic, disease results and may lead to deterioration or death. Man's structure and function are determined by his legacy, for each person is a unique medley of nearly numberless variables of form and action. Accretions of change from the physical events and memory traces of his past and the race's past are impinged on continuously by stimuli, great and small, sure and unsure, heard and unheard, inside and out. One's life is process, operating in time and in a finite place. We react to and impinge on our own environment, and both change.

Though it would be desirable to eliminate unhealthy and disastrous environments such as those characterizing the whole growth and decay of cities and life with the industrial revolution, concomitant elimination of a large quantity of disease would not be assured. Obviously the general level of life should improve by diminishing certain preventable disorders, but other forms of illness seem to fill any vacuum produced by changes in the environment.

IV. DISCUSSION

This brief survey indicates that the medicine of any period in history has been a child of the times. The limitations of its practitioners are the intellectual, ideological, economic, social, and environmental limitations of the age. Any explanation of medical phenomena must be in terms of contemporary knowledge. Medicine is thus, by definition, provisional. A society's attitude toward illness, toward the sick person, and toward its responsibilities to that person varies in time and place. But it is the nature of civilized man to create his own diseases and, as time goes on, to modify them. Up to the present, such creation and modification has been largely accidental or circumstantial. The question for the future is whether, by exercising more wisdom than he has been able to harness in the past, man will be able to direct the future by a constructive and creative attack on the trials, tribulations, dangers, and damages of life. Control might enable him to approach closer to but never reach Utopia. Without pain and without disease, life would not be Utopian, but it might be such that preventable difficulty is averted and that which cannot be prevented is faced rationally and courageously.

Nosography is built on the natural history of medicine, which is determined by observations of persons in nature. Observation, for a time at least, is simply looking and seeing. The next phase is the active examination of the patient by the physician. In the early stages, this examination stops at the bedside. Then it is extended by invention of technical machinery involving instruments and procedures of all kinds. A further important extension carries the fluids, secretions, excretions of the patient to the laboratory. Ultimately groups of cells and bits of tissue are removed for examination. The precision and cost of modern medical technology restrain, erratically but nontheless vigorously, the technology that otherwise would include doing all tests on all patients.

Though the succession splash was known to Hippocrates and sounds of an open chest wound, pneumothorax, creaking joints, borborygmi and the expulsion of flatus, or belching gave some crude notions of what went on inside, real advance did not occur until Auenbrugger developed percussion and Laennec devised the stethoscope. Harvey, a great naturalist and biologist, added experimentation to biological observation and reduced thereby the time and energy wasted on detached speculation. The introduction of an active examination into a process that hitherto had been mere observation and description set modern medicine on its feet. The whole arena on medicine began to change in a way far more radical than its pioneers could have understood. The development of physical examination as technique was encouraged by repeated corrections that occurred when the predictions about the nature and lesions during terminal diseases were corrected and extended by the findings at autopsy.

A concept of cause, an automatic relation of antecedent to subsequent event or process, and an understanding of the relationship in a chain of events occurring in sequence have developed to some degree in all sentient creatures. The predictive value of these relations enabled man to find his way in the perils of a hostile world. Empirically he has often succeeded because he developed a rough rule of thumb to deal with many circumstances and situations in which he found himself. Without our ability to react to stimuli and to learn by experience, we could not survive. But when we come to the more complex matters of intellectual comprehensions of causality, we are frustrated. Everything and every action has properties and processes that are incalculable. Every happening is contingent on or related to every other happening. A comprehensive and instantaneous understanding of cause surpasses the strait limits of human intellect.

To get at causality we must use words in symbolic thought. Once a concept is frozen in words or printed as a statement, it acquires an artificial finality that sharply limits its usefulness. Maxims and aphorisms are inadequate as guides for action because they lack the necessary specifications or have numerous exceptions. Laws of nature represent not so much the essence of things as the frequency of symbols in a distribution curve. Variations and exceptions reveal the essentially arbitrariness of nature's laws. They are unnatural matings of separate elements in a biological and philosophical bed of Procrustes. The laws of nature are made by man for his convenience. As understanding increases, they are changed. Our rules as well as our concepts are provisional but at the same time must be operational, for they are the only maps we have. We correct them as we move on and see new terrain from a new vantage. As science advances, we hope that it will give us more and more exact maps. In its nature, however, the practice of medicine consists of reading inevitably incomplete or erroneous maps. Yet the lay of the land seemingly goes in a certain direction. The most marvelous maps, if unread, can be of no help. The most exquisite map will never do the job for us but can only tell us whither and to some extent how a journey might go.

An inevitable effect of a commitment to a belief in any a priori system of medicine is that it disqualifies the mind for correct observation. No one with a crotchet in his mind is to be trusted. He will find what he expects to find and will fail to find what he believes not to be present. It is not that he is willfully falsifying the evidence; it is simply that his machinery for vision is inadequate. Every object he sees is distorted through the astigmatism of his own biased lenses. The view is not achromatic or true. As Bartlett says:

The art of observation is always a very difficult art but nowhere is it more so than in the science of medicine. It is one of the rarest accomplishments. The annals of medical science are crowded with the names of the men who are famous for their learning, for experiments or for their reasoning and speculative power, but very few are remembered as distinguished observers.

The inherent variability of man, the biological and structural uniqueness of every different individual, present formidable obstacles to the understanding of disease processes and particularly in generalizing them. We assume that some external agents that cause, influence, or set going the process of disease have specificity within fairly narrow lines. Presumably, however, microorganisms share the variability of man. When one uses an experimental animal, precisely measured doses, clear control of environment, and a pure strain of animal—which may be further brought toward homogeneity by using litter mates or physical parabiosis—individual variations still prevail. Statistics cancel some of them. Even the quantitative aspects of environmental heat or cold, the important problem of nutritional controls, all militate against the derivation of sound general concepts to help us understand the mechanisms of disease.

This hodgepodge summary may merely serve to demonstrate how little we really comprehend of health or disease. We talk of treating the whole person of the patient. We use the catch name holism, not for its real substance but to float yet more cults with more zealots, organizers, and money-raisers as the ignorant gull the innocent. Nor will a Christian Scientist's denial keep him from having an offending cancer or an appendix operated on and removed. Nonetheless, a realization that a man exists with a specific heredity, finite structure, and measurable physiological state in a given environment impinged upon by particular and partly defined stimuli at least defines the problem of illness as one aspect of the broader problem of ecology.

The answers we seek are a clearer perception of man and his place in nature.

REFERENCES

Ackerknecht, E. H. (1955). "A Short History of Medicine," p. 258. Ronald Press, New York.
Bartlett, E. (1844). "An Essay on the Philosophy of Medical Science," pp. 205-206. Lea and Blanchard, Philadelphia.
Bean, W. B. (1953). Caritas medici. *Arch. Intern. Med.* **92,** 153-161.
Bean, W. B. (1955). Vitamania, polypharmacy and witchcraft. *Arch. Intern. Med.* **96,** 137-141.
Bean, W. B. (1957). Careers in medicine: some inquiry into "why we study medicine" and "why we specialize." *Arch. Intern. Med.* **99,** 847-858.
Bean, W. B. (1958a). Embryon truths in verities yet in their chaos. *Arch. Intern. Med.* **102,** 179-188.
Bean, W. B. (1958b). William Harvey. *Arch. Intern. Med.* **102,** 149-154.
Bean, W. B. (1961a). A patient's pilgrimage through medical history. *Arch. Intern. Med.* **108,** 548-558.

Bean, W. B. (1961b). Some historic sidelights on medicine's forgotten man, the patient. *Trans. Assoc. Life Insur. Med. Directors Ann. Meet., 69th* **45**, 138-154.

Bean, W. B. (1962a). Greek experience. *Arch. Intern. Med.* **110**, 411-413.

Bean, W. B. (1962b). The humanities in medicine: the medical and scientific significance of the seemingly small, trivial and insignificant (The Groedel Lecture for 1961). *Am. J. Cardiol.* **9**, 1-11.

Bollet, A. J. (1964). On seeking the cause of disease. *Clin. Res.* **12**, 305-310.

Cahill, K. M. (1963). Platonic concepts of hepatology. *Arch. Intern. Med.* **111**, 819-822.

Clements, F. E. (1932). Primitive concepts of disease. *Univ. Calif. Pub. Am. Archeol. Ethnol.* **32**, 185-252.

Dorn, H. F. (1959). Some problems arising in prospective and retrospective studies of the etiology of disease. *N. Engl. J. Med.* **261**, 571-579.

Engel, G. L. (1952). Homeostasis, behavioral adjustment and the concept of health and disease. *In* "Midcentury Psychiatry, An Overview" (R. Grinker, ed.), pp. 33-46. Thomas, Springfield, Illinois.

Garrison, F. H. (1964). "An Introduction to the History of Medicine." Saunders, Philadelphia, Pennsylvania.

Hudson, R. P. (1966). The concept of disease. *Ann. Intern. Med.* **65**, 595-601.

Major, R. H. (1954). "A History of Medicine in Two Volumes." Thomas, Springfield, Illinois.

Menninger, K. (1977). The physical concept of illness: treatment by manipulation. *In* "The Vital Balance: The LIfe Process in Mental Health and Illness," pp. 58-59. Penguin Books, Baltimore, Maryland.

Mettler, C. C. (1947). "History of Medicine, A Correlative Text Arranged According to Subject." Blakiston, Philadelphia, Pennsylvania.

Middleton, W. S. (1956). The natural history of disease. *Arch. Intern. Med.* **98**, 401-408.

Richard, M. J., and Harper, D. M. (1958). Evolution and illness. *Lancet* **ii**, 92.

Riese, W. (1963). "The Conception of Disease, Its History, Its Versions and Its Nature." Philosophical Library, New York.

Sigerist, H. (1951). "A History of Medicine: Primitive and Archaic Medicine," Vol. 1, p. 564. Oxford Univ. Press, London and New York.

Sigerist, H. (1961). "A History of Medicine: Early Greek, Hindu and Persian Medicine," Vol. 2, p. 352. Oxford Univ. Press, London and New York.

Singer, C. (1928). "A Short History of Medicine Introducing Medical Principles to Students and Non-medical Readers." Oxford Univ. Press, London and New York.

Singer, C., and Underwood, E. A. (1962). "Short History of Medicine," 2nd ed. Oxford Univ. Press, London and New York.

Virchow, R. (1849). *De Einheitsbestrebunger in der wissenschaftlichen Medizin*. G. Reimer, Berlin.

Wolf, S. (1963). A new view of disease. *J. Am. Med. Assoc.* **184**, 129-130.

3
Culture, Biology, and the Study of Disease

HORACIO FABREGA, JR.

53

BIOCULTURAL ASPECTS OF DISEASE
Copyright © 1981 by Academic Press, Inc.
All rights of reproduction in any form reserved.
ISBN 0-12-598720-X

I. INTRODUCTION

This volume and its overall organization reflect a rather classic Western biomedical perspective. In that perspective, "disease" generally refers to physical changes that produce interferences in function, and "culture" refers to any group or population of people among whom one is likely to find specific diseases or frequencies of diseases that differ from those of other groups. One obvious aim of such a volume is to inform the clinician or public health specialist about the medical problems he or she is likely to be concerned with. A basic postulate of anyone looking at medical problems from a biological standpoint must be that the biomedical sciences provide a true and realistic portrait of medical problems seen in social–cultural space. By that it is meant that the sciences in question are held to rest on units of analysis, modes of classifying, and rules of interpretation that are unproblematic and that provide a valid and "real" description of medical diseases as they distribute among populations.

In this chapter "culture" and medical problems or "diseases" are looked at somewhat differently. First, the epistemological assumptions of the biomedical perspective will be examined. Second, the way in which biomedical concepts are used and the kind of insights about disease they produce, and also ignore, will be examined. In this discussion, culture is not considered as population or society, but rather as something symbolic or conventional—a rule system, as it were. The implications of looking at disease and culture in this way will be discussed. I will try to relate this discussion to contemporary biologic and social theory. In terms of the metaphor of a biomedical portrait of medical problems, one can say that in this chapter we shall scrutinize and look beyond the biomedical portrait of disease and inquire about its units of analysis and how they acquired their configuration.

II. BASIC CONCEPTS

A. Definition of Culture

The term culture has a broad meaning. It can refer to groups and mean such things as a group's religion, values and attitudes, ritual practices, family structure, language, and mode of social organization. The possible role of these factors in disease is complex. The vagueness and generality of culture begs the question of which specific factors influence disease frequency and expression. A related problem has been that social scientists often use culture in a general sense as a contrast to biologic–organic, a strategy that is not satisfactory (see below). Indeed, a basic biologic capacity of man is developing and using culture, and, moreover, if one takes a historical and population frame of reference (i.e., studies the evolution and movements of populations), the connection between the cultural (regardless of how defined) and the neuro-organic is direct. This is so because a "group's way of life," a traditional component of culture, encompasses mating rules, dietary habits and practices, activity cycles and patterns, and modifications of microclimate, all of which are classically thought to have physiologic or organic effects and to have evolved for successfully coping with ecologic factors that pose biologic threats.

An important contemporary definition of culture, and one that we shall adopt here, involves a group's system of social symbols and their meanings (Geertz, 1973). A sine qua non of human action is its expressiveness, and social symbols figure importantly in what such actions mean and the role they play in behavior. That the meanings of social symbols can only be inferred from a group's mode of life prompts a definition that will be used here. Culture refers to the symbolic properties discernible in a people's social and psychologic behaviors.

B. Culture and Behavior

One is led to posit a concept like culture as a way of explaining parsimoniously the differences in the observed behaviors among peoples. The idea behind culture is thus linked to human behavior in an elemental way. The student of culture may look at behavior in two ways. Social behaviors refer to activities such as gestures, demeanor, facial displays, and simple or coordinated actions (including the performance aspects of language and speech) that are viewed in an interindividual context. The appropriate performance of a social role belongs in this behavior category.

Behaviors that reflect internal discriminative processes and that correlate with observable social behaviors are here termed psychological. They often imply learning and, in humans, the internalizations of symbols and rules that are shared. Each category of behavior (i.e., social and psychological) logically implies the other. Psychological behaviors embrace such things as thinking, perceiving, interpretation of actions, rules for expressing actions, remembering, and problem-solving. Although "psychological" implies conscious or deliberate, many psychologic behaviors cannot easily be considered to be either.

An additional aspect of behavior needs to be singled out: the "sensorimotor." In looking at behavior from that aspect one emphasizes the sequences of more or less coordinated muscular contractions and changes therein. Reflexes, postural changes, muscular tone, the coordination of finely graded muscular contraction, and changes in sensation, when viewed purely as physical phenomena, constitute sensorimotor behaviors as do covert ("hidden") vegetative responses involving the viscera, blood vessels, and organs. These three categories of behavior are considered later in the chapter.

C. Culture and the Nature-Nurture Question

I have defined culture as a special type of environmental factor or influence. A system of social symbols (i.e., meanings) refers to people's understanding, something they learn that is somehow linked to language and thought. A cultural anthropologist examines the various ways in which culture operates in a given context and he seeks ways of understanding the "reality" to which the people subscribe. The logic, structure, and rationale of social activity viewed symbolically (i.e., symbolic behavior) and purely for its own sake—and regardless of other determining factors—is what will claim his or her interest. If one were to find a mythical group whose members operated without brains, livers, or hearts, the cultural anthropologist's interest in culture would in no way weaken, for the relevance of physical organs to his domain of interest is not critical.

We, however, are interested in behavioral organization and functioning seen in relation to persons with brains, livers, and hearts. As observers interested in separating out different types of influences operating on a given phenomenon (in this instance, disease and behavior), we seem driven to distinguish among environmental influences, both physical (things like diet or altitude) and nonphysical (social, cultural, or symbolic), and also between environmental influences and nonenvironmental ones, specifically genetic factors. To the claim of the cultural anthropologist that "behaviors of a certain type reflect culture," we often counter that they really reflect genetic influences or organic factors.

Exchanges such as these illustrate the nature-nurture quandary that is integral to the study of biologic phenomena, especially human social and psychologic behavior. We have little difficulty in understanding that eye color or blood groups (phenotypes) are mainly genetically determined. Even colorblindness we unproblematically accept as being genetic, although we would be prepared to accept that the intrauterine environment of the fetus might contribute some variance to this phenotype. The possible role of cultural factors in affecting such phenomena seems remote indeed, if not nonsensical.

Yet in one way culture as symbolic phenomena could be made relevant. If one could show that eating preferences and social living habits (i.e., symbolic phenomena) affected maternal nutritional status and health and that these in turn influenced dramatically the intrauterine environment of a pregnant mother, then a way would be open for a discussion of possible cultural influences in eye color or color vision. A seeming competition between culture and physical environmental factors—and indeed between environment and genes—can in fact be said to be inherent in analysis of most biologic phenomena whose form or structure varies from person to person. Precisely because "competitions" of this type are so integral to explanations of phenomena like human social and psychologic behavior are we forced to give up the quest for either/or solutions to the problem of understanding their bases or causes. In the study of certain aspects of disease and behavior, reducing analysis to either/or perspectives may not be feasible or appropriate, whereas acknowledging an indeterminacy of sorts, and indeed a complementarity, may be. Because of the inseparability of biological and cultural sources of human variation one can use the term biocultural.

D. Definition of Disease

We use the term disease frequently and mean by it an impairment in health and well-being. All peoples have ideas of disease that are generally analogous. However, because my purposes have been to explore the theoretical and scientific implications of this idea, I have adopted rigorous definitional criteria: disease refers to a negative (i.e., unwanted) discontinuity or deviation in the condition of a person. The condition of a person is assessed from his verbal reports (e.g., pain, body functioning), the observation of others, and/or information obtained in applying various procedures. The assessment (i.e., diagnosis) involves determining whether a person's condition deviates, and two types of norms seem to be used to establish that this deviation is present: norms set by the person across time (i.e., personal norms) and norms set by a relevant group to which the person belongs during the present period (i.e., group norms). I have indicated elsewhere that from a social standpoint this stipulation constitutes a necessary condition for claiming that someone is diseased (Fabrega, 1974). The class of diseased persons of a society is a subset of those classed as deviant. Cultural conventions about well-being and health are used to measure deviations. When preliterate people use the idea of disease, they usually have in mind changes in the (sick) person's behavior and functioning. In modern nations, behavior and functioning are important, but more and more abstract attributes of the person (e.g., physiochemical, anatomical, physiological) are implied. When the latter attributes are salient, I say that the idea or concept of disease in biomedical.

III. CULTURE AND BIOLOGIC PROCESSES

In contemporary biologic theory, observed behavioral differences are considered part of the phenotypes and are judged to represent expressions of genotypic factors that have been influenced or modulated by the environment. In this chapter, phenotypic patterns of psychosocial behavior of a people are partially equated with culture. The behavior patterns noted reflect rules and programs (i.e., symbolic phenomena) that have a neural representation of some sort and that are operative throughout a person's life. Such rules and programs can influence a number of biologic processes. In this section, the complementarity between biologic and cultural phenomena is illustrated.

A. Neonate Behaviors

The work of Brazelton (1977) among the Maya Indians of Zinacantan in the highlands of Chiapas, Mexico, serves as an example of the ways in which child development has been studied cross-culturally and also illustrates one aspect of the complementarity between culture and biology. Contrary to approaches used by social scientists who study child development, Brazelton, a pediatrician, emphasized neurological findings in his work. He performed neurological examinations and unstructured observations of neonates at birth and in the first week of life.

The Zinacantan Maya are an agricultural group that has retained its traditional indigenous ways despite strong efforts by the national government to encourage Western values and principles. Brazelton noted that among these people individual self-expression is not a goal and that instead conformity is highly valued and respected. The Zinacantecos show a high incidence of disease and illness; about 30% of children die before age 4, half of that group in infancy. Subclinical malnutrition is widespread, although severe malnutrition, which might permanently damage the infant central nervous system, is not present. Brazelton reported that among the Zinacantecos no pharmacologic agents are given during delivery and no obstetrical techniques are used. The infant is swaddled after birth and is soon thereafter carried by the mother in a rebozo, a small blanket that she wraps around her shoulder. This mode of carrying ensures that infants have a higher level of kinesthetic and tactile stimulation during the first year. During that year, infants are neither propped up to enable them to look around nor are they talked to or stimulated by eye contact. Similarly, infants are not generally placed on the floor to allow them to explore, and the mothers rarely try to elicit social responses from them. Finally, mothers frequently respond to activity of the infant by breast-feeding the child.

From observations made soon after delivery, Brazelton reported that the size of Zinacanteco neonates appeared to be much like premature babies in the United States, although they showed no jerky movements or snapback of limbs as do the U.S. prematures. In appearance and behavior, the Zinacantecos appeared mature and seemed to show a high level of regulation and control of the autonomic nervous system. They were quiet, having relatively limited motor activity, but displayed a striking sensory alertness. Compared with Caucasian controls, Zinacanteco infants were distinguished by a higher freedom and fluidity of movement, low output of spontaneous movement, and no overshooting or overreaction to stimuli like U.S. infants. The Zinacanteco's muted level of response noted at birth was maintained through the first week. The U.S. infants showed an increase in the intensity of their responses. Among Zinacantecos, spontaneous startles were rare and the general disorganization and lack of coordination usually seen in days 1 and 2 in U.S. newborns were not observed. A quiet and alert mental state was maintained for long periods, with slow smooth transitions from state to state. Thus, the Zinacanteco child's apparent control of motor behavior and mental state appeared to be of higher order, permitting repeated and prolonged responses to auditory, visual, and kinesthetic stimuli during the first week.

Observations during their first year revealed a paucity of vocalizations among Zinacanteco infants; cries were brief and promptly terminated by mother's quieting activities. Infants rarely mouthed their hands and never sucked their fingers, and no pacifiers were used. Zinacantecos appeared quieter and less demanding than middle-class U.S. infants of comparable ages. During formal testing, Zinacantecos met novelty with impassive faces and showed little exploration or experimental play. Estimations of mental and motor ages of Zinacantecos lagged behind by about 1 month those of American babies, but no increasing decrement with age was observed. The Zinacanteco infants passed through the same developmental milestone sequences as did U.S. infants and also at about the same rate.

Brazelton concluded that U.S. neonates are motoric, and that among them reflex motor responses interfere with alertness. On the other hand, the mental states of Zinacanteco neonates appear to be less labile and peaks of sleep and awake states are leveled off. These differences in behavior were related to cultural styles of adult behavior and could result from genetic differences and/or environmental factors. Thus, the great amount of regular physical activity of pregnant females in Zinacantan and the subclinical malnutrition that prevails might have produced slow liquid movements and what appeared to be a superb state of motorsensory control. The Zinacantecos showed a possible auditory or visual precocity, but that could have resulted from a lack of competition from motor activity. At the same time, it appeared to Brazelton that the mother set up a mode of contingent responsiveness to infant's needs before he or she expressed a need or made demands. Thus, Zinacantecos seemed to have no experience during infancy that might lay the framework for a sequence of self-motivated demand, frustration, and then gratification. Zinacanteco child-rearing emphasis on subdued motor activity and on averting demand–response patterns was noted during testing, for when infant motor activity was elicited, the breasts of their lactating mothers leaked milk. Such a "letdown" response follows the baby's cry in U.S. mothers. Results of Brazelton's study suggest that the "mothering responses" of Zinacantecos reinforce the quiet passivity and limited motor activity that was already present in early neonatal interactions and that is valued among adults. In Zinacantan a fussy baby is, in fact, judged to be ill and to be in need of a curing ceremony. Contrariwise, quiet nondemanding babies are a desideratum and child-rearing influences seem to contribute to their production. Thus Brazelton, while emphasizing cultural factors, was also arguing for a possible fit between biologic–organic factors (i.e., genes, subclinical infection) and symbolic ones (e.g., values, preferred styles of behavior).

B. Basic Neurobiologic Processes

A line of research directly suggesting genetic "racial" differences in sensorimotor behaviors is that reported by Freedman (1974). He matched groups of Chinese-American and European-American newborns for age, sex, mean Apgar scores, mean hours of labor, age of mothers, and whether mothers had received medication during labor. Furthermore, behavior scales and neurological examination were used to screen for neural damage. The behaviors of newborns were observed using categories such as temperament, sensory development, autonomic and central nervous system maturity, motor development, and social interest and response. Neonates were tested hours after delivery. Multivariate analysis of variance indicated that on total performance the two groups were significantly different; the main difference stemmed from items measuring temperament and a variable termed excitability–unperturbability. These differences in infant behaviors are consistent with cultural norms and traits linked to Oriental culture. Important to note is the substantial overlap in range on all scales found between the Chinese and Caucasian infants. Quantitative differences thus distinguished the two groups. These results were attributed to differences in gene pool between the respective populations. In conformance with the results of Freedman's study are the observations of Wolff (1977), who studied the vasomotor responses to alcohol in Caucasoid and Monogoloid infants. Group differences were observed, independent of geographic boundary or previous exposure to alcohol. Wolff tentatively concluded that group differences among newborns may indicate differences in autonomic nervous system reactivity having a genetic basis.

Studies of pitch discrimination among infants show their discriminations are adultlike and probably continuous (Eimas et al., 1970). This finding parallels others involving the perception of luminance (Bornstein, 1978). Coincidentally, preverbal infants perceive speech sounds like adults in that they can discriminate meaningful units (termed phonemes) discontinuously. For example, they are able to tell the difference in acoustical properties that account for phonemic distinctions between /b/ and /p/. This type of perception parallels that of wavelength regions as colors (Bornstein et al., 1975). Discrimination of phonemes thus gives rise to perceptual features for the infant as they do in the adult. More specifically, infants show clear-cut between-phonemic-category discriminations but no within-phonemic-category discrimination. From these results one cannot, of course, conclude that infants are processing acoustic variations as though they "had meaning," but one can hypothesize that mechanisms underlying speech perception are innate. Categorical perception in infants in the auditory mode has also been demonstrated with nonspeech musical sounds (Cutting et al., 1976). Because similar categorical perception exists in adults, these studies emphasize the ontogenetic stability of this perceptual capacity.

Studies involving color and speech perception point to the universal and neurobiologic nature of discriminability. Regions of the continua of voice-onset time and wavelength wherein acute discriminations are possible represent points of transition among perceptual features. The latter thus reflect discontinuity in the operating characteristics of these particular sensory systems vis-à-vis particular physical continua. Sensory systems can thus be said to provide an infant with a kind of innate knowledge. The properties of sensory systems involving speech and hue have been studied in infrahuman species and found to be similar in certain respects to those of man, pointing to their evolutionary origins (Petersen *et al.*, 1978; Waters and Wilson, 1976; De Valois and De Valois, 1975; Zoloth *et al.*, 1979).

Recently Bornstein (1980) critically reviewed empirical data in infant sensory physiology and discussed its implications, and the following account draws heavily from his analysis. As he indicated, an important question in behavioral biology concerns the possible universality (i.e., pancultural distribution) of feature perception. Related to such universality is whether the neurologic substrates of feature perception are plastic and their development is influenced by selective environmental experiences. With respect to universality of feature perception, babies have been noted to be able to discriminate speech sounds that are intrinsic to some languages different from their native languages, but not from others. In other words, the evidence shows that infants are born with the capacity for categorical perception and can make many more discriminations than are actually used in their immediate language community. Conversely, adult perception is not necessarily congruent with infant perception, indicating that new discriminations can be learned as a result of selective experiences. Because perceptual features can be added to the infant's endowed repertoire, initial discriminative capacities do not constrain him. At the same time, in some spheres, adults retain the ability to distinguish features not capitalized in their language community; the neurologic machinery for these perceptions thus persists in the absence of relevant selective or reinforcing experiences, indicating that natural properties of the auditory and visual sensory systems are not easily eroded. General experience with a wide range of colors and sounds thus appears sufficient to maintain "native" feature sensitivities. In summary, "feature perception is ontogenetically canalized, and its pancultural validity biases the newborn system in the direction of mature perceptual analysis. Feature perception is adaptive, moreover, and during ontogeny it is subject to tempered modification, addition or attrition, but under somewhat rigid constraints" (Bornstein, 1980).

Bornstein points out that discontinuous discriminability of energy in the environment gives rise to perceptual contrasts and opposition that structure impressions into usable "chunks" of information that are stable and can be further organized by the organism. This reduction of variance, which facilitates information encoding, is the basis of categorization that itself underlies cognitive activity. Categorization speeds encoding time and facilitates recognition. Perceptual constancies made possible by innate capacities for categorical perception provide an initial guidance for the emergence of rules for communication and elementary cognitive behavior. In this way, perceptual constancies in vision and audition may be viewed as elementary visual and auditory concepts that facilitate learning, serve as templates for thinking, and form an *"Anlagen* for mature conceptual behavior and the treatment of transformations or variations of other stimulus sets" (Bornstein, 1980). Neurobiologic constancies built into the human apparatus are here seen to lay the groundwork for later cultural learning.

Studies involving global aspects of the sensorimotor behaviors of newborns suggest an even more pervasive uniformity or universality rooted in the sociobiology of man. Thus, observations of neonate interaction with caretaker have shown that infant whole-body movements synchronize with the articulatory elements of adult speech as early as the first day of life. From studies of adult behavior that rely on an ethological frame of reference, Condon and Sander (1974) derived the concept of "interactional synchrony," which refers to the configurational organization of units of a listener's body motions that synchronize with the speaker's speech. Interactional synchrony occurs out of awareness of the interactant. Condon and Sander applied their techniques of measurement of microbody movements to newborns. Their study focused on interactional synchrony between sound segments of adult speech and points of change in the configuration of neonate movements. They found that the infant responds in a patterned and organized manner to adult speech. Segments of movements were synchronous with the adult speech, indicating a precise and sustained concurrence. No such concurrence was demonstrated when random neonate movements, filmed during silence, were analyzed in relation to adult sounds. These findings indicated that the correspondence was not due to a random fitting together of patterns of infant movement with patterns of adult speech. Furthermore, audiotapes containing English and Chinese were presented to American neonates and a clear correspondence between speech sounds and neonate movement emerged in both instances. Disconnected vowel and tapping sounds did not produce the correspondence associated with natural rhythmic speech, suggesting that meaningful speech was the organizing variable.

That study thus suggests that infants (at least those in the United States) are born with a general capacity to orient and relate organismically to human language in speech regardless of its morphology and syntax. Early in life the infant thus begins to move in a precise and rhythmic fashion with the organization of the speech structure of his culture. A developmental sociobiologic entrainment process appears to be set up between the body (and its motions activities) and the linguistic system of a culture. Rhythm, syntax, and paralinguistic nuances are interlocked with body motion styles and responses. This pattern of neonate responsivity no doubt prepares and helps shape operational formats for later speech and may be held to provide a conditioning context for internal and external body activities with respect to nonverbal, but still linguistic, aspects of communication. Language, speech, and, by extension, culture are here seen to connect into bodily rhythms and processes and illustrate one aspect of the complementarity between culture and biology.

C. Culture and Internal Bodily States

The term internal bodily states will be used to denote patterns of visceral muscular responses that are viewed in physical terms (which in principle could correlate with subjective states given cultural significance). In physiological anthropology this class of responses is the one that has been of greatest interest to anthropologists investigating group differences in behavior with the aim of linking these to nervous system functioning. The area of work known as environmental physiology is concerned with similar kinds of problems.

Several observations can be made about this area of study. The first is the importance given to the idea of physiological adaptation. The researcher assumes and searches for response patterns indicating that the person's physiological system is changed in some special way that implies a better adapted fit to the environment. Another important question is that of separating genetically determined versus environmentally acquired response patterns. A third general feature of this area of study is that, when acquired influences are documented, physical environmental variables (to which a particular cultural group is exposed) are usually seen as producing the differences in responses. Conversely, symbolic influences are rarely proffered in the explanations for any observed differences. At most the indirect or passive aspect of culture is held important: rules of the group may cause the individual to be exposed to a different constellation of physical environmental variables. A fourth feature of this field is that nervous system parameters are ordinarily not directly studied and often are not even invoked in explanations, the researchers concentrating instead on the gross physiological response per se. When physiological anthropologists do (indirectly) invoke neural explanations, it is the "lower" level of the nervous system that is represented. Reflex phenomena and other forms of automatic and nonvolitional (i.e., "nonsymbolic") factors are used to account for an observed effect, for example, peripheral nerve functioning or reflex adjustments in the spinal cord or brainstem.

In line with this general trend in physiological anthropology (for researchers to focus on more or less automatic and peripheral aspects of nervous system function), one observes a relative paucity of interest in psychophysiology. In this field, one finds principles and concepts that implicate "culture" and thus should have an inherent appeal to anthropologists. As an example, Mandler (1967) distinguished between psychologically functional physiological variables and physiologically functional psychological variables. The former refer to physiological responses that control psychological events and processes; the latter (which on intuitive grounds should appeal to anthropologists) refer to psychological or behavioral events that control physiological responses. To the extent that psychological states are affected by cultural influences, they may control physiologic responses. Additional topics in psychophysiology that relate to anthropological questions devolve from the ideas of Engel (1972) vis-à-vis "response specificities" and those of Schachter (1971) on interpretation of "emotional" states. Because anthropologists have been attracted to the notion of personality and character as internalized correlates of culture, one would think that the idea of individuals and groups showing distinctive hierarchies of autonomic responses would have a similar appeal. In short, it is theoretically plausible that, just as cultural groups show differences in physiological adaptation to physical environmental factors, they can show differences in (psycho)physiologic adaptation to their social environment.

The ability of a person to consciously modify the functioning of his autonomic nervous system through contingent reinforcement of responses fed back to him is an established generalization in the field of psychophysiology. Just as it is reasonable to expect that groups may differ in (psycho)physiological responsivity, one may expect that they may differ in their ability to control this responsivity and that these differences can be traced to acquired (and also, of course, genetic) influences. In this category of behavior, one may well find correlates of culture that persons more or less consciously learn or that at least they acquire passively as a consequence of unique social experiences. As an example of this line of research, Japanese subjects studied in a laboratory situation were compared with U.S. subjects and showed a more general stress response to films than did Americans (Lazarus et al., 1966). That study suggested that cultural and/or genetic factors accounted for differences in autonomic reactivity. In another study, Japanese subjects showed operant self-control of their skin potentials similar to that of Americans. This control appeared to be more immediate in the Japanese, however (Shapiro and Watanabee, 1972). (See Schwartz and Shapiro, 1973, for a review of this literature.)

Subjects belonging to different ethnic groups have been compared for their reactions to pain (Sternbach and Tursky, 1965; Tursky and Sternbach, 1967; Weisenberg, 1977). In the study of pain, threshold discrimination of pain sensation and of tolerance for pain are usually emphasized. A study by Sternbach and Tursky (1965) failed to show differences in the way ethnic groups estimate the magnitude of pain, reflecting a uniformity in the way pain is evaluated from a sensory point of view. Ethnic differences were noted in measures involving pain tolerance, which are judged to reflect the motivational–reactive component of pain. Attitudes and anxiety levels in subjects belonging to different ethnic groups are ordinarily invoked in explanations of differences in pain tolerance. Ethnic differences in pain responses have also been explained in terms of psychophysical and autonomic functioning, for example, as reflected in habituation to pain stimuli.

Since cultural factors apparently can influence some aspects of pain, an internal state having behavioral correlates, one is left to wonder whether similar factors might influence other visceral states, specifically emotions of different types. The role of culture language in the description of emotional terms is a staple theme in cross-cultural psychology (see e.g., Tanaka-Matsumi and Marsella, 1976; Marsella *et al.*, 1973), and the work of Schachter (1971) points to ways in which cultural influences may affect the meaning and labeling of internal states. At the same time, the influence of culture on the facial expressions that accompany emotion have been carefully analyzed (Ekman, 1973, 1977; Ekman *et al.*, 1972). The work of Ekman points to pancultural factors in the way certain "basic" emotions are registered in the face, leading him in fact to posit a facial affect program, the neurological substrate of which is probably located subcortically. Although that body of work constitutes yet another line of evidence that points in the direction of biological uniformities, Ekman has described cultural differences in the way emotions are masked and elaborated. However, the (psycho)physiologic correlates of emotions constitute a topic that has not been systematically studied cross-culturally.

D. Conceptualizing Culture Neurobiologically

1. *Cultural Influences and Brain Function*

Culture refers to symbols, rules, and/or conventions that a group has about such things as the world, the self, others, and social life itself. The way in which culture could affect brain function can be conceptualized in three ways. First, cultural conventions involving behavior and child-rearing may, in a purely mechanical sense, influence which physical environmental stimuli (and to what degree) impinge on the newborn and the developing infant. Such stimuli typically are studied by neural scientists, and to varying degrees many (given sufficient underload or overload conditions) can affect neural development and function and, by implication, behavior. Whether human infants are ordinarily subject to analogous levels of "under" or "over" stimulation is questionable. Nonetheless, on logical grounds alone, one should allow for the possibility. Cultural conventions can also be conceptualized dynamically as a code that is internalized by the infant and then helps regulate which level or pattern of stimuli is attended to, selected, processed, and integrated in the higher levels of the nervous system. This influence might take place not in primary sensory areas, but rather in secondary association areas wherein intermodal integrations and transformations are believed to occur. Initially nonverbally (i.e., "emotively," through cooing, touch, fondling, directing), and later through the acquisition of actual language and speech, stimuli from the environment may be viewed as "packaged" or ordered in a meaningful way. This effect of culture on brain functioning is clearly evident prelinguistically and during the acquisition of language and may play a role in music recognition, in emotional expression, and in the way other brain capacities come to be realized, such as those for taste, emotional experience, and the patterning and labeling of internal bodily states. In contemporary interpretations of human brain organization, emphasis is given to the various "brains" (e.g., protomammalian, limbic) that are seen as somehow fused together. In these accounts, emphasis is given to the role language and culture play in modifying the functions of the "ancestral" brain.

A third way in which one can conceptualize cultural influences is by considering an adult who migrates to a new social group and comes to adopt its social practices. Such a person will no doubt learn a great deal simply by observation and imitation, and his native language system would obviously play an influential role in the process (e.g., through verbal introspection, rehearsal, and training). A better understanding of the conventions of the group would follow from learning its language. In both instances, neurolinguistic substrates play a critical mediating role. How and to what extent other structures and levels of the nervous system participate in this type of "enculturation" is not known. The literature dealing with recovery of aphasia among polyglots contains hints that emotion and language performance are linked in complex ways.

2. Neurologic Substrates of Culture

A review of literature involving culture and behavior points to uniformities underlying much of the behavior studied by anthropologists. Moreover, even when cultural differences are singled out, one can say that culture as a symbol system influences and patterns behavior, provided that the behavior is looked at in symbolic (i.e., cultural) terms. Although a tautology of this form is often reflected in the way culture and behavior are conceptualized, so-called symbolic behaviors are the outcome of (produced by) brain programs or routines of some sort. How is one to understand cultural differences in terms of neural substrates?

Neuropsychologists speak of the engram as the physical brain substrate of memory. Although not often mentioned explicitly, it is likely that part of what social scientists have in mind when speaking of "culture," and "symbolic" can be equated with the engrams of the semantic memory system. As described by Tulving (1972) and illustrated by Warrington (1975), that system presumably embodies the repository of knowledge and beliefs that a person acquires as he learns his culture. Information of the semantic memory system may be judged to embrace such overlearned things as role prescriptions, attitudes, and values as well as beliefs, all of which constitute the data of social scientists. In summary, one brain analogue of culture can be thought of as involving protein changes that influence conduction properties of synapses and populations of neurons and that serve as substrates for the posited semantic memory system. Molecular changes of this type may also be equated with the modules of Mountcastle and Edelman (1978); obviously, understanding how these molecular changes operate is at present beyond the reach of neuroscientists.

Another brain analogue of culture (and also not explicitly mentioned as such in the literature) can be equated with what neuroscientists mean when they speak of "motor programs" (Turvey, 1975; Heilman *et al.*, 1975; Rosenbaum, 1977; Deuel, 1977; Miles and Evarts, 1979), that is, physical changes (again involving molecular arrangements, patterns of synaptic transmission, neural nets, etc.) in the brain that mediate or organize sequences of coordinated skeletal and visceral muscle movements. Motor programs are posited so as to account for the execution of organized human action, including neuromuscular activity, nonverbal communication, the expression of affect, emotion, and speech, all of which are linked to internal bodily states. Speech is an example, par excellence, of a form of human motor activity that is dominated and coordinated by thought processes. Complex motor actions like those involving speech are generally thought of as coordinated by hierarchical structures, the uppermost or executive structure of which has little or no direct control over actual motor output. The executives in charge of speech are defined as sensorimotor ideas or concepts (McNeill, 1979). These are outgrowths of sensorimotor action schemas that in infants generate movement and constitute the earliest forms of cognitive activity. Thus, at an early stage of development sensorimotor ideas are viewed as simultaneously part of action and meaning, serving as the basis of sensorimotor behavior and cognition. These ideas and schemas are viewed as the earliest templates for speech and as providing a motor basis for thought and awareness.

The neurological literature suggests that motor programs for speech may partially embody knowledge, though the information discussed above (as semantic memory) is best thought of as being represented in a physically separate manner (Geshwind *et al.*, 1968). Clearly, the location, neural organization, and mode of operation of these motor programs vis-à-vis memorial, cognitive, and visceral systems are beyond understanding at present. Nevertheless, motor programs in the brain can also be thought of as constituting neurologic substrates of culture, though neuroscientists handle these programs as universal, disregarding the question of cultural specificity and differences.

A review of the literature in the field of brain behavior indicates that when neurologically oriented researchers explicitly invoke "cultural factors" they refer to such things as patterns of cerebral asymmetry and/or relative amounts of brain tissue of a certain type that might be required (for cultural reasons) to carry out specific psychologic functions. A basic assumption, in other words, is that the brain is like a vector of connected centers and processes, each of which is organized and functions in a uniform way across the species. This "vector" is judged as a potential that social experiences can draw on. Cultural influences are equated with the way entries in this vector are used, i.e., overemphasized or underemphasized. Neurologically, then, culture is linked to special emphases to which brain regions are put and to the overall pattern and arrangement that results from such differential emphases. However, the tendency is to view much of the behavior linked to culture as reflecting universals in the underlying ''hardware'' of the brain.

E. Comment

The material reviewed in this section involving biologic processes seemingly bears little relation to culture-symbolic factors and points directly at uniformities that are built into the organism. The similarities these mechanisms have with corresponding processes in infrahuman groups raise the question of biological determinism. Behaviors which we may wish to qualify as cultural are, as it were, constrained by (or must conform to) the biologic processes outlined. However, as acknowledged by most of the writers (e.g., Bornstein, Brazelton, Condon, Freedman), such behaviors can also be said to be elaborated into a pattern that makes sense only when viewed socially and culturally. This complementariness between the neurobiologic and cultural linguistic dimensions of behavior leads some anthropologists to speak about the biocultural unity of human social behavior. The expression ''biocultural'' can also be given an evolutionary meaning. It is now held that, at different points in the evolutionary time scale, prevailing social conditions served as factors that helped select for neurologic structures and changes; behavioral adaptations made possible by these changes had the effect of modifying the social conditions of man, thereby yielding a new context for natural selection (Fox, 1975; Washburn, 1961; Wilson, 1975). These arguments imply a connection between social conditions and neurobiologic traits. This connection between social and neurobiologic factors in the evolutionary process is held to account for possible similarities in the social and cognitive behaviors of man and other primates and also to explain why the precise origins and meanings of culture are problematic. A consequence of the connection is that higher cerebral functions of man must be continuous with those of humanoid groups and might be with those found in the species most akin to man, the apes (Eisenberg and Dillon, 1971; Washburn and Moore, 1974; Napier, 1973; Young, 1974).

In summary, in this section I have argued that internal physical processes and bodily mechanisms are influenced by symbolic or cultural factors. A basic theme has been the biocultural unity of man. My intention has been to suggest that concrete expressions of disease in a society—phenomena to which we shall presently turn—involve persons who are ''programmed'' by *both* biology and culture. In succeeding sections I will try to show that disease can also be interpreted from the complementary perspectives of biology and culture.

IV. ILLNESS AND DISEASE IN BIOLOGIC THEORY

A. General Statement

What we refer to by a term such as disease is a universal occurrence in social groups. The phenomena referred to by this term is ubiquitous and recurring. All peoples develop diseases but they also, it seems, want to be rid of them.

Disease can also be seen from a purely biologic standpoint. The conditions for disease are prescribed by the synthetic theory of evolution; key concepts of evolutionary biology, such as genetic variability, environment, adaptation, and natural selection are sufficient to explain occurrences of disease. In a strict biological evolutionary sense, disease is a factor that influences the operation of natural selection. It is one of the sources of adaptive variability that determines which organisms are selected, and, if genetic factors underlie the disease (in evolutionary theory, the expression of a poor organism–environment fit), these will be underrepresented in future generations.

B. The Concept of Disease in General Biology

Because man is a member of the class of living animals, one would think that the idea of disease would have scientific utility in general biology. However, though the idea is used, its meaning is ambiguous and its explanatory power can be questioned. For example, in the mathematical study of populations, disease and its effects are constantly being considered. Here the idea is used to mean factors, often genetic, that are harmful to the population. The condition of deviations that is central to the use of the concept in human communities (see Section III, D) seems far removed. Moreover, one can envision states of a population that an evolutionary biologist might describe as involving disease but which would not meet the condition involving deviations. Thus, members of a previously stable population whose size is not decreasing because they are showing evidence of poor adjustment (e.g., because of genetic defects, acquired metabolic or physiologic disturbances) could not easily be diagnosed as diseased. Many "successful" populations have probably gone through such phases, but developments during them could not have been explained by means of the idea of disease if the condition about deviations posited earlier had been required. In other words, one would be forced to say that the minority of the population did not have the disease that proved lethal to the majority, a claim that thoroughly discredits the condition of deviation from group norms that seemed to be needed to articulate and apply the idea in the first place. Many genetic diseases pose similar logical problems, if the condition of deviation from past personal norms of the individual is required, because organisms may fail to adapt and reproduce, although biologic measures that account for this may show no changes (i.e., deviations) from earlier values.

The idea of disease is often used to point to one of the selective influences of the environment. An ecologically differentiated environment, as an example, is said to pose more hazards involving parasitic diseases than one less differentiated. When used in this way, the idea appears to refer to potentially harmful attributes of the physical environment itself (e.g., along with others such as altitude and availability of foodstuffs). At other times, the idea of disease is used to qualify acquired characteristics of the organisms that limit or militate against its capacity to reproduce or survive. As an example, the effect of crowding and inadequate diet or water supply are said to pose health hazards and to interfere (through disease) with the survival of a group. Implicit in these uses of the idea is the view that the behavior and adaption of the organism are compromised by physiological and/or structural changes. However, it is the cumulated effects on reproduction and survival that are critical, not the social–behavioral changes of the organisms.

Many observations of biologists deal with organisms with acquired defects and diseases. It is generally assumed that diseased members are shunned if they are unable to keep up with the group because they can attract predators (Bramblett, 1967; Harlow and Harlow, 1965). However, Berkson (1974) has indicated that in some instances physically compromised members are protected and dealt with in special ways, and this was, of course, noted by Darwin (1914). One can thus see behaviors that are outgrowths of "disease" and that co-members "notice," and "do something about," in the process seeming to suspend the selfish pursuits expected on the basis of evolutionary theory. Berkson suggested that the ecology of these defects and diseases can be used as clues of what the environment is currently selecting for. In other words, if (as an example) visually handicapped organisms are found in a particular group, then the environment of the group is said not to be selecting for visual acuity. Here, then, it is acknowledged that disease is linked to a maladaptation of the organism, but its survival is explained as a socially constructive group effort made possible by the valence of other selective factors. Social–behavioral changes in the diseased or defective members and in co-members have been explained in terms of ideas of social bonding, social support, dependence, and, ultimately, parent–offspring interactions (Hinde, 1974). These types of behaviors are integral to the idea of disease when we use it to qualify happenings in human groups, but similar behaviors in animal groups seem not to warrant the idea because concepts and principles linked to the sciences of social biology and ethology suffice.

The material reviewed in this section leads me to conclude that when the idea of disease is used in general biology, it can have several different meanings, some of which are not usually implied when the idea is used in a human practical framework. Moreover, states of disease in animals can be linked to changed social behaviors, some of which can elicit support; however, these behaviors are not included in the meaning of the idea of disease when it is applied to animals.

As already indicated above, the synthetic theory of evolution has available many ideas whose meanings embrace much of what one has in mind when using the idea of disease. Ideas such as organism development, genetic variation, fitness, natural selection, and environment seem sufficient to explain many of the phenomena linked to disease. The explanatory power of these ideas and the seemingly motivated and expressive aspects of behaviors linked to disease in humans are thus factors that create tensions when the idea of disease is used in a general frame of reference.

C. The Separate Meanings of Disease

The discussion thus far suggests to me that a general definition stating the conditions for using the idea of disease in a human-practical as well as in a general biological frame of reference may not be possible. One needs to make explicit specific kinds of phenomena that require explanation and develop guidelines for using ideas with reference to them. I propose that we give the general idea of disease alternative meanings. In some circumstances these meanings would be separated and in others fused.

The idea of disease as "illness" may be used to signify purely behavioral changes. In a general anthropological sense, it is a set of behaviors, judged as undesirable and unwanted in a culture, that is considered as having medical relevance. Changes in the behavioral sphere in the form of symptoms initially concern members of a social group and lead them to seek help. Relief from these unwanted behaviors is often the end-point of treatment. Disease as illness, then, may serve as a suitable idea for explaining certain changes that are of special significance to human groups. Because it refers to properties of an individual and is used in a present-oriented time-frame, the condition of deviations from past personal norms and prevailing social norms (of behavior) can be stipulated and met.

An idea or concept is also needed in general biology to describe an emergent set of changes in the structures and internal processes of living forms that underlie and account for their failure to adapt. The biomedical meaning of disease seems useful here. Because this idea of disease also refers to properties of an individual and requires diagnosis, the condition of deviations, this time involving abstract attributes of the individual (and not behaviors), still seems relevant. However, if a stipulation about reproduction and survival is included, disease as deviation from personal and group norms is difficult to sustain, because in that instance the future of the organism is implied. I also indicated earlier that in an unbounded time frame, the condition of deviation from current group norms was problematic; the criteria for establishing group deviations would not hold up when clear-cut interferences in functioning existed among most members of a population. I also indicated that genetic diseases made the condition of deviation from personal norms problematic. Moreover, in a strict evolutionary sense, the meaning of disease as a "harmful" interference in internal structures and processes that subserve living and reproduction of an organism really does require consideration of genetic material as well as future course. In addition to the difficulty of specifying future states of affairs, it is hard to see how one could equate harm between altogether differing levels of phenomena (e.g., between whole structures and genes) (Lewontin, 1974). I note, in summary, that application of strict logical criteria about deviations is problematic in the case of our biomedical disease.

In referring to abstract (e.g., chemical, molecular) structures and internal processes that underlie and account for failures in adaptation and reproduction, the biomedical idea of disease can be used to describe organisms of any type. Because of its special meanings and the fact that it is used with reference to all types of living forms, the idea of a biomedical disease has a restricted utility in a human social and valuational frame of reference. The biomedical "disease" may be especially relevant for explanations about biologic evolution, whereas the social-medical "illness" seems relevant for explanations about the complementary process of social evolution.

D. The Concept of Illness Applied to Nonhuman Organisms

I have suggested that the idea of illness applies principally to human groups and operates in a social-practical framework. Nonetheless, it seems useful to search for analogues among nonhumans. Because through illness an individual communicates disability and dysfunction, and group members respond by offering help and support, highly socialized groups and motivated actions are presupposed. That fact points me in the direction of our closest relatives, the nonhuman primates. For heuristic reasons, I will stipulate that states of (biomedical) disease can give rise to illness behaviors and lead to reciprocated ("altruistic") responses by other group members. Illness behaviors will be judged as communicative and functional, a product of natural selection. What kinds of questions and problems are raised by this stipulation?

The first set of issues involves a consideration of the conditions under which so-called illness behaviors and reciprocated actions of others occur. Intuitively compelling is the fact that a weak and diseased animal who emits distress signals poses a hazard to its group, for predators can also be drawn by the signals. In addition, should others heed this call, they themselves are rendered less mobile and less able to forage for food, which can blunt their competitiveness. Both of these consequences of heeding a diseased member's calls are disadvantageous and suggest that group members will avoid responding to, and in fact will shun, sick members. On the other hand, behaviors that attract and link members together clearly are prominent among nonhuman primates. Maternal-offspring attachments and, later, kinship bonds are powerful socializing influences that consolidate a group and facilitate coping and adaptation. Behaviors that promote such bonds could be activated during episodes of disease. It is well known that primates send and receive messages by means of facial displays that inform about the valuational quality of situations, and thus communications linked to (unpleasant, undesirable) states of disease are realistic possibilities (Miller, 1971). From these considerations I posit that states of disease bring into play conflicting tendencies and behaviors, and ecological factors may well influence which of the tendencies will predominate. Obviously this whole problem needs further research.

Another set of issues needing consideration has to do with whether "illness behaviors" are merely similar or actually equivalent to those linked to helplessness, dependence, and parent–offspring interaction. Evolution is by definition a conservative process, and common sense leads me to believe that natural selection did not forge a special class of illness behaviors (reflecting internal biomedical disease processes) if behaviors already in the repertoire of a species could serve similar ends. Yet the cost of hastily concluding that illness behaviors are merely those of social support and analogues of parent–offspring interactions is high indeed, because one would miss exploring a facet of adaptation that may contain useful insights.

Until this question is resolved by empirical research, I will assume, as have others, that the behaviors generated when organisms have a defect, or biomedical disease ("illness behaviors"), are in essence those of helplessness, dependence, care-giving and -seeking, and parent–offspring situations. This assumption raises two sets of questions. The first is why the evolutionary process allows neurological routines that subserve these behaviors to persist beyond the time when they are most critical for survival. In other words, parent–offspring-related care-seeking and care-giving seem "natural to" and critical during a specified development period. Once that period is passed and the special survival pressures are mastered, one would think that the evolutionary process might reuse elements of the neural routines for others purposes more critical to the organism, in the process modifying the integrity of the routines. Instead, the potential for such dependence and helplessness behaviors seems to remain "in" the organism, the neural routines subserving them being reasonably coherent but dormant. To explain these behaviors in adults, re-examining the role disease plays in the social behaviors of an infraprimate group seems useful.

The second set of questions raised by the assumption that illness behaviors are those natural to helplessness, dependence, and care-seeking and care-giving involves the mechanism of how they are elicited or released. One must assume that dormant neurological substrates are somehow activated, but the question here is how this activation is accomplished. A biomedical disease process can involve the dysfunction of neuroendocrine systems directly or through the mediation of toxins or inflammatory products, all of which may alter brain cell thresholds and neural circuits subserving potential illness behaviors. In the case of permanent defects, the mechanism is less clear, although the dehydration and/or undernutrition of the organism that is a consequence of the defect may be a factor. Those who posit a degree of ''self-awareness'' and motivated actions in animals might develop interesting clues about this topic were they to study behaviors of higher primates during conditions of disease (Griffin, 1976). If something resembling illness is found and it has a motivated and communicational function, then the mechanisms that trigger the illness behaviors and the reciprocated responses in a group need to be studied.

The preceding discussion leads me to suggest that, at least in nonhuman groups, the existence of a biomedical disease could be a necessary condition for a (behavioral) state of illness (i.e., it can ''trigger'' that state). But because I am also dealing with the (reciprocated) responses of other group members, I am forced to enquire as to the mechanisms and conditions that account for such responses. An obvious necessary condition for the responses of other group members to occur is the presence of illness behaviors in the first place. In addition, others in the group must somehow be provided with a target to which to respond and also somehow decide whether, in light of selective pressures, it is prudent to engage in (altruistic) responses vis-à-vis the sick member. At this point the requirement for the definition of illness comes to mind, namely, that of a deviation from past personal and prevailing social norms. Let me elaborate on its possible significance.

The behaviors that realize a state of illness differ in kind from those ordinarily descriptive of an organism's identity. In other words, organisms are individuated, among other things, on the basis of their social rank, age, sex, and— important to my theme—style of behavior. It is to this whole that co-members are locked in during group activities. For an organism to show illness and have it be recognized by others, his behavior must deviate from the accustomed norm of behavior set by him in the past. Speaking anthropomorphically, the organism has to signal that he is changed. The stipulation that illness involves a deviation from an organism's past personal behavior norms may be viewed as also providing a condition for having illness behavior recognized by others. This is, of course, a hypothesis that could be tested under field conditions.

I have indicated that a state of illness also appears to require that the behavior of the organism in question deviate from the prevailing (social) norms set by a relevant group or subgroup to which the organism belongs presently. I will suggest that the condition of social norm violation is also a factor that plays a role in eliciting reciprocated responses, specifically in the evaluation by others in the group of whether it is prudent to engage in reciprocal (altruistic) responses toward the sick organism (Trivers, 1971). In other words, when behaviors that can potentially elicit reciprocated (altruistic) responses are infrequent in the group (they constitute a deviation from group norms), members in the group are provided with a distinguishable target toward which it may be safe to behave altruistically. This point can be stated differently. If a disease process affects most of the members of a group, then it may well not be in the interest of the nondiseased group members (now a minority) to respond altruistically. The fact that under such conditions the behaviors of the diseased members may not in fact constitute a deviation from group norms (i.e., not on social grounds constitute an illness) is a factor that may mar their visibility and effectiveness as signals for altruistic responses. In summary, deviations from observable social norms, an apparent feature of illness behaviors, may constitute a condition for the occurrence of reciprocated responses from co-members. Observations in the field would clarify whether (or under what conditions) this deviation–reciprocation, in fact, takes place.

V. ILLNESS AND DISEASE IN SOCIAL THEORY

A. General Statement

Illness has been defined as a disvalued state or condition of the individual considered as a whole being. It is something manifested concretely in behavior adaptation. Illness is conceptualized as different from a possible underlying disorder or disease process that is physical. Instead, illness is judged as a discontinuity in the life arc of a person. It involves an impairment in function and hence a deviation. In all groups, a state of illness is associated with a relative failure to perform basic expected tasks. The person acknowledges—implicitly or explicitly—his "ill" state, namely, he shows it in behavior overtly, covertly, and/or symbolically in words. For example, he reports it, displays it, is unable to perform, stays in bed. The social group usually validates or certifies a claim of illness. This validation is a fairly general observation, though it is not true in our culture. Our system of medicine allows positing that someone who claims to be ill is really not diseased.

B. Illness and Its Interpretation

Illness poses a problem with which all societies grapple. The basic directives are to prevent and treat illness and to provide a means for minimizing its social impact. In the process of trying to control the problems associated with illness, societies develop an understanding of their sources, their manifestations and consequences, and of the actions (whether in the form of procedures, medicines, symbols, or psychosocial influences) that are necessary to prevent and treat them effectively. The total organized effort a society generates to control illness is reflected in the workings of its medical care system (MCS): a composite of knowledge, personnel, established medical practices and resources, behavioral expectations of practitioner and patient, and even the spatial configuration of physical settings where illness is studied and treated. MCS, it should be noted, is a component of the society's culture, but it also reflects the social structure, level of development, and mode of ecologic coupling.

Not only in a historical sense, but also in a practical sense, the targets of any MCS are occurrences of illness. To accomplish its objectives, MCS has available what one can term a "theory of illness." Through such theories, causes of illness are explained and treatment programs implemented. That "theory of illness" refers to a cultural trait should be re-emphasized. In other words, the theory is an attribute of the social system—specifically, of the MCS of a particular society. The theory of illness is what the experts of the society use and develop to treat illness. This formal body of knowledge can be distinguished from the "informal" system for understanding illness that the lay populace rely on. Hypotheses about the relations between these two facets of a group's MCS have been proposed (Fabrega, 1976a,b, 1977).

The discussion to this point applies to all types of societies regardless of how primitive or advanced they may be. An emphasis on the society as a social and cultural structure leads one to appreciate that political, economic, and ethical overtones exist in the way illness is defined and handled. Because of this, one is allowed to make moral judgments about whether the criteria of a particular illness are sound, good, proper, practical, and useful. A society's theory of illness and its MCS obviously change with time. The processes of variation, selection, and retention that are judged as integral to biologic evolution can, when applied to social evolution, be seen as involving medical cultural traits of a society.

C. Theories of Illness Viewed from the Standpoint of Information

In light of the discussion so far, explanations of illness can be seen as formulas produced by means of the group's theory. Each "formula" contains measures that derive from the domains of the theory. An explanation of illness may be judged to reflect "cultural information" about a medical problem.

Each occurrence of illness may be judged to pose a variable degree of uncertainty to a group. The occurrence, which is problematic and disruptive, requires identification and resolution; the explanation (arrived at via the theory) in a sense accomplishes this: the explanation is the group's way of making understandable that occurrence and in so doing provides a rationale for treatment. This conceptualization of the way a theory of illness functions should in principle be measurable. One might then see the explanation, when suitably "quantified," as expressing how much uncertainty was implicit in the occurrence of illness and thereby "removed" in that particular group at that particular time. Alternatively, one could say that an occurrence of illness in space and time contains a variable amount of information that members of the group or culture can use and interpret, and that in fact they do so in diverse ways by means of their theories of illness. In view of the matter, the explanation, when suitably quantified, expresses how richly the group or culture has availed itself of the occurrence, that is, the extent to which group members have delved into the occurrence and ferreted out information that they judge is present and that then guides their attempts at resolving the occurrence.

Ordinarily, illness occurrences are visualized as involving chemical and physiological changes and as occasioning such things as pain, disability, and emotional problems. It is important that one keep separate these matters from those involving what has been described as the uncertainty and/or information implicit in the occurrence. The former set of issues involves the concrete burdens of illness to an individual and by extension to his group. On the other hand, the notion of information or uncertainty contained in an illness occurrence implicates the functioning mode of the illness theory and the group's social system of medicine—that is, how the theory is used to explain and arrive at a course of action to resolve the occurrence. In this instance, the occurrence of illness is viewed as a point source of difficulty in the group, once necessitating interpretation and to be dealt with symbolistically in the group.

D. On the Functions of a Medical Care System (MCS)

A group's MCS can be viewed macroscopically, which is to say as a social structure. This system includes practitioners, organizations of practitioners, ways in which these do their work, places or physical structures where they practice and see persons with illness and disease, institutionalized ways of certifying and passing judgment on the quality of practitioners, legally binding and politically grounded forms of medical practice regulations, and the like. The MCS of a group is situated within a larger social collectivity. In the language of systems theory, the MCS of a group constitutes a subsystem (together with transportation, economics, politics, communication, and the like) of a more inclusive social system that is regulatory and more general in its purposes. A higher regulatory system can be seen as related to the medical care system cybernetically in the sense that questions of policy, regulation, and other reference values for the MCS are carefully set and in such a manner that they take into account and affect developments in that particular subsystem and also other subsystems (e.g., political, economic). All subsystems are tied together in a more or less functionally interdependent manner, and all are to some extent monitored in relation to the others by the higher regulatory system. Similarly, insofar as social paths may be said to characterize the way in which social groups evolve and change, the respective paths inherent in the way MCS's develop and change should likewise be explained. As an example, all groups entrust the care of the sick to others; but different types of other persons may be available to undertake this function, be they elders, headmen, shamanistic practitioners of various types, or general physicians. Whichever types of personnel are available, one must assume that distinct relations exist among them and that organizations of such personnel may exist with types of (legally?) certified sanctions, recruitment criteria, and standards of performance. The manner in which they are recompensed and the means by which clients obtain their services (referral processes) and then pay for them vary. In short, the MCS of a group is itself organized in some determinate manner. Furthermore, occurrences of illness and medical care activities become costs and resources respectively of the social group. How these matters are economically resolved relates to the requirements and outputs of the remaining institutions subsystems of the group. The whole of this, of course, can be expected to vary across types of social groups. Evolving sets of priorities probably underlie the different stages of growth of social groups, and these also should be brought into relation with health and medical issues. Key factors are the means by which sociological processes take place and the role medical institutions play in them. That this level of study of medical systems merges with a general theory of social systems should be obvious.

An important question in the comparative study of MCS is how successful a social group functions vis-à-vis burdens posed by illness and disease in light of its prevailing theory of illness and the MCS it has managed to develop. Included in this problem area are how well illness and disease are controlled and also how well the group itself functions. Thus, the health of the members of the group and the functional efficiency of the MCS (i.e., its health) would constitute focal points of inquiry. Relevant questions would be: In light of existing cultural definitions and/or in light of an external (i.e., observer-developed) form of accounting, how healthy are group members in the social group? What is their level of illness and disease? How productively do individuals function? How responsible, equitable, and widely distributed are the resources of the system of care? How efficiently are its resources utilized? What are its costs to the individual? What are the economic, social, and medical costs that have to be balanced with the benefits of medical treatment? What incidence and prevalence figures of illness characterize the social group? How good is the quality of medical care? How are the creative and productive energies of group members and of the group itself furthered by the theory of illness and by the care practices that it entails? What is the level of achievement of the group given the benefits provided by the system of care?

VI. SOCIAL ECOLOGICAL CONTEXT OF DISEASE AND ILLNESS

A. Disease in Egalitarian Societies

An assumption of the physical anthropologist is that biological characteristics of man were forged in a simplified, elementary form of social setting. This type of social group was probably standard during human evolution. Groups classified as egalitarian or bands are small and migratory, and their members highly interdependent; environmental pressures are jointly experienced. All facets of human life have a social and shared basis. The effects of disease, then, are visible to co-members, and the latter share in the tribulations of those diseased. In such social settings, an occurrence of disease does not simply incapacitate or eliminate a person in some mechanical sense. Rather, it affects the person's capacity and performance as a participating member of a highly interdependent group. Only at this point, when it comes to affect individual behavior, does disease assume relevance as a biological phenomenon.

All extant egalitarian groups have articulated beliefs and explanations about disease, and the likelihood is high that such beliefs and explanations have been the case since soon after the emergence of man as a species. Belief systems explain causes of disease and rationalize treatment actions; moreover, they also pattern the expectations of the sick person and of those around, resulting in a host of behaviors designed to help the sick person and his family.

With regard to biologic sources of disease among egalitarian societies, the following generalizations can be offered (Boyden, 1970):

Disease forms among these people were importantly influenced by exposures to and infections with microorganisms and parasites common to the animals that they came into direct contact with.

What are termed today typically human infections—those with acute onset, which are short lived, yield lasting immunity, and have no apparent animal reservoir (e.g., polio, measles, influenza)—were probably nonexistent among egalitarian groupings due to the fact that the respective microorganisms require a large enough human population to provide a pool of noninfected susceptibles and the size of bands was simply too small for such a pool.

Infections characterized by a long latency and recurrence that were essentially chronic and in which reinfection was possible provided a large proportion of the conditions for the forms of disease found among egalitarian groupings.

Infections that could be propagated vertically across generations (which meant a symbiotic relation between agent and infected host) may have been prominent.

The diet of peoples of very small-scaled societies (i.e., "bands") was probably balanced, adequate in quantity, but poor in highly palatable items that yield highly refined carbohydrate sources, and this dietary adequacy has suggested to many that the conditions for caries and obesity may have been less prevalent.

Life was physically demanding, level of activity was high, obesity was probably uncommon, but leisure time for group activity was ample; these conditions may have involved fewer changes that are thought of today as stressful and are believed to lead to chronic degenerative changes. Forms of disease among egalitarian groupings were no doubt affected by these conditions.

Chronic biological changes that are commonly seen in the elderly were probably rare in part because of factors already mentioned and in part because the life span of people of egalitarian groups was believed to be rather short for such changes to develop.

Death due to cannibalism, infanticide, sacrifice, geronticide, head hunting, and trauma were probably high among prehistoric egalitarian peoples.

Chronic skin infections were probably common.

Due to the nomadic way of life, fecal–oral infection routes were not prominently implicated as factors contributing to disease forms.

B. Disease in Ranked Societies and States

With larger societies, classified as ranked, one finds more complex forms of social organization, a division of labor that extends beyond strictly sexual lines, a greater degree of role specialization, early forms of institutions, and extended interconnected families whose members are able to acquire household items and properties. With a settled form of social life, particularly when population density reaches a high figure such as to allow for microbial persistence and noninfected susceptibles (as one finds in urban settlements), comes the possibility of human epidemics (e.g., measles, smallpox). These infections act as influences that can yield new disease forms in ranked societies. Irrigation systems often mean a common water supply, and hence the possibility of fecal–oral transmission, setting the stage for further changes affecting patterns of disease forms. Microorganisms from nondomesticated animals may have been expected to affect people less easily because of the greater "distance" from a pristine physical habitat. Changing agricultural practices, however, set the stage for the risk propagation of vectors of microorganisms as well as new patterns for infection routes.

Settled groupings in the absence of developed sanitary practices also means that carrier members can directly infect others through fecal–oral modes of transmission. Among some early ranked societies, the possibility that a diet consisted mainly of vegetable foods is a distinct possibility. Among many such groupings, however, mixed diets no doubt prevailed. Some people came to depend mainly on cereals and root crops. It is believed that a bulk of root vegetables providing about 2500 calories complemented with significant amounts of great leaves would have provided members of ranked societies with a nutritionally adequate diet. The bulk and water content of such diets would have yielded a slow sustained absorption of nutrients. These features of the diet must be presumed to have affected physiologic patternings, energy balances, and metabolic and biochemical profiles. Because social differentiation becomes a striking feature in ranked societies, altogether different forms of personal relations may have complicated social life, in the process modifying the earlier family-oriented and egalitarian society. Social differentiation also means social inequality and more heterogeneous forms of life-styles. This life-style heterogeneity in turn suggests that physical activity, leisure-time allotments, sedentary pursuits, and a complex distribution of type and quality of food prevailed among members of ranked societies. The preceding conditions must be seen as correlated with, if not producing, a higher level of individual differences in psychobiologic types. These differences in turn provide sources of altogether different kinds of health profiles compared with those of egalitarian band societies, whose members led a much more homogeneous life.

An important dimension of medical problems in contemporary society is the high prevalence of disease conditions that appear to be at least partly the outcome of the life-style in these societies. We may illustrate this by considering hypertension.

Intense competitiveness is a central feature of a specific behavior pattern, called type A, that has been linked to an increased likelihood of hypertension and coronary heart disease (CHD). According to Rosenman and Friedman (1974), the type A person tends to be competitive, aggressive and hostile, hard-driving and ambitious, and restless and impatient. In style and manner, the person exhibits brisk speech and body movements, fist-clenching, taut facial muscles, and explosive speech. The type A person acts as though he is in a chronic "struggle with time," ever attempting to accomplish more and more in less and less time, and in a chronic struggle with those around him. His life-style is to live more rapidly and aggressively than his peers. Type A behaviors are reportedly elicited more readily by some environmental conditions (deadlines, interruptions or delays, competitive challenges) than by others. According to many, type A behaviors are more typical of evolved and complex social systems (Eyer, 1975). Persons living in less disturbed, more organized, and simpler social conditions tend to show more normal blood pressures and less CHD despite similarities in diet and salt intake that are also held to be important influences in the genesis of these conditions.

Much research on the type A behavior pattern has led to a specific formulation of man–environment factors in hypertension and CHD. Certain cultural conditions (competitive challenges, deadlines) must combine with certain susceptible persons (type A, whom one should view as more typically formed under certain cultural conditions) to produce changes (e.g., excess sympathetic response, reduced blood clotting time) that, if repeated sufficiently often, cause permanent damage to the cardiovascular system. In essence one could say that adverse cultural conditions can lead to permanent maladaptative nervous system responses; the fixing of these is associated with increased levels of morbidity and mortality. All four parts of this model have been researched to some degree. According to the model, a limited part of the human environment, combining with susceptible people, is translated through the central nervous system into neurologic, neuroendocrine, and biochemical adaptations that contribute to hypertension and CHD. Important to the theme of the chapter is the fact that this disease is partly a consequence of our historically unique ecology and life-style.

In summary, rival perspectives in biomedicine draw attention to two facets of a medical problem: the biologic substrates of disease and the social and psychological aspects of what has been termed illness. Both of these perspectives when overdrawn tend to play down the connection between cultural and biological aspects of illness of all types, that is, the fact that illness is an inevitable outcome of the process of social adaptation and that both its prevalence and manifestations make sense is an ecologic and sociobiologic frame of reference. Habits related to diet, leisure, and exercise are examples in the case of hypertension and diabetes. Seemingly, the way of life in modern societies creates conditions that help these diseases "surface" as illnesses. In the case of psychiatric illnesses, such as depression, attention has at different times focused on object losses, child-rearing influences, personality types, and life-change events. As with diabetes or hypertension, one can ask whether the way of life in Western societies has played a role in producing depression (e.g., by changing the structure of the family). A basic point is that culture contributes to the formation of a distinctive ecology, including social conditions, physical–environmental factors and genetic structures, which combine to yield diseases and illnesses of various types.

C. Systems of Medicine in Egalitarian and Ranked Societies

In previous publications I have described and discussed characteristics of the social orientations toward disease/illness as well as the medical care practices of egalitarian (band) and more complex (ranked), but still nonliterate, societies (Fabrega, 1980, also unpublished data). In this section I summarize this information and draw from it generalizations for discussion. Analyses such as these can serve as background for comparisons involving the systems of medicine of larger states and civilizations.

In both types of nonliterate groups the lay persons themselves serve as the first line of defense against disease/illness. Lay persons share among themselves broad knowledge about medical problems and initiate treatments when symptoms arise. The responses to illness including attempts at its treatments are more public and visible in egalitarian or band societies, seeming to have what one could term a communal basis, whereas in ranked societies responses tend to be private and contained within the family.

In band societies, theories of illness emphasize causal agencies and forces outside the person. Among people of ranked societies, although these agencies remain important, aspects of the person and "mechanisms" or "substances" inside him seem to become more prominent in explanations of cause. This internalization of cause suggests that the theories of illness in ranked societies people are more elaborate. In band societies, medical treatment involving a practitioner tends to occur in an open setting and in a large group that includes many co-members; in the ranked societies, by contrast, a more closed setting is preferred, and the members of the ill person's family are the main participants. Treatment of disease appears to be an occasion for re-establishing group health in egalitarian societies, whereas it is more individuated and focused (on the sick person and his family) in ranked societies. Family units and kin groups generally appear to be the managers of treatment in ranked societies, whereas in egalitarian societies the group as a whole seems to function as manager.

In contrast to band societies, in most ranked societies one finds persons whose functions are clearly medical. These persons have specialized knowledge of illness and its tangible attributes. They often undergo official certification and/or have special clothing and equipment that sets them apart physically; moreover, they are highly distinguishable from co-members on social behavioral criteria. A differentiation of practitioner types exists in ranked societies, each showing specialization of types of treatment (or phases of the treatment process), illness types, or causes. Having elaborate and specialized worldly knowledge about illness manifestations, mechanisms of causation, and effects of specific medicines appear to distinguish practitioners of ranked societies. These practitioners are also known for their spiritual and preternatural expertise. However, among band groups, practitioners can be described as more totally concerned with purely preternatural causes and their significance.

Among band societies, severe illnesses that require practitioner intervention appear to be judged as undifferentiated wholes: illness behaviors subserve a general symbolic or metaphoric function and specific manifestation disabilities of illness are played down. Although there are exceptions, among the more complex ranked societies, these types of illnesses appear to be judged in a more differentiated way; that is, the actual properties of the illness tend to be specified and the illness is handled in a more discrete, and tangible, way. Possibly the actual behaviors of sick persons among the ranked societies draw emphasis to types of manifestations and levels of constraints, and bodily awareness and experience are more important and diversified. Information directly supporting this is not available, though descriptions of curers' actions suggest this.

People of ranked societies differ in that they tend to remunerate their medical practitioners. In most of the groups examined, the payment was considered an instrument of cure rather than a fee for the services of the curer, though the curer was personally enriched by these offerings. The curer has a broad range of power and prestige and he often is comparatively wealthy. What one could term a "private and materialistic" approach to medical care (e.g., contract between parties, fee for service) is observed among some of the groups studied, something that is simply not seen among the band societies. In the latter, the medical practitioner seems to have little special prestige, does not benefit economically from curing, and does not administer care privately.

Because ranked societies have specialist types of practitioners and even a hierarchy of sorts, practitioner–client relations can be said to be more focused and individuated than in band groups, where no differentiation exists and where the group as a whole is the focus and setting of treatment. One assumes that issues of trust, obligations, bargaining, entitlements, payments or remuneration, disaffection, dependence on part of patients, and the like all become significant elements of client–practitioner relations among people of ranked societies. In brief, among the latter, medical treatment becomes more focused, individuated, secularized and worldly; client–practitioner relations heightened, intensified, and made more complex; and therapy management groups concerned to resolve among competing interpretations about disease treatment.

D. Points of Contrast With Western Civilizations

The emerging discipline of the social history of (Western) medicine provides information one can use as a general contrast to the mode of operation of the systems of medicine of small scale (non-Western) societies (Cartwright, 1977; Cipolla, 1973). A striking and obvious difference is the existence of a centralized policy about health and disease, and with such policy a structurally distinct social institution of medicine. This difference can be related in large part to the evolution of the state (eventually, modern civilization). This was associated with urbanization leading to increased size and density of populations. The latter social developments provide the conditions for new infectious diseases linked to patterns of contagiousness. The prevalence of these diseases, in turn, lead to social policy changes in the evolving Western system of medicine. Additional factors linked to the evolution of the Western system of medicine include (1) the accumulation of written texts about disease and medicines, which provides a common body of knowledge that people and practitioners draw on; (2) growth of cities, trade communications, educational centers, schools of medicine (and with them formal education of physicians and eventually their identification as a corporate profession); (3) evolution of centralized authorities and governing bodies that increasingly come to articulate a social public health policy and to regulate licensing and eventually the practices of medicine; and finally (4) the emergence of science and technology with obvious effects on understanding disease causes, mechanisms, modes of prevention, and therapeutics. The above factors, together, are among the ones that constrain the perspective toward illness and disease and the way they are handled in modern nations. A comparison of how people of modern nations versus small-scale societies orient to medical problems and cope with them obviously involves taking into account the practical as well as attitudinal consequences of these demographic and sociological changes.

As an example, we may consider the effects related to the demographic transition. Especially relevant are the effects of large-scale epidemics, such as plague and smallpox. Each of these epidemics was to some extent made possible by the new ecologies of the state/civilization. Efforts linked to the control of epidemics were instrumental in fostering a ''public health'' orientation and with it the idea of state controlled agencies with policies about health and medical care. In late Medieval Renaissance times, centralized control and/or local governments already saw fit to create health boards empowered to institute public health measures necessitated by the then prevailing medical problem, bubonic plague. The growth of state regulatory agencies concerned with public health problems is linked to attempts to control other key infectious diseases (e.g., smallpox, cholera, leprosy, tuberculosis, and syphilis).

In many ways, our modern view of disease as a tangible and worldly ''thing'' that disrupts a naturally healthy body—and creates social problems—grows out of the upheavals linked to epidemics. Many things have obviously contributed to a secularized view of man, nature, and disease. The effects of epidemics on attitudes toward disease, health, and mortality is one such factor that set the groundwork for a physical approach to the body and its scientific investigation. The growth of hospitals as settings for care and the consolidation of the professions of surgery, medicine, and pharmacy are developments linked to a growing socialized and secular view of disease. All of these developments come to play increasing roles in the organization of the social system of medicine of Western states.

In earlier historical eras, state interventions in public health have affected transportation of people and merchandise and led to the quarantine of suspected patients, the fumigation of their belongings, and the imposition of medical care and hygienic practices regarding sanitation and food intake (Cartwright, 1977; Cipolla, 1973). In contemporary times, infectious diseases are much less burdensome and problems such as cardiovascular disease and cancer loom as significant. Given these types of diseases and the precedent of state intervention in public health, a logical outcome would appear to be campaigns against smoking and drinking, the promulgation of healthy diets and regular exercise, and now the encouragement of ''correct'' principles of social and family relations, principles derived from government-supported research. All of these treatment rationales are aimed at the posited causes of disease that are predicated by our theory of illness.

VII. COMMENT

The medical system of a society may be described as the composite of traditions, beliefs, practices, and institutions for dealing with disease. In small scale societies, medical systems are not clearly differentiated from other systems of the society, for example, the religious or political. What this means is that in those societies disease is understood and dealt with in terms of ideas and practices that also have religious and political overtones. Given the mode of functioning of such societies, one could say that what from our standpoint are medical phenomena, in small-scale societies is socialized (or politicized, etc.).

A striking feature of our modern and evolved medical system is its relative independence from other social systems. The processes of diagnosis and treatment of disease in modern societies constitute enterprises that involve knowledge and practices having fewer immediate religious and political overtones, relatively speaking. The relative independence of our medical system from that of other social systems can be seen as one consequence of the processes of modernization, the growth of science, and general secularization. Nevertheless, often in modern societies phenomena that we judge as social, such as deviance, or personal, such as personal worry, are judged and handled as medical. From that standpoint, one could say that, in modern societies, social phenomena are medicalized. I believe that a logical error is inherent in this characterization of medical and social phenomena.

Disease is a universal and recurring human problem that poses a threat to a social group. All societies can be seen as challenged by disease, the conditions for which are partly dictated by its size, structure, and organization. We can restate this point and say that the biology and ecology of disease are partly influenced by sociological and historical factors. The societies' approach to disease—their way of understanding and dealing with it—will be conditioned by these biological and ecological factors, and also by related factors involving their social history and culture. These factors determine what diseases prevail, how they are thought of, and how they are dealt with concretely in the society.

At any time when we examine how a society is viewing and handling illness and disease, we are examining a problem that, in a concrete sense, is conditioned by its ecology, history, sociology, and culture—and, moreover, a problem that, in an analytic sense, is construed in terms of symbols and conventions that grow out of (and are based on) the same ecological, historical, sociological, and cultural influences. Given this interconnection between disease prevalence and disease symbolization (more generally, culture, social perspectives, and ecology) we would be highly ethnocentric were we to say that certain societies medicalize social happenings more than others or, conversely, that some societies differentially "socialize" (or politicize or religiously color) medical happenings. In brief, approaches to disease and approaches to other problems and concerns are cast in the same social mold: what we label as disease or treatment is in many ways as much a social phenomenon as anything else. Conventional wisdom may today handle "disease" and "medical" as intrinsically different from other concerns or problems. However, it is somewhat ethnocentric to reason as though our distinctions are correct and universal, or as though other societies operated with misguided ones.

VIII. ILLNESS, DISEASE, AND MEDICAL PRACTICE

A. Illness Behavior

The discussion so far implies that the cultural orientation of the person and of the group to which he belongs plays a critical role in how illness will be interpreted, explained, responded to, and dealt with. An illness does not convey this information, for an illness is essentially a state of impairment in well-being. A people's culture (their system of social symbols and their meanings) furnishes the name, explanation, and treatment rationale for an illness. The raw data of illness, then, is a person showing dysfunction, often linking it to changes in his body. Obvious uniformities exist in the physical changes underlying this condition and in sensorimotor behavior changes that make up the illness. But even these changes are abstracted out of the illness picture via cultural conventions (see below).

It follows from the above that the manner in which a person believes himself to be constructed or formed (his view of his self, body) will influence how he reports or explains his illness, and how he goes about treating it. Thus, in an anthropological sense, a person's conception of self-person and his or her conceptions of illness are locked together and influence illness behavior and explanation. As stated earlier, all societies furnish people with culturally specific conceptions about behavior, about why and how they get ill, how illness changes the person, and what being ill implies about the person.

Among some peoples of the world, illness of the self ("of the whole me") is distinguished from illness of "my leg" or of "my joint." This distinction raises an interesting point about the interpretation of illness behaviors. A part of a person is both an anatomical fact and a social fact. Anatomically, all persons have brains, livers, hearts, and nerves. From a cultural standpoint, however, only Western peoples describe themselves as having minds, brains, nerves. In other words, features of their knowledge base lead them to make these distinctions. In our culture a person who is ill can state that his liver is bad, that his nerves are overactive, or that he has a brain tumor. In another culture, these complaints may not be possible because the concepts are not part of their knowledge of the body. Instead, other peoples, when ill, will report pain due to a coldness or to an object that has "entered" the body; and weakness may be explained by a supernatural "robbing" of the spirit. Clearly, the explanation of the cause of the symptom or illness will influence the behavior of the ill person.

B. The Biomedical Theory of Illness

As indicated earlier, Western societies have evolved what one can term a biomedical care system. In the biomedical theory of illness, importance is given to physical, chemical, and physiological changes that occur in a person's systems. This emphasis points to the special biomedical concept we have termed disease (D_i), which refers to disorders of chemistries, physiologies, and anatomies. In contrast to illness that refers to whole persons, has a structure and appearance that is behavioral and that is assessed using psychosocial and symbolic criteria, disease has a structure and appearance that is biophysiologic and it is assessed using physical (physiological and chemical) criteria.

In biomedicine, a disease is held to "cause" illness. More specifically, disordered bodily organ systems (i.e., disease) transform to changes in behavior and function (i.e., illness). This transformation is partly determined by the nature of the organ systems that are diseased and by the nature of the cultural system that provides symbolic conventions and codes vis-à-vis behavior. The appearance of illness involves brain–behavior interactions and cultural factors are operative in some way.

C. Factors That Influence the Structure of Illness

One may point to a number of factors that need to be handled in an analytically separate manner for studying illness. These are disease processes or conditions; physical signs of disease; level of awareness and well-being (or state of the self); bodily perceptions; sociocognitive orientations; illness theories; theories of personhood; medically relevant environmental happenings; and illness (or illness behavior).

Disease conditions consist of changes we observe and/or identify by means of principles and methods of biomedicine, such as electrical devices or chemical examination of urine or of the blood. The term disease, then, is used to qualify physical changes in the structure of the body. Disease conditions can produce local–specific physical changes in the body (e.g., displacement, destruction, secretion) and distal–general physical changes in the central nervous system.

Information on local physical changes is transmitted to the central nervous system directly by peripheral nerves or indirectly by the bloodstream.

The signs of disease are outcomes of disease changes in the various organ systems of the body. Signs of disease include changes visible on the surface of the body, changes involving emanations from body orifices, or sensorimotor behavior changes that register impairments in body function. Signs of disease are viewed as more or less obligatory physical effects of disease. By convention, signs of disease are thought of as overt and visible to an observer, but one should understand that they are logically equivalent to the internal covert physical changes uncovered by technical procedures (e.g., X rays, blood analyses). The latter, then, are also signs of disease. Behaviors, when looked at from a physical standpoint (so-called sensorimotor behaviors), may be seen as signs of disease.

The effects of disease include two types of phenomena: changes in the sense of awareness and well-being, and bodily perceptions. By sense of awareness and well-being, one means general assessments by the person about his or her self and correlated general characteristics of his or her cognitive functions (e.g., mental clarity, discrimination, alertness). Disease conditions typically can change how the person evaluates himself and his life situation and how discriminating are his responses to his environment.

Bodily perceptions are private, subjective experiences the person links to his or her body. Persons have bodily perceptions and report them through language. All languages provide users with a means of describing bodily perceptions, the original "data" for this description being changes in the peripheral and central nervous system (a product of pancultural uniformities in the way the body is structured anatomically and neurologically).

The language used for describing body changes relates somehow to cognitions about illness and the self that are acquired by the individual from his social group. Cognition refers to the manner of orienting or interpreting and not (in the Piagetian sense) to operations or structures. Generally, a person's cognitive orientations reflect uniformities in the perceptual system and the organization that exists in nature. Cognitive orientations are also partly symbolic, that is, they reflect cultural conventions. Cognitive orientations pattern, order, and regulate the way persons perceive their physical and social environment and the way they behave socially.

Cognitive orientations about illness and the self are influenced by the theories about illness that a group endorses and also by their theory of personhood, each of which draws on, and is complementary to, the other. Both types of theories can be seen as systems of meanings grounded in symbolic conventions. They are thus products of the person's culture and social experiences. Persons from different social backgrounds would be assumed to endorse different theories about self and about illness, and these theories influence how they behave and act when ill and what they expect of practitioners, doctors, and the like.

Medically relevant environmental happenings also impact on the illness-related experiences of a person. These happenings are proximal or distal in time and are linked either to the physical or social environment, and their importance is partly dictated by the native theories of illness and personhood. In other words, what is happening to a person currently and what has happened to him in the past can affect how a person behaves when ill; it can affect what he thinks of the illness, what he worries about, and how he will respond. And, of course, how a person interprets social happenings is influenced by his culture, social position, education, and other circumstances—the same kinds of factors that influence the theory of illness and of personhood.

Cognitive orientations about illness and the self, the central nervous system physical effects of disease, the signs of disease, and medically relevant environmental happenings are what influence the structure and content of illness. In the biomedical theory, these factors together help explain the chain from disease to illness.

In summary, "illness" refers to the totality of social and psychologic behavior changes (including any signs or physical effects of disease) that on conventional grounds is judged to have "medical" significance in a particular society (e.g., it is disvalued, requires corrective action). A society identifies many different types of illnesses. From a biomedical standpoint, the structure and content of any one type of illness results from biophysical as well as social cultural factors.

D. The Clinical Analysis of Illness Behaviors

A basic aim of the physician is to establish whether a person shows evidence of illness and, if so, to decide whether treatment might be useful. Toward that aim, one must come to understand and evaluate the behavior of another person and how biologic processes influence this behavior. A principal mode of access to the behavior of another person is by means of the medical interview. During this interview one obtains direct information from the person about his or her past life, recent experiences, and current functioning.

A basic task that one faces on completion of a medical interview is to determine whether the person interviewed is showing evidence of illness. At the most general level, the task of determining whether a person shows illness can be formulated as a question: does the person at this time show an impairment or disruption in his or her adaptation and function? Impairments can be manifest in the spheres of psychological (e.g., thinking, emotions, worries) and/or social (e.g., work, family) and/or bodily (e.g., digestion, motion) functions. A different query aimed at the same issue is the following: is the person showing changes in the psychosocial and/or bodily sphere that are disruptive of, or interfering with, his or her capacity to function and obtain satisfaction in life? A "yes" answer to these questions can be taken as evidence for the presence of illness, in which case the task of the interviewer changes.

A person adjudged as not showing evidence of illness may nonetheless show evidence indicating a disease process. Determining the presence or absence of a condition of disease is best thought of logically as involving a separate enterprise from that of determining whether a condition of illness is present. In most instances, one will find evidence for the coexistence of illness and disease, but, though this coexistence is so contingently or empirically, it is not always the case. Evidence for disease comes from three sources: (1) physical examination of the person, (2) laboratory examination of person's body fluids or physiologic systems, and (3) type and pattern of behavioral changes of illness. These comments are obviously true in the case of ("asymptomatic") disease conditions such as cancer or hypertension, and they are equally true in the case of some psychiatric disease conditions that may not have produced behavior changes of a type or level that interferes with adaptation-function (i.e., that may not add up to a state of illness).

In summary, a basic traditional aim of a medical inquiry is to assess and explain a condition of illness that troubles a person and about which he or she seeks help. Another basic and traditional aim is to conduct an inquiry so as to help prevent a possible future condition of illness. When I say basic and traditional, I mean that inquiries of this type seem to be universal in human societies regardless of whether they are preliterate or modern. In each of the two instances, the practitioner who conducts the inquiry will be initially guided by assessments of a person's psychological, social, and sensorimotor behaviors. Once having determined that a person is ill, which means that he or she is showing evidence of a failure or impairment of adaptation in any of three areas (i.e., psychologic, social, bodily), the practitioner uses his theory to explain the illness and eventually to administer treatment. If no actual illness is present and instead the possibility of a future illness is to be avoided or minimized, the practitioner will use his theory of illness as a basis for further examinations and recommendations. In the biomedical system of medicine, procedures involving technology will be used to uncover possible "hidden phenomena" (related to disease). In the "non-literate" small-scale system of medicine, social and ritual procedures will be used to uncover possible "hidden" phenomena (related to the preliterate theory of illness).

In contemporary Western medicine, the emphasis given to technology, to the physiological–chemical, and to the molecular often has the effect of obscuring the fact that illness is the basic datum of any medical-care system. In other words, physical parts are emphasized at the sacrifice of whole persons. From a comparative social science point of view, the centrality of illness is obvious, since all systems of medicine, viewed as entities *sui generis,* seem geared to prevent, control, and eliminate concrete instances of a medical problem (i.e., illness) that are realized in persons. This centrality is also true from a comparative clinical science point of view, since persons who are sick or those in fear of it are the ones who seek medical care from a practitioner. Emphasizing that a physician should see himself as conducting two separate and independent inquiries may serve to reinforce the centrality of illness and whole persons (biocultural entities) to medicine.

REFERENCES

Berkson, G. (1974). Social responses of animals to infants with defects. *In* "Origins of Behavior" (M. Lewis and I. Rosenblum, eds.), Chap. 11. Wiley, New York.

Bornstein, M. H. (1978). Visual behavior of the young human infant: relationships between chromatic and spatial perception and the activity of underlying brain mechanisms. *J. Exp. Child Psychol.* **26,** 174–192.

Bornstein, M. H. (1980). Perceptual development: stability and change in feature perception. *In* "Psychological Development from Infancy" (M. H. Bornstein and W. Kessen, eds.). Erlbaum Assoc. Hillsdale, New Jersey.

Bornstein, M. H., Kessen, W., and Weiskoff, S. (1975). The categories of hue in infancy. *Science* **191,** 201–202.

Boyden, S. V., ed. (1970). "The Impact of Civilization on the Biology of Man." Univ. of Toronto Press, Toronto.

Bramblett, C. (1967). Pathology in the Darajani baboon. *Am. J. Phys. Anthropol.* **26,** 331–340.

Brazelton, T. B. (1977). Implications of infant development among the Mayan Indians of Mexico. *In* "Culture and Infancy: Variations in the Human Experience" (P. H. Leiderman, S. R. Tulkin, and A. Rosenfeld, eds.), pp. 151–188. Academic Press, New York.

Cartwright, F. F. (1977). "Social History of Medicine." Longmans, Green, New York.

Cipolla, C. (1973). "Christofano and the Plague: A Study of the History of Public Health in the Age of Galileo." Univ. of California Press, Berkeley.

Condon, W. S., and Sander, L. W. (1974). Neonate movement is synchronized with adult speech: interactional participation and language acquisition. *Science* **183,** 99–101.

Cutting, J. E., Rosner, B. S., and Foard, C. F. (1976). Perceptual categories for musiclike sounds: implications for theories of speech perception. *Q. J. Exp. Psychol.* **28,** 361–378.

Darwin, C. (1914). "The Descent of Man." Random House (Modern Library), New York.

Deuel, R. K. (1977). Loss of motor habits after cortical lesions. *Neuropsychologia* **15,** 205–215.

De Valois, R. L., and De Valois, K. K. (1975). Neural coding of color. *In* "Seeing" (E. C. Carterette and M. P. Friedman, eds.), Handbook of Perception, Vol. 5. Academic Press, New York.

Eimas, P. D., Siqueland, E. R., Jusczyk, P., and Vigorito, J. (1970). Speech perception in infants. *Science* **171,** 303–306.

Eisenberg, J. F., and Dillon, W. S., eds. (1971). "Man and Beast: Comparative Social Behavior." Random House (Smithsonian Inst. Press), New York.

Ekman, P. (1973). Cross-cultural studies of facial expression. *In* "Darwin and Facial Expression (A Century of Research in Review)" (P. Ekman, ed.), pp. 169–220. Academic Press, New York.

Ekman, P. (1977). Biological and cultural contributions to body and facial movement. *In* "The Anthropology of the Body" (J. Blacking, ed.), pp. 39–84. Academic Press, New York.

Ekman, P., Friesen, W. V., and Ellsworth, P. (1972). "Emotion in the Human Face." Pergamon, New York.

Engel, B. T. (1972). Response specificity. *In* "Handbook of Psychophysiology" (N. S. Greenfield and R. A. Sternbach, eds.), pp. 571-576. Holt, Rinehart, New York.

Eyer, J. (1975). Hypertension as a disease of modern society. *Int. J. Health Serv.* **5,** 539-558.

Fabrega, H., Jr. (1974). "Disease and Social Behavior: An Interdisciplinary Perspective." MIT Press, Cambridge, Massachusetts.

Fabrega, H., Jr. (1976a). The biological significance of taxonomies of disease. *J. Theor. Biol.* **63,** 191-216.

Fabrega, H., Jr. (1976b). The function of medical care systems: a logical analysis. *Perspect. Biol. Med.* **20,** 108-119.

Fabrega, H., Jr. (1977). The scope of ethnomedical science. *Cult., Med. Psychiatry* **1,** 201-228.

Fabrega, H., Jr. (1980). Elementary systems of medicine. *Cult., Med. Psychiatry.*

Fox, R. (1975). Primate kin and human kinship. *In* "Biosocial Anthropology" (R. Fos, ed.). Malaby Press, London.

Freedman, D. G. (1974). "Human Infancy: An Evolutionary Perspective." Erlbaum Assoc., Hillsdale, New Jersey.

Geertz, C. (1973). "The Interpretation of Cultures (Selected Essays)." Basic Books, New York.

Geschwind, N., Quadfasel, F. A., and Segarra, J. M. (1968). Isolation of the speech area. *Neuropsychologia* **6,** 327-340.

Griffin, D. R. (1976). "The Question of Animal Awareness." Rockefeller Univ. Press, New York.

Harlow, H., and Harlow, M. (1965). Affectional systems. *In* "Behavior of Non Human Primates" (A. Schrier, H. Harlow, and F. Stollnitz, eds.). Academic Press, New York.

Heilman, K. M., Schwartz, H. D., and Geschwind, N. (1975). Defective motor learning in ideomotor apraxia. *Neurology* **25,** 1018-1020.

Hinde, R. (1974). "Biological Bases of Human Social Behavior." McGraw-Hill, New York.

Lazarus, R. S., Tomita, M., Opton, E. M., Jr., and Kodama, M. (1966). A cross cultural study of stress-reaction patterns in Japan. *J. Pers. Soc. Psychol.* **4,** 622-633.

Lewontin, R. (1974). "Genetic Basis of Evolutionary Change." Columbia Univ. Press, New York.

McNeill, D. (1979). "The Conceptual Basis of Language." Erlbaum Assoc., Hillsdale, New Jersey.

Mandler, G. (1967). The conditions for emotional behavior. *In* "Biology and Behavior: Neurophysiology and Emotion" (D. C. Glass, ed.), pp. 96-102. Rockefeller Univ. New York.

Marsella, A. J., Kinzie, D., and Gordon, P. (1973). Ethnic variations in the expression of depression. *J. Cross-Cult. Psychol.* **4,** 435-458.

Miles, F. A., and Evarts, E. V. (1979). concepts of motor organization. *Annu. Rev. Psychol.* **30,** 327-362.

Miller, R. E. (1971). Experimental studies of communication in the monkey. *In* "Primate Behavior: Developments in Field and Laboratory Research" (L. A. Rosenblum, ed.), p. 139. Academic Press, New York.

Mountcastle, V. P., and Edelman, G. M. (1978). "The Mindful Brain." MIT Press, Cambridge, Massachusetts.

Napier, J. (1973). "The Roots of Mankind." Harper Torch Books, New York.

Petersen, M. R., Beecher, M. D., Zoloth, S. R., Moody, D. B., and Stebbins, W. C. (1978). Neural lateralization of species-specific vocalizations by Japanese Macaques (*Macaca fuscata*). *Science* **202,** 324-327.

Rosenbaum, D. A. (1977). Selective adaptation of "command neurons" in the human motor system. *Neuropsychologia* **15,** 81-91.

Rosenman, R., and Friedman, M. (1974). Neurogenic factors in pathogenesis of coronary heart disease. *Med. Clin. North Am.* **58,** 269-279.

Schachter, S. (1971), "Emotion, Obesity and Crime." Academic Press, New York.

Schwartz, G. E., and Shapiro, D. (1973). Social psychophysiology. *In* "Electrodermal Activity in

Psychological Research'' (W. F. Prokasy and D. C. Raskin, eds.). Academic Press, New York.

Shapiro, D., and Watanabe, R. (1972). Reinforcement of spontaneous electrodermal activity: a cross-cultural study in Japan. *Psychophysiology* **9**, 340–344.

Sternbach, R. A., and Tursky, B. (1965). Ethnic differences among housewives in psychophysical and skin potential responses to electric shock. *Psychophysiology* **1**, 241–246.

Tanaka-Matsumi, J., and Marsella, A. J. (1976). Cross-cultural variation in the phenomenological experience of depression. *J. Cross-Cult. Psychol.* **7**, 379–396.

Trivers, R. (1971). Evolution of reciprocal altruism. *Q. Rev. Biol.* **46**, 35.

Tulving, E. (1972). Episodic and semantic memory. *In* "Organization of Memory" (E. Tulving and W. Donaldson, eds.). Academic Press, New York.

Tursky, B., and Sternbach, R. A. (1967). Further physiological correlates of ethnic differences in responses to shock. *Psychophysiology* **4**, 67–73.

Turvey, M. T. (1975). "Preliminaries to a Theory of Action With Reference to Vision," Status Rep. Speech Res. SR-41. Haskins Lab.

Warrington, E. D. (1975). The selective impairment of semantic memory. *Q. J. Exp. Psychol.* **27**, 635–657.

Washburn, S. L. (1961). "Social Life of Early Man." Aldine, Chicago, Illinois.

Washburn, S. L., and Moore, R. (1974). "Ape into Man: A Study of Human Evolution." Little, Brown, Boston, Massachusetts.

Waters, R. S., and Wilson, W. A. (1976). Speech perceptions by Rhesus monkeys: the voicing distinction in synthesized labial and velar stop consonants. *Percep. Psychophys.* **19**, 285–289.

Weisenberg, M. (1977). Pain and pain control. *Psychol. Bull.* **84**, 1008–1044.

Wilson, E. O. (1975). "Sociobiology: The New Synthesis." Belknap Press, Cambridge, Massachusetts.

Wolff, P. H. (1977). Biological variations and cultural diversity: an exploratory study. *In* "Culture and Infancy: Variations in the Human Experience" (P. H. Leiderman, S. R. Tulkin, and A. Rosenfeld, eds.), pp. 357–384. Academic Press, New York.

Young, J. Z. (1974). "An Introduction to the Study of Man." Oxford Univ. Press, London and New York.

Zoloth, S. R., Petersen, M. R., Beecher, M. D., Green, S., Marler, P., Moody, D. B., and Stebbins, W. (1979). Species-specific perceptual processing of vocal sounds by monkeys. *Science* **204**, 870–872.

4

Genetic Polymorphisms and Human Disease

WILMA B. BIAS

I. INTRODUCTION

The simultaneous occurrence of two or more forms or alleles of a gene in a population is a genetic polymorphism. Such an occurrence may be balanced or

95

BIOCULTURAL ASPECTS OF DISEASE
Copyright © 1981 by Academic Press, Inc.
All rights of reproduction in any form reserved.
ISBN 0-12-598720-X

transient. As defined by Ford (1940), a balanced polymorphism has a proportion of alleles such that the rarest cannot be maintained by mutation alone. This definition implies that under appropriate environmental conditions one allele confers better fitness than the other or, alternatively, the prevailing environment favors the heterozygote. A transient polymorphic state exists while one allele is being replaced by another through selection or random genetic drift. Although the transient and balanced states may be distinguished for short-lived organisms such as *Drosophila,* they cannot in man. Nevertheless, the most compelling evidence of Ford's hypothesis comes from man, namely, the relationship between malaria and hemoglobins A and S.

Ford suggested that the test of his hypothesis would come through determining the distribution of the alleles of polymorphic systems in various disease states. At that time, the only human polymorphism known was the ABO system and many disease association studies had already been carried out (Hirszfeld, 1928) with unimpressive results.

One important advance leading to the recognition of new polymorphisms was the introduction of zone electrophoresis, using a variety of supporting media coupled with appropriate staining methods. This technological breakthrough uncovered a wealth of variations in serum proteins and red blood cell enzymes.

About one-third of the enzymes studied in man have electrophoretically detectable variants. Harris *et al.* (1973) estimated that the average heterozygosity per individual for the recognized polymorphic enzyme loci is about 8%. Extrapolating data from several species, including man, Kimura (1974) estimated the average heterozygosity, over *all* loci of a single individual in a large human population, to be about 10%. Although a fundamental of Darwinism is that natural selection can operate only if genetic variation occurs, the genetic load imposed by 10% heterozygosity is too great, even if all the polymorphisms are maintained by modest selection. Kimura suggested, therefore, that many alternative forms of genes are functionally equivalent, and that polymorphism results from random genetic drift.

For some exceptional systems, such as the hemoglobins, glucose-6-phosphate dehydrogenase (G6PD), and the ABO, Rh, and Duffy blood groups, selective forces seemingly operate to maintain the balance. For most systems, however, survival of a new gene is probably a matter of chance. Early in human history, when effective population size was small, grossly deleterious mutations would have been quickly eliminated by selection. Those that were only slightly deleterious or neutral, however, would have been affected more profoundly by random genetic drift. As agriculture developed and populations became larger, the selection process became proportionately more effective, showing a trend toward the mutation–selection balance Ford (1940) hypothesized. Probably the genetic constitution of most modern human populations has been altered more drastically by gene flow (inward migration) than by the influence of disease. The few remaining aboriginal groups that have not experienced genetic admixture are so small that, like early man, their gene frequencies are influenced more by chance than by selection.

Nevertheless, logic dictates that certain polymorphic systems should be associated with disease. These include the ABO system, the immunoglobulin allotypes, and HLA. This chapter will consider selected associations and the possible biochemical and immunologic processes by which they occur.

II. THE BLOOD GROUP SYSTEMS

A. The ABO System

1. History

The science of genetics did not exist in 1900 when Karl Landsteiner published his discovery of the human ABO blood group system (Landsteiner, 1900). His observations, reported in the same year that Mendel's laws governing heredity were rediscovered, served as the benchmark for other immunologic studies. Landsteiner's simple experiments of mixing the red blood cells of one person with the serum of another were prompted by the earlier observations that erythrocytes of one animal species can be agglutinated by the serum of another. Landsteiner decided to see whether this phenomenon might occur within a species and chose to study man. His choice was fortunate, because isoagglutination is rare in the commonly used laboratory animals, although it is observed in dogs, cats, goats, pigs, and horses.

Landsteiner found that his experimental sample assorted into three groups, according to whether their cells were agglutinated by the sera of the groups to which they did not belong. Cells from Group I were not agglutinated by the sera of Groups II or III; however, Group I sera agglutinated the cells of the other two groups. Groups II and III were reciprocal in their agglutination patterns. Soon his co-workers (von Decastello and Sturli, 1902) found subjects whose red blood cells corresponded to those of both Groups II and III, leading Landsteiner to generalize that two components of human blood exist that can appear singly or together, or be absent altogether. In addition, the serum never contains autoantibodies, but always has antibodies against the absent components.

The practical applications of blood typing for transfusions were immediately apparent, but another 10 years passed before von Dungern and Hirszfeld (1910) showed that the blood groups are inherited as simple Mendelian traits. Determining the blood groups of parents and children of the Heidelberg faculty, they concluded that two genes are responsible, one for Group II and one for Group III, and that Group I had neither gene but is doubly recessive. They also proposed

changing the designations of the groups to A, B, AB, and O, with O corresponding to Landsteiner's Group I. Later, Bernstein (1924) demonstrated mathemati-
cally, from population data, that the groups belonged to a single genetic system,
thus introducing the concept of multiple alleles.

The extensive blood typing necessitated by World War I enabled Hirszfeld and
Hirszfeld (1918-1919) to show that the frequencies of the ABO groups varied
significantly among different populations. In addition to recognizing the importance of blood groups to anthropological studies, those investigators anticipated
Ford's hypothesis and pioneered in studying the relationship of the ABO groups
and their susceptibility to disease (Hirszfeld *et al.*, 1924). More than 25 blood
group and disease studies from most of the countries of Europe and Asia were
reviewed by Hirszfeld (1928) and were found to be essentially inconclusive. The
exception was that of the effects of maternal-fetal incompatibility on infant survival and health (Hirszfeld and Zborowski, 1925). The data revealed an excess of
A offspring from matings of O fathers with A mothers as compared with the
reciprocal mating type. Two decades later, after the discovery of the Rh system,
these observations were confirmed by Levine (1943), who recognized that ABO
incompatibility could result in early abortion and stillbirth.

The early efforts at analyzing the genetics, immunology, anthropology, and
disease asociations of the ABO blood groups have their counterpart today in the
plethora of similar studies of the HLA system. *Plus ça change, plus c'est la
méme-chôse!*

Antigens similar to those of the ABO system are ubiquitous. They are found
on the red blood cells of anthropoid apes and in the plasma of a variety of
animals, where they are absorbed passively onto the red blood cells.

2. Immunochemistry and Genetics

Glycoproteins bearing determinants of the ABO system were discovered in
human body fluids by Lehrs (1930) and Putkonen (1930), enabling recovery of
sufficient quantities of soluble material for immunochemical studies and for
determining the structure of the blood group substances. Certain plant lectins
capable of agglutinating human red blood cells were found to be selectively
inhibited by the glycoprotein secreted by group O subjects. The secreted macromolecule from O subjects was designated H, for hemagglutinating substance.
H substance is not only secreted by group O persons but also in varying amounts
by A, B, and AB persons as well; however, about 25% of all persons, regardless
of blood group, do not secrete A, B, and H substance. The ability to secrete is
determined by another gene, *Secretor* (Schiff and Sasaki, 1932), inherited independent of the ABO system.

Both secretors and nonsecretors may secrete another macromolecule, called
Lewis substance, which can be absorbed passively onto red blood cells and be
typed with anti-Lewis antisera. Persons may be Lewis-positive or negative,

depending on whether or not they inherit the *Lewis* (*Le*) gene (Mourant, 1946), which is also unlinked to *ABO* or to *Secretor*.

Immunochemical studies (reviewed in Watkins, 1972) have shown that the A, B, H, and Lewis antigenic determinants reside on the same molecule and result from the sequential addition of sugar residues to a precursor glycoprotein. The *Le* and *H* genes encode two different α-fucosyltransferases that attach α-fucose to two adjacent glycosyl residues on the precursor macromolecule to confer Lewis and H specificities. The Lewis system is polymorphic, and the presence or absence of the Lewis-specific fucose does not affect the biosynthesis of A, B, or H. However, the H-specific fucose is required for the action of the glycosyl-transferases encoded by the *A* and *B* genes. An extremely rare ABH variant, called the Bombay phenotype (Bhende *et al.*, 1952), is of the genotype *hh*. Although pedigree analysis shows that *hh* persons have the *A* or *B* gene and that their sera contain the specific A or B glycosyltransferase, their red blood cells do not react with anti-A or anti-B.

Subjects of the *hh* genotype who are also *Lewis* (*lele*) negative secrete a glycoprotein that cross-reacts with a capsular antigen of *Pneumococcus*, type XIV. Treating A or B substance with certain carbohydrases yields H substance plus the A- or B-specific sugar residue. Further hydrolytic treatment of the H substance removes fucose and degrades both H and Lewis substances to the same material that reacts with the antipneumococcal antiserum. This cross-reactivity further attests to the ubiquity of these macromolecular structures.

The product of the *Secretor* gene, *Se*, is unknown, and its action is not fully understood. Perhaps it is required for active transport of the macromolecules across the cell membrane. Apparently either free diffusion or some other transport mechanism operates until the H-specific sugar is added to the growing chain, inasmuch as the percursor molecule and Lewis substance are found in the body fluids of nonsecretors.

The ABH antigens have been detected on virtually all tissues, the exceptions being lymphocytes and tissues of the nervous system. Given this widespread distribution and the possible cross-reactivity with microorganisms, it is most unlikely that the population distribution of the alleles of this system is the product of chance alone.

3. Disease Associations

The literature on blood groups and diseases has been thoroughly reviewed by Mourant *et al.* (1978) and it would be presumptuous as well as redundant to attempt to repeat their efforts. Rather, I have used their excellent volume as a resource for the examples to be discussed in this and subsequent sections of this chapter.

The search for evidence that polymorphisms are maintained by selective pressure should focus on the infectious or malignant diseases that take their toll during infancy or childhood, i.e., before the age of reproduction. Ideally, such studies would be carried out prospectively in populations having high infant mortalities and morbidities from infectious diseases. Few such studies have been reported; most data are retrospective and derive from advanced or relatively advanced populations.

The first unequivocal association between blood group and disease was that between group A and gastric carcinoma (Aird *et al.*, 1953). The neoplasias reviewed by Mourant *et al.* (1978) include only solid tumors and, in general, show an association of malignancy with group A and, to a lesser extent, with group B. No significant association of disease with secretor status has been reported, except for salivary gland cancer in which the ratio of secretors is excessive. Although these diseases of adult onset are unlikely to affect reproductive fitness, the data may be instructive in terms of immune surveillance. The somewhat increased occurrences of malignancy in groups A and B suggest that surveillance may be somewhat impaired in those groups or somewhat enhanced in group O.

Recent data on ABO associations with infectious diseases are hardly more conclusive than those reviewed in 1928 by Hirszfeld. Perhaps the most interesting and convincing are the relationship of the system of α-hemolytic streptococcus infections. In this case, the various studies looked at different parameters of infection and immune response to it, and the findings were rather consistent. In summary, group A persons had a lower incidence of scarlet fever but a higher incidence of positive reactors to the Dick test than did persons in other groups. Among rheumatic fever patients the association with groups A and B was higher than expected, and this increased frequency is even greater in those with rheumatic heart disease. Rheumatic fever is a consequence of the normal, but perhaps enhanced, immune reponse to the infection. Therefore, one might speculate that carriers of groups A and B can mount a more effective immune response to α-hemolytic streptococcus as revealed by the development of rheumatic fever or a positive Dick test, whereas group O remains susceptible to infection from this class of organism. Also of interest are the findings that the number of secretors having rheumatic fever and carrying the type A strain, which is responsible for scarlet fever, was fewer than expected. Perhaps the soluble H substance in some way acts as a carrier or activator for the organism or for a product of the infectious process.

Data on the viral diseases are scanty, indeed. Unfortunately, the reports on smallpox contain many discrepancies and contradictions. Nor can conclusions be drawn from the few studies concerned with influenza. However, the results from polio studies are somewhat more conclusive. Among patients having the disease, groups A and B had a somewhat lower than expected frequency than did group O. When group ratios for paralytic polio were compared with those for nonparalytic disease, the deficiency of groups A and B was significant. Unfortunately, no data are available on secretor status. Nonetheless, with polio as with α-hemolytic streptococcus, group O appears to be more susceptible to infection.

Additional indirect evidence that infectious disease may have exerted selective pressure on the ABO system comes from the observations by Eichner *et al.* (1963) that "naturally occurring" antibodies to bacterial antigens having no apparent cross-reactivity with ABO are not randomly distributed among the human blood groups. For example, they found that antibody titers against *Escherichia coli* 086:B7 were lowest in persons of blood group O.

An ABO relationship to thromboembolic disease was first reported by Dick *et al.* (1963). They found a highly significant deficit of group O in a series of 461 patients in Tübingen. The importance of this observation became apparent when results of an international study on young women (Jick *et al.*, 1969) confirmed the findings. Bates (1971) examined the London records of maternal deaths from 1963 to 1968 and found blood groups recorded for 53 of 150 women who had died of pulmonary embolism. Again, the number of group O women was strikingly low. Although group O appears to confer somewhat increased susceptibiltiy to infectious disease, it seems to be protective against thromboembolism. This particular advantage of group O may be further enhanced since the advent of oral contraceptives.

B. The Rh System

1. History

The Rhesus system was so named because of the antiserum produced by Landsteiner and Wiener (1940) from a rabbit immunized to rhesus monkey erythrocytes. The antiserum, when tested against human red blood cells, agglutinated those of about 85% of blood donors. These subjects were designated as Rhesus positive.

Several species of apes had been shown to have red blood cell components indistinguishable from the human ABO system (Landsteiner and Miller, 1925a), and, although the sera of rhesus monkeys contained anti-A (Landsteiner and Miller, 1925b), their erythrocytes did not appear to have groups A or B. Thus, if a xenogeneic antibody* were produced against rhesus cells, it should not be specific for the ABO system, but it might react with some other component shared by rhesus and human red blood cells.

The success of this experiment coincided in time with the discovery by Levine and Stetson (1939) of an antibody in the serum of a woman whose child was stillborn as a result of erythroblastosis fetalis, or hemolytic disease of the newborn. They reasoned correctly that the antibody was pregnancy induced and

---

*Xenogeneic antibody—cross-species immunization.

showed that it agglutinated the red blood cells of the woman's ABO compatible husband. Unfortunately, Levine and Stetson did not name their new blood group, so that when their antiserum was found to react similarly to anti-Rh there was no competing choice of name. Similar antibodies were also found by Wiener and Peters (1940) in the sera of patients who has suffered transfusion reactions. Then, the definitive report by Levine *et al.* (1941) establishing maternal–fetal Rh incompatibility as the major cause of hemolytic disease of the newborn left no doubt as to the clinical importance of the system.

The recognition that blood group antibodies could be induced by pregnancy and transfusion paved the way for the discovery of many new blood groups, including a large number belonging to the Rh system. The new Rh antibodies that were found revealed a genetic and serologic complexity that is still far from undersood. On the one hand is the system proposed by Fisher and elaborated by Race (1948), of three closely linked loci each with multiple alleles. With few exceptions the genetic and serologic data are compatible with this hypothesis. On the other hand, the data are also consistent with a single locus system with a large number of alleles whose products have multiple immunodominant determinants. The remarkable number of Rh variants led Rosenfield *et al.* (1962) to develop a numerical system based strictly on serology with no regard to genetic hypotheses. As of 1973 the Rh variants numbered 35 (Rosenfield *et al.*, 1973), rivaling the HLA system, which was known at that time to comprise two serologically defined loci.

Ironically, the anti-rhesus antibody originally produced in rabbit has subsequently been found not to be identical to the allogeneic antibody. The xenogeneic antibody is now called anti-LW (after Landsteiner and Wiener).

2. Hemolytic Disease of the Newborn

The genetic basis of Rh hemolytic disease is an Rh-negative mother whose mate is Rh positive. If the father is homozygous, all the children from the union will be Rh positive; if he is heterozygous, half will be Rh positive. Maternal–fetal incompatibility that leads to selection against the fetus does not aid in the maintenance of polymorphism. On the contrary, it works against such maintenance because selection is against the heterozygote. While this selection results in the loss of both alleles, the rarer will be eliminated at a greater rate than the more common one, with a tendency toward fixation of the common allele in the absence of a counteracting mechanism to maintain the polymorphic state. One possible counteracting mechanism is reproductive compensation in which the mother experiences a greater than average number of pregnancies to produce the desired number of offspring. Since the live-born children will be Rh negative, thus replacing every lost Rh-positive gene with its Rh-negative allele, the trend would be toward an increase in the frequency of Rh negative, except that the mothers with Rh-positive homozygous mates have no opportunity for compensation.

Hemolytic disease of the newborn results from the normal immune response of the mother to an incompatible blood group "transfused" from her child. The pathology occurs when the antibody she produces diffuses through the placenta into the fetal circulation and destroys the fetal red blood cells. The fetal liver is incapable of removing the accumulated waste products so that, at best, the newborn is jaundiced and, at worst, he is stillborn or severely ill and mentally retarded.

Under perfect conditions the placenta is impermeable to the passage of cells between the fetus and mother. Whether or not perfect conditions are maintained during pregnancy, at parturition it is common for fetal blood to cross the placenta into the maternal circulation. This event, at the end of the first incompatible pregnancy, is usually the primary immunologic challenge. Because the quantity of red blood cells that leak across the placenta during pregnancy is insufficient to immunize, hemolytic disease rarely occurs in first-born infants. The quantity of blood transfused by the transplacental hemorrhage appears to govern whether or not the mother mounts a primary response. Less than 4% of mothers are immunized by their first pregnancy if the transplacental hemorrhage is less than 0.2 ml, as compared with about 20% if it is greater. On average, about 10% of Rh-negative mothers with incompatible babies are immunized by the first pregnancy; about 30% are immunized by the end of the second pregnancy. Thus, the third and later pregnancies experience substantial risk.

An Rh-negative mother is protected against Rh immunization if she is also ABO incompatible with her fetus (Levine, 1943). The ABO incompatible fetal cells that pass into the mother's circulation are removed by her "naturally occurring" anti-A or anti-B before they can be recognized by her immune system. About 13% of Rh incompatible pregnancies will also be ABO incompatible. After discounting ABO incompatibility, and Rh-negative status of the fetus because the father is Rh negative or is heterozygous, about 50% of the Rh-negative mothers are at risk of immunization. Before 1971, the incidence of Rh hemolytic disease of the newborn among Caucasians was 1 in 200 births.

3. Prevention of Rh Immunization

The first step in the prevention of a disease is the understanding of its cause. The cause of hemolytic disease of the newborn became clear almost immediately after the discovery of the Rh system in 1940. The first approach to prevent the disease was exchange transfusion of the infant immediately after delivery. Even that approach was too late in severe cases, so techniques were developed for intrauterine transfusion. Those procedures involved replacing the infant's Rh-positive red blood cells with those from an Rh-negative donor that would be safe

from attack by the maternal antibodies. Although these were important achievements, the problem could not be solved until methods could be found to prevent
immunization of the mother.

The knowledge that the "naturally occurring" isoagglutinins of the ABO
system afforded protection against RH immunization suggested that the passive
administration of anti-Rh before primary immunization occurred might accomplish the same thing in the ABO compatible pregnancy (Finn, 1960). Rh-
negative male volunteers were recruited to participate in the experiments required
to test the proposed methods. The protocols involved injection of various quantities of Rh-positive erythrocytes labeled with radioactive chromium, followed
by the administration of anti-Rh, and determining whether the antibody cleared
the Rh-positive cells from circulation and prevented immunization.

"Naturally occurring" isoagglutinins are IgM molecules that cannot cross the
placenta; therefore, anti-Rh of that class was used initially in the experiments.
This antibody did, indeed, destroy the radiolabeled cells, but it did not prevent
immunization. Antibodies of the IgG class were successful in both removing the
Rh-positive cells and in preventing antibody synthesis. However, those antibodies are the ones that cross the placenta and provoke the disease one is
attempting to prevent.

Under the assumption, based on empirical evidence, that the transplacental
passage of fetal red blood cells during pregnancy is insufficient to immunize,
clinical trials were begun in 1965 in which the anti-Rh was given shortly after
delivery. By 1971 the number of mothers in the collaborative studies who had
produced second babies was sufficiently large to determine that the incidence of
immunization was less than 2%, an overall reduction of about 90% (Clarke,
1973). The 10% failure rate probably has two explanations. A certain number
could be attributed to previous unreported Rh-positive pregnancies terminated by
abortion. The remainder are probably primary failures due to predelivery immunization. A trial of prophylaxis during the last trimester was carried out in
Canada (Bowman, 1978) with no adverse effects on the fetus. Consequently, in
that country the practice is to administer one dose of anti-Rh IgG at 28 weeks
gestation, a second dose at 34 weeks, and a final dose after delivery.

Since 1971 Rh prophylaxis has become routine for Rh-negative women who
bear Rh-positive children or who undergo abortions.

4. Other Disease Associations

That the Rh system would relate to any other diseases seems too much to
expect; in fact, only the report of Paciorkiewicz (1970) provides data for Rh
association with infectious diseases. That investigator found a deficiency of Rh
positive in cases of typhoid, paratyphoid, tuberculosis, sarcoidosis, mumps,
infectious mononucleosis, and viral meningitis.

C. Other Blood Group Systems

1. History

Between the discoveries of the ABO and Rh systems, efforts to identify new human blood groups returned to the production of xenogeneic antisera. In 1927 Landsteiner and Levine (1927a,b) identified the MN and P systems using antisera raised in rabbits. As with all the human blood groups systems, allogeneic antisera were later found for the major groups of the MN and P systems as well as for many variants. These two systems are good polymorphisms of primary interest to geneticists and anthropologists and have minimal clinical impact.

Antigens similar to P_1, the common P allele, are ubiquitous. For example, a glycoprotein found in copious amounts in hydatid cyst fluid from sheep shows P_1 reactivity. The P system is of some further interest, not because of its antigenic variation, but because antibodies to various of its specificities have been found in several pathologic conditions, the most prevalent being anti-P_1 appearing as an autoantibody in paroxysmal nocturnal hemoglobinuria (Levine et al., 1963).

According to the latest edition of the splendid reference work of Race and Sanger (1975) more than 160 red blood cell antigens belonging to more than 30 systems are now identifiable. Almost all have been implicated in transfusion reactions or hemolytic disease of the newborn. With the exception of the Duffy antigens, none has been shown to be associated with disease. Perhaps, as Kimura (1974) postulated, the alleles of these systems are functionally equivalent and the polymorphisms are chance phenomena.

2. The Duffy System

The Duffy antibody, designated as anti-Fy^a, was found in 1950 in a multi-transfused patient (Cutbush et al., 1950). Anti-Fy^b, recognizing an allelic specificity, was reported one year later by Ikin et al. (1951). The gene frequencies in Caucasians are 0.43 for Fy^a and 0.56 for Fy^b (Race and Sanger, 1975). The frequency distribution is different in blacks. The Duffy null genotype, $FyFy$, occurs in about 95% of West Africans but is rare in other populations (Mourant et al., 1976). Coincidentally, the West Africans are resistant to Plasmodium vivax but are susceptible to other malaria species (Bray, 1958). While searching for erythrocyte receptors for malaria parasites, Miller et al. (1975) found that Duffy null red blood cells are resistant to infection by Plasmodium knowlesi, a simian malaria parasite that can also infect man. Fy^{a}Fy^a, Fy^{b}Fy^b, and the Fy^{a}Fy^b heterozygous cells are not resistant but could be made resistant by enzymatic removal of the Duffy antigens from their membrane surfaces. These observations suggested that the high frequency of the Fy allele results from selection pressure against Fy^a and Fy^b by vivax malaria.

These serendipitous observations represent the first evidence that a blood group antigen can function as a receptor for a pathogenic organism.

III. THE HEMOGLOBINS

A. Background

Human biochemical genetics can be said to originate with the demonstration by Pauling *et al.* (1949) that an abnormal hemoglobin, now designated HbS, was responsible for the sickling phenomenon exhibited by the erythrocytes of a certain proportion of persons of African descent. Neel (1949) and Beet (1949), working independently, showed that persons having sickle cell anemia are homozygous for HbS whereas those with sickle trait are heterozygotes.

The electrophoretic method for detecting hemoglobin variants is simple and requires no staining procedures, so, as would be expected, considerable effort was invested to detect new forms of this important protein. As a result, more than 100 hemoglobin variants are known. Most are rare and have been observed only in the heterozygous state.

The globin moiety of adult hemoglobin, HbA, is a tetramer of two α chains and two β chains. A minor component, HbA_2, is $\alpha_2\delta_2$. There are also fetal and embryonic hemoglobins that have γ and ϵ chains, respectively, in place of β chains. A developmental sequence of gene action occurs in which ϵ production ceases in favor of γ and γ diminishes as β synthesis begins. The ϵ, γ, β, and δ genes are tightly linked on the same chromosome and probably arose by gene duplication early in speciation.

There is evidence that the α-chain gene is also duplicated (Kan *et al.*, 1975a), but the gene products are both identifiable as α, suggesting that this duplication is recent relative to those of the partner series.

The hemoglobin variants range from single amino acid substitutions to nonhomologous crossing-over between the β and δ genes, creating a "hybrid" polypeptide (Hb Lepore) or a deleted chain (Hb Gun Hill). They also include abnormally elongated α chains resulting from mutation in the terminating codon [Hb Constant Spring, Icaria, Koya Dora, and Seal Rock (Weatherall and Clegg, 1975)] and complete deletions of the α-chain sequences (Clegg and Weatherall, 1976).

Most of the variants observed in homozygous state are deleterious, and one group of mutants produces unstable products that are deleterious in single dose. One should keep in mind, however, that because of the manner in which the data are obtained the benign forms are under-reported.

B. The Hemoglobinopathies

1. Hemoglobin S

The sickle shape assumed by erythrocytes in the HbS homozygote occurs under low oxygen tension. The abnormal cells are rapidly cleared from the circulation, resulting in chronic hemolytic anemia. Before their destruction, however, the relatively rigid deformed cells block small vessels, causing infarcts in various organs, painful crises, and, ultimately, premature death.

Why so deleterious a gene had such a high incidence in tropical Africa remained unclear until the epidemiologic data of Allison (1954) clearly showed that HbAS heterozygotes were more resistant to falciparum malaria that HbA homozygotes. Thus, the loss of two HbS alleles in the homozygotes to sickle disease was offset by the loss of two HbA alleles to malaria. The selective advantage of the AS heterozygote represents the classical example of balanced polymorphism.

The frequency of the HbS allele should be decreasing in the United States and other nonmalarial countries to which Africans have migrated since the selective pressure on HbA homozygotes has been removed.

2. The Thalassemias

Thalassemia is a heterogeneous collection of 50 different genetic disorders characterized by ineffective erythropoiesis producing severe anemia, fever, hyperuricemia, and skeletal deformities (Weatherall and Clegg, 1972). The Mediterranean background of the patients is implicit in the name of the syndrome as it was first described, although now the thalassemias are known not to be limited geographically.

In thalassemia the rate of one or more of the globin chains, either α or β, is reduced, which leads to a relative excess of the partner chains of the polymer. The pathologic events are a consequence of the precipitation of the unpaired chains.

Three basic types of mutations are responsible for the α thalassemias. One type of mutation results in a complete absence of alpha chains. In infants homozygous for this form, the gamma chains form tetramers (Hb Bart's) that can function as hemoglobin but have a reduced half-life and abnormal oxygen-binding properties. This defect appears to be caused by deletion of both the α-chain genes (Ottolenghi et al., 1974; Taylor et al., 1974). The second mutant class has partially reduced α-chain production apparently due to deletion of one of the α genes (Kan et al., 1975a). In the third type, the α chain has 31 extra amino acid residues at the C terminal end (Hb Constant Spring) that causes synthesis to be impaired. Clinically, the latter two syndromes are less severe than Hb Bart's syndrome since α chains are not completely absent.

The β thalassemias are also a heterogeneous group of disorders. In all cases studied so far, none gives evidence for deletion of the β gene (Tolstoschev et al., 1976). These syndromes have been reviewed by Weatherall and Clegg (1976), who reported that the common denominator is a reduced amount of messenger RNA.

In the Sicilian and Greek form of δ-β thalassemia and in the hereditary persistence of fetal hemoglobin a large segment of the β gene has been deleted (Kan et al., 1975b; Ottolenghi et al., 1976).

Following the lead of Allison (1954), Carcassi et al. (1957) suggested that malaria acts as a selective agent favoring the thalassemia heterozygote in the Mediterranean region. Although there is no direct evidence supporting this hypothesis, given the severity of disease in thalassemia homozygotes, the genes could not have reached the observed high frequencies in the absence of rather significant advantage to the heterozygotes.

IV. RED BLOOD CELL ENZYMES

A. Glucose-6-Phosphate Dehydrogenase

During World War II, a significant proportion of American black soldiers were found to have acute hemolytic crises when given the synthetic antimalarial drug, primaquine (Hockwald et al., 1952). Carson et al. (1956) showed that the hemolysis was caused by a deficiency of G6PD, the first enzyme utilized in the metabolism of glucose via the hexose monophosphate shunt. The gene for G6PD is located on the X chromosome; therefore, the deficiency occurs more frequently in males than in females. Unlike other enzyme deficiencies, the deficient state for G6PD is sufficiently frequent that the quantitative variability constitutes a polymorphism.

Other quinoline-derived antimalarial drugs and the sulfonamides also induce hemolysis in G6PD-deficient subjects, as does ingestion of the fava bean, a diet staple in many Mediterranean countries.

Two electrophoretic variants of G6PD, A and B, are common, and deficient states for both exist. The normal A gene and its deficient allele are rare, except in blacks. In addition, the World Health Organization (1967) reported a total of 28 electrophoretic or quantitative variants from many regions of the world. Some variants are associated with chronic hemolytic anemia because of their instability, whereas others appear relatively benign.

As with HbS and thalassemia, the geographic distribution of G6PD deficiency follows that of malaria. Allison and Clyde (1961) were able to show a correlation between G6PD deficiency and resistance to malarial infection in African children. That proliferation of the parasite might be inhibited in G6PD-deficient red blood cells has been suggested (Motulsky, 1964). This explanation is inadequate for the maintenance of the polymorphism, however, because both the A allele with normal enzymatic activity and A^- allele with no enzymatic activity have a high frequency in Africa.

B. Other Enzymes

The catalogue of erythrocyte enzyme polymorphisms has become extensive (Giblett, 1969; Mourant *et al.*, 1976), but disease associations are rare except for the deficiency states. The enzyme polymorphisms are especially useful to the anthropologist and to the geneticist interested in chromosome mapping, the establishment of paternity, or zygosity status of twins.

A recent application of the hemopoietic markers, i.e., the blood groups, enzymes, and immunoglobulin allotypes, is the documentation of bone marrow engraftment. Good engraftment will result in a shift from recipient type to donor type for the markers that are genetically different in recipient and donor. This process, or its failure to occur, is useful as an early indicator of graft outcome.

A typical repertoire of red blood cell enzymes that would be typed by a comprehensive genetic marker laboratory includes G6PD, 6-phosphogluconate dehydrogenase, adenosine deaminase, adenylate kinase, phosphoglucomutase, acid phosphatase, uridine monophosphate kinase, esterase-D, and glyoxalase-1. These enzymes are genetically polymorphic in man. None but G6PD have shown convincing disease associations. The rare deficiency states of other enzymes result in deleterious inborn errors of metabolism.

V. SERUM PROTEINS

A. Immunoglobulin Allotypes

As with the blood groups, population studies have shown racial and geographic differences in allotype* distribution. Given the biologic importance of the immunoglobulins and the great diversity of isotypes† that differentiate classes and subclasses, idiotypes that characterize the products of single clones, and the high degree of allotypic polymorphism that distinguishes genetic differences between members of the species, one must conclude that the system is the product of exquisite selective forces.

Polymorphic determinants, or allotypes, of immunoglobulins (Ig) are designated as Gm if they reside on the γ heavy chain, as Am if they are on the α heavy chain, and Km for κ light chain variants. No λ light chain variants have been observed, and presently used methods cannot detect IgM polymorphisms.

Antibodies to the immunoglobulins are regularly found in the sera of patients with rheumatoid arthritis. Often these are autoantibodies and somewhat

---

*Allotype: genetically determined variation within a species.

†Isotype: a characteristic of an immunoglobulin (Ig) class. Isotypes reside in the constant regions of heavy chains.

nonspecific in their reactivity. We have found anti-Ig antibodies developing during pregnancy or early in the postpartum period; however, they are transient and broadly reacting (W. B. Bias, unpublished data). Specific antibodies to Gm and Km antigens occur in low frequency in the sera of normal persons, some of whom have experienced no known immunizing event. My laboratory's most fruitful search for anti-Ig reagents came from screening sera of male inmates in a local penitentiary. Many of the subjects were drug addicts, leading me to hypothesize that the sharing of improperly cleaned hypodermic needles resulted in repeated small immunologic challenges of Gm and Km antigens sufficient to induce specific antibodies of high titer.

The antibodies to Ig allotypes are of the IgM class and are identified by a hemagglutination technique. Rh-positive red blood cells are reacted to anti-D (Rh_0) of the IgG class. The monovalent (incomplete) anti-D "coats" the erythrocytes but cannot cause agglutination unless an antiglobulin reagent is added. For ordinary blood grouping a xenogeneic anti-human globulin (Coomb's reagent) is used. For allotyping, however, one adds the human serum suspected of containing anti-Gm or anti-Km. If the anti-D has the allotypic determinant recognized by the anti-Ig serum, agglutination will occur. In that event, one now has a typing system, i.e., an anti-D of specific Gm or Km type and an antiglobulin that recognizes it. Typing of unknown sera can now be done. This is carried out by an agglutination–inhibition procedure. Serum to be typed is incubated with the various anti-Gm and anti-Km reagents, after which the appropriate anti-D-coated red blood cells are added. If agglutination does not occur, the person being typed has the allotype of the inhibited anti-D.

Although the methodology is relatively simple, the acquistion of reagents has always been difficult, especially now that Rh immunization is routinely prevented by anti-D prophylaxis. Because the allotyping reagent systems are not generally available, few disease association studies have been carried out.

In a small study of Italian children with thalassemia major, Vierucci (1965) found 43% with anti-Gm antibodies, presumably because of frequent transfusions, but their allotype distributions did not differ from the normal population in the same district. Podliachouk et al. (1965) typed 168 patients with ankylosing spondylitis, 477 with rheumatoid arthritis, and 118 with other articular disease for Gm(a), Gm(b), Gm(x), and Gm-like, now called Gm-1, Gm-5, Gm-2, and Gm-6, respectively. While they observed Gm(a) to be somewhat decreased in ankylosing spondylitis and Gm(x) to be slightly increased in rheumatoid arthritis, the findings are generally not impressive.

In a study of 164 malignant melanoma patients that included typing for ABO, Rh, haptoglobin, group-specific component, Gm-1 and Gm-2, a significant increase in Gm-2 was reported by Jorgensen and Lal (1972).

Blake and Greally (1975) typed sera from 136 Irish myeloma patients for Gm-1, -2, -4, -12, and for Km-1 and compared the distributions with a series of

294 normal Irish subjects reported by Walter and Palsson (1973). Patients and controls did not differ in the frequencies of Gm-1, -2, and -12; however, the patient group had a striking deficiency of Gm-4. The frequency in patients was only 41% as compared with 90% in the normal subjects. The authors do not suggest a genetic or immunologic explanation for their findings. Rather, they expressed concern that the difference may be technical. It is important that this interesting finding in a malignant disease of antibody biosynthesis be confirmed.

B. Haptoglobin

Haptoglobin is a glycoprotein synthesized by the liver with a specific affinity for free hemoglobin. Its normal function is unknown, but a common belief is that it may aid in the conservation of iron. Smithies (1955) demonstrated three common electrophoretic phenotypes of haptoglobin, Hp 1-1, Hp 2-1, Hp 2-2, controlled by a diallelic genetic system (Smithies and Walker, 1956). Studies of the molecular structure of haptoglobin revealed two kinds of polypeptide chains, α and β. The β chains appeared to be invariant (Cleve *et al.*, 1967), but structural differences in chains (Smithies *et al.*, 1966), designated Hpα1S (slow) and Hpα1F (fast), were detectable under certain conditions of electrophoretic separation. Whereas the Hpα1F and Hpα1S polypeptides each has a molecular weight of about 900, the Hpα2 chain was found to be almost twice as large (Smithies *et al.*, 1962). Peptide fingerprint patterns and amino acid sequencing indicated that the *Hp 2* gene arose as a product of unequal crossing over, so that a *Hpα1F* gene was fused end to end with a *Hpα1S* gene.

Similar haptoglobin characteristics have not been found in primates (Parker and Bearn, 1961), suggesting that the gene duplication occurred after hominid evolution.

In most human populations the *Hp 2* allele is more frequent than *Hp 1* (Kirk, 1968), indicative of selective advantage; yet Hp 1 is more efficient at binding free hemoglobin. That the hemoglobin binding capacity is not the major selective factor for maintaining the polymorphism is apparent, because variants that result in virtual absence of serum haptoglobin are phenotypically normal (Giblett and Steinberg, 1960).

C. Group-Specific Component

Group-specific component (Gc) is an α-globulin with two common alleles, *Gc-1* and *Gc-2*, that until recently had no known function. Schanfield *et al.* (1975) discovered that Gc serves as a carrier for vitamin D. The geographic distribution of the alleles can be explained on the basis of this function. According to Mourant *et al.* (1978), the frequency of Gc-1 is higher in sunny climates and Gc-2 is prevalent in less sunny regions, suggesting that availability of vitamin D has been a selective force in determining the allele frequencies. No studies have been reported on Gc typing of patients with rickets.

D. Protease Inhibitor

Serum α_1-antitrypsin is a polymorphism of a locus designated Pi with one common allele, Pi_M, and at least 20 infrequent variants (reviewed in Giblett, 1969). The polymorphism of Pi was discovered after Laurell and Eriksson (1963) showed that deficiency of α_1-antitrypsin was a causal factor in a small proportion of cases of pulmonary disease. Sharp *et al.* (1969) also demonstrated liver disease attributable to deficiency for this protease inhibitor. Kueppers and Bearn (1966) suggested that the function of the protein might be to prevent the digestion of tissue during an inflammatory process. The genetic variants are both qualitative and quantitative. Most exhibit some degree of decreased activity, usually with accompanying disease. However, sibs of the same Pi genotype may differ in disease manifestation, indicating the importance of environmental interaction with this system.

VI. PTC TASTE RESPONSE

It was shown by Fox (1931) that persons could be classified according to whether or not they found phenylthiocarbamide, PTC (thiourea), to have a bitter taste. Family studies have shown that PTC taste response is inherited as a Mendelian dominant trait (Blakeslee and Salmon, 1931).

Numerous studies (reviewed in Mourant *et al.*, 1978) have shown goitrogenic properties of thiourea and related compounds, some of which are found in foods of the cabbage family. Harris and Kalmus (1949) showed that these substances act as thyroid inhibitors and that PTC tasters find them all similarly bitter. Harris *et al.* (1949) found fewer tasters among patients with nodular nontoxic goiters than among normal subjects, whereas an increased frequency of tasters was observed by Kitchin *et al.* (1959) in patients with diffuse toxic goiter. Widström and Henschen (1963) showed that PTC tasters have a higher level of protein-bound iodine than do nontasters.

In their early review, Harris and Kalmus (1949) suggested that PTC tasters fix iodine more efficiently and that the frequency of the taster allele would increase in environments with low iodine content or an abundance of thyroid inhibitors and would decrease under the opposite conditions, resulting in a balanced polymorphism for this genetic system.

VII. HLA, THE MAJOR HISTOCOMPATIBILITY SYSTEM IN MAN

A. History

In a series of animal and human experiments, Medawar (1944, 1958) obtained evidence that a first allogeneic skin graft enjoys a latent period of well-being before rejection occurs. Further, he found that a second skin graft from the same donor was rejected in a much shorter time than was the first and that this rejection response was donor specific. He further showed that an injection of donor leukocytes before grafting could also induce accelerated graft rejection, thus demonstrating that the leukocytes shared antigens with the grafted skin.

The classical studies in the mouse by Snell and Gorer (reviewed in Klein, 1975) demonstrated that circulating antibodies could be produced by graft challenge or by blood transfusions. These antibodies appeared to recognize antigens belonging to a single genetic system, which they designated *H-2*. The letter H signified *histocompatibility,* and, to date, more than 30 H systems have been identified in the mouse.

Dausset (1958) produced the first defined histocompatibility antiserum in man by immunizing one blood donor with the leukocytes of another. The resulting antiserum agglutinated the white blood cells of about 60% of his Parisian blood donor panel. Dausset called the antigen recognized by his antiserum MAC, and the antiserum was designated anti-MAC.

At about the same time, Payne and Rolfs (1958) observed that the sera of many multiparous women contained leukoagglutinins. The discovery that these antibodies were produced as a result of pregnancy challenge was as important for the histocompatibility field as it was for the red blood cell blood grouping field. The sera of healthy multiparous women would provide a source of reagents for a new area of immunogenetics.

The human white blood cell blood groups did not yield to genetic analysis readily. Many of the antisera apparently contained multiple antibodies, and, furthermore, the reactions were not always reproducible. Van Rood and van Leeuwen (1963) approached the first problem by a computerized sorting of the reaction patterns obtained with a large number of antisera against a panel of 100 cells. This sorting resulted in several groups of sera that correlated positively or negatively with each other. One system that appeared diallelic was designated by van Rood and van Leeuwen as *Four,* with the alleles being *4a* and *4b*. Payne *et al.* (1964) similarly described a triallelic system, which they called *LA*. Family studies supported the computerized evidence for a single immunogenetic system (Histocompatibility Testing, 1965, 1967). The Fourth International Workshop (Histocompatibility Testing, 1970) results provided clear evidence for a genetic system of two closely linked loci, each with multiple alleles. The data from that workshop suggested the possibility of a third locus in the complex, a suggestion subsequently confirmed by Kissmeyer-Nielsen *et al.* (1971).

The letters HLA, for human leukocyte antigens, were chosen for the emerging human histocompatibility system. The *LA* and *Four* series were renamed *HLA-A* and *HLA-B*. It is important to note that the original 4a and 4b are diallelic specificities on the HLA-B molecule that recognize determinants separate from the HLA-B "private" antigens. A similar "public" system has not been defined for the A locus, although the specificities of both the A and B loci cluster in cross-reacting groups (called Cregs).

The problem of reproducibility of HLA typing was solved largely by Terasaki and McClelland (1964). They developed a complement-dependent cytotoxicity test for lymphocytes that are less prone to nonspecific clumping than granulocytes and also developed laboratory "tools" that greatly simplified the method.

The early experiments of Medawar clarified the relevance of histocompatibility testing to organ transplantation and, once the tools were available for routine typing, laboratories were established worldwide.

B. Genetics

1. The HLA Map

The HLA gene complex occupies a segment about 2 centimorgans (cM)* in length of the short arm of chromosome 6. This region is about 25 cM from the centromere in the proximal half of band 6p21 (Francke and Pellegrino, 1977). Also within this band is the gene for the red blood cell enzyme, glyoxalase-1 (GLO), which maps about 5 cM toward the centromere from HLA (McBreen *et al.*, 1977). At least eight loci can be assigned with some confidence to the HLA region and all play some role in immune function. Three loci are serologically well-defined—HLA-A, -B, and -C—and two loci are defined by reactivity in the mixed lymphocyte response (MLR) test—HLA-D and the weak MLR locus. HLA-D can also be recognized serologically; however, it is not yet clear whether the antigenic determinants are the same gene products as the HLA-D determinants defined by MLR. For this reason, the serologically defined D region specificities are designated as HLA-DR, or D related. Also within the complex are loci that determine the structure of C2, the second component of complement, and C4, for the fourth component. Another locus, *Bf*, is the structural gene for properdin factor B, an enzyme of the alternate complement pathway. A gene that controls the biosynthesis of 21-hydroxylase maps between HLA-DR and

*1 cM≈1% recombination.

HLA-A (Bias *et al.*, 1981). The close linkage to HLA was first reported by Dupont *et al.* (1977). Deficiency for this enzyme causes congenital virilizing adrenal hyperplasia.

The HLA complex is the most polymorphic of all known human systems. More than 20 alleles have been identified at the A locus and more than 40 at the B locus. The C and D loci are less well understood and are currently defined by only 8 and 12 alleles, respectively (Histocompatibility Testing, 1980). Given the large number of alleles at each of the loci, and assuming D and DR are identical, the possible number of haplotypic combinations exceeds 20 million.

2. Diseases Linked to HLA

a. **Complement Deficiencies.** The genes for C2 and C4 were identified when deficiency states for those two components of complement were found to segregate in families with particular HLA complexes (haplotypes) (Fu *et al.*, 1974; Ochs *et al.*, 1977). Later, electrophoretic variants for both C2 and C4 were observed that also segregated with HLA, establishing the HLA-linked loci as structural genes and the null alleles, responsible for the deficiency syndromes, as amorphs or deletions (Alper, 1976; Teisberg *et al.*, 1976). In man, complement deficiencies are associated with increased susceptibility to infection or lupus-like syndromes (Alper and Rosen, 1976).

Deficiency for properdin factor B has not been observed; however, at least one family study can only be explained by invoking the inheritance of a Bf null allele (L. U. Lamm, personal communication).

b. **Congenital Adrenal Hyperplasia.** Congenital adrenal hyperplasia is an inborn error of metabolism that may be due to deficiency of one of several hydroxylases involved in hormone physiology. Dupont *et al.* (1977) and Levine *et al.* (1978) presented evidence that the gene controlling the biosynthesis of 21-hydroxylase maps in the interval between the genes for glyoxalase-1 and HLA-A. In cases of recombination between HLA-A and B, the 21-hydroxylase deficiency allele segregated with the B end of the haplotype, as it did in the GLO-HLA recombinants. One of seven families studied in our laboratory that had two intra-HLA recombinants permitted more precise localization of the 21-hydroxylase gene (Bias *et al.*, 1981). In both recombinant subjects the deficiency gene segregated with HLA-B rather than HLA-D, thus localizing it inside the HLA-A to D interval. It will be necessary to find segregation with HLA-D or HLA-A to determine whether the gene is to the left or right of HLA-B.

C. HLA and Disease Associations

The first study of HLA and disease association was carried out by Amiel (1967) on Hodgkin's disease. Amiel's interest was not in testing the hypothesis of

E. B. Ford (1940) but in determining whether major histocompatibility complex (MHC)-linked control of susceptibility to a malignant disease could be demonstrated for man similar to that observed by Lilly *et al.* (1964) in the mouse. Because viral pathogenesis had long been suspected in Hodgkin's disease, it was a logical choice for such a study—although premature, considering the state of the art of histocompatibility testing in 1967. Nevertheless, an association with the 4c (HLA-B5) cross-reacting group was found that was later confirmed by others (Forbes and Morris, 1970).

Further interest in searching for HLA and disease associations was stimulated by the demonstration by McDevitt and Sela (1967) of *H-2* control of immune response to synthetic polypeptides. They showed that C57 mice carrying the *H-2b* haplotype gave a low antibody response to the branched multichain polymer of histidine, glutamic acid, alanine, and lysine [abbreviated (H,G)-A-L)], whereas the CBA mouse of *H-2k* haplotype gave a high response. When histidine was replaced by tyrosine in the polymer, the responses were reversed, with C57 giving high and CBA low responses. The F_1 hybrids all gave high responses, showing that high response is inherited as a dominant trait. Studies of intra-*H-2* recombinant mice showed that the gene-controlling response was separable from the serologically defined *H-2D* and *H-2K* loci and that it mapped in the general region of the gene controlling mixed lymphocyte responses. The immune response gene was designated as *Ir-1* (McDevitt *et al.*, 1971). Further studies revealed that multiple genes within the *H-2* complex control immune response. The linear array of these genes constitutes the *I* region of *H-2* and is considered to be homologous to the *D* region of *HLA*.

The investigators searching for disease associations with HLA reasoned that disease-susceptibility (*DS*) genes should map in a region homologous to the *I* region of mouse, and the serologically defined (SD) specificities HLA-A, -B, and -C, should serve as markers to identify them. Because the human MHC comprises a genetic distance of only about 2 cM, any *DS* gene mapping within the complex should be associated in the population with a particular allelic specificity because of linkage disequilibrium. It is important to note, however, that population associations would break down for any gene mapping at a distance greater than about 5 cM. This point will be discussed later.

The appropriate intra-HLA recombinants with and without particular disease traits that permit fine-structure mapping have not been identified; consequently, it is not yet possible to state with certainty, as McDevitt *et al.* (1971) did for the mouse, that the disease susceptibility gene is *not* the same as the associated HLA marker gene. However, in keeping with the mouse model, the greatest likelihood is that multiple loci along the HLA chromosomal segment influence specific immune responses. It is of some relevance to determine whether the marker specificity is the controlling element in susceptibility, because, in such cases, the antigen–antibody reaction can be used as a probe to elucidate disease pathogenesis.

Perhaps the best candidate for a serologically defined allele being a disease susceptibility gene is the best known association, that of HLA-B27 and ankylosing spondylitis. The data supporting *B27* itself as being the disease susceptibility (*DS*) gene include the following:

1. Ankylosing spondylitis (AS) is associated with B27 in all ethnic groups. If the *DS* gene were another locus, it would not likely be in linkage disequilibrium with *B27* in diverse populations. Furthermore, in general, the incidence of AS is higher in populations with the highest B27 frequencies.

2. Non-B27 patients more often than not have a cross-reacting specificity (Arnett *et al.*, 1977). In this report, 10 of 44 patients with Reiter's syndrome were B27 negative. Of these, seven (70%) had another B locus antigen in the B7 cross-reacting group: two were B7, four were Bw22, and one was Bw42.

3. There is some evidence of cross-reaction or interaction between B27 and *Klebsiella* cell wall antigens, suggesting that this organism may be implicated in disease pathogenesis. Ebringer *et al.* (1976, 1977, 1978) observed an increased incidence of excretion of *Klebsiella pneumoniae* in AS patients as compared with healthy controls. They also had some evidence indicating cross-reactivity between *B27* and *Klebsiella* cell wall antigen. Following this lead, Seager *et al.* (1979) studied *in vitro* lymphocyte responses to *Klebsiella*. They found that lymphocytes of B27-positive AS subjects responded significantly lower than B27-positive or negative healthy controls. They further observed that antibody against *Klebsiella* raised in rabbit lysed lymphocytes of the B27-positive patients but not those of B27-negative patients or healthy B27-positive or B27-negative controls. These data suggest that infection may produce antigen modification in the B27-positive patients.

4. Data from the Third American Workshop suggest that B27 can be "split" into two or more components; however, the components appear equally frequent in B27-associated disease (Hopkins *et al.*, 1979). This equal frequency indicates that the relevant DS determinant on the B27 molecule is shared by the different components. One might further assume that this DS determinant is shared, at least in part, by other specificities of the HLA-B7 cross-reacting group. Recent experiments of Schwartz *et al.* (1979) provide evidence for a determinant on the HLA-B molecule that is shared by the B7 Creg specificities but is distinct from the "private" antigenic determinants. This determinant would account for the cross-reactivity, and the gene controlling it might be the *DS* gene.

Cross-reactivity between HLA antigens and microorganisms was first reported by Hirata and Terasaki (1970). They were able to inhibit lymphocytotoxic reactions of HLA antisera with the M protein component of a particular strain of

Streptococcus. From such observations in man and animal has come the concept of "molecular mimicry." Molecular mimicry may occur when a microorganism has antigens structurally similar to those of the host and thereby escapes detection by the host immune system. Disease susceptibility resulting from molecular mimicry would be inherited as a dominant trait.

The other side of the coin from molecular mimicry is the receptor mechanism. While receptor function has not been demonstrated for any particular HLA and disease association, the concept is supported by the findings of Helenius *et al.* (1978) that both H-2 and HLA antigens serve as receptors for the Semliki Forest virus. As illustrated by the association between Duffy blood group and vivax malaria, susceptibility attributable to an antigenic receptor would also be inherited as a dominant trait.

In contrast to molecular mimicry and the receptor mechanism, susceptibility to Gross leukemia virus is a recessive trait possessed by relatively few mouse strains (Lilly *et al.*, 1964), i.e., resistance is "normal." Therefore, one would assume a different immunologic mechanism is operating. Evidence for other mechanisms comes from several sources. Aoki *et al.* (1966) observed that strains resistant to Gross virus produce higher titer of antibodies to the virus than animals homozygous for the *H-2* linked susceptibility gene. This observation points to MHC control over antibody production, either directly on B cell function or via T-B interaction.

In studies with Friend leukemia virus (FV), Blank *et al.* (1976) found that resistant animals can generate a cell-mediated lympholysis (CML) response against FV-induced tumor cells whereas susceptible animals cannot. Meruelo (1979) refined these observations in a radiation-induced leukemia virus (RadLV) system. The gene conferring resistance to RadLV maps in the *H-2D* region of the mouse (Meruelo and McDevitt, 1978). After animals were infected with RadLV, Meruelo *et al.* (1978) observed a considerable increase in H-2D antigen expression on thymocytes of resistant, but not susceptible, animals. Meruelo (1979) further observed that augmentation of antigen is required for the generation of the CML response to virus-infected cells. In a human system, McMichael (1978) found HLA-A2 to be associated with poor CML responses against influenza virus-infected targets, in contrast to good lysis with other specificities. His observation supports the notion that HLA-A2 may be a "susceptibility" gene for influenza. Meruelo and Edidin (1979) suggested that one mode of action of the MHC in viral disease resistance is the enhancement of cell-mediated immune response through modification of the expression of cell surface antigens. Increased resistance via the augmentation of cell surface antigen expression, as well as by increased antibody synthesis, would be inherited as a dominant trait.

In the foregoing discussion, I pointed out whether resistance or susceptibility should be inherited as a dominant or recessive trait for each immunologic mechanism. Yet, even in the case of anklylosing spondylitis, which exhibits extremely close association with B27, about 6–10% discordance occurs between presence of antigen and disease. Any of several factors may be responsible.

First, the necessary environmental factors may be lacking. Certainly, exposure to the appropriate agent is necessary in infectious diseases. The study of monozygotic twins discordant for disease can aid in elucidating the relative contributions of unknown environmental components.

Second, the disease in question may exhibit heterogeneity, i.e., the same syndrome may be caused by more than one agent, each with separate genetic requirements. For example, juvenile diabetes mellitus (JDM) has been associated with both HLA-B8 (or Dw3) and B15 (or Dw4) (summarized in Svejgaard et al., 1975). It has been reported that the onset of JDM may follow infection with one of several different viruses, including mumps, rubella, and Coxsackie B4 (Gamble et al., 1973; Steinke and Taylor, 1974). That one of the causative agents may interact with B8 and another with B15 is not unlikely.

Third, the expression of disease may require the interaction of other gene loci, namely, the trait is polygenic. This interaction is certainly the case with IgE-mediated immune response to allergens. Although we have shown several associations between specific responses to highly purified pollen allergenic components and certain HLA specificities at the population level, we cannot demonstrate concordant transmission of responses in families, even with relatively uniform environmental exposure (Black et al., 1976; Bias et al., 1979). We have determined that one of the interacting loci controls the basal levels of IgE (Marsh et al., 1974). Other genes, as yet unidentified, functioning at the level of antigen processing and presentation, are probably also required.

As discussed above, HLA-associated disease susceptibility genes may be the serologically defined specificities themselves or may be other loci mapping within or close to the *HLA complex*. Association of linked genes at the population level can occur only if the two loci are extremely close together and show linkage disequilibrium. For instance, the loci for the Lutheran blood group and ABH-Secretor trait are separated by only 8 cM, yet their alleles show no association in population studies. It is inappropriate to assume, therefore, that absence of disease in a sib carrying the associated specificity, or presence of disease in the absence of the relevant antigen, is evidence that recombination has occurred between *HLA* and the *DS* gene. In the case of ankylosing spondylitis, such an assumption would place the *DS* gene at a minimal distance of 6–10 cM outside the *HLA* complex. Such localization is too distant to observe population association between AS and B27.

D. Generation of HLA Polymorphism

This discussion of HLA and disease associations began with the concept of how genetic polymorphisms are maintained in populations. I have not yet dealt with the question of how they arose. Understanding the evolution of the major histocompatibility complex is not conceptually difficult. The similarity of structure between *H-2D* and *H-2K* of mouse and their sequence homologies with *HLA-A* and *HLA-B* of man indicate that the region evolved via a series of gene duplications similar to the hemoglobins and immunoglobulins and, like the loci for the Ig heavy chains, have remained closely linked because of functional necessity. Although it is likely that this process occurred before mammalian evolution, since all mammalian MHCs appear to be homologous, the generation of polymorphism had to have occurred independently for each species. Therefore, the capacity for variation must be inherent within the MHC. I have assumed that polymorphism of the MHC is necessary for a species to respond effectively to the assault of pathogens. But how did the species survive during the period of polymorphism generation? One possible explanation is that the generation of variation occurred rapidly, namely, the MHC is a highly mutable region. Another possibility is that the emerging species had a gene that conferred ''good'' generalized immune responsiveness that enabled that species to survive during the period required for the generation of polymorphism. Ideally, these two conditions would coexist. The latter condition will be discussed first.

In human, HLA-B8 has been associated with a multiplicity of immunopathic disorders (Svejgaard *et al.*, 1975). Marchalonis *et al.* (1974) offered the explanation that B8 may act to amplify the immune response. Data from our laboratories of HLA relationships to response to purified pollen components tend to support this hypothesis. We found several specific associations, e.g., HLA-B7 with ragweed allergens Ra5 and HLA-A2 with Ra3 (Marsh *et al.*, 1973, 1977). In addition, we found B8 to be associated with IgE response to several allergens, including rye grass groups I and II (Marsh and Bias, 1977; Marsh *et al.*, 1980). To look at many components simultaneously, Marsh *et al.* (1980), carried out crossed radioimmunoelectrophoresis (CRIE) in polyacrylamide gels of a set of common environmental antigens and reacted the gels with sera from study subjects drawn from a population unselected for allergy. In this study group, the frequency of HLA-B8 was significantly increased in responders as compared with that of nonresponders irrespective of allergen. The B8 association with response was especially striking in the 10 ragweed allergic subjects included in the analysis. The geometric mean IgE levels were higher in the responders than in nonresponders. Our interpretation of these data is that B8 confers a generalized hyperresponsiveness that, in individuals with the genotype for high IgE biosynthesis, enhances response to many different allergens. Whether a characterisitic of B8 activity is the augmentation of IgE biosynthesis is not yet clear.

An antithetical association with poor immune function has been suggested for HLA-B7 (Svejgaard *et al.*, 1975). Support for this relationship comes from Petranyi *et al.* (1974), who associated B7 with poor cell-mediated cytotoxic responses and from Persson *et al.* (1975), who found that HLA-B7 is associated with sarcoidosis, but only in a subgroup of patients who were tuberculin skin test negative.

In 1977, I postulated that a pair of allelic genes, one conferring increased and the other decreased immune responsiveness to environmental pathogens, might readily become established as a balanced polymorphism (Bias and Chase, 1977). Such a diallelic system, perhaps similar to HLA-B7 and B8, might be marginally sufficient in conferring disease resistance until further variation could be superimposed.

By what mechanism could polymorphism be generated rapidly before an epidemic eliminated an emerging species of limited breeding size? An attractive hypothesis is that put forward by Meruelo and Edidin (1979). They suggested that the MHC might have evolved, and indeed, if they are correct, is still evolving, via the integration of viral genomes into germinal cells in a fashion similar to lysogeny in bacteria. Transcription of portions of the incorporated viral genome, together with portions of the pre-existing host genome would lead to synthesis of a "mutant" antigen that may or may not have altered function.

The possibility that the MHC is a viral intergration site was first proposed by Bailey (1966) as an explanation for the relatively high spontaneous mutation rate for histocompatibility (H) loci in mice, and for the fact that 138 of 142 detected H mutations were of the gain or loss-and-gain types. Bailey pointed out that virus genome incorporation would result in the appearance of new H antigens in the cell membrane of the somatic cells descending from the "infected" germ cells. Bailey further noted that the H mutation rate is higher in animals maintained in a "less isolated," i.e., more likely to be infected, environment (Bailey, 1966), a factor that appears to have no influence over the rate of mutation at non-H loci (Searle, 1972).

Viral integration within the H-2D region would explain Meruelo's (1979) observations of marked and prolonged increases in H-2D synthesis following RadLV infection. Meruelo and Edidin (1979) pointed out that increased H-2D expression would be expected because, after viral genome integration, transcription would be under virus control and would preferentially transcribe viral genome sequences and the adjacent H-2D sequences.

Other evidence in support of the MHC as a site for viral genome integration is provided by the somatic cell hybrid data of Gazdar et al. (1977) and Ruddle et al. (1978) that localized murine leukemia virus integration sites to mouse chromosomes 5, 15, 17. The mouse MHC maps on chromosome 17 as does TLa, a locus controlling the expression of thymus leukemia antigen. Conversion from TL-negative to TL-positive phenotype occurs only in conjunction with the appearance of malignancy (Stockert et al., 1971). Antigen gain accompanied by malignant transformation lends credence to the notion that TLa is a viral integration site.

Thus, following the above reasoning, the evolutionary sequence of events leading to the generation of a highly polymorphic genetic complex such as the MHC would be as follows:

1. Gene duplication of one or more primordial genes in an early ancestral species followed by the mutational events that led to the development of functions now exhibited by the mammalian MHC, e.g., antigen recognition, cell–cell interactions, complement structures.

2. Transmission of the prototype complex during phylogeny: The maintenance of structural and functional homology of the complex throughout mammalian speciation indicates that disruption of the complex would be incompatible with species survival.

3. Generation of polymorphism: A single initial mutation, whether by viral genome integration or by one or more DNA base pair substitutions, produced a basic diallelic system of at least one locus in the complex. Additional alleles at this locus would arise rapidly if the locus is a viral integration site. Because the entire complex probably arose by gene duplication, it is reasonable to assume that multiple genes in the complex are capable of viral integration. Thus, the expectation would be a linear array of closely linked multiallelic loci, as observed for the MHC. One could postulate that perpetuation of the original diallelic system with the properties of generalized weak response in carriers of one allele and hyperresponsiveness in the other, as suggested for HLA-B7 and B8, is advantageous to the species. The retention of these alleles would leave intact a "back-up" immune response system to act nonspecifically in pathogenic encounters for which an optimal immune response gene is not present.

Determining whether MHC genes are viral integration sites should be possible by more precise mapping of these sites on chromosome 17 of the mouse. If the hypothesis is correct, specificity of the different loci for particular viruses can be tested for both mouse and man by *in vitro* infection of cell lines carrying known MHC alleles in various combinations.

We can expect a clearer understanding of MHC relationships to disease as data emerge from studies that test the relative effects of alleles controlling antigen recognition, the generation of T-suppressor and T-effector cells, and T-B interaction in the presence of pathogens or components of pathogens. The mechanism by which resistance or susceptibility to a particular disease is conferred may determine which MHC locus is associated with disease susceptibility. An understanding of basic mechanisms should lead to effective utilization of HLA associations in diagnosis and management of disease.

VIII. SUMMARY

The genome of the human species has been conservatively estimated to consist of at least 50,000 structural loci and that about one-third of them are polymorphic. Furthermore, each individual of the species is heterozygous at about one-third of the polymorphic loci, or for about 10% of the entire genome.

Polymorphisms may be transient, namely, the alternative alleles exist together in a population temporarily until selection pressure or random genetic drift eliminates the rarer variant. Polymorphisms that are more or less permanent exhibit a balance between the frequencies of alternative alleles. Ford (1940) hypothesized that balanced polymorphisms result from heterozygote advantage or differential environmental effects on the various phenotypes. Polymorphisms maintained by selective forces may be the bases for human disease; however, the genetic load imposed by 10% heterozygosity for minimally deleterious genes is too great for species survival. Therefore, Kimura (1974) reasoned that most polymorphisms are selectively neutral.

Numerous studies (reviewed in Mourant *et al.*, 1978) indicate that several human polymorphic systems have been maintained by selection, most notably some of the blood groups, hemoglobins, and HLA.

Investigations of blood group and disease associations suggest that, in general, persons of blood group O may be more susceptible to infectious disease but more resistant to malignancies and thromboembolism. Since the data on thromboembolism were partially derived from young women of child-bearing age, this information provides some evidence of how natural selection may operate in maintaining a polymorphism. Mourant *et al.* (1978) made the interesting point that the available data also suggested that viral diseases tend to attack the null phenotype of both the ABO and Rh systems.

Because of gene flow and dramatic environmental change characteristic of modern human history, it is unlikely that any polymorphism is in a state of equilibrium. The environmental changes have eliminated or reduced the selection pressure on many polymorphic systems. An outstanding example is the reduction of selection by malaria brought about by the use of DDT and the quinoline drugs. Of importance is that the selection pressure of DDT on the mosquito and of the quinoline drugs on the *Plasmodium* has resulted in increased frequencies in these two organisms of genes conferring resistance to these agents.

One must also realize that whenever a trait is protected from the direct action of natural selection, mutations will accumulate in the population and that random genetic drift will allow "degeneration" to occur. The ability to synthesize ascorbic acid is a case in point. Most animals, with the exception of primates, the guinea pig, and the Indian fruit bat, can synthesize the enzyme that hydrolyzes uridine diphosphoglucuronic acid, the nucleotide precursor of ascorbic acid, to glucuronic acid. The diets of these species provide ascorbic acid, thereby allowing the gene for enzyme deficiency to accumulate in the population, through random drift, to the point of fixation.

More recent examples of reduced selection pressure included myopia and color blindness. These two visual defects, which today exist as polymorphisms in the human population, were surely deleterious to hunting and gathering societies. Development of urbanization shielded myopic and color-blind persons from the action of natural selection so that in modern societies the traits are merely inconveniences.

Environmental changes also include medical intervention. A classic example is insulin-dependent juvenile diabetes mellitus. The use of insulin has permitted reproduction of many diabetics who would not have survived to reproductive age. Although reproductive fitness remains low, juvenile onset diabetes illustrates, nevertheless, that environmental change in the form of medical intervention can influence gene frequencies to the extent that a rare inborn error of metabolism may become a genetic polymorphism.

REFERENCES

Aird, I., Bentall, H. H., and Roberts, J. A. F. (1953). A relationship between cancer of the stomach and the ABO blood groups. *Br. Med. J.* **1**, 799–801.

Allison, A. C. (1954). Protection afforded by the sickle cell trait against subtertian malarial infection. *Br. Med. J.* **1**, 290–294.

Allison, A. C., and Clyde, D. F. (1961). Malaria in African children with deficient erythrocyte glucose-6-phosphate dehydrogenase. *Br. Med. J.* **1**, 1346–1349.

Alper, C. A. (1976). Inherited structural polymorphism in C2: evidence for genetic linkage between C2 and Bf. *J. Exp. Med.* **144**, 1111–1114.

Alper, C. A., and Rosen, F. S. (1976). Genetics of the complement system. *Adv. Hum. Genet.* **7**, 141–188.

Amiel, J. L. (1967). Study of the leucocyte phenotypes in Hodgkin's disease. *In* "Histocompatibility Testing 1967" (E. S. Curtoni, P. L. Mattiuz, and R. M. Tosi, eds.), pp. 79–81. Munksgaard, Copenhagen.

Aoki, T., Boyse, E. A., and Old, L. J. (1966). Occurrence of natural antibody to the G (Gross) leukemia antigen in mice. *Cancer Res.* **26**, 1415–1419.

Arnett, F. C., Hochberg, M. C., and Bias, W. B. (1977). Cross-reactive HLA antigens in B27-negative Reiter's syndrome and sacroiliitis. *Johns Hopkins Med. J.* **141**, 193–197.

Bailey, D. W. (1966). Heritable histocompatibility changes: Lysogeny in mice? *Transplantation* **4**, 482–487.

Bates, M. M. (1971). Venous thromboembolic disease and ABO blood type. *Lancet* **1**, 239.

Beet, E. A. (1949). The genetics of the sickle-cell trait in a Bantu tribe. *Ann. Eugen.* **14**, 279–284.

Bernstein, F. (1924). Ergebnisse einer biostatistischen zusammenfassenden Betrachtung über die erblichen Blutstrukturen des Mechen. *Klin. Wochenschr.* **3**, 1495–1497. (Translation *in* "Selected Contributions to the Literature of Blood Groups and Immunology." U.S. Army Med. Res. Lab., Ft. Knox, Kentucky, 1966.)

Bhende, Y. M., Deshpande, C. K., Bhatia, H. M., Sanger, R., Race, R. R., Morgan, W. T. J., and Watkins, W. M. (1952). A "new" blood group character related to the ABO system. *Lancet* **1**, 903–904.

Bias, W. B., and Chase, G. A. (1977). Genetic implications of HLA and disease association. *Transplant. Proc.* **9**, 531–542.

Bias, W. B., Hsu, S. H., Meyers, D. A., Goodfriend, L., and Marsh, D. G. (1979). HLA associations with chemically-defined ragweed pollen components. *Transplant. Proc.* **11**, 1853–1857.

Bias, W. B., Urban, M. D., Pollard, M. K., Migeon, C. J., Hsu, S. H., and Lee, P. A. (1981). Intra-HLA recombinations localizing the 21-hydroxylase deficiency gene within the HLA complex. *Hum. Immunol.* **2**, 139-145.

Black, P. L., Marsh, D. G., Jarrett, E., Delespesse, G. J., and Bias, W. B. (1976). Family studies of association between HLA and specific immune responses to highly purified pollen allergens. *Immunogenetics* **3**, 349-368.

Blake, P. J., and Greally, J. F. (1975). Gm and Inv markers in whole myeloma sera in an Irish population. *J. Immunogenet.* **2**, 147-149.

Blakeslee, A. F., and Salmon, M. R. (1931). Odour and taste blindness. *Eugen. News* **16**, 105-108.

Blank, K. K., Freedman, H. A., and Lilly, F. (1976). T-lymphocyte response to Friend virus induced tumor cell lines in mice of strains congenic at H-2. *Nature (London)* **260**, 250-252.

Bowman, J. M. (1978). Prevention of maternal Rh immunization. *In* "Genetic Issues in Public Health and Medicine" (B. H. Cohen, A. M. Lilienfeld, and P. C. Huang, eds.), pp. 401-421. Thomas, Springfield, Illinois.

Bray, R. S. (1958). The susceptibility of Liberians to the Madagascar strain of Plasmodium vivax. *J. Parasitol.* **44**, 371-373.

Carcassi, U., Ceppellini, R., and Pitzus, F. (1957). Frequenza della talassemia in quattro popolazioni sarde e suoi rapporti con la distribuzione dei gruppi sanguigni e della malaria. *Boll. Ist. Sieroter. Milan.* **36**, 206-218.

Carson, P. E., Flanagan, C. L., Ickes, C. E., and Alving, A. S. (1956). Enzymatic deficiency in primaquine-sensitive erythrocytes. *Science* **124**, 484-485.

Clarke, C. A. (1973). The prevention of Rh isoimmunization. *In* "Medical Genetics" (V. A. McKusick and R. Claiborne, eds.), pp. 263-270. HP Publ. Co., New York.

Clegg, J. B., and Weatherall, D. J. (1976). Molecular basis of thalassemia. *Br. Med. Bull.* **32**, 262-269.

Cleve, H., Gordon, S., Bowman, B. H., and Bearn, A. G. (1967). Comparison of the tryptic peptides and amino acid composition of the beta polypeptide chains of the three common haptoglobin phenotypes. *Am. J. Hum. Genet.* **19**, 713-721.

Cutbush, M., Mollison, P. L., and Parkin, D. M. (1950). A new human blood group. *Nature (London)* **165**, 188.

Dausset, J. (1958). Iso-leuco-anticorps. *Acta Haematol.* **20**, 156-166.

Dick, W., Schneider, W., Brockmuller, K., and Mayer, W. (1963). Thromboembolische Erkrankungen und Blutgruppenzugehorigkeit. *Med. Welt* **24**, 1296-1298.

Dupont, B., Oberfield, S. E., Smithwick, E. M., Lee, T. D., and Levine, L. S. (1977). Close genetic linkage between HLA and congenital adrenal hyperplasia (21-hydroxylase deficiency). *Lancet* **2**, 1309-1312.

Ebringer, A., Cowling, P., Ngwa, S. N., James, D. C. O., and Ebringer, R. E. (1976). Crossreactivity between Klebsiella aerogenes species and B27 lymphocyte antigens as an aetiological factor in ankylosing spondylitis. *In* "HLA and Disease" (J. Dausset and A. Svejgaard, eds.), p. 27. INSERM, Paris. (Abstr.)

Ebringer, R., Cooke, D., Cawdell, D. R., Cowling, P., and Ebringer, A. (1977). Ankylosing spondylitis: Klebsiella and HLA-B27. *Rheumatol. Rehabil.* **16**, 190-196.

Ebringer, R. W., Cawdell, D. R., Cowling, P., and Ebringer, A. (1978). Sequential studies in ankylosing spondylitis. Association of Klebsiella pneumoniae with active disease. *Ann. Rheum. Dis.* **37**, 146-151.

Eichner, E. R., Finn, R., and Krevans, J. R. (1963). Relationship between serum antibody levels and ABO blood group polymorphism. *Nature (London)* **198**, 164.

Finn, R. (1960). Erythroblastosis. *Lancet* **1**, 526.

Forbes, J. F., and Morris, P. J. (1970). Leukocyte antigens in Hodgkin's disease. *Lancet* **1**, 849–851.

Ford, E. B. (1940). Polymorphism and taxonomy. *In* "The New Systematics" (J. Huxley, ed.), p. 493. Oxford Univ. Press (Clarendon), London.

Fox, A. L. (1931). Six in ten "taste blind" to bitter chemical. *Sci. News Lett.* **19**, 249.

Francke, U., and Pellegrino, M. A. (1977). Assignment of the major histocompatibility complex to a region of the short arm of human chromosome 6. *Proc. Natl. Acad. Sci. U.S.A.* **74**, 1147–1151.

Fu, S. M., Kunkel, H. G., Brusman, H. P., Allen, F. H., Jr., and Fotino, M. (1974). Evidence for linkage between HLA histocompatibility genes and those involved in the synthesis of the second component of complement. *J. Exp. Med.* **140**, 1108–1111.

Gamble, D. R., Taylor, K. W., and Cumming, H. (1973). Coxsackie viruses and diabetes mellitus. *Br. Med. J.* **4**, 260–262.

Gazdar, A. F., Oie, H., Lalley, P., Moss, W., Minna, J. D., and Francke, U. (1977). Identification of mouse chromosomes required for murine leukemia virus replication. *Cell* **11**, 949–956.

Giblett, E. R. (1969). "Genetic Markers in Human Blood." Blackwell, Oxford.

Giblett, E. R., and Steinberg, A. G. (1960). The inheritance of serum haptoglobin types of American Negroes: evidence for a third allele Hp^{2M}. *Am. J. Hum. Genet.* **12**, 160–169.

Harris, H., and Kalmus, H. (1949). Genetical differences in taste sensitivity to phenylthiourea and to anti-thyroid substances. *Nature (London)* **163**, 878.

Harris, H., Kalmus, H., and Trotter, W. R. (1949). Taste sensitivity to phenylthiourea in goitre and diabetes. *Lancet* **2**, 1038–1039.

Harris, H., Hopkinson, D. A., and Robson, E. B. (1973). The incidence of rare alleles determining electrophoretic variants: data on 43 enzyme loci in man. *Ann. Hum. Genet.* **37**, 237–253.

Helenius, A., Morin, B., Fries, E., Simons, E., Robinson, P., Schirrmacher, V., Terhorst, C., and Strominger, J. I. (1978). Human (HLA-A and HLA-B) and murine (H-2K and H-2D) histocompatibility antigens are cell surface receptors for Semliki Forest virus. *Proc. Natl. Acad. Sci. U.S.A.* **75**, 3846–3850.

Hirata, A. A., and Terasaki, P. I. (1970). Crossreactions between streptococcal M proteins and human transplantation antigens. *Science* **168**, 1095–1096.

Hirszfeld, H., and Hirszfeld, L. (1918–1919). Essai d'application des methods serologiques au probleme des races. *Anthropologie* **29**, 505–537.

Hirszfeld, H., Hirszfeld, L., and Brokman, M. (1924). On the susceptibility of diphtheria with reference to the inheritance of blood groups. *J. Immunol.* **9**, 571–591.

Hirszfeld, L. (1928). "Konstitutionsserologie und Blutgruppenfurschung." Springer-Verlag, Berlin. (Translation *in* "Selected Contributions to the Literature of Blood Groups and Immunology." U.S. Army Med. Res. Lab., Ft. Knox, Kentucky, 1969, v. 3.)

Hirszfeld, L., and Zborowski, H. (1925). Gruppenspezifische Beziehungen zwischen Mutter und Frucht und elektive Durchlassigkeit der Placenta. *Klin. Wochenschr.* **4**, 1152–1157.

"Histocompatibility Testing" (1965). *N. A. S. N. R. C., Publ.* No. 1229.

"Histocompatibility Testing 1967" (1967). (E. S. Curtoni, P. L. Mattiuz, and R. M. Tosi, eds.). Munksgaard, Copenhagen.

"Histocompatibility Testing 1970" (1970). (P. I. Terasaki, ed.). Munksgaard, Copenhagen.

"Histocompatibility Testing 1980" (1980). (P. I. Terasaki, ed.). U.C.L.A. Tissue Typing Laboratory, Los Angeles.

Hockwald, R. S., Arnold, J., Clayman, C. B., and Alving, A. S. (1952). Status of primaquine. IV. Toxicity of primaquine in Negroes. *J. Am. Med. Assoc.* **149**, 1568–1570.

Hopkins, K. A., Enlow, R. W., Arnett, F. C., and Bias, W. B. (1979). Serologic evidence for at least two components of HLA-B27. *Annu. Meet. Am. Assoc. Clin. Histocompat. Test, 5th* p. A58. (Abstr.)

Ikin, E. W., Mourant, A. E., Pettenkofer, H. J., and Blumenthal, G. (1951). Discovery of the expected hemagglutinin anti-Fy[b]. *Nature (London)* **168**, 1077.

Jick, H., Slone, D., Westerholm, B., Inman, W. H. W., Vessey, M. P., Shapiro, S., Lewis, G. P., and Worchester, J. (1969). Venous thromboembolic disease and ABO blood type. *Lancet* **1**, 539–542.

Jorgensen, G., and Lal, V. B. (1972). Serogenetic investigations on malignant melanoma with reference to the incidence of ABO system, Rh system, Gm, Inv, Hp and Gc systems. *Humangenetik* **15**, 227–231.

Kan, Y. W., Dozy, A. M., Varmus, H. E., Taylor, J. M., Holland, J. P., and Lie-Injo, L. E. (1975a). Deletion of alpha globin genes in haemoglobin-H disease demonstrates multiple alpha globin structural loci. *Nature (London)* **225**, 255–256.

Kan, Y. W., Holland, J. P., Dozy, A. M., Charache, S., and Kazazian, H. (1975b). Deletion of the beta globin structure gene in hereditary persistence of foetal hemoglobin. *Nature (London)* **258**, 162–163.

Kimura, M. (1974). Gene pool of higher organisms as a product of evolution. *Cold Spring Harbor Symp. Quant. Biol.* **38**, 515–524.

Kirk, R. L. (1968). "The Haptoglobin Groups in Man." Karger, Basel.

Kissmeyer-Nielsen, F., Svejgaard, A., and Thorsby, E. (1971). Human transplantation antigens. The HL-A system. *Bibl. Haematol.* **38**, 276–281.

Kitchin, F. D., Howel-Evans, W., Clarke, C. A., McConnell, R. B., and Sheppard, P. M. (1959). P.T.C. taste response and thyroid disease. *Br. Med. J.* **1**, 1069–1074.

Klein, J. (1975). "Biology of the Mouse Histocompatibility-2 Complex." Springer-Verlag, Berlin and New York.

Kueppers, F., and Bearn, A. G. (1966). A possible experimental approach to the association of α_1-antitrypsin deficiency and pulmonary emphysema. *Proc. Soc. Exp. Biol. Med.* **121**, 1207–1209.

Landsteiner, K. (1900). Zur Kenntis der antifermentativen, lytischen und agglutinierenden Wirkungen des Blutserums und der Lymphe. *Zentralbl. Bakteriol. Abt. 1* **27**, 357–362. (Translation *in* "Selected Contributions to the Literature of Blood Groups and Immunology." U.S. Army Med. Res. Lab., Ft. Knox, Kentucky, 1966. p. 1–10.)

Landsteiner, K., and Levine, P. (1927a). A new agglutinable factor differentiating individual human blood groups. *Proc. Soc. Exp. Biol. Med.* **24**, 600–602.

Landsteiner, K., and Levine, P. (1927b). Further observations on individual differences of human blood. *Proc. Soc. Exp. Biol. Med.* **24**, 941–942.

Landsteiner, K., and Miller, P. (1925a). Serological studies on the blood of primates. II. The blood groups in anthropoid apes. *J. Exp. Med.* **42**, 853–862.

Landsteiner, K., and Miller, P. (1925b). Serological studies on the blood of primates. III. Distribution of serological factors related to human isoagglutinogens in the blood of lower monkeys. *J. Exp. Med.* **42**, 863–872.

Landsteiner, K., and Wiener, A. S. (1940). An agglutinable factor in human blood recognized by immune sera for rhesus blood. *Proc. Soc. Exp. Biol. Med.* **43**, 223.

Laurell, C. B., and Eriksson, S. (1963). The electrophoretic α-globulin pattern of serum in α_1-antitrypsin deficiency. *Scand. J. Clin. Lab. Invest.* **15**, 132–140.

Lehrs, H. (1930). Über gruppenspizifische Eigenschaften des menschlichen Speichels. *Z. Immunitaets forsch. Exp. Ther.* **66**, 175–192. (Translation *in* "Selected Contributions to the Literature of Blood Groups and Immunology." U.S. Army Med. Res. Lab., Ft. Knox, Kentucky, 1970. pp. 4–24.)

Levine, L. S., Zachman, M., New, M. I., Prader, A., Pollack, M. S., O'Neill, G. J., Yang, S. Y., Oberfield, S. E., and Dupont, B. (1978). Genetic mapping of the 21-hydroxylase-deficiency gene within the HLA linkage group. *N. Engl. J. Med.* **299**, 911-915.

Levine, P. (1943). Serological factors as possible causes in spontaneous abortions. *J. Hered.* **34**, 71-80.

Levine, P., and Stetson, R. E. (1939). An unusual case of intragroup agglutination. *J. Am. Med. Assoc.* **113**, 126-127.

Levine, P., Celano, M. J., and Falkowski, F. (1963). The specificity of the antibody in paroxysmal cold hemoglobinuria (P. C. H.). *Transfusion* **3**, 278-280.

Levine, P., Katzin, E. M., and Burnham, L. (1941). Pathogenesis of erythroblastosis fetalis: Statistical evidence. *Science* **94**, 371-372.

Lilly, F., Boyse, E. A., and Old, L. J. (1964). Genetic basis of susceptibility to viral leukaemogenesis. *Lancet* **ii**, 1207-1209.

McBreen, P., Engel, E., and Croce, C. M. (1977). Assignment of the gene for glyoxalase 1 to region p21 pter of human chromosome 6. *Cytogenet. Cell Genet.* **19**, 208-214.

McDevitt, H. O., and Sela, M. (1967). Genetic control of antibody response. II. Further analysis of the specificity of determinant-specific control, and genetic analysis of the response to (H, (H,G)-A--L in CBA and C57 mice. *J. Exp. Med.* **126**, 969-978.

McDevitt, H. O., Shreffler, D. C., Snell, G. D., and Stimpfling, J. H. (1971). Genetic control of the antibody response: Genetic mapping studies of the linkage between the H-2 and Ir-1 loci. *In* "Immunogenetics of the H-2 System" (A. Lengerova and M. Vojtiskova, eds.), pp. 69-75. Karger, Basel.

McMichael, A. (1978). HLA restriction of human cytotoxic T-lymphocytes specific for influenza virus. Poor recognition of virus associated with HLA-A2. *J. Exp. Med.* **148**, 1458-1467.

Marchalonis, J. J., Morris, P. J., and Harris, A. W. (1974). Speculations on the function of immune response genes. *J. Immunogenet.* **1**, 63-67.

Marsh, D. G., and Bias, W. B. (1977). Basal serum IgE levels and HLA antigen frequencies in allergic subjects. II. Studies in people sensitive to rye grass group I and ragweed antigen E and of postulated immune response (Ir) loci in the HLA region. *Immunogenetics* **5**, 235-251.

Marsh, D. G., Bias, W. B., Hsu, S. H., and Goodfriend, L. (1973). Association of the HL-A7 crossreacting group with a specific reaginic antibody response in allergic man. *Science* **179**, 691-693.

Marsh, D. G., Bias, W. B., and Ishizaka, K. (1974). Genetic control of basal serum immunoglobulin E level and its effect on specific reaginic sensitivity. *Proc. Natl. Acad. Sci. U.S.A.* **71**, 3588-3592.

Marsh, D. G., Goodfriend, L., and Bias, W. B. (1977). Basal serum IgE levels and HLA antigen frequencies in allergic subjects. I. Studies with ragweed allergen Ra3. *Immunogenetics* **5**, 217-233.

Marsh, D. G., Hsu, S. H., Hussain, R., Meyers, D. A., Freidhoff, L. R., and Bias, W. B. (1980). Genetics of human immune response to allergens. *J. Allergy Clin. Immunol.* **65**, 322-332.

Medawar, P. B. (1944). The behavior and fate of skin autografts and skin homografts in rabbits. *J. Anat.* **78**, 176-200.

Medawar, P. B. (1958). The homograft reaction. *Proc. R. Soc. (London), Ser. B* **148**, 145-166.

Meruelo, D. (1979). A role for elevated H-2 antigen expression in resistance to neoplasia caused by radiation-induced leukemic virus. Enhancement of effective tumor surveillance by killer lymphocytes. *J. Exp. Med.* **149**, 898-904.

Meruelo, D., and Edidin, M. (1979). The biological function of the major histocompatibility complex: Hypotheses. *Contemp. Top. Immunobiol.* **9**, 231-253.

Meruelo, D., and McDevitt, H. O. (1978). Recent studies on the role of the immune response in resistance to virus-induced leukemias and lymphomas. *Semin. Hemat.* **15**, 399-419.

Meruelo, D., Nimelstein, S., Jones, P., Lieberman, M., and McDevitt, H. O. (1978). Increased synthesis and expression of H-2 antigens on thymocytes as a result of radiation leukemia virus infection. A possible mechanism for *H-2* linked control of virus-induced neoplasia. *J. Exp. Med.* **147**, 470–487.

Miller, L. H., Mason, S. J., Dvorak, J. A., McGinniss, M. H., and Rothman, I. K. (1975). Erythrocyte receptors for (*Plasmodium knowlesi*) malaria: Duffy blood group determinants. *Science* **189**, 561–563.

Motulsky, A. G. (1964). Hereditary red cell traits and malaria. *Am. J. Trop. Med. Hyg.* **13**, 147–158.

Mourant, A. E. (1946). A "new" human blood group antigen of frequent occurrence. *Nature (London)* **158**, 237.

Mourant, A. E., Kopec, A. C., and Domaniewska-Sobczak, K. (1976). "The Distribution of the Human Blood Groups and Other Polymorphisms," 2nd ed. Oxford Univ. Press, London and New York.

Mourant, A. E., Kopec, A. C., and Domaniewska-Sobczak, K. (1978). "Blood Groups and Diseases." Oxford Univ. Press, London and New York.

Neel, J. V. (1949). The inheritance of sickle cell anemia. *Science* **110**, 64–66.

Ochs, H. D., Rosenfeld, S. I., Thomas, E. D., Giblett, E. R., Alper, C. A., Dupont, B., Scholler, J. G., Gilliland, B. C., Hansen, J. A., and Wedgwood, R. J. (1977). Linkage between the gene (or genes) controlling the synthesis of the fourth component of complement and the major histocompatibility complex. *N. Engl. J. Med.* **296**, 470–475.

Ottolenghi, S., Lanyon, W. G., Paul, J., Williamson, R., Weatherall, D. J., Clegg, J. B., Pritchard, J., Pootrakul, S., and Boon, W. H. (1974). Gene deletion as the cause of alpha-thalassemia: The severe form of alpha-thalassemia is caused by a haemoglobin gene deletion. *Nature (London)* **251**, 389–391.

Ottolenghi, S., Comi, P., Giglioni, B., Tolstoshev, P., Lanyon, W. G., Mitchell, G. J., Williamson, R., Russo, G., Musumeci, S., Schilliro, G., Tsistrakis, G. A., Charache, S., Wood, W. G., Clegg, J. B., and Weatherall, D. J. (1976). Delta-beta thalassemia is due to a gene deletion. *Cell* **9**, 71–80.

Paciorkiewicz, M. (1970). The correlation between blood groups and some infectious diseases in children. *Pediatr. Pol.* **45**, 943–950.

Parker, W. C., and Bearn, A. G. (1961). Haptoglobin and transferrin variation in humans and primates: two new transferrins in Chinese and Japanese populations. *Ann. Hum. Genet.* **25**, 227–240.

Pauling, L., Itano, H. A., Singer, S. J., and Wells, I. C. (1949). Sickle cell anemia, a molecular disease. *Science* **110**, 543–548.

Payne, R., and Rolfs, M. R. (1958). Fetomaternal leukocyte incompatibility. *J. Clin. Invest.* **37**, 1756–1763.

Payne, R., Tripp, M., Weigle, J., Bodmer, W. F., and Bodmer, J. (1964). A new leukocyte iso-antigen system in man. *Cold Spring Harbor Symp. Quant. Biol.* **29**, 285–295.

Persson, I., Ryder, L. P., Staub Nielsen, L., and Svejgaard, A. (1975). The HL-A7 histocompatibility antigen in sarcoidosis in relation to tuberculin sensitivity. *Tissue Antigens* **6**, 50–53.

Petranyi, G. G., Benczur, M., Onody, C. E., Hollan, S. R., and Ivanyi, P. (1974). HL-A 3, 7 and lymphocyte cytotoxic activity. *Lancet* **1**, 736.

Podliachouk, L., Jacqueline, F., and Eyquem, A. (1965). The serum factors Gm(a), Gm(b), Gm(x) and Gm-like in patients with chronic rheumatic affections. *Vox Sang.* **10**, 188–194.

Putkonen, T. (1930). Über die gruppenspezifischen Eigenschaften Verschiedener Korperflussigkeiten. *Acta Soc. Med. Fenn. Doudecim* **14**, 1–113. (Translation *in* "Selected Contributions to the Literature of Blood Groups and Immunology." U.S. Army Med. Res. Lab., Ft. Knox, Kentucky, 1970, pp. 25–161.)

Race, R. R. (1948). The Rh genotypes and Fisher's theory. *Blood* **3**, Suppl. 2, 27-42.

Race, R. R., and Sanger, R. (1975). "Blood Groups in Man," 6th ed. Blackwell, Oxford.

Rosenfield, R. E., Allen, F. H., Swisher, S. N., and Kochwa, S. (1962). A review of Rh serology and presentation of a new terminology. *Transfusion* **2**, 287-312.

Rosenfield, R. E., Allen, F. H., and Rubinstein, P. (1973). Genetic model for the Rh blood group system. *Proc. Natl. Acad. Sci. U.S.A.* **70**, 1303-1307.

Ruddle, N. H., Conta, B. S., Leinwand, L., Kozak, C., Ruddle, F., Besmer, P., and Baltimore, D. (1978). Assignment of the receptor for ecotropic murine leukemia virus to mouse chromosome 5. *J. Exp. Med.* **148**, 451-465.

Schanfield, M. S., Giles, E., and Gershowitz, H. (1975). Genetic studies in the Markham Valley, northern Papua New Guinea: gamma globulin (Gm and Inv), group specific component (Gc) and ceruloplasmin (Cp) typing. *Am. J. Phys. Anthropol.* **42**, 1-7.

Schiff, F., and Sasaki, H. (1932). Der Ausscheidungstypus, ein auf serologischem Wege nachweisbares mendelendes Merkmal. *Klin. Wochenschr.* **11**, 1426-1429. (Translation *in* "Selected Contributions to the Literature of Blood Groups and Immunology." U.S. Army Med. Res. Lab., Ft. Knox, Kentucky, 1970, pp. 336-346.)

Schwartz, B. D., Luehrman, L. K., and Rodey, G. E. (1979). A public antigenic determinant on a family of HLA-B molecules—a basis for crossreactivity and a possible link with disease predisposition. *J. Clin. Invest.* **64**, 938-947.

Seager, K., Bashir, H. V., Greczy, A. F., Edmonds, J., and de Vere-Tyndall, A. (1979). Evidence for a specific B27-associated cell surface marker on lymphocytes of patients with ankylosing spondylitis. *Nature (London)* **277**, 68-70.

Searle, A. G. (1972). Spontaneous frequencies of point mutations in mice. *Humangenetik* **16**, 33-38.

Sharp, H. L., Bridges, R. A., Krivit, R. A., and Freier, E. F. (1969). Cirrhosis associated with alpha-1-antitrypsin deficiency: a previously unrecognized inherited disorder. *J. Lab. Clin. Med.* **73**, 934-939.

Smithies, O. (1955). Zone electrophoresis in starch gels: group variations in the serum proteins of normal human adults. *Biochem. J.* **61**, 629-641.

Smithies, O., and Walker, N. F. (1956). Notation for serum protein groups and the genes controlling their inheritance. *Nature (London)* **178**, 694-695.

Smithies, O., Connell, G. E., and Dixon, G. H. (1962). Chromosomal rearrangements and the evolution of haptoglobin genes. *Nature (London)* **196**, 232-236.

Smithies, O., Connell, G. E., and Dixon, G. H. (1966). Gene action in the human haptoglobins. I. Dissociation into constituent polypeptide chains. *J. Mol. Biol.* **21**, 213-224.

Steinke, J., and Taylor, K. W. (1974). Viruses and the etiology of diabetes. *Diabetes* **23**, 631-633.

Stockert, E. L., Old, L. J., and Boyse, E. A. (1971). the G_{IX} system. A cell surface alloantigen associated with murine leukemia virus: implications regarding chromosomal intergration of the viral genome. *J. Exp. Med.* **133**, 1334-1335.

Svejgaard, A., Platz, R., Ryder, L. P., Staub-Nielsen, L., and Thomsen, M. (1975). HLA and disease association—a survey. *Transplant. Rev.* **22**, 3-43.

Taylor, J. M., Dozy, A. M., Kan, Y. W., Varmus, H. E., Lie-Injo, L. E., Ganesan, J., and Todd, D. (1974). Genetic lesion in homozygous alpha thalassemia (hydrops fetalis). *Nature (London)* **251**, 392-393.

Teisberg, P., Akesson, I., Oliasen, B., Gedde-Dahl, T., Jr., and Thorsby, E. (1976). Genetic polymorphism of C4 in man and localization of a structural C4 locus to the HLA gene complex of chromosome 6. *Nature (London)* **264**, 253-254.

Terasaki, P. I., and McClelland, J. D. (1964). Microdroplet assay of human serum cytotoxins. *Nature (London)* **204**, 998-1000.

Tolstoschev, P., Mitchell, J., Lanyon, G., Williamson, R., Ottolenghi, S., Comi, P., Giglioni, B.,

Masera, G., Modell, B., Weatherall, D. J., and Clegg, J. B. (1976). The presence of the gene for β-globin in homozygous β^0 thalassemia. *Nature (London)* **259**, 95-98.

van Rood, J. J., and van Leeuwen, A. (1963). Leukocyte grouping. A method and its applications. *J. Clin. Invest.* **42**, 1382-1390.

Vierucci, A. (1965). Gm groups and anti-Gm antibodies in children with Cooley's anemia. *Vox Sang.* **10**, 82-83.

von Decastello, A., and Sturli, A. (1902). Über die Isoagglutinine im Serum gesunder und kranker Menschen. *Muench. Med. Wochenschr.* **49**, 1090-1095. (Translation *in* "Selected Contributions to the Literature of Blood Groups and Immunology." U.S. Army Med. Res. Lab., Ft. Knox, Kentucky.)

von Dungern, E., and Hirszfeld, L. (1910). Ueber Vererbung gruppenspezifischer Structuren des Blutes. *Z. Immunitaets-Forsch. Exp. Ther.* **6**, 284-292. (Translation *in* "Selected Contributions to the Linkage of Blood Groups and Immunology." U.S. Army Med. Res. Lab., Ft. Knox, Kentucky.)

Walter, H., and Palsson, G. (1973). The incidence of some genetic markers in Ireland. *In* "Symposia of the Society for the Study of Human Biology" (D. F. Roberts and E. Sutherland, eds)., Vol. 12, p. 161. Taylor & Francis, London.

Watkins, W. M. (1972). The biochemical basis of human blood group ABO and Lewis polymorphism. *In* "Annual Report, The Lister Institute of Preventative Medicine." pp. 12-29.

Weatherall, D. J., and Clegg, J. B. (1972). "The Thalassemia Syndromes," 2nd ed. Blackwell, Oxford.

Weatherall, D. J., and Clegg, J. B. (1975). The alpha chain termination mutants and their relationship to the alpha thalassemias. *Philos. Trans. R. Soc. London, Ser. B* **271**, 411-455.

Weatherall, D. J., and Clegg, J. B. (1976). Molecular genetics of human hemoglobin. *Annu. Rev. Genet.* **10**, 157-178.

Widström, G., and Henschen, A. (1963). The relation between P.T.C. taste response and protein bound iodine in serum. *Scand. J. Clin. Lab. Invest.* **15**, Suppl. No. 69, 257-261.

Wiener, A. S., and Peters, H. R. (1940). Hemolytic reactions following transfusions of blood of the homologous group, with three cases in which the same agglutinogen was responsible. *Ann. Intern. Med.* **13**, 2306-2322.

World Health Organization (1967). Standardization of procedures for the study of glucose-6-phosphate dehydrogenase. *W.H.O. Tech. Rep. Ser.* No. 366.

5

Geography of Disease: Purpose of and Possibilities from Geographical Medicine

DENIS P. BURKITT

I. THE ROLE OF GEOGRAPHICAL MEDICINE

Although most disease results from environment, genetic factors influence the susceptibility of individuals or different ethnic groups to various potentially harmful factors in the environment.

Diseases that result predominantly from environment will affect members of all racial groups in a community to a comparable extent, depending on their exposure to the causative factors. As a consequence, members of different racial groups will all suffer from maximal incidences of a disease where its causative factors are maximal. and from minimal incidences where these factors are minimal.

The converse of this is that if a disease is observed to be common in all racial groups in one area, and rare in all groups in another, one can deduce that a major

133

BIOCULTURAL ASPECTS OF DISEASE
Copyright © 1981 by Academic Press, Inc.
All rights of reproduction in any form reserved.
ISBN 0-12-598720-X

causative factor is present to a high degree in the former and only to a low extent, if present at all, in the latter.

Studying the distribution of a disease, not only geographically, but also socioeconomically and chronologically, has proved to be a highly effective method for identifying causative factors. This method in fact is the basis of the science of geographical medicine.

It must be emphasized that a demonstrated association between a disease and some environmental factor does not necessarily imply that the factor is causative. A relationship between the prevalence of lung cancer and the number of television sets sold does not, for example, indicate that television viewing causes lung cancer.

Although observed associations do not *prove* a cause-and-effect relationship, the absence of any consistent relationship between the prevalence of a disease and some postulated causative factor disproves the hypothesis. Thus, studies of the distribution of a disease not only provide grounds for formulating a hypothesis of causation, but can eliminate, one by one, hypotheses that are not consistent with the epidemiological features of the disease and reduce the number deserving of experimental testing.

II. HISTORICAL CONQUESTS IN GEOGRAPHICAL MEDICINE

The first illnesses investigated by this means were the infective diseases, that is, those induced by pathogenic organisms or parasites.

One of the first to give up its secrets to this approach was cholera, illustrated by the classic observations and subsequent deductions of John Snow in 1854. On a street map, he plotted the location of cases occurring in a London epidemic and then sought some factor that was common to each case. He found that all sufferers used the Broad Street water pump. Suspecting that the water delivered by this pump might somehow be implicated, he successfully petitioned the local council to remove the handle, a measure that was followed by subsidence of the epidemic. Although sewage-contaminated water was found to be responsible, the offending organism, the cholera vibrio, was not discovered until much later. This fact emphasizes the scientifically unwarranted and morally unjustifiable approach that demands proof of causation and understanding of mechanisms involved before measures are taken to reduce or eradicate environmental factors shown to be consistently related to the occurrence of a disease.

The discovery of the various causes of nearly all the great tropical epidemics depended largely on the study of their distribution and the search for potentially causative factors in the areas, or within the communities in which a given disease was most prevalent. Thus was the *Anopheles* mosquito, and later the parasite it transmitted, implicated in the cause of malaria. The tsetse fly was likewise identified as the vector of trypanosomiasis (sleeping sickness), and rodents were shown to be the vectors of fleas carrying the organisms responsible for plague.

A similar approach showed that yellow fever was caused by a virus transmitted by a mosquito, and that onchocerciasis (which causes river blindness, only one of its manifestations) was caused by a parasite (*Onchocercus volvulus*) transmitted by the river fly *Simulium damnosum*.

One intriguing detectivelike tracking of the cause of a disease by examining the areas in which it occurred, in recent years, was the successful identification of the virus responsible for Lassa fever and the animal that acts as its intermediate host. Much has been written on the geographical distribution of infective diseases, so the remainder of this chapter will be devoted to the geographical distribution and other epidemiological features of noninfective diseases.

Historical Examples

Geographical medicine was recognized as a potent tool to unravel the cause of various types of cancer before it was used to any great extent to find an explanation for the enormous contrasts in prevalence observed with respect to the so-called "degenerative" diseases. As will be emphasized later, epidemiological studies have rendered this designation no longer tenable.

Early in the last century British surgeon Sir Percival Pott recognized that many of the men who consulted him suffering from cancer of the scrotum had been chimney sweeps when they were boys. At that time, children were used to climb and clean chimneys. Pott had recognized an association between soot and cancer long before the carcinogenic effects of hydrocarbons became known.

At about the same time, skin cancer became associated with the oil-soaked clothes that were a feature of those operating the mules in the Lancashire cotton mills. Oil, like soot, contains hydrocarbons.

At a much later date, workers in aniline dye factories were shown to be at increased risk of developing cancer of the bladder, and, later still, cigarette smoking was shown to be closely related to the risk of suffering from cancer of the lung. The latter was a classic story of how the study of a disease's distribution can lead to an understanding of its causative factors. This form of cancer was shown to be almost limited to smokers, more common in heavy than in light smokers, and more common in men than women, who at that time smoked much less. As more women smoked, the incidence of lung cancer among them grew. Among nonsmoking communities within a Western culture, the Seventh Day Adventists and Mormons were found to have an almost nil incidence of lung cancer unless they had been converted to one of these religious groups later in life. The evidence is far too comprehensive to even attempt a summary here. Early workers included Ernest Wynder in North America and Sir Bradford Hill and Sir Richard Doll in Britain. Again, the close association between lung cancer and cigarette smoking is more than sufficient to justify recommendations to abandon the practice without waiting for an understanding of the mechanisms involved.

A study of disease distribution has also played a major role in the discovery of vitamin deficiency as the cause of several disorders. Lind's recognition that lemons provided protection against scurvy, a disease associated with conditions that precluded fresh fruit from the diet, is the most obvious example. Yet another was the discovery of vitamin B, which emanated from an astute observation that the chickens outside the wire fence surrounding a prison were in better condition than those on the inside. Both had been fed with scraps of human food, and this observation prompted a comparison between the food of inmates with that of outsiders. As a result, a dietary deficiency was recognized and vitamin B was eventually isolated. Not until later was it shown that the cause was a group of substances and not a single entity.

III. SPECIFIC DISEASES

Diseases whose distribution, geographical, and other, have recently been or are presently being investigated for clues that might lead to identification of causative factors will now be discussed.

A. Cancer

Well over 80% of all cancer is believed to result primarily from environmental factors.

Only in a few relatively rare forms of cancer has heredity been shown to play a major role. One example is multiple polyposis of the colon; however, even in that disease the genetic defect appears to be expressed only in the presence of certain environmental factors. The disease, virtually unknown in Africans, occurs in black Americans, though to a lesser degree than in whites.

1. Skin Cancer

Associations between skin cancer and hydrocarbons have already been alluded to. Two other potent causes of cancer of the skin are X rays and sun radiation. This form of cancer was tragically common in those working with X rays before protective clothing and other precautions became obligatory. The highest incidence in the world of skin cancer is found in Eastern Australia, where Caucasians lacking the pigmented skin that protects dark-skinned races, tend to expose themselves excessively in sport and work. Fortunately, this form of cancer is easily cured in most cases by X-ray treatment.

2. Cancer of the Cheek

This common form of cancer occurs only where a concoction of various ingredients is wrapped in a pan leaf and chewed. The concoction is the Asian equivalent of chewing gum. In the parts of Asia, for example, South India and New Guinea, where this custom is practiced, buccal (cheek) cancer is one of the commonest forms of cancer observed.

It is analogous to lung cancer caused by cigarette smoking in Western countries, and is nowhere commonly observed in communities not addicted to the chewing habit.

3. Cancer of the Nasopharynx

The back of the mouth, where the oral and nasal cavities meet, is a common site for cancer in some parts of the world but extremely rare in others. Chinese populations in Southeast Asia have maximal prevalences of this tumor, the most frequent form of cancer encountered in their men. It is also common in some rather restricted areas in Africa, notably in the Nandi tribe in the highlands of Kenya (Clifford, 1970).

Although unraveling the respective part played by genetic endowment and by traditional customs is difficult, a genetic component does seem implicated in this form of cancer. Even after emigration to North America the Chinese remain much more susceptible to this tumor than do Americans of other ethnic groups.

Substantial evidence now exists that one causative factor may be the Epstein–Barr virus (EBV) (Epstein and Achong, 1977; Epstein, 1978), first identified in tissue from a patient with Burkitt's lymphoma (described below) (Epstein et al., 1964). Antibodies in the blood against this virus are consistently much higher in African patients with Burkitt's lymphoma and with nasopharyngeal cancer than in the rest of the population. In both tumors some other factor must be working in cooperation with the EBV, since this virus is ubiquitous.

4. Cancer of the Esophagus

With the single exception of primary cancer of the liver, which is 500 times as common in Lorenco Marques (Mozambique) as it is in Bombay (India), no form of cancer shows such extreme contrasts in frequency or changes in incidence within short distances.

In Europe, highest rates are found in Britanny in northern France (Tuyns and Masse, 1975), where the tumor is 20 times as common as it is in Holland, only 400 miles away.

In Africa very high rates are observed in the Transkei district in South Africa, in eastern Rhodesia and southern Malawi, and near Durban (Bradshaw and Schonland, 1974). Another high incidence area exists in Western Kenya, particularly around Kavirondo Bay on the east side of Lake Victoria (Cook and Burkitt,

1971). From there the incidence falls off steeply toward the north and south but less so toward the east.

It appears from examination of earlier records that the prevalence of esophageal cancer in parts of South Africa has been increasing over the past 40 years and that the area of high incidence has been gradually extending in a northern direction. In this region various alcoholic drinks have been incriminated in the causation of the tumors.

The highest rates in the world are reported from the region east of the Caspian Sea, and the tumor gets progressively less common from east to west along its south coast. It is 70 times as common on the east as it is on the west of the sea (Kmet and Mahboubi, 1972). These people are Moslems, and there is no evidence that drinking or smoking play a role in the causation of the disease.

Although, as indicated, communities have been identified showing enormous contrasts in their risk of developing esophageal cancer, no single environmental factor has been identified that is common to all situations. In northern France, alcohol has been incriminated, in Africa beer made from maize (Cook, 1971). In the region of the Caspian, tumor incidence is inversely related to rainfall. No satisfactory hypothesis of causation has yet been formulated, and different factors, possibly a combination of many, may be responsible in different areas.

5. Cancer of the Stomach

As with cancer of the esophagus, the incidence of stomach cancer varies greatly in different localities, yet no satisfactory hypothesis of its cause has been formulated.

The highest rates in the world occur in Japan and Korea. Other high-incidence areas include eastern Finland, and the adjacent part of Russia, and the mountainous regions, but not the coast, in Colombia, South America. In Africa this form of cancer is particularly common in the Nile–Congo watershed, which includes eastern Zaire, Rwanda, Burundi, and extreme southwest Uganda. Another high-frequency area is around the slopes of Mount Kilimanjaro, Africa's highest mountain (Hutt and Burkitt, 1978). Patients with pernicious anemia have a four to five times greater risk of developing gastric cancer than the others.

When Japanese emigrate to America, their rates of stomach cancer fall, but even in the second generation they have a higher risk than other Americans of developing this tumor (Haenzel and Kurihara, 1968).

In North America and Britain, the incidence of gastric cancer is falling.

One current suggestion is that nitrosamines, known to be carcinogenic, may play a role.

6. Intestinal Cancer

By far, most intestinal tumors occur in the large bowel, which includes the colon and the rectum.

This tumor is the most common cause of cancer death in North America and western Europe, with the exception of lung cancer from cigarette smoking. Bowel cancer is actually more common than lung cancer, but the latter is more often fatal.

No other form of cancer so closely associates with economic development and modern Western culture. Maximal incidence occurs in economically developed countries and minimal in rural communities in developing countries (Wynder *et al.*, 1969; Burkitt, 1971).

Unlike cancer of the esophagus and stomach referred to above, which have patchy distributions throughout the world, large-bowel cancer is rare in tribal societies everywhere and is common in all Western societies, although less common in certain groups within Western culture. For example, it is about one-third less common in Seventh Day Adventists, who are predominantly vegetarians (Wynder and Shigematsu, 1967), and in Mormons (Lyon, 1975), who are not vegetarians, than in other Americans. It is only a quarter as common in rural Finns as in Copenhagen Danes (MacLennan *et al.*, 1978) or New Yorkers (Reddy *et al.*, 1979).

Jews who emigrated to the new state of Israel from Yemen and North Africa after World War II had low rates of bowel cancer, but those who emigrated young now have rates approaching that of those born in Israel.

Today black and white Americans have similar rates (Doll, 1969), whereas 40 and more years ago blacks had much higher rates than did whites (Quinland and Cuff, 1940). Moreover, one must assume that when African slaves were brought to America their bowel cancer rates were at least as low as those of rural Africans today, which are only about one-tenth of those of North Americans.

Colon cancer, formerly rare among Japanese, is increasing in prevalence in urban communities in Japan. After emigration to Hawaii and California, second-generation American–Japanese develop a risk of developing this form of cancer comparable to that of other Americans (Stemmerman, 1966).

The geographical distribution of polyps, nonmalignant tumors of the bowel, are rare where cancer is rare and exceedingly common where cancer is common, being present in up to 20% of adults in some Western countries. They are so rare in situations where cancer is rare that in a 2000-bed hospital in South Africa only six were found in all autopsies and specimens removed surgically over a 13-year period.

It is now generally accepted not only that benign and malignant tumors of the bowel share a common cause, but that most bowel cancers, at least in Western countries, develop in pre-existing polyps. One of the major defects in cancer registration is the omission of nonmalignant tumors, for an understanding of the causation of these might well provide clues as to the origins of cancers in the same organs.

That large-bowel cancer is related to diet is now generally accepted, and the most widely accepted concept is that excessive fat in the diet, and animal fat in particular, is a causative factor (Wynder and Reddy, 1975) and that adequate fiber in the diet may provide protection (Burkitt, 1975a). The fat content and the fiber content are almost invariably inversely related. Consumption of fiber protects both through diluting carcinogens in the larger stool volume associated with fiber-rich diets and by shortening intestinal transit time and thus reducing contact between carcinogens and intestinal mucosa.

Other forms of cancer, the incidences of which are directly related to fat consumption, are tumors of the breast, prostate, and endometrium. These four types of cancer are closely associated epidemiologically with a number of other diseases characteristic of economically developed communities and collectively referred to as "Western diseases."

Food is not thought to be directly carcinogenic, but to alter bacterial activity in the feces. The responsible carcinogens may well be results of such activity.

A prudent protection would appear to be a reduction in fat and an increase in fiber in our diet.

7. Liver Cancer

Primary cancer of the liver, as distinct from secondary deposits that have spread from tumors in other sites, is uncommon in Western countries but is the overall most frequently observed cancer across subsaharal Africa from the Indian to the Atlantic oceans. It is uncommon in North Africa.

The concept of causation that best fits in with available epidemiological evidence is that the cause is associated with both a toxin (aflatoxin) produced by a fungus (*Aspergillus flavus*) growing on crops stored in moist, warm conditions, and also with infection caused by a virus, hepatitis B (Coady, 1976). Avoiding infection with the latter may not be possible, but improved methods of food storage could reduce the growth of *Aspergillus flavus*. The presence of this fungus and its associated toxin in food has been shown to have a distribution similar to that of liver cancer.

8. Burkitt's Lymphoma

This bizarre form of cancer only occurs commonly in limited areas of the world. It mainly affects children, and one of its most frequent manifestations is the development of jaw tumors that are so characteristic they cannot easily be overlooked (Burkitt, 1970). This fact greatly facilitated the study of the geographical distribution of the tumor that was the initial and basic work on which many international studies of the the tumor's nature have been built.

Burkitt's lymphoma has proved such a notable example of the role of geographical medicine in unraveling disease etiology that the progressive steps that have led to the incrimination of a virus will be summarized. The initial event was the recognition in Uganda that a number of tumors observed in different parts of the body, and previously considered to be different pathological entities, were but different manifestations of a single tumor process. This fact was deduced first from the observation that the tumor tended to be associated with different anatomical sites in individual patients and also from their geographical association (described below). This multifocal tumor presenting in different guises was found to be almost limited to children and to have a characteristic age distribution.

Soon the fact became apparent that, whereas this was the most common form of childhood cancer in certain parts of Africa, it was unknown in other areas. The geographical distribution of the tumor was consequently studied, initially by means of a questionnaire accompanied by illustrations of the clinical features of the tumor, which was widely distributed throughout Africa. Subsequently, more detailed information was obtained by extensive safaris to enable personal visits to medical units throughout the continent. The latter enabled details of distribution of the disease to be extended after personal discussions with numerous physicians and provided the opportunity to encourage an active search for the occurrence of this tumor in as many places as possible.

These geographical studies disclosed that the tumor was limited to a belt across Africa between about 10 degrees north and 10 degrees south of the equator, but with a tail down the east coast (Burkitt, 1962, 1963). Within this belt were tumor-free areas, and these were recognized as being areas more than 5000 ft above sea level near the equator and more than 3000 ft 1000 miles south of the equator. Eventually the tumor was determined as occurring in Africa only in regions where the temperature never fell below about 60°F and the rainfall was above 20 inches a year (Haddow, 1964). Similar observations were later made in New Guinea and elsewhere.

This climatic dependence suggested that some insect vector was implicated. Attention was turned to the possibility that some vectored virus might be responsible, in which case this could be the first human cancer to be shown to be virus induced. A virus, which has subsequently become world renowned as the Epstein–Barr virus, was in fact identified in a piece of tumor sent to England from Uganda (Epstein *et al.*, 1964). Later studies, however, showed that although the virus is apparently implicated in causing the tumor, it is not in fact vectored and has a ubiquitous distribution throughout the world. The characteristic geographical distribution of the tumor coincides with that of the particularly intense and continuous malarial infestation referred to as "holoendemic malaria." Both the EBV and malaria apparently act in cooperation with one another to give rise to this tumor (Kifuko and Burkitt, 1970).

B. Diseases Affecting the Alimentary Tract

1. Constipation

Many will be surprised to learn that constipation has a geographical distribution. Appreciating that fact is essential, because the diseases discussed below are in part directly or indirectly the result of constipation. By constipation, in this context, is meant the slow passage of intestinal content through the large bowel, and its small volume and firm consistency. Unless stool weight and intestinal transit time are measured, the word "constipation" is a subjective and unreliable estimate of bowel behavior.

People in Third World countries living in a largely traditional manner void on average 300–500 g of stool daily. Normally the stool is soft, and food residue takes about 30 hours to transverse the alimentary tract from mouth to anus. In communities characterized by North America and Great Britain, only about 80–120 g of stool is voided daily; often it is firm, and intestinal transit times take about 72 hours in young healthy adults and often more than 2 weeks in the elderly (Burkitt *et al.*, 1973). The importance of constipation has only become adequately recognized since the study of the geographical distribution of certain diseases that are characteristic of modern Western culture in an effort to determine their causes. The consistency, bulk, and transit time of intestinal content relates directly to the amount of fiber, and of cereal fiber in particular, in the diet.

2. Diseases Believed to Be Causally Related to Constipation

The geographical distribution of the diseases outlined below is for the most part the geography of diets depleted in fiber.

Those that affect the alimentary tract include the following: (a) appendicitis; (b) diverticular disease of the colon; (c) cancer of the colon and rectum; (d) hiatus hernia, which is an upward protrusion of the top of the stomach through the esophageal hiatus in the diaphragm; and (e) hemorrhoids.

a. Appendicitis. Invariably rare in tribal societies, this disease is common in all economically more developed countries, and is one of the first of the characteristically Western diseases to emerge after impact with Western culture. During the last 20 years, its frequency has been rising in urban communities in Africa in which Western-type foods have been replacing traditional diets. It became much less common in enemy-occupied countries in Europe during World War II. It emerged for the first time in units of African soldiers after they were attached to British units and shared their rations (Burkitt, 1975b). The only hypothesis concerning its cause that is consistent with the epidemiological features of the disease is that blockage of the lumen of the appendix is the initial factor. This blockage can be caused directly by the presence of a firm fecal particle or result from exaggerated activity of the muscle in the appendix wall due to the presence of solid fecal matter. Either of these conditions can block the lumen of the appendix. The inflammatory process supervenes on the initial obstruction.

The presence of solid fecal material in the appendix is believed to be responsible for the start of this train of events, and only in Western communities consuming fiber-depleted diets is the appendicular content commonly solid.

b. Diverticular Disease.   Not only is this disease exceedingly rare outside the economically most developed countries, such as in northern and western Europe, North America, and Australia and New Zealand, but it was uncommon even in those communities until after World War I. The disease is almost unknown in subsaharal Africa, but is the most common disorder of the intestine in North America, black and white Americans being comparably affected.

It is now believed to result from raised intraluminal pressures within the colon occasioned by the contractions of muscle in the colon wall, which are required to propel forward fecal content that is small in volume, resistant to movement, and firm (Painter and Burkitt, 1971; Painter, 1975).

c. Hiatus Hernia.   Among the last of the characteristically Western diseases to emerge in developing countries, hiatus hernia is still exceedingly rare, even in urban communities in subsaharal Africa, and is uncommon in Asia (Burkitt and James, 1973). The disorder is believed to result from the increased intraluminal pressures generated during the abdominal straining necessitated for the evacuation of small, firm feces. Pressures generated below the diaphragm are much in excess of those above it (Fedail *et al.*, 1979). Some investigators have postulated that these pressures force the upper end of the stomach upward through the hiatus in the diaphragm that transmits the esophagus. The mechanism is believed to be similar to that whereby squeezing a ball filled with water will impel the water through a hole in its wall. Once again the presence of firm feces is incriminated in the cause of this common complaint.

d. Hemorrhoids.   Persons in Western countries inadequately appreciate that hemorrhoids are much more prevalent in Western than in Third World communities.

The traditionally accepted concept that hemorrhoids are varicosities of the anal veins analogous to varicose veins in the legs has been challenged (Thomson, 1975). Now they are believed to be normal vascular submucosal cushions that surround the upper part of the anal canal to maintain continence of feces. Hemorrhoids result when these cushions are forced down the canal by a combination of their venous engorgement due to abdominal straining and the shearing stress of hard fecal masses passing through the anal canal. Once more, the presence of small, firm feces due to fiber-depleted diets is thought to be the most important underlying cause.

3. Cholelithiasis (Gallstones)

Most gallstones in Western communities are largely composed of cholesterol. They are in fact but the tip of the iceberg, representing the presence of what is referred to as lithogenic bile, that is, bile having a tendency to form stones. The likelihood of stone formation depends on the relative proportions of the chrystoid substance, cholesterol, and the bile acids that act as solvents. Most gallstones do not cause symptoms and consequently remain undetected during life. Incidence increases with age, and various populations are affected to different extents.

The highest frequencies have been reported from the Pima Indians in the southwestern United States and from the Swedes. A radiological survey showed no less than 73% of Pima Indian women aged 25–34 years to have gallstones. In the entire group, including men and women aged 15–74 years, nearly 50% had gallstones (Sampliner *et al.,* 1970).

In an autopsy series in Sweden, stones were present in the gallbladder in more than 50% of women and 30% of men over age 20 years (Heaton, 1973).

Gallstones are found at autopsy in rather less than 10% of adult women in England, but a much higher figure has been reported from Australia (Heaton, 1973). For the United States, the estimate of the annual number of gallbladder removals, now the most frequently performed abdominal operation, is 330,000.

Although 30 and more years ago the disease was much less frequent in black than in white Americans, recent reports show a comparable incidence today. When black and white Americans live in a similar environment, that they have a comparable risk of developing gallstones seems likely.

In contrast, gallstones are exceedingly rare throughout subsaharal Africa. In a large teaching hospital in Uganda, only 15 out of 61,000 admissions were for gallstones (Shaper and Patel, 1964). Only 27 patients with gallstones were admitted to another large teaching hospital during a 5-year period in West Africa (Parnis, 1968). In earlier years gallstones were even less common, for Edington (1957) found none in more than 4000 autopsies in Ghana.

Burkitt and Tunstall (1975) sent a questionnaire to 130 hospitals in Africa monthly for two years trying to estimate the number of patients admitted with gallstones. In 13 countries 84 hospitals sent regular replies and only 15 of those saw even a single case during that period. On average, less than one case was seen per hospital per year, which represents about 1 in every 3000 admissions.

As with other diseases, many factors are likely to be involved, but one is almost certainly dietetic. Adequate fiber in the diet is thought to confer protection by reducing the lithogenicity of the bile (Heaton, 1978).

4. Ulcers

a. Duodenal Ulcer. The geographical variations in the distribution of duodenal ulcer are much more pronounced than are those of gastric ulcer, and only the former will be considered here.

Even in Western countries, duodenal ulcer was uncommon before the present century. Before World War II, it was predominantly a disease of men, having a male to female sex ratio of 4.5:1. By 1970, that ratio had fallen to 1.9:1.

The type of duodenal ulcer occurring in Western countries and becoming increasingly common in urban communities in developing countries is different from that which is particularly prevalent in certain rural communities in Africa and Asia. The most frequently encountered complications in the former type are hemorrhage and perforation and, in the latter, pyloric stenosis (Tovey, 1974, 1977). The former type appears to be somehow related to changes in life associated with economic development.

b. Stenosing Duodenal Ulcer. A very common complaint in South India, spreading up the west side as far as Bombay, and on the east coast as far as Calcutta, stenosing duodenal ulcer is also common in Kashmir, Assam, West Bengal, and Bangladesh. In contrast, it is uncommon in much of North India and, in particular, in the Punjab and Rajasthan.

This type of ulcer is about 15 times more common in men than in women, and, in the regions where it occurs commonly, duodenal ulcer is about 20 times as frequent as gastric ulcer.

The Western type of duodenal ulcer is relatively common in large urban communities in both North and South India.

In Africa, an area of extremely high incidence of stenosing duodenal ulcer is the Nile-Congo watershed, which includes Rwanda, Burundi, and eastern Zaire. The disease, uncommon throughout most of the rest of East and Central Africa, appears to be rather common in the central region of Ethiopia.

Duodenal ulcer is also common along the moister southern parts of all West African countries, but its incidence falls toward the dry savannah in the northern parts of those territories. As in India, the Western type of ulcer is becoming more common in urban and otherwise westernized communities in Africa.

The causes of the Western and urban type of ulcer, with its tendency to bleed or perforate, must differ from those responsible for the stenosing variety, which has an entirely different geographical distribution. Probably protective factors and causative factors exist, and, although many factors have been suggested to account for its cause, no consensus has yet been reached. Further studies of the geographical distribution of this disease may well throw light on its etiology.

C. Diseases of the Circulatory System

1. Ischemic Heart Disease (IHD)

In many economically advanced Western countries, one man in three and one woman in six dies of ischemic heart disease.

The prevalence of this disease is much lower in Southeast Europe, and in subsaharal Africa this disease is still almost nonexistent.

In the past this disease has been less common in western Ireland than in North America. A recent study (Brown *et al.*, 1970) compared IHD rates in more than 1000 pairs of brothers, one of whom had stayed in Ireland and the other gone to live in Massachusetts and adopted that way of life, in particular, the dietary customs of North America. Although both brothers in each pair were from the same genetic stock, those living in America were found to have IHD nearly twice as often. Trowell (1975a) suggested that the greater consumption of potatoes and brown bread in Ireland supplied fiber that provided protection.

a. Africa. IHD remains almost unknown in subsaharal Africa, and only occasional cases are observed even in urban situations. Between 1960 and 1972, only 30 patients were seen with this disease in Baragwanath Hospital, the largest hospital in Africa, admitting 40,000 patients a year (Seftel *et al.,* 1973). Many of these patients had for long been eating semi-westernized diets.

b. The Indian Subcontinent. Here IHD is universally more common in urban or otherwise westernized communities than it is in rural communities. The prevalence is intermediate between the prevalences in Africa and North America.

c. Historical Aspects. Even in North America and western Europe this disease was considered rare until the latter 1920s. Although the electrocardiogram was not available, angina was well described as a clinical symptom but not commonly seen.

Even 30 years ago IHD was much less common in black than in white Americans, but both races appear to have comparable risks of developing the disease today (Trowell, 1975a).

d. Cause. Many factors are believed to contribute to the cause of this disease. Risk factors include: (1) smoking—heavy cigarette smoking doubles the risk; (2) fat—high intakes of fat, particularly animal fat, are associated with a high incidence; (3) obesity and diabetes—both increase the risk of developing IHD, but whether the increase occurs because these diseases contribute to the cause of IHD or because all three diseases share common causative factors is not clear; (4) sedentary occupations.

e. Protective Factors. Fiber associated with starchy foods such as cereals, tubers, and legumes appears to confer protection against IHD, as does exercise.

2. Hypertension

This disorder is rare in primitive communities such as the aborigines in Australia, the bushmen in the Kalahari desert in South Africa, and in parts of New Guinea. It was uncommon in East Africans 40 or more years ago but is common today (Trowell, 1978).

Probably the highest rates in the world occur in Japan and Taiwan.

The prevalence of hypertension is closely related to salt intake. Primitive people eat only about 3 g a day. In most Western countries, persons consume 10–15 g. The average intake in the North Island of Japan is about 28 g.

Several medical clinics are not having good results treating patients who have hypertension with diets low in salt.

3. Venous Thrombosis

Venous thrombosis is more common in westernized than in tribal communities.

Pulmonary embolism, the possibility of which is ever in the minds of Western surgeons, is rare in Third World countries. Regional difference holds despite the fact that operative and anesthetic techniques are often identical. Some evidence suggests that dietary factors alter the tendency for blood to clot, and fiber-rich foods may be protective (Trowell, 1978).

4. Varicose Veins

In Western countries, this disorder is exceedingly common. A large survey in North America showed varicose veins present in 45.8% of women and 29.5% of men between the ages of 40 and 60 years (Coon *et al.*, 1973).

In contrast varicose veins are much less prevalent in communities in the Third World still living in a largely traditional manner. Most surveys in Africa and India have shown prevalences of about 10% in adults who have had significant contact with Western culture and less than 5% for those in tribal communities.

The disorder certainly depends more on environmental than on genetic factors, and there is evidence that diet may play an important role. Raised intra-abdominal pressures caused either by straining at stool or by certain occupations have been implicated (Burkitt, 1976).

D. Diseases of the Endocrine System

1. Diabetes

Diabetes is yet another disease closely related to modern Western civilization. About 2% of persons over age 50 years in Britain and North America are known to have diabetes, and probably more than 15% have undetected abnormalities in their ability to metabolize sugar than can be considered as hidden diabetes.

Diabetes is almost unknown in hunter–gatherers, such as the traditionally living Australian aborigines and South African bushmen.

The disease was rare in East Africa before World War II (Trowell, 1960) but has been increasing since.

It is about ten times as prevalent in Durban Indians as it is among the inhabitants of South India, from where these people emigrated early in the century (Cleave, 1976).

Rare in Eskimos in their traditional surroundings, the disease increases in prevalence after adoption of Western dietary customs.

The highest incidence known is that in the Pima Indians in the southwestern part of North America (Comess *et al.*, 1969). The high incidence is thought to be due to a genetic susceptibility together with the fact that these people suddenly changed from their traditional diets to the modern diets of North Americans. A similar situation has been observed in desert rats, who never develop diabetes or obesity even in captivity when fed ad libitum the fibrous plants that are their customary diet. When fed more refined carbohydrate foods, they fatten and develop diabetes.

The people of the small island of Nauru in the Pacific quickly became immensely wealthy when it was recognized that the island was covered with phosphates. As a result they began to import Western-type foods, and today more than 30% of the whole population over age 15 years suffer from diabetes (Zimmett *et al.*, 1978).

The evidence is good that the fiber in food affords protection against diabetes and that the prevalence of this disease relates to the consumption of refined carbohydrate foods.

2. Goiter

Goiter is an enlargement of the thyroid gland. It is a good example of a disease that relates to a particular environmental factor and that can be controlled by altering the environment responsible for its cause. It is disfiguring but not usually serious, although it can cause difficulty in breathing because of pressure on the trachea.

The disease, now known to be due to a deficiency of iodine in the soil, can be prevented by adding iodine to the water so that a sufficient amount is drunk to compensate for the deficiency.

The disease has a geographical pattern in that the areas most affected are mountainous. In those regions, iodine has been washed away with the water passing down the hills.

In Africa, the disease is most prevalent in Ethiopia and in the Nile–Congo watershed (consisting of Rwanda, Burundi, and extreme eastern Zaire), both of which are mountainous areas.

E. Urologic Disorders

Urinary Stones

Stones may develop in the upper urinary tract, and be found in the kidneys or ureters, or in the lower tract, and found in the bladder or urethra.

Before the present century, stones were much more common in the lower than in the upper urinary tract in western European countries. The situation has since been reversed, with kidney stones now much more common than bladder stones.

Bladder stones are found more commonly in parts of rural Thailand than anywhere else in the world, but in the capital city, Bangkok, the frequency of bladder and kidney stones is about equal (Anderson, 1968).

Throughout subsaharal Africa, stones in any part of the urinary tract are rare, but the situation changes dramatically from Southern to Northern Sudan. In the former, populated by black Nilotic tribes, stones are almost nonexistent, but in the latter, with a semi-Arab population and culture, both renal and bladder stones are relatively common.

IV. CONCLUSIONS

Although only a limited number of diseases have been discussed, the evidence that most if not all disease is attributable to various extents to environmental factors is overwhelming. This in no way belittles the fact that genetic inheritance also plays a role, rendering certain individuals and different ethnic groups more or less susceptible to various environmental factors.

These observations impel the inescapable conclusion that much disease could be drastically reduced if not totally prevented if factors predominantly responsible for its causation could be identified and then reduced or eliminated.

We cannot alter the genetic constitution that we have inherited, but we can modify our environment.

Curative or therapeutic medicine can be likened to the stationing of an ambulance at the foot of a cliff to rescue casualties occasioned by people falling over the edge, and conveying them to efficient, but expensive, medical establishments. This service is necessary, but it is surely better to erect a fence round the top of the cliff. We can erect our own fences by such measures as refraining from smoking, being abstemious with alcohol, wearing seat belts when driving, and eating a prudent diet, which means less fat, more fiber-rich foods, and less sugar.

The fruits of geographical medicine become apparent when people are willing to personally apply the knowledge acquired.

REFERENCES

Anderson, D. A. (1968). The incidence of urinary calculi. *Hosp. Med.* pp. 1024–1033.
Bradshaw, E., and Schonland, M. (1974). Smoking, drinking and oesophageal cancer in African males of Johannesburg, South Africa. *Br. J. Cancer* **30**, 157–163.
Brown, J., Burke, G. J., and Gearty, G. F. (1970). Nutritional and epidemiologic features relating to heart disease. *World Rev. Nutr. Diet.* **12**, 1–42.
Burkitt, D. P. (1962). A tumour safari in Eastern Central Africa. *Br. J. Cancer* **16**, 379–386.

Burkitt, D. P. (1963). A childrens' cancer related to climate. *New Sci.* **17**, 174–176.

Burkitt, D. P. (1970). Geographical Distribution. *In* "Burkitt's Lymphoma" (D. P. Burkitt and E. H. Wright, eds.), pp. 186–197. Livingstone, Edinburgh.

Burkitt, D. P. (1971). Epidemiology of cancer of the colon and rectum. *Cancer (Philadelphia)* **28**, 1–13.

Burkitt, D. P. (1975a). Large bowel cancer: an epidemiologic jigsaw. *J. Natl. Cancer Inst.* **54**, 3–6.

Burkitt, D. P. (1975b). Appendicitis. *In* "Refined Carbohydrate Foods and Disease" (D. P. Burkitt and H. C. Trowell, eds.), p. 87. Academic Press, New York.

Burkitt, D. P. (1976). Varicose veins: facts and fantasy. *Arch. Surg.* **111**, 1327–1332.

Burkitt, D. P., and James, P. A. (1973). Low-residue diets and hiatus hernia. *Lancet* **2**, 128–130.

Burkitt, D. P., and Tunstall, M. (1975). Gallstones, geographical and chronological features. *J. Trop. Med. Hyg.* **78**, 140–144.

Burkitt, D. P., Walker, A. R. D., and Painter, N. S. (1974). Dieting fiber and disease. *J. Am. Med. Assoc.* **229**, 1068–1074.

Cleave, T. L. (1976). "The Saccharine Disease." Wright, Bristol, England.

Clifford, P. (1970). On the epidemiology of nasopharyngeal carcinoma. *Int. J. Cancer* **5**, 287–309.

Coady, A. (1976). Tropical sclerosis and hepatomas. *J. R. Coll. Physicians London* **10**, 133–134.

Comess, J., Bennett, P. H., Birch, T. A., and Miller, M. (1969). Congenital abnormalities and diabetes in the Pima Indians of Arizona. *Diabetes* **18**, 471–477.

Cook, P. (1971). Cancer of the oesophagus in Africa. *Br. J. Cancer* **25**, 853–880.

Cook, P. J., and Burkitt, D. P. (1971). Cancer in Africa. *Br. Med. J.* **27**, 14–20.

Coon, W. W., Willis, P. W., and Keller, J. B. (1973). Venous thrombo-embolism and other venous diseases in the Tecumseh County Health Study. *Circulation* **48**, 839–846.

Doll, R. (1969). The geographical distribution of cancer. *Br. J. Cancer* **23**, 1–8.

Edington, G. M. (1957). Observations on hepatic diseases on the Gold Coast with special reference to sclerosis. *Trans. R. Soc. Trop. Med. Hyg.* **51**, 48–55.

Epstein, M. A. (1978). An assessment of the possible role of viruses in the aetiology of Burkitt's lymphoma. *Prog. Exp. Tumor Res.* **21**, 72–99.

Epstein, M. A., and Achong, B. G. (1977). Recent progress in Epstein–Barr virus research. *Annu. Rev. Microbiol.* **31**, 421–425.

Epstein, M. A., Achong, B. G., and Barr, Y. M. (1964). Virus particles in cultured lymphoblasts from Burkitt's lymphoma. *Lancet* **1**, 702–703.

Fedail, S. S., Harvey, R. F., and Burns-Cox, C. J. (1979). Abdominal and thoracic pressures during defaecation. *Br. Med. J.* **1**, 91.

Haddow, A. J. (1964). Age incidence in Burkitt's lymphoma syndrome. *East Afr. Med. J.* **41**, 1–6.

Haenzel, W., and Kurihara, M. (1968). Studies of Japanese migrants: 1. Mortality from cancer and other diseases among Japanese in the United States. *J. Natl. Cancer Inst.* **40**, 43–68.

Heaton, K. W. (1973). The epidemiology of gallstones and suggested etiology clinics. *Gastroenterology* **2**, 67–83.

Heaton, K. W. (1978). Are gallstones preventable? *World Med.* July 12, 21–23.

Hutt, M. S. R., and Burkitt, D. P. (1978). Epidemiology of cancer in the colon. *Recent Adv. Med.* **17**, 1–22.

Kifuko, G. W., and Burkitt, D. P. (1970). Burkitt's lymphoma and malaria. *Int. J. Cancer* **6**, 1–9.

Kmet, J., and Mahboubi, E. (1972). Oesophageal cancer in the Caspian Littoral of Iran. *Science* **175**, 846–853.

Lyon, J. N. (1975). Cancer incidence in Mormons and non-Mormons. *N. Engl. J. Med.* **294**, 129–131.

MacLennan, R., Jensen, O. M., Mosbeth, J., and Vuori, H. (1978). Diet, transit time, stool weight and colon cancer in two Scandinavian populations. *Am. J. Clin. Nutr.* **10**, Suppl. 31, 239–242.

Painter, N. S. (1975). "Diverticular Disease of the Colon." Heinemann, London.

Painter, N. S., and Burkitt, D. P. (1971). Diverticular disease of the colon: a deficiency disease of western civilization. *Br. Med. J.* **ii**, 450–454.

Parnis, R. (1968). The abnormal gall-bladder in Nigeria: a ten year study 1957–67. *St. Luke's Hosp. Gaz.* **4**, 87–91.

Quinland, W. S., and Cuff, J. R. (1940). Primary carcinoma in the negro: Anatomic distribution of three hundred cases. *Arch. Pathol.* **30**, 393–402.

Reddy, B. S., Hedges, R., Laaks, O. K., and Wynder, E. L. (1979). Metabolic epidemiology of large bowel cancer, faecal bulk and constituents of high-risk North American and low-risk Finnish populations. *Cancer (Philadelphia)* **142**, 2832–2838.

Sampliner, R. K., Bennett, P. H., Comess, L. J., Rose, S. A., and Birch, T. A. (1970). Gall-bladder disease in Pima Indians: demonstration of high prevalence and early onset by cholecystography. *N. Engl. J. Med.* **283**, 1358–1364.

Seftel, H. C., Spitz, M. G., Bersoon, I., Goldin, A. R., Jaffe, B. I., Rubenstein, A. H., and Metzger, B. E. (1973). Metabolic features of Johannesburg Bantu myocardial infarction. *S. Afr. Med. J.* **47**, 1571–1575.

Shaper, A. G., and Patel, K. M. (1964). Diseases of the biliary tract in African and Ugandans. *East Afr. Med. J.* **41**, 246–250.

Stemmerman, G. N. (1966). Cancer of the colon and rectum discovered at autopsy in Hawaiian Japanese. *Cancer (Philadelphia)* **19**, 1567–1572.

Thomson, W. H. C. (1975). The nature of haemorrhoids. *Br. J. Surg.* **62**, 542–552.

Tovey, F. I. (1974). The geographical distribution of possible factors in the etiology of peptic ulcer. *Trop. Doct.* **1**, 17–21.

Tovey, F. I. (1977). Geographical aspects of peptic ulcers surgery. *World J. Surg.* **1**, 47–73.

Trowell, H. C. (1960). Diabetes mellitus. *In* "Non-Infective Disease in Africa" (H. C. Trowell, ed.), p. 306. Arnold, London.

Trowell, H. C. (1975a). Ischaemic heart disease, atheroma and fibrinolysis. *In* "Refined Carbohydrate Foods and Disease" (D. P. Burkitt and H. C. Trowell, eds.), p. 195. Academic Press, New York.

Trowell, H. C. (1975b). Hypothesis of the etiology of diabetes mellitus. *Diabetes* **24**, 762–765.

Trowell, H. C. (1978). *In* "Recent Developments in Dietary-Fibre Hypothesis. Dietary Fibre: Current Developments of Importance to Health" (K. W. Heaton, ed.), pp. 1–8. New Publ., London.

Tuyns, A. J., and Masse, G. (1975). Cancer of the oesophagus in Britanny: an incidence study in Ille-et-Villaine. *Int. J. Epidemiol.* **4**, 55–59.

Wynder, E. L., and Reddy, B. S. (1975). Dietary fat and colon cancer. *J. Natl. Cancer Inst.* **54**, 7–10.

Wynder, E. L., and Shigematsu, T. (1967). Environmental factors of cancer of the colon and rectum. *Cancer (Philadelphia)* **20**, 1520–1561.

Wynder, E. L., Kajitan, I. T., Ishikaw, A. S., Dodo, H., and Takanoa, A. (1969). Environmental factors of cancer of the colon and rectum. *Cancer (Philadelphia)* **23**, 1210–1220.

Zimmett, P. Z., Whitehouse, S., Jackson, L., and Thoma, K. (1978). High prevalance of hyperuricemia and gout in urbanised micronesian population. *Br. Med. J.* **1**, 1237–1239.

6

Disease, Political Events, and Populations

ROBERT S. ROBINS

I. INTRODUCTION

Natural selection, by causing the differential survival of some genotypes at the expense of others, is considered to be the most significant of all factors in evolution. Other factors, such as climate and natural variability, are well documented and also known to be important, but one influence that is often overlooked is that of political relations and events. Individuals or groups can greatly enhance their genetic contribution by exercising political dominance;

153

BIOCULTURAL ASPECTS OF DISEASE
Copyright © 1981 by Academic Press, Inc.
All rights of reproduction in any form reserved.
ISBN 0-12-598720-X

conversely, a genetically associated advantage (e.g., an inherited resistance to certain diseases) can facilitate a group's rise and maintenance of power.

Viewed politically, disease, through its effect on a leader or as it causes differential mortality of large numbers of persons, may affect a population. In the first set of circumstances a disease can change the distribution of political power when a key person suffers from an illness, the illness changes his behavior, and that behavior affects politics. A notable example is George III's porphyria-induced madness, which greatly frustrated his efforts to restore the royal peroga-tive (Macalpine and Hunter, 1969). Had George III not suffered from this metabolic disorder, the already difficult road to a popularly based Parliament in the next century would have been far more violent and drawn out. Ivan IV's syphilis (Grey, 1964), St. Joan's hallucinations (MacLaurin, 1922), Woodrow Wilson's stroke (Weinstein, 1967), and Winston Churchill's arteriosclerosis (Moran, 1966) are examples of disease affecting shifts in political power through the agency of an important leader. "Political" refers to those arrangements, for the most part enforced by institutions such as churches and armies, that permit one group to dominate another.

The question of disease affecting politics through one person will not be reviewed here because analyses of the role of the person in history would be necessary and would inevitably extend into biographical and psychological evaluations. What will be examined is the influence of widespread, high-mortality diseases as selective agents. The weakening of the pre-Colombian civilizations by measles and smallpox, the Black Death of the fourteenth cen-tury, and endemic malaria in classical Rome are examples in which disease clearly affected political, ethnogenetic, and cultural relationships and thus evolu-tionary trends.

II. HISTORICAL EVENTS, SOCIETAL EFFECTS

Health disasters have not been rare. Cipolla (1962) in "The Economic History of World Population" showed statistically that the "sudden disappearance of a fifth of the population or a third or even half, was, every once in a while, a recurrent catastrophe of local experience." Haldane (1949) emphasized that infectious diseases probably have been the major agent of natural selection of man during recorded history. Such disasters in the ancient world were largely unrecorded, though mythic reflections of what must have been actual events survive. The pestilence that led to the freeing of the Hebrews from Egyptian bondage was probably genuine. Among authenticated early disasters was the pestilence (probably typhus or the bubonic or pneumonic plague) that vitally weakened Athens in the Peloponnesian War about 450 BC leading eventually to the rise of Macedonian and then Roman power. As these two examples illustrate, the effect of a disease may be sudden and dramatic or extremely slow in its consequences. It is also likely to be one factor among several. In any event, the disease is likely to have genetically differential consequences. Large and established groups in conflict are not likely to be genetically identical. Often they are distinct.

The crucial factor is not the disease's severity, its incidence, or its duration. What matters is whether the disease acted as an independent and identifiable force in pushing power toward certain groups or institutions. Diseases such as tuberculosis in the nineteenth century or syphilis in Europe in the sixteenth century decimated populations, but their effects were so general that whether they had any political, cultural, or ethnogenetic importance is impossible to determine, human disasters though they were.

III. DISEASE AS A WARTIME ENEMY OR ALLY

A. Napoleon's Russian Campaign

The most common way in which disease affects politics is when one group is weakened more than its opponents. Battles, sieges and campaigns are all likely to be affected by disease. In most cases one battle, one campaign, or one siege is not likely to make much difference. Certain events in history, however, may have produced disproportionate consequences. One of the severest military blows disease ever struck, with the greatest long-term consequences, is often overlooked because other aspects of the story were more dramatic. In June 1812, Napoleon had assembled an international army of from 500,000 (Marshall-Cornwall, 1967) to more than 600,000 (Cartwright, 1972) soldiers, the greatest army the world had ever seen, for his invasion of Russia. He wanted to be sure that the military advantage would be his because he was well aware of the difficulties of supply (Marshall-Cornwall, 1967). The Russian army of that time consisted of only 258,000 troops, some of whom were fighting the Turks. Irregulars would also come to the Russsian army's aid, but they were not likely to be decisive except against a disorganized and demoralized opponent. As is well known, Napoleon's one-half-million-strong Grand Army had been reduced to only 40,000 by the time of its return, and, reportedly, only 1000 of these were ever again fit for service. Unquestionably, the decline of French power in Europe dated from that disaster.

The general interpretation of the French catastrophe is that the Russians, under General Kutusov, cleverly drew Napoleon into Russia, avoiding battles and fighting (for that period) only relatively small engagements at Smolensk and Borodino. After Napoleon retreated from Moscow, the Russians attacked. Flanking raids by Russian troops and partisans savaged the French, but even more important, the argument goes, the Grand Army was unable to cope with the rigors of the Russian winter and the immensity of the Russian land. Certainly the retreat was one of the most horrific in military history, and certainly Kutusov must be recognized as a great general for exploiting geography and weather to gain victory over a larger, better trained, and better staffed army. Not generally known, however, is that Napoleon's army had declined to only 65,000 troops (Marshall-Cornwall, 1967) when it began its retreat from Moscow. It had already suffered casualties of about 90% during a largely unopposed campaign in an unseasonably mild autumn. Certainly neither General Kutusov nor "General Winter" was responsible for so many casualties before the retreat began—the culprit was "General Typhus."

Typhus, a disease carried by lice, caused by *Rickettsia prowazekii*, and encouraged by dirty and crowded environments, was endemic in Poland and Russia, but Napoleon's armies had largely not experienced it before the invasion (Cartwright, 1972). The disease first broke out in the third week of July in Vilna, now Lithuania, Soviet Union (Prinzing, 1916). By late July 1812, about 80,000 troops had died or had been invalided. Dysentery—aggravated by the scarcity of water in the crowded bivouacs that the French had to resort to because of Kutusov's "scorched earth" policy—added to the health problem. The diary of one of Napoleon's lieutenants speaks not only of the extraordinary "filth and vermin" (Vossler, 1969), but of having to cook with a "brackish liquid scooped from stinking wells and putrid ponds" (Vossler, 1969). The Russian autumn that year was especially warm and dry.

The disease progressed rapidly. When Napoleon's troops drew up for the only major battle of the campaign, Borodino, on September 5, 1812, his strike force had already been reduced to 130,000. That was the only battle in which casualties were heavy: the French lost 28,000 and the Russians, 40,000 (Marshall-Cornwall, 1967). Typhus and dysentery continued to ravage the army and were the principal cause of tens of thousands of additional casualties before Moscow was reached. When Napoleon decided to abandon Moscow and begin his long march back to France on October 19, many of the sick had to be abandoned in the city. Many more were to be left along the way.

The Russians too suffered from disease, including typhus. They had, however, some immunity, and in any event did not suffer major infection from the disease in its most virulent form until they entered Vilna while pursuing the defeated "Grande Armee."

Disease played at least as large a role in defeating Napoleon's army as did Russian soldiers, Russian weather, and Russian space. Did France's defeat in Russia lead to its defeat in Europe? That is more difficult to assess. Napoleon was able to raise another army of 300,000 even before the full knowledge of the Russian disaster reached France. Yet after the Russian defeat, Napoleon had to fight a two-front war, having lost many of his most experienced officers and men (many with great experience in the Peninsular Wars), having allies that were similarly weakened, and, most important for this military genius who had terrorized the greatest armies in Europe for more than a decade, having lost a major campaign. That defeat had profound psychological consequences. Those who wanted to overthrow Napoleon were encouraged to ally themselves to Britain, eventually creating the alliance that destroyed Napoleon at Waterloo.

Although the effect of disease was clear concerning political and military events, its effect on genetic factors is not so readily described. A significant segment of a generational cohort was eliminated, especially among the upper classes of France. France's allies were similarly affected. There was also an expansion of Russian, especially Great Russian, peoples into what is now Poland. These events affected the genetic distribution in those areas.

B. Athens versus Sparta and Pestilence

Twenty-two centuries earlier, a disease, possibly also typhus, had been a crucial factor in the conflict between two widely different cultures, those of Athens and Sparta. In the early years of the fourth century BC, Sparta and several other Greek city-states considered themselves threatened by Athens' imperialistic democracy. By 430 BC an army of the Spartan-led Peloponnesian League was pressing toward Athens, preparing to make siege. At about the same time a disease broke out in the countryside near Athens. Thucydides (1959), who nearly died of it himself, wrote that the pestilence first broke out in the port city of Peiraeus, and spread rapidly. Danger from the Peloponnesian forces in the vicinity had, at about the same time, led Athens to open its walls to refugees. Soon, about 400,000 persons were crowded within the walls (Prinzing, 1916).

As Ehrenberg wrote, "The effects of the disaster on the war were immediate and far reaching" (Ehrenberg, 1967). "Athens never regained the advantages in numbers which she had at the start of the war" (Bowra, 1971). At first the Peloponnesian invaders fled when they heard of the pestilence, but they soon realized that the disease was not affecting them. They quickly returned to the attack, and the war, which was a vicious one, continued for 20 years. Not only had the plague eliminated Athens' numerical advantage, it had more subtle, but perhaps no less important, results. It was the indirect cause of the great Pericles' fall and the direct cause of his death. More important, as Sir Maurice Bowra argues (Bowra, 1971), was that the suffering and degradation of the pestilential conditions undermined the Athenians' sense of honor. They saw their countrymen, under the stress of privation and disease, put self-interest before family ties, before civic responsibility, and before military honor. Thus they lost the sense of self-confidence and self-respect that is necessary for any people to accomplish great things.

Did it really matter, politically or genetically, that one group of Greeks achieved dominance over another? Politically, the defeat was important because Athens had been an empire (though a loose one, by later standards). If Athens had unified the Hellenic world, it would have been in a better position than the Peloponnesian League to block Macedon and then Rome. The defeat of Athens was even more important culturally because it destroyed not only Athenian political power, but also the brightest of Greek civilization (Bowra, 1971). Thus ended one of the three or four golden ages of Western man. Of course, like all things, it would have ended eventually, somehow. But without the pestilence of 430 BC, the Golden Age of Greece would have lasted longer and grown even greater.

Genetically, the fall of Athens, by clearing the way for the rise of Macedon and especially Rome, facilitated the genetic interaction that these empires permitted. Indeed, the Roman Empire was the first great political institution in the West that not only permitted, but also encouraged, the ready movement of genetically dissimilar peoples.

IV. PROLONGED UNDERMINING OF A SOCIETY

So far we have seen how disease can change societies by affecting a specific event, a campaign, a siege. Another way that disease can affect populations, politics, ethnogenic patterns, and culture is through a general undermining of an entire society during a substantial period (e.g., the disruption of the Amerindian civilizations by European-introduced diseases). Two complementary and little-known effects of disease subtly weakened the Roman Empire in its later years.

A. Decline of Rome via Malaria and Lead Poisoning

Rome declined for a variety of reasons: increased external pressures, secessionist tendencies, and overburdening taxation (Jones, 1966). The population, too, had become increasingly uninterested in its own defense. "No one who reads the scanty records of the collapse can fail to be struck by the apathy of the Roman population from the highest to the lowest" (Jones, 1966). Various causes of this lethargy have been suggested. The overregulation of the population and the otherworldly teachings of Christianity are frequently cited (Jones, 1966). Two other factors that deserve consideration are the influence of malaria in the Roman Campagna and the effect of lead on the aristocracy. Both undermined the will and ability of those at the heart of the empire, in Rome itself, to resist the forces of disintegration.

1. Malaria

The area around Rome was endemic for malaria until the twentieth century. From Cato to Cavour, Italian governments encouraged or attempted to force citizens to farm in what is apparently a rich agricultural area near a wealthy and populous capital city. Even as late as 1933, the Italian scholar Celli could still exclaim "How was it that Rome, twice Queen of the world, for more than thirty years capital of the third Italy, was the only metropolis situated in the midst of a desert?" (Celli, 1933). Until malaria was better understood, the explanation given for this "desert" were unsatisfactory, emphasizing political factors that could just as well apply to London or Paris, Florence or Naples. With the discovery of the mosquito's role in transmitting malaria, the periodic nature of malarial outbreaks, and the role of a silting river in establishing and enhancing the *Anopheles* mosquitoes' breeding grounds, the influence of malaria in undermining Roman society first became a matter for speculation.

Malaria is insidious. The normal primary defenses against illness—good nutrition, clean surroundings, adequate clothing—are not defenses against malaria. Furthermore, acquired immunity is rare. The plasmodic variety attacks the red corpuscles during several years, causing fever, tumors in the spleen and liver, anemia, and sometimes death. Even the mildest forms weaken the will and body of the sufferer. Not only does it attack people—usually in well-watered and rich river-bottom areas of great agricultural potential—but also a variant affects horses and stall cattle as well. People tend to leave such malarial areas (the Solonge in France and the Fen region of England were formerly such areas) and populate nearby towns.

We know that malaria was endemic in the Campagna in the late Roman period, but whether its incidence increased is unclear (Brunt, 1971). The depopulation of the Campagna, the silting of the relevant rivers (improving the breeding grounds for *Anopheles*), and the increasing reports of extraordinary lethargy among the Romans are indirect evidence of the increasing severity of malaria in the region. The evidence suggests that malaria played a significant role in the weakening of Rome in the period of its worst decline.

2. Lead Poisoning

The effect of malaria on population is well known, and that the disease could undermine even a capital city is not difficult to see. Within the past 20 years, however, another and not uncomplementary hypothesis has been suggested to explain the remarkable decline of the Romans' ability to defend themselves. Basically the hypothesis traces the weakening of Roman leadership to a weakening of the aristocracy, and the weakening of that aristocracy to chemical pollution.

The Romans were well aware of the danger of lead poisoning. Vitruvius and Pliny both warned of the dangers of taking lead internally. Poisoning among workers in the lead mines of Italy and Britain was notorious. Victims developed palsy and other symptoms of lead toxicity. The disease was not restricted to lead mines. Records tell of lead poisoning epidemics as late as the seventh century AD (Waldon, 1973). The disease appears to have affected the upper class of Rome much more than the rest of the population (except for miners and craftsmen working with lead) for two reasons. First was the use of lead pipes for plumbing. Water absorbed lead salts from the pipes, which were most likely used to supply drinking water to the well-to-do. This form of lead ingestion, however, probably affected the health of the upper class only minimally.

Apparently much more dangerous was their adoption of the Greek method of making and preserving fruit juices and wine, the so-called "Greek wine" introduced by Greek slaves of the aristocracy. At first, they boiled down the wine or grape juice to a syrup in bronze or copper vessels, but those metals transmitted an unpleasant taste to the liquid. The vessels also tended to oxidize, and any verdigris could ruin the syrup. If the vessels were coated lightly with lead, the syrup was found to be without the unpleasant taste and (by lead's antienzyme action) the wine or juice was better preserved (Waldon, 1973). In fact, wine was sometimes "doctored" with lead to improve its flavor. This practice was largely confined to the upper classes who could afford Greek servants.

S. C. Gilfillan, by examining human bones of that period and also inspecting records on the birth rates and level of birth defects of the later Roman period, argued that each generation of the Roman upper class was about a fourth of the previous one (new recruits presumably coming from below) and that this decline in fertility was due to lead poisoning among aristocratic women of childbearing age (Gilfillan, 1964, 1965). Sterility, miscarriages, stillbirths, high infant mortality, and mental impairment of children are all associated with lead poisoning. Gilfillan pointed out that the fertility level of the Roman poor did not similarly decline. He also suggested that the same process might have occurred earlier in Greece.

The argument is plausible, though other scholars are not as confident as Gilfillan as to the importance of the phenomenon (Waldon, 1973). If one assumes the aristocrats were genetically superior, the argument that their decimation damaged Rome holds up well, but that is a questionable assumption. Mazzarino (1959) in "The End of the Ancient World" denies the importance of genetic decline in the aristocracy as a cause of Rome's fall. He argues that as many, if not more, great men lived in the late period as in any other (Mazzarino, 1959). Nevertheless, genetic considerations aside, a society cannot absorb a 75% loss of its ruling class every generation without its government being severely damaged. Ruling classes are effective partly because of their patterns of formal and informal education, their family and other group alliances and arrangements, and their general training in social skills. They offer a continuity with the past and promise continuity for the future. The inclusion of new groups is necessary, but a 75% elimination of the ruling class is excessive. The evidence on this controversy is not all in, but if lead poisoning can be shown to play as large a role as Gilfillan claims, then it must be considered a major cause in the decline of Rome. Even at this point, it must be considered a contributing factor.

The ethnogenetic and cultural effects of the fall of Rome were, of course, profound. No other highly developed civilization of antiquity was as nearly destroyed as that of Rome. Large numbers of persons of different ethnic stocks and diverse cultural backgrounds streamed into western and southern Europe and became integral parts of that society. Culturally, a centralized empire gave way to monarchies and feudalism, the God-centered and bureaucratic religion of Christianity replaced the largely private humanism of the ancients. Disease among the Romans was evidently one of the factors that facilitated these genetic and cultural changes.

B. Colonization of America Aided by Disease

Whereas one must be somewhat hesitant in hypothesizing about malarial and lead poisoning effects on the ability of the late Romans to resist disintegration, no such hesitation is necessary when discussing the magnitude of the effect of disease on Amerindian efforts to resist their European invaders. Just how great the disaster was is controversial (Denevan, 1976), but that it was a great disaster to Amerindians, weakened them, and aided the domination of the European race and European culture is not.

Typhoid, diphtheria, the common cold, influenza, measles, chicken pox, whooping cough, tuberculosis, yellow fever, scarlet fever and other streptococcus infections, gonorrhea, and smallpox were all diseases for which the Amerindians had no natural immunity and which were all introduced to them by the Europeans in the early days of the conquest (Martin, 1976). Syphilis, tularemia, anthrax, pneumonia, and mumps, at least in their most virulent forms, should probably also be added to the list (Cook, 1973; McNeil, 1976). One wonders how the Indians were able to resist. Not only did they lack natural immunity, but also their social and hygienic patterns increased their vulnerability. Indians spread infection within the tribe by commonly living close together. They spread infection to other tribes by their custom of traveling about and visiting. Their treatment for the diseases seldom were effective. Indeed, a common method of "treating" a disease was by making the influenza- or smallpox-ridden victim sweat and then plunging him into the coldest water available. Other cultural practices, such as severe dieting, fasting, exposure to the elements, and general lack of nursing, were unfortunately common (Stearn and Stearn, 1945).

The effect on the size of the population was immediate and great. The island of Haiti, for example, lost two-thirds of its population, principally from disease, in the 3 years after Columbus' landing. Cortez's invasion of central Mexico about 20 year later was preceded by a fearsome epidemic "In most districts half the population died, towns became deserted," and the indigenous leadership was more than decimated. The experience was repeated among the Quiche-Cakchequel in Guatemala about 1521–1522 and as late as 1589 in Paraguay.

Reliable statistics from 1707 on the impact of a similar group of diseases on the indigenes of Iceland indicate that an initial mortality of slightly more than a third of the population is likely in such an exposed population (Stearn and Stearn, 1945). Even by the nineteenth century, epidemics among Indians in certain areas created a death rate of from 55 to 90%. Entire tribes and villages were probably destroyed. Parallel with these dramatic catastrophes, certain newly introduced diseases—especially those such as tuberculosis and syphilis—produced a low-level, continuing attack on the population, weakening the Indians' vigor and lessening their numbers. Cook, in a careful and ingenious examination of mortality statistics, estimates that nonepidemic diseases of European origin resulted in a mean annual population loss of 1.6% among the New England Indians (Cook, 1973). Compounded over only a few generations, this endemic factor would have more than halved the Indian population. There is also evidence that the Europeans brought diseases and strains of diseases that adversely affected most of the wildlife on which the Indians depended (Martin, 1976). Tularemia, anthrax, and sylvan plague may have caused epidemics among wild animals such as beaver and deer. In some cases these diseases would also have been transmitted to man through their animal hosts.

What diseases were most damaging? Smallpox was probably the principal epidemic killer (Stearn and Stearn, 1945). Even among the Europeans in the New England colonies in the early 17th century, about 13% of all deaths were due to smallpox (Winslow, 1974), though in children it was often confused with measles. Among the endemic diseases, tuberculosis and syphilis probably did the greatest harm.

The Europeans had a number of advantages for penetration that the Indians did not have for resistance. Enjoying at least some immunity and having developed some techniques for control and treatment, Europeans' resistance to infection was much better than that of the Indians. Of course, the Europeans also had great advantages in other fields, principally military technology and political organization. Yet, they had only intermittent incentive, until the late seventeenth century at the earliest, for colonization. If the Europeans had immigrated more slowly, perhaps the Indians could have better protected their holdings. North America might then have become a multiracial society, like Mexico, and many Latin American countries might have been multiracial, with Indians dominant.

A somewhat different view, however, is suggested by one of the best known experts on the topic:

> The elimination of certain tribes and the decimation of many others greatly facilitated colonial expansion. Indirectly, smallpox saved both lives and property [of the colonists] which would otherwise have been expended in warfare with the Indians (Duffy, 1953).

Without disease to weaken his natural opponents, the colonist would have had to wage more wars and even more bitter relations between the races might have resulted. The expansion of one people into another's territory has always been a violent and deadly process. How would the political institutions and cultural ideals of America differed if the push West had been one principally of warfare against a different race? The Russians had an experience somewhat of this sort when they pushed their frontier eastward in the eighteenth and nineteenth centuries.

Disease, then, was a major factor in facilitating the dominance of the western hemisphere by European stock and European culture. History records no other event of such ethnogenetic, political, and cultural importance as the seizure and domination of the western hemisphere by Europeans. Cipolla (1962) estimated that about 22% of the world population was Caucasian in 1800; by 1930 that figure had grown to 35%. Not all, but much, of this increase was due to settlement of the New World. The shift in ethnogenetic composition was most striking, of course, in the Western Hemisphere: in 1492 the population was virtually 100% Amerindian; by the mid-twentieth century probably no more than one-third of the population was native, and that percentage was concentrated in a few areas.

Disease meant that in most areas of the Americas the colonists had nature as their principal enemy, not other people. It also meant that the region (especially North America) would be rapidly settled during the eighteenth and nineteenth centuries, in the early stages of the Industrial Revolution. Without the epidemic and endemic diseases, the European domination of the New World would have been slower, less complete, and of a different nature.

C. Colonization of Africa Thwarted by Disease

In the colonization of the Americas, disease facilitated conquest. What would have happened had the Amerindians had the relative advantage, i.e., if the Europeans had had to pass through exotic pestilences that halved their numbers? Such a situation did exist elsewhere, in subsaharan Africa.

Europeans had colonized North Africa in classical times, and established regular sea contact of the more southerly coastal regions (especially West Africa) by the sixteenth century. Geography certainly discouraged penetration: the Sahara Desert inhibited invasion from the north, and forest and swamps hampered penetration along the coast. Yet caravans and explorers regularly crossed the Sahara, and several rivers—most notably the Congo—were good routes into the interior. On other continents, early modern explorers overcame more forbidding physical obstacles (Burns, 1969). In Africa, disease kept the explorers, the military, and the merchants from settling in certain regions. For centuries Africa, especially West Africa, was known as the White Man's Grave and the mortality of expeditions and attempted settlements confirmed this reputation (Hazzledine, 1969).

The Scots explorer Mungo Park was among the first to attempt to find the source of the Niger. In 1805, he set out with an expedition of 44 Europeans; all but five or six died of disease. In 1837, James Tuckey of the Royal Navy tried to discover the source of the Congo; in mild weather on a calm and broad river, his expedition suffered 37% mortality in 3 months (Cartwright, 1972). The survivial data improved only slightly in the mid-nineteenth century. Table I shows the effect of disease on European employees—most of whom were healthy young men—of the British Company of Merchants on the Gold Coast (Morgan and Pugh, 1969).

Such mortality was not confined to commercial employees and adventurous explorers. Between February 1825 and June 1828, the British colony of Sierra Leone had five governors, each dying in service (Morgan and Pugh, 1969). Soldiers under military discipline living in the best situation available suffered as much. Of the 199 soldiers who, in May 1825, arrived in The Gambia, 160 had died of disease by the end of that December. Sea duty in the region was not much better, if the base was African. The antislavery cruisers out of Freetown, Liberia, were known as the Coffin Squadron because their crews' death rate was so high.

Although the situation was extremely bad in West Africa, it was not much better in most other areas. Europeans were eager to settle anywhere, and the areas were few in which some sort of settlement was not attempted. Where health conditions permitted, they succeeded. South Africa and the East African uplands quickly acquired large and vigorous populations of European settlers. A move into Central Africa was first attempted in the seventeenth century by the Portuguese (Gelfand, 1953), but disease frustrated their efforts. Disease long prevented even the great riches of the Cooper Belt in the Central African Zambesi Valley from being developed (Watson, 1957). In that region the death rate from disease (again among initially healthy and fairly young Europeans) was 13.2/1000 as recently as 1930 (Watson, 1957).

What were the diseases that prevented, if not European imperialism, at least European settlement? The diseases that were so destructive of human life were

TABLE I

Effects of Disease on Europeans Working on Africa's Gold Coast

Year	Deaths/1000	Invalided/1000
1887	54	208
1888	55	555
1891	32.7	175
1897	76.6	155

principally those carried by vectors, especially insects and worms, that thrive in wet, humid, and warm climates. Table II shows the most damaging diseases and their principal vectors (Watson, 1957).

Of course, other diseases were damaging, especially smallpox, syphilis, and influenza, but they were not as widespread for as long a period. The most effective diseases in preventing European penetration were malaria and sleeping sickness (infections with *Trypanosoma gambiense*). Malaria, discussed earlier in relation to the Roman Campagna, was probably a greater impediment to the Europeans than was sleeping sickness. The African variety of malaria differed sufficiently from the European to permit only a partial immunity, and it was more lethal (Cartwright, 1972). Sleeping sickness did not appear in Europe (a related disorder, Chagas disease, exists in Brazil and Venezuela), and was not only frequently fatal, but had socially disturbing symptoms. After being infected, the victim became alternatingly drowsy and violent, experienced tremors and paralysis, and eventually died (Cartwright, 1972). The disease was recognized by the early slavers who named it "Negro lethargy" (Ackernecht, 1965). Not only did it disable and kill many of the European would-be settlers, it also did the same to their horses and cattle.

Three related points should be made here. First, the overall effect of these diseases was probably as great on the Africans as on the Europeans. The newly arrived Europeans had, as adults, the same mortality as the African infant as well as the normal adult mortality (Curtin, 1964; Hoeppli, 1959). American blacks who "returned" to Africa in the nineteenth century suffered from disease at about the same rate as their European counterparts (Curtin, 1964). Second, for the Africans the coming of the Europeans created even worse conditions by introducing new diseases and new strains of established diseases. Third, greatly

TABLE II

The Most Damaging Diseases Affecting Europeans in Africa

Disease	Vector
Malaria, yellow fever, dengue fever, elephantiasis	Mosquito
Bubonic plague, viral typhus	Flea
Sleeping sickness	Tsetse fly
Kala azar	Sand fly
Cholera, typhoid, and dysentery	House fly
Relapsing fever	Tick
Viral typhus	Louse
Viral jungle typhus	Mite

expanded communication, due to European trade and to waterborne traffic, spread many African diseases into new areas. For example, Stanley's expedition of 1888 to the Congo introduced West African sleeping sickness into several areas, with resulting large-scale loss of life. About 12 years later, diseases of African origin but exotic to the Congo accounted for about 500,000 deaths (Ackernecht, 1965). According to some reports, two-thirds of the population of Uganda died at about the turn of the century from a sleeping sickness epidemic of West African origin but introduced through European penetration (Ackernecht, 1965).

The situation, therefore, was not that the indigenes were relatively healthy while the "invaders" were being decimated. Rather it was that the diseases tended to affect both Europeans and Africans. The Europeans had some choice in where they could live, did not choose to press forward with settlement, and so were slow to establish political authority.

Disease prevented subsaharan Africa from becoming an extension of Europe, as largely occurred in the Americas—with all that that implies for political power, ethnogenetic domination, and cultural presence. Indeed, subsaharan Africa would have been a more likely target for European colonization than was Latin America: the indigenous political organizations were often less developed, the populations were smaller, and the area was closer to Europe. Where the opportunity presented itself, as in South Africa, the Europeans were quick to take advantage of it. From the standpoint of African political independence, ethnogenetic distinctiveness, and cultural individuality, the mosquito, the fly, and the worm were Africa's most effective defending warriors. Ironically, the long-term effect of the European interlude—especially the application of medical science and political organization—has been to greatly lessen the prospects of subsaharan Africa ever again being so vulnerable to external domination.

V. CHANGES FROM WITHIN OR WHOLE-SOCIETY EFFECTS

The examples discussed so far show how disease may harm one group to the benefit of another, with significant political, cultural, and ethnogenetic consequences. Diseases can also profoundly disrupt an entire society, with extremely widespread and pervasive consequences, but not to the advantage or disadvantage of any external group.

A. The Black Death

The most striking example of such a profound disease-caused disruption is that of the Black Death of the fourteenth century. The Black Death was the greatest disaster that Europe ever experienced. Only a general outbreak of atomic warfare among all the European powers—sporadically extending over a half century— could suggest today what the Black Death meant in human suffering in the fourteenth century. Its first outbreak occurred in England in 1349, followed by an almost equally severe one 12 years later, and then a series of others until 1405. Even then the plague prevailed; no 5-year period up to 1670 was free of a major outbreak somewhere in England (Mullett, 1956). Good, though not conclusive, evidence exists to support the belief that genetic selection creates plague bacilli-resistant genotypes (Sokhey and Chitre, 1937). The increasing dominance of such genotypes may explain the weakening of the plague's severity.

In the first major outbreak—when it was most severe and disruptive—from one-fourth to three-fourths of the population of England perished (Mullett, 1956). Incomplete, ambiguous, and obscure records, complicated by the plague's varying severity among different groups and in different places, make estimates difficult. One-third to one-half of the population is probably as accurate an estimate as we can make. Unquestionably, many villages and even districts were nearly depopulated. Not only was the disease highly infectious but its manner of attack was gruesomely dramatic: a well person would suddenly be striken, often experiencing shafts of pain as if by fiend-sent arrows and (in the bubonic form) agonizing swellings in the groin and armpits. The victim remained conscious during most of the ordeal, facing an 80% certainty of his own death, often abandoned by his family, or died with the sight of his family being wracked by the same malady. The medical details of the illness do not concern us greatly here, but the rapid spread of the pestilence and the characteristic black "bruis-ing" that was reported indicate that the principal form of the disease was proba-bly pneumonic, though the bubonic form was also present (Shrewsbury, 1970; Cartwright, 1972).

What was the political effect of the catastrophe? How did it affect the distribu-tion of power within society? Curiously, it had little effect on politics. No boundary change can be traced to the plague; no nation gained over another because of it. Even a more superficial level where generalized effects—such as a mass religiosity—can be traced, the manifestations were often contradictory. In some plague areas the population turned to a fanatical religion of flagellation and hysteria; in others they mocked the Church and let licentious passions free; in still others they became apathetic. In some areas the power of the state gained and became oppressive over a weak and demoralized society, and in others the lord's power waned for as much as a generation (Deaux, 1969).

The effect of the plague was interactive, creating nothing itself of lasting note, but crucially compounding some preexisting trends and mitigating others. To understand the plague's social consequences, one must ask how it affected what was basic and essential to medieval society: the system of labor exchange by which agriculture was carried on, and the institution of the Catholic Church.

Viewed this way, when not just the outbreak of 1349 but also outbreaks following to 1405 are considered, the Black Death clearly reinforced certain already present trends and deflected others to vitally undermine the medieval synthesis. In this way, it facilitated the emergence of what we call the beginning of the modern world after 1500.

B. Decline of Serfdom

The agricultural system of England (and much of Europe) was characterized by persons having familial obligations to labor for their overlord. A person might, for example, be expected to plant and harvest 8 acres as such a service. The overlord himself would have certain reciprocal obligations, but the advantage in the relationship was his. Nevertheless, for a variety of reasons and before the Black Death outbreak, commutation (abolition) of these services was an established and growing practice. Under this procedure a person owing such services could purchase (or perhaps be granted) freedom from this obligation. Henceforth, the lord would have to pay—not always, but often, at least partly in money—for the serf's labor. With commutation, the laborer gained at least legal freedom to move about and offer his labor to the highest bidder. Of course, the opportunity for real mobility was rare and the opportunity for bargaining limited, but from time to time such opportunity did arise. Although commutation was well underway before 1349, the sudden decrease of the labor supply after that date made labor far more valuable (Cowie, 1972). Serfs saw the improved situation of those who could sell their labor, they sometimes inherited means to buy their freedom, and, most important, if their overlord did not commutate their obligation they could move off. They could simply squat on the great amount of vacant land then available or move to another lord's holding, where their labor would be accepted and they would be well compensated with no questions asked. Despite such efforts as the Statute of 1351, which attempted to set wages at preplague levels, the price of labor remained higher than it had been and the trend toward commutation continued so strongly that "peasant" and "serf" ceased to describe any group of Englishmen (Cartwright, 1972).

The release of the poorer rural population from the most restrictive aspects of serfdom was one precondition for the rise of parliamentary democracy and liberal capitalism, and the Black Death was one of several factors that facilitated the destruction of the English peasantry system. Had the Black Death not occurred, the Middle Ages as we know them would have continued longer, capitalism would have developed later, and parliamentary democracy might have appeared, if it came at all, by an altogether different route.

C. Weakening of the Church

The other institution vitally weakened by the Black Death was the Catholic Church. Whereas the weakening of the peasantry system was evident at the time, the effect on the Church was largely hidden, indeed often even disguised by an enhanced prosperity.

Some damage was obvious, however. Mortality among priests was substantially higher than that among the rest of the population, and this difference affected the quality of the priesthood. Men inferior in learning and in vocational zeal replaced the dead priests (Ziegler, 1969). The tendency toward the use of English rather than Latin and Norman French in education and government was greatly accelerated by the decreasing number of those who could teach the two languages (Ziegler, 1969; Cowie 1972). This decline of Latin and Norman French also facilitated the access to government by the common man. An example of this movement was the Act of Parliament of 1362, by which English replaced Norman French as the language to be used in the courts. Use of the vernacular was also an essential precondition to the growth of general literacy, which also meant that the Church no longer had a necessary monopoly on education or its officers a necessary function in the governing of the state.

Both the Church as an institution and its members as a body emerged from the Black Death period with severely damaged reputations. Although the catastrophe undoubtedly made many fear the wrath of God more, they respected the Church less. After all, the plague did occur; the Church did not warn them of its coming (though many false warnings had been given at the time of the millenium of Christ's birth 350 years before); the Church was unable to lessen the plague's impact; and the plague struck down the clergy with greater severity than those not in religious orders. Although one would think the Church would have received some respect for the sufferings its priests and monks had experienced, this was not the case. Some priests fled their parishes for safety or better livings, some demanded large sums of money for doing their duties, and some simply did not attend to their duties (Mullett, 1956). These were the exceptions, but not rare ones, and the people apparently remembered the misdeeds best. The picture one gets is of the clergy for the most part doing its duty, but with hesitation and reluctance. As we would expect, those priests who sacrificed most, who worked hardest and exposed themselves the most, suffered the highest mortality. The good suffered more than the bad, thus lowering the quality of those who remained (Ziegler, 1969). Not only were those left behind often morally inferior to those who died, but many of the new clergy, i.e., the laymen who entered it in large numbers after the first outbreak, clearly were inferior in learning, strength of vocation, and administrative skill to those they replaced (Mullett, 1956).

Also adverse was the material effect on the Church, not because it grew poorer, but because it grew wealthy well beyond its needs. The first effect of the plague on the Church, as on other institutions, was impoverishment; with the decline in population and the disruption in agriculture, tithes radically declined and far fewer remained to till the Church's land (Ziegler, 1969). That reversal, however, was brief. Many persons left property to the Church, some gave it out of piety, and others brought it with them when they entered holy orders. Moreover, in the civil unrest that followed the epidemics, the (greatly enriched) ruling class saw the Church as a bulwark of stability, and so it was given many gifts.

To say that the Church grew wealthy is not to say that it grew more powerful. What existed was a wealthy and showy institution that had a decreasing role in society aggravated by a decreasing level of public trust and respect (Robins, 1976). When social strains sharpen, such institutions become vulnerable to attack and profitable to destroy. This process is precisely what began in the following century and a half. The Black Death was a major factor in undermining the economic system of the Middle Ages and in weakening its principal institution. What happened in Europe from 1500 on—the rise of Protestantism, capitalism, parliamentary democracy, centralized monarchy, secular bureaucracy, and nationalism—all probably would have occurred without the plague, but they would have come later and in a moderated form. Without the Black Death the modern world would be less modern and, in some ways that cannot be guessed at, different.

VI. FUTURE HEALTH DISASTERS?

The sudden decline of disease can profoundly affect a society's or world cultural and ethnogenetic composition as can a pandemic like the Black Death. Since World War II, modern methods of hygiene, food production and distribution, vector control, and inoculation have greatly lowered the death rate in Africa and Asia. The effect of these humane improvements has been to increase vastly the rate of population growth, an increase that is beginning to restore the racial and political proportions that existed before the great European expansion. The sudden increase of population, with its distortions of age distribution, changes in relative strength of groups within and between nations, and pressures on emigration, is having major cultural and political consequences and will have even greater ones as the trend continues.

Has disease, like famine, become one of those formerly central phenomena that henceforth will be only marginal to history? Or will someone 100 years from now have to add a few more pages to this essay?

VII. PERSPECTIVES OF THE PRESENT

There are some grounds for optimism. The last major pandemic was a little more than a half century ago, the influenza pandemic of 1918–1919. About 20 million persons died and about 500 million were infected (Clarke, 1968). The death rate among those infected was not particularly high, about 4%, with the largest loss of life among the weak and old. Nevertheless, a larger-than-average number of young men also died (World Health Organization, 1970). Of course, compared with the Black Death (in which about one-third of the population in the affected area died and the mortality was 90% among the infected), the 1918 influenza pandemic was not a great killer. In the context of the other diseases we have been discussing, no major ethnogenetic, political, or cultural consequences can be identified. Another killer strain of influenza could possibly cause a pandemic. The virus lives in wild animals and apparently becomes dangerous to man when it infects domestic animals in close contact with man (Beveridge, 1977). Still, modern methods of immunization and treatment would likely lessen its impact even below that of the last pandemic, at least among the more advanced countries. Individuals and even groups would suffer, but the social fabric would probably not be affected. Of course, any large-scale breakdown of sociopolitical institutions would make diseases such as influenza, cholera, smallpox, plague, and yellow fever as unmanageable as they ever were.

Future large-scale health disasters are, however, not likely to be due to chance but to man's efforts in the laboratory. Lethal biological agents may be used in warfare, such agents may accidentally escape from warfare laboratories, or they may accidentally escape from laboratories doing benign research.

What is the likelihood that someone would deliberately use a disease or combination of diseases in warfare? No record exists of biological warfare being practiced, though, as is well known, several governments do extensive research and perhaps testing on such agents (McCarthy, 1970). A major reason for its not having been used is that biological agents are much more awkward to use than conventional weapons. To be effective, a biological weapon must be stable, resistant to antibiotics, resistant to natural antigens, rapid-acting, and capable of mass production, and the sending power must ensure that its own population and allies will not be similarly affected (Clarke, 1968). As far as we know, no natural biological agent fits all these characteristics. The danger, of course, is that through recently developed methods of genetic engineering, a custom-made bacterium or virus could be developed (probably based on an influenza virus or a rickettsia). The aggressing country could immunize its population and then attack others. Also, a country facing its own extinction in a war might possibly release such agents to destroy everyone else as well.

Such events are fortunately outside our experience, and guessing the consequences would be extremely difficult. Perhaps the human race would be wiped out, or reduced to a few thousand living on out-of-the-way islands; perhaps only some areas would be destroyed. For example, such an outbreak in the Middle East might lead the western hemisphere to quarantine itself until its population was immunized. Thus, the disease might be "confined" to Africa and Eurasia. Predicting the behavior of bacterial and viral agents, once they are out of the laboratory and into a large biological pool, is difficult. They might shift their effects on humans from rapid death to incapacitation or chronic illness; they might turn out to result in long-term effects through carcinogenesis, immediate or future birth defects, or sterility (World Health Organization, 1970). New foci of infectious disease might be established, or the disease might affect nonhuman forms of life adversely, upsetting the ecological balance (World Health Organization, 1970). Also, after an initial pandemic, perhaps no more severe than the influenza one of 1918–1919, the disease might be brought under control.

The danger is not only present in connection with an outbreak of war. Unconfirmed rumors have spread of the escape of biological agents from military laboratories and storage facilities (McCarthy, 1970). Contamination may also come from nonmilitary research laboratories. In 1976, smallpox virus escaped from a research laboratory in London, and in 1978 an infection of smallpox from a Birmingham, England, laboratory resulted in one death.

One can speculate on all sorts of outbreaks, caused by terrorists, lunatics, and natural disasters. The danger of such an outbreak is constant; the consequences are largely unknown.

VIII. THROUGH THE PAST, DARKLY

Part of the problem about predicting the future is that we poorly understand the past. In all the instances described, the effect of disease on political relationships was evident. In several of the cases, however (Napoleon's Russian campaign, the Black Death, malaria in the Campagna), the political event's effect on genetic distribution within the population cannot be determined. This is not to say that there was no effect. Whenever a group genetically interacts with itself more than with other groups for several generations, it becomes genetically differentiated. If that differentiated group changes in political status, that change is likely to have consequences for that group's genetic expansion or contraction. In some cases, such as the winning of the New World by Europeans, the effect is obvious in degree and form. In other circumstances—e.g., Napoleon's defeat in Russia—it is not.

Pursuing the impact of disease on history has never been academically fashionable. The influence of great personalities, economic determinism, climate, geography, the independent power of ideas—all have had their vogue. Our understanding of history today is at best the refined residue of these excesses. Fortunately, no one has been so simplistic as to try to add health and disease to this list of reductionist arguments. But because there have been no excesses, the valuable residue has not been created; otherwise worthwhile studies of the European settlement of the Americas hardly mention epidemics among the Indians, and otherwise good essays on the decline of feudalism largely ignore the Black Death. A recent book devoted to extinction and survival in human populations gives scant attention to the effect of disease (Laughlin and Brady, 1978). In a small way, I have tried here to suggest how disease has conditioned and perhaps will continue to condition the way populations are distributed, which groups exercise power, and the form the culture takes. Sometimes the effect has been great.

ACKNOWLEDGMENT

I thank the professional staff and the Governors of the Library of the Wellcome Institute for the History of Medicine, London, for their assistance.

REFERENCES

Ackernecht, E. (1965). "History and Geography of the Most Important Diseases." Hafner, New York.

Adcock, F., and Mosley, D. J. (1975). "Diplomacy in Ancient Greece." Thames & Hudson, London.

Beveridge, W. I. B. (1977). "Influenza: The Last Great Plague." Heinemann, London.

Bowra, C. M. (1971). "Periclean Athens." Weidenfeld & Nicolson, London.

Brunt, P. S. (1971). "Italian Manpower, 225 BC–14 AD." Oxford Univ. Press, London and New York.

Burns, A. (1969). "History of Nigeria." Allen & Unwin, London.

Campbell, A. M. (1931). "The Black Death and Men of Learning." Columbia Univ. Press, New York.

Cartwright, F. F. (1972). "Disease and History." Hart-Davis, MacGibbon, London.

Celli, A. (1933). "The History of Malaria in the Roman Campagna." Bale & Danielsson, London.

Cipolla, C. M. (1962). "The Economic History of World Population." Penguin Books, London.

Clarke, (1968). "We All Fall Down: The Prospect of Biological and Chemical Warfare." Lane, London.

Cloudsley-Thompson, J. L. (1976). "Insects and History." Weidenfeld & Nicolson, London.

Cook, S. F. (1973). The significance of disease in the extinction of the New England Indians. *Hum. Biol.* **45,** 485–508.

Cowie, L. W. (1972). "The Black Death and the Peasant's Revolt." Wayland, London.

Cumpton, J. H. L. (1914). "The History of Smallpox in Australia, 1788–1908." Gov. Printer, Melbourne.

Curtin, P. D. (1964). "The Image of Africa: British Ideas and Actions, 1780–1850." Univ. of Wisconsin Press, Madison.

Deaux, G. (1969). "The Black Death." Hamish, London.

Denevan, W. M., ed. (1976). "The Native Population of the Americas in 1492." Univ. of Wisconsin Press, Madison.

Duffy, J. (1953). "Epidemics in Colonial America." Louisiana State Univ. Press, Baton Rouge.

Ehrenberg, V. (1967). "From Solon to Socrates: Greek History and Civilization During the Sixth and Fifth Centuries BC." Methuen, London.

Gelfand, M. (1953). "Medical Victory: An Account of the Influence of Medicine on the History of Southern Rhodesia." Juta, Cape Town.

Gilfillan, S. C. (1964). Roman culture and dysgenic lead poisoning. *Mankind Q.* **5,** 131–148.

Gilfillan, S. C. (1965). Lead poisoning and the fall of Rome. *J. Occup. Med.* **7,** 53–60.

Grey, I. (1964). "Ivan the Terrible." Lippincott, New York.

Haldane, J. B. S. (1949). Disease and evolution. *Ric. Sci., Suppl.* **19,** 68–76.

Hazzledine, G. D. (1969). "The White Man in Nigeria." Negro Univ. Press, New York. (Orig. publ. 1904.)

Henschen, F. (1966). "The History of Diseases." Longmans, Green, London.

Hobson, W. (1963). "World Health and History." Wright, Bristol, England.

Hoeppli, R. (1959). "Parasites and Parasitic Infections in Early Medicine and Science." Univ. of Malaya Press, Singapore.

Howe, G. M., ed. (1977). "A World Geography of Human Diseases." Academic Press, New York.

Jones, A. H. M. (1966). "The Decline of the Ancient World." Longmans, Green, London.

Jones, W. H. S. (1907). "Malaria, a Neglected Factor in the History of Greece and Rome." Cambridge Univ. Press, London.

Jones, W. H. S. (1909). "Malaria and Greek History." Manchester Univ. Press, Manchester.

Laughlin, C. D., Jr., and Brady, I. A., eds. (1978). "Extinction and Survival in Human Populations." Columbia Univ. Press, New York.

Macalpine, I., and Hunter, R. (1969). "George III and the Mad-Business." Pantheon, New York.

McCarthy, R. D. (1970). "The Ultimate Folly." Gollancz, London.

MacLaurin, C. (1922). "Post-Mortem." Doran, New York.

McNeill, W. H. (1976). "Plagues and Peoples." Blackwell, Oxford.

Marshall-Cornwall, J. (1967). "Napoleon as Military Commander." Van Nostrand, Princeton, New Jersey.

Martin, C. (1976). Wildlife diseases as a factor in the depopulation of the North American Indian. *West. Hist. Q.* 47–61.

Mazzarino, S. (1959). "The End of the Ancient World." Faber & Faber, London.

Moran, C. (1966). "Winston Churchill: The Struggle for Survival, 1940–1965." Constable, London.

Morgan, W. B., and Pugh, J. C. (1969). "West Africa." Methuen, London.

Mullett, C. F. (1956). "The Bubonic Plague and England." Univ. of Kentucky Press, Lexington.

Post, J. D. (1976). Famine, mortality, and epidemic disease in the process of modernization. *Econ. His. Rev.* **29,** 14–36.

Prinzing, F. (1916). "Epidemics Resulting from Wars." Oxford Univ. Press (Clarendon), London.

Robins, R. S. (1976). "Political Institutionalization and the Integration of Elites." Sage, Beverly Hills, California.

Russell, J. C. (1948). "British Medieval Population." Univ. of New Mexico Press, Albuerqueque.

Shrewsbury, J. F. D. (1970). "A History of Bubonic Plague in the British Isles." Cambridge Univ. Press, London and New York.

Siegel, R. E. (1960). Epidemics and infectious diseases at the time of Hippocrates: their relation to modern accounts. *Gesnerus* **17,** 77–98.

Sokhey, S. S., and Chitre, R. B. G. D. (1937). L'immunite des rats sauvages de L'Inde vis-a-vis de la peste. *Bull. Off. Int. Hyg. Publique* **29,** 2093–2096.

Stearn, E. W., and Stearn, A. E. (1945). "The Effect of Smallpox on the Destiny of the Amerindian." Humphries, Boston, Massachusetts.

Thucydides (1959). "The Peloponnesian War" (T. Hobbes, transl.; D. Grene, ed.). Univ. of Michigan Press, Ann Arbor.

Vossler, H. A. (1969). "With Napoleon in Russia: 1812" (W. Wallich, trans.). Folio Soc., London.

Waldon, H. A. (1973). Lead poisoning in the ancient world. *Med. Hist.* **17,** 391–399.

Watson, M. (1957). "African Highway: The Battle for Health in Central Africa." Murray, London.

Weinstein, E. A. (1967). Denial of presidential disability: a case study of Woodrow Wilson. *Psychiatry* **30**, 376–391.

Winslow, O. E. (1974). "A Destroying Angel: The Conquest of Smallpox in Colonial Boston." Houghton, Boston, Massachusetts.

World Health Organization (1970). "Health Aspects of Chemical and Biological Weapons." WHO, Geneva.

Ziegler, P. (1969). "The Black Death." Collins, London.

7
Ethnic Groups: A Paradigm

HENRY ROTHSCHILD

I. INTRODUCTION

In his "On Airs, Waters, and Places," written about 400 BC, Hippocrates counseled us about the value to medicine of such factors as the seasons, winds, waters, urbanization, topography, and the "mode in which the inhabitants live." Since that time, the association of geographic, climatic, and sociological factors and disease continued to be stressed, culminating in August Hirsch's (1883–1886) "Handbuch der geographischen und historischen Pathologie" toward the end of the nineteenth century. Later, as technology advanced, scientists were no longer content with mere descriptions of environment–disease associations, and they took up a reductionistic quest for principles to explain the pathogenesis of diseases. Thus, medical inquiry shifted its focus because, as Ackerknecht (1965) noted, "spectacular discoveries in bacteriology seemed to make all further research in other directions utterly superfluous."

As instrumentation and experimental design—and with them, data validity—improved, the chasm between ignorance and the understanding of disease pathophysiology narrowed. As scientists learned more of the inciting organism's molecular structure and of the host's physiological milieu, their knowledge of

177

infectious diseases expanded. As they probed the atom and unraveled the double helix, they made great strides in advancing the understanding of hormonal influences in metabolic diseases and gene mutations in simple monogenic disease. Optimistically, they began to believe that the understanding of most diseases lay just beyond their reach, blocked only by the ignorance that could be resolved by a few imminent discoveries in molecular biology.

Yet understanding of common but probably more complex diseases, such as coronary artery disease and diabetes, continues to elude us. Despite the unprecedented amount of money and research that have been channeled into studying these diseases, their pathogenesis and effective treatment remain obscure.

Perhaps some of the difficulties encountered in delineating the web of factors contributing to the pathogenesis of some diseases may be resolved by concentrating our studies on a properly chosen human model. Thus diseases which have resisted definition by study of isolated cases, families of various sizes, or cross sections of the population may be more amenable to study in genetically and/or environmentally homogeneous groups. Study of properly chosen ethnic groups— ones in which the prevalence of given diseases is either high or low—may enable us to understand the pathogenesis of some of these hitherto poorly understood diseases.

Finding the appropriate ethnic group, whether racial, national, religious, or geographic, may be becoming an increasingly difficult task. Peoples of similar genetic and cultural heritages have increasingly diverged, become mixed, and have altered their internal and external environments. The twentieth century has witnessed a remarkable transformation in the pattern and magnitude of world migration, a movement of people that has profoundly changed the demographic order. Increasing mobility has dispersed and mixed breeding isolates. Except in isolated pockets of the world, ''inbreeding'' now rarely occurs. Therefore, knowledge of the gene pool and environmental factors, including the presence of physical, chemical, and infectious vectors, cultural ceremonials, climate, and geography, may be as essential for understanding some of the complex disease processes as is knowledge of the molecular biology of the process. Cited here are a few instances where, either by accident or by design, such knowledge has been fruitful or may be helpful in our understanding of diseases.

II. LESSONS FROM THE PAST

A. Etiology

Awareness of the cultural customs and rituals of an ethnic group was critical to delineating the cause and pathogenesis of a group of human neurological diseases. Until about a decade ago, chronic progressive neurological diseases were labeled simply as degenerative. Gajdusek (1978) and colleagues, however, by thorough study of the rites of a small isolated group, demonstrated that unconventional (slow) viruses can cause chronic neurological diseases.

While studying among the endocannibalistic Fore people, an isolated mesolithic culture in the Eastern Highlands of Papua, New Guinea, Gajdusek learned of kuru, a fatal brain disease that had been prevalent among the group for a half century. The disease, confined to 19 adjacent villages, involved 11 culturally and linguistically distinct populations in the mountainous interior. Common in children of both sexes and in women, but rare in men, kuru was the group's major cause of death. In some villages among the Fore, about 90% of all deaths in adult women were attributed to kuru.

Originally, the disease was thought to be genetically determined (Gajdusek and Zigas, 1957), and, from pedigree data, Bennett *et al.* (1959) proposed a single-gene hypothesis. Epidemiological studies of kuru had given no evidence of contagiousness; no outsiders to the Fore region ever developed kuru after residence in the area. Furthermore, the disease had developed in some Fore natives years after they left the region for schooling or work.

Knowledge of the target population's customs, and awareness that not all members had equal access to nutritional resources, directed the investigators to the conclusion that the mechanism of spread was undoubtedly contamination from dead relatives during the cannibalistic rite of respect and mourning. Among the Fore, the butchering of dead kinsmen was left to the women. The mourning rite, in which close contact with the corpse was maintained and all tissues were cooked and eaten, thus resulted in the infection of most women and many of the small children. Boys, however, left the female society at 4-6 years of age and generally did not take part in the cannibalistic rites, thereby usually avoiding contamination. Men rarely ate the flesh of dead kuru victims. This avoidance by males accounted for the observed difference in incidence by sex, the disease having occurred preponderantly in women.

With cessation of the cannibalistic ritual during the last two decades kuru has virtually disappeared from New Guinea; no one born since the ritual ceased has ever developed the disease. All childhood kuru has thus been eliminated.

The notable fact is, however, that understanding of the disease process is insufficient to establish cause if it is not supplemented with laboratory information. For kuru, once the mechanism of transmission was established, laboratory investigations then showed the disease was caused by an unconventional (slow) virus. Work with kuru and Creutzfeldt–Jakob disease (another human disease), scrapie and transmissible mink encephalopathy (two animal diseases)—classed together as subacute spongioform encephalopathies—has shown they are caused by filterable viruslike agents that cause diseases with long latency periods.

B. Genetic Heterogeneity

Study of disease variation in specific ethnic groups has also been helpful in differentiating diseases that have similar phenotypic manifestations but are actually caused by different mechanisms. Common examples of this phenomenon are the hemolytic anemias, which, until the turn of the century, were lumped together as one disease. Now we know there are multiple causes of hemolysis. Our knowledge about some of the causes, e.g., sickle hemoglobin, thalassemia, glucose-6-phosphate dehydrogenase (G6PD) deficiency, was enhanced by studying these defects in specific ethnic groups.

As long ago as the sixth century BC the Greek philosopher Pythagoras warned his followers against eating the fava bean, or even against walking through fields in which it was growing. Later it was noted that only certain persons whose heritage was from around the Mediterranean and who ate raw or partly cooked fava beans (or breathed the pollen from a flowering plant) became ill. Everyone else—those without the genetic defect or those unexposed to the environmental agent—was unaffected. Later, hemolysis was also seen to occur after those having the genetic defect were exposed to infection or had ingested any of several drugs. Neither the environmental factor nor the gene defect alone is sufficient to produce the effect.

The inherited defect was subsequently found to be due to a deficiency of an X-linked red blood cell enzyme (Dern *et al.*, 1954). Different variants of the enzyme have been found in high frequency throughout the world, especially in a wide belt of tropical Africa, the Near East, India, Southeast Asia, South America, China, Arabia, the Philippines, and around the Mediterranean—all areas with a high incidence of malaria. Numerous variants of the enzyme were found; some were not associated with clinical signs or symptoms, whereas others were associated with chronic hemolytic anemia, some in the absence of exogenous agents and others necessitating the presence of those agents.

Two clinically important types of deficient enzyme are GdA⁻, found mainly in blacks, and Gd Mediterranean, found primarily in groups originating in the Mediterranean basin. Drug-induced hemolytic anemia is more severe in persons with Gd Mediterranean than with GdA⁻, and under a given oxidant stress there may be inadequate compensation in the former and yet a compensated hemolytic state in the latter.

C. Evolutionary Insights

G6PD deficiency distribution in ethnic groups exemplifies another use of biocultural interactions in the study of human disease. G6PD, when present in the homozygous state, may be detrimental, or even lethal, but in the heterozygous state may provide the carrier with a selective advantage.

Despite the disadvantage of such a gene, its continued prevalence can possibly be explained by the correspondence in geographic distribution of G6PD deficiency and falciparum malaria. Motulsky (1960) and Allison (1960) suggested that being heterozygous for this genetic trait provides resistance to malaria. The trait does not necessarily protect against malarial infection, but it may confer at least partial resistance to malaria. This resistance, expressed primarily in childhood, was found to differ significantly between carriers and persons with normal variants. The proportion of parasite carriers among female heterozygotes is similar to that of the normal population, but their infections are usually milder, and the frequency of infection is less than might be expected. The level of parasitemia, however, is sometimes greater among carriers than in most persons without the gene and may persist long enough to produce gametocytes.

A possible explanation for the advantage of the G6PD heterozygotes may be the use of common enzymatic pathways by the parasite and the host. *Plasmodium falciparum* and possibly *P. malariae* may use the oxidative pathway of carbohydrate metabolism, which may involve a rate-limiting enzyme needed for the parasite to proliferate.

Parenthetically, study of the distribution of this polymorphic enzyme in heterozygous females has provided evidence in human beings for the concept of X inactivation that Lyon (1961) demonstrated in mice (Beutler *et al.,* 1962). According to this hypothesis, only one X chromosome is "active" in a given cell, and, therefore, females with genes for GdB and GdA⁻, for example, have clones of cells that are either normal (B) or deficient (A⁻) rather than cells all of which have intermediate activity.

D. Disease Variation

The spectrum and variability of diseases that may be caused by the Epstein–Barr virus (EBV), exemplifies not only the complexity of the biocultural interactions in the pathogenesis, but also the use of ethnic groups to observe variation in reactions to an inciting agent.

Although the structure of EBV and its interaction with the host are fairly well understood, we are only beginning to understand the role of the virus in causing variation in disease. Response to the virus varies with the age, socioeconomic status, and genetic constitution of the host, and with the geographic location of the affected person. Apparently, to understand the diversity of disease attributable to EBV, one must delineate not only the molecular biology of the virus but also the biocultural interactions with the host.

The virus is ubiquitous; antibody to EBV is evident in every population thus far tested, including populations living in such remote areas that even measles and influenza antibodies are often undetectable. Although infection with the virus is common, resultant disease is not only rare but also varied, different ethnic groups manifesting different diseases.

EBV is unique among human pathogens in that it infects B lymphocytes in preference to other types of blood cells (Pattengale *et al.*, 1974), with some noteworthy exceptions (zur Hausen *et al.*, 1970). The virus stimulates repeated rounds of cell division of B lymphocytes. This response is specific in the sense that only B lymphocytes respond in this way because they possess a receptor for EBV on their surfaces. However, most of the atypical lymphocytes in the blood of patients with infectious mononucleosis are T cells. Some may be cytotoxic toward EBV-containing B cells and others inhibit the activation and proliferation of B cells (Tosato *et al.*, 1979).

EBV causes infectious mononucleosis, an acute, usually benign lympho-proliferative disease of adolescents and young adults in industrialized countries. The virus is also intimately associated with, and probably causes, two different neoplasms, Burkitt's lymphoma and nasopharyngeal carcinoma. Although the virus can induce malignant lymphoma in nonhuman primates, it has not been established that it is the causative agent in these neoplasms; it may merely colonize the cells of these tumors.

Socioeconomic status correlates empirically with infectious mononucleosis incidence. In lower but not upper socioeconomic groups, infection is usually acquired during early childhood. In the United States, the prevalence of EBV antibody in children less than 6 years old is about 80% in lower socioeconomic groups, but only about 15% in those of higher socioeconomic levels (Andiman, 1979). Children, however, rarely show the classical clinical picture of fever, sore throat, lymphadenopathy, and lymphocytosis with atypical lymphocytes. About 10–15% of those persons without antibodies who become college freshman (and, therefore, considered to be in the higher socioeconomic group) become infected and manifest the disease. Evans *et al.* (1968) noted that in Connecticut during a period of rapid industrial development from 1948 to 1967, the annual incidence of infectious mononucleosis increased 25-fold. Although more than 80% of the children become seropositive for EBV before 2 years of age in developing countries, clinical infectious mononucleosis is extremely rare. However, as hygienic conditions and socioeconomic levels improve in the developing countries, the incidence of classical infectious mononucleosis has increased.

One may infer, therefore, that the infectious pattern corresponds to antibody profiles of infants, which may be the result of differences in living conditions. In lower socioeconomic groups, younger children are likely to be exposed to the virus. Early antibody development thereby limits the infection in adolescence, when the virus is associated with morbidity. However, this is not the complete explanation, as African children develop antibodies to EBV early in infancy but subsequently develop Burkitt's lymphoma.

Although no relationship between infectious mononucleosis and increased risk of cancer has been shown, EBV infection has been associated with two malignant tumors that affect primarily two different ethnic groups. Because those manifestations of EBV infection are less easily explained, other biocultural factors must be implicated. That nasopharyngeal carcinoma and African or endemic Burkitt's lymphoma are caused by EBV, for example, has not been proved, although the circumstantial evidence is considerable. The virus, first discovered in a biopsy specimen taken from a child with Burkitt's lymphoma (Epstein *et al.*, 1964), causes tumors in nonhuman primates, and multiple copies of the viral genome have been found in human tumor cells (zur Hausen *et al.*, 1970).

As described by Burkitt (see Chapter 5), the malignant tumor that now bears his name affects primarily the jaw and affects children between the ages of 1 and 14 years, with the highest incidence occurring between ages 6 and 8 years. Burkitt's lymphoma has a limited geographical distribution in the hot, wet lowland of equatorial Africa (Burkitt, 1962). The disease is endemic in several regions of both East and West Africa and New Guinea, and its occurrence is sporadic and infrequent outside those areas. Burkitt's lymphoma accounts for as much as 60% of all childhood cancers in Nigeria.

Because most nonendemic cases are EBV-genome negative, Burkitt's lymphoma may in effect be another example of disease heterogeneity, two diseases manifesting with similar phenotypes. Nonendemic cases also differ from African Burkitt's lymphoma in age distribution and tumor sites. Otherwise both endemic and nonendemic Burkitt's lymphomas appear to be clinicially indistinguishable; both originate from B lymphocytes, have similar histology, and have a unique cytogenetic abnormality; a small segment of chromosome 8 is translocated to the long arm of chromosome 14, and a small segment of chromosome 14 to chromosome 8. Both show good clinical response to chemotherapy.

Practically all children in the endemic areas have antibodies to the EBV by age 3 years. Like the endemic cases, a small but significant number of nonendemic cases, including those found in the United States, are associated with a wide range of serum antibodies to EBV-determined antigens, including viral DNA and nuclear membrane neoantigens. The genome-positive endemic form is relatively frequent, but the genome-positive nonendemic form is rare.

As was suggested by Burkitt (1962), the expression of African Burkitt's lymphoma may require both the virus and a climate-dependent cofactor, the distribution of which determines the endemic zones. During the late 1950s Burkitt concluded, from careful clinical observations, that the distribution of the tumor is influenced by geographical factors associated with temperature and rainfall. The tumor occurs in areas that have an elevation of less than 1800 m, an annual rainfall of 60 cm, and an average temperature of more than 16°C. These circumstances suggested that an arthropod vector might be the carrier of an oncogenic virus. Moreover, analysis of the epidemiological data indicated a geographical association between the incidence of malaria, which occurs in a well-defined tropical belt of Africa, and that of Burkitt's lymphoma. Malaria has been suggested as the essential geographically restrictive cofactor enabling the emergence of target cells capable of malignant transformation by interaction with EBV. This explanation, however, is insufficient to account for the other types of disease caused by EBV in other areas where malaria abounds.

At present, there is no apparent explanation for the ethnic distribution of nasopharyngeal carcinoma, a squamous cell carcinoma with lymphocytic infiltration of the epithelial lining. The tumor affects mostly adults, with a peak incidence at age 40. It has its highest incidence in southern China, especially in Guandong Province, where it has an overall frequency as high as 39.9 per 100,000 persons per year, which is about 40 times that of whites living in California. The tumor's incidence is also high among Chinese living in other areas. In Singapore the age-standardized incidence per 100,000 per year is 18.7 for Chinese men and 7.1 for Chinese women, with variation among the major Chinese dialectic groups (29.1 and 11.0 among Cantonese, 17.4 and 5.9 among Teochews, and 13.7 and 4.4 among Hokkiens) (Shanmugaratnam, 1977). For other peoples of Southeast Asia, e.g., Thais, the rates appear intermediate. The tumor has also been frequently found among natives in Kenya, especially the Nandi tribe (Clifford, 1970). Apparently the carcinoma is rare in Northern China, Japan, western Europe, the United States, and elsewhere in the world. No EBV-genome-negative samples have yet been reported.

The explanation for its ethnic distribution appears to be neither wholly genetic nor wholly geographic. Among first-generation immigrants to the United States from South China, the high frequency of nasopharyngeal carcinoma declines somewhat but remains considerably above that of the white population. The incidence of this tumor among emigrants of this ethnic group, whether to other parts of China or to the United States, remains higher than among other ethnic groups (Buell, 1974). For offspring of mixed marriages between South Chinese and other ethnic groups, the tumor frequency is intermediate.

Infection with EBV in areas endemic for Burkitt's lymphoma and nasopharyngeal carcinoma occurs at an early age, similar to that found in the lower socioeconomic populations in the United States. However, the antibody titers in the patients with these tumors are 10- to 15-fold higher than in the respective control population in each locale. Thus, unlike protection against infectious mononucleosis, in these ethnic groups or locales early antibody response appears to be associated with tumor formation.

Some investigators have suggested that the protean manifestations and the diverse ethnic response to the virus could be due to the geographic distribution of different strains of viruses. That does not, however, appear to be the explanation, because all strains of EBV, from whatever source, have remarkably uniform structure and biological behavior (Rymo et al., 1979). The one variant of EBV that has been isolated was probably the result of laboratory manipulations, as the parent virus from which the apparent virus was derived was antigenically similar to the other viruses.

Again the point is emphasized: one must know not only the inciting agent but also the gene pool and the environment of the target population. Furthermore, by observing the differences in diseases produced by an inciting organism among the ethnic groups, we may not only be able to understand better the virus–host interactions but also to begin to gain insight into oncogenic transformation in humans.

E. Benefit of Hindsight

We may even be able to learn more about disease mechanisms by studying disease distribution that obtained among ethnic groups in times past. The discovery of the cause of rickets and tetany and the distribution of these diseases and hysteria may help us to understand how knowledge of the environment, including the diet, habitat, and working conditions of ethnic groups, can give us insight into the pathogenesis of diseases that were prevalent in the past. Consider, for example, that in latitudes where ultraviolet solar radiation is not intense, such as in parts of Europe, a pale skin lets enough ultraviolet light penetrate to produce adequate amounts of vitamin D for growth (Loomis, 1967). Of the neolithic Europeans whose diet consisted largely of cereals (which contain the precursors of vitamin D but not the vitamin itself) and little animal protein, the most likely to survive and procreate were those who were deficient in skin pigmentation.

During the Industrial Revolution in England, when the rural population became urbanized, lived in dark slums, and worked in factories during the day, tetany and rickets became prevalent. As was later understood, the change in the work and living patterns of the society allowed the new group of diseases to appear.

Between 1880 and 1895, the working classes of European cities had an epidemic of hypocalcemic tetany that may be attributable to these environmental factors. The cause of that plague of tetany was not understood at the time because the role of calcium in tetany had not been established. Screening out the sun prevented the vitamin D precursors from converting to the active form of the vitamin in sufficient quantity. More recently, cases of rickets have been reported in immigrant Pakistanis who migrated to England and had working and housing conditions similar to those available to workers at the end of the eighteenth century.

The epidemic of rickets and/or tetany—precipitated by constraints of custom, economy, food, dress, working hours, and access to open spaces and lighting, not only among working people but also among all classes in late nineteenth century Europe—coincided with the popularization of hysteria as a psychiatric diagnosis in this population. During the early twentieth century, the general amelioration of social conditions and the discoveries of the value of sunlight, milk, and vitamin D-containing foods were accompanied by greatly reduced frequencies of rickets, tetany, and hysteria. Thus, one may ask whether the study of the physiological milieu of hypocalcemia of Europeans during that period would not have revealed a conditioning factor in hysteria.

III. CONCLUSION

Increasingly appreciated is the fact that no single discipline can provide the methods for study, the knowledge necessary for interpretation of data, or the breadth of vision that are needed for understanding the complex pathogenesis of some of the common diseases. Does the biologist ever give credence to motive as a cause? Does the psychologist ever analyze trace elements in the soil? Without abandoning *Drosophila* and *E. coli* altogether, let's back off a bit in our collective view to see a larger, albeit more complex, model—that of biocultural interactions.

Perhaps because we have peered so long through the microscope, our view has become microscopic. The study of complex diseases will necessitate revitalizing the historical and geographic approach to disease that once formed the groundwork of medical knowledge. Unfortunately, that approach was deemphasized with the advent of the laboratory. While fully recognizing the advantages of molecular biology, we must appreciate the macro-influences, placing the study of ethnogenic, social, and ecological factors on a parity with the study of laboratory-pursued factors.

REFERENCES

Ackerknecht, E. H. (1965). "History and Geography of the Most Important Diseases." Hafner, New York.

Allison, A. C. (1960). Glucose-6-phosphate dehydrogenase deficiency in red blood cells of East Africans. *Nature (London)* **186**, 531–532.

Andiman, W. A. (1979). The Epstein–Barr virus and EB virus infections in childhood. *J. Pediatr.* **95**, 171–82.

Bennett, H. G., Pholes, F. A., and Robson, H. N. (1959). A possible genetic basis for kuru. *Am. J. Hum. Genet.* **11**, 169–187.

Beutler, E., Yeh, M., and Fairbanks, V. F. (1962). The normal human female as a mosaic of X-chromosome activity: studies using the gene for G-6-PD-deficiency as a marker. *Proc. Natl. Acad. Sci. U.S.A.* **48**, 9–16.

Buell, P. (1974). The effect of migration on the risk of nasopharyngeal cancer among Chinese. *Cancer Res.* **34**, 1189–1191.

Burkitt, D. (1962). Determining the climatic limitations of a children's cancer common in Africa. *Br. Med. J.* **ii**, 1019–2310.

Clifford, P. (1970). A review on the epidemiology of nasopharyngeal carcinoma. *Int. J. Cancer* **5**, 287–309.

Dern, R. J., Weinstein, I. M., LeRoy, G. V., Ralmage, D. W., and Alving, A. S. (1954). The hemolytic effect of primaquine. I: The localization of the drug-induced hemolytic defect in primaquine-sensitive individuals. *J. Lab. Clin. Med.* **43,** 303–309.

Epstein, M. A., Achong, B. C., and Barr, Y. M. (1964). Virus particles in cultured lymphoblasts from Burkitt's lymphoma. *Lancet* **1,** 702–703.

Evans, A. S., Niederman, J. C., and McCollum, R. W. (1968). Seroepidemiologic studies of infectious mononucleosis with EB virus. *N. Engl. J. Med.* **279,** 1121–1127.

Gajdusek, D. C. (1978). Unconventional viruses. *In* "Human Diseases Caused by Viruses" (H. Rothschild, F. Allison, Jr., and C. Howe, eds.), pp. 231–258. Oxford Univ. Press, London and New York.

Gajdusek, D. C., and Zigas V. (1957). Degenerative diseases of the central nervous system in New Guinea; the endemic occurrence of "kuru" in the native population. *N. Engl. J. Med.* **257,** 974–978.

Hirsch, A. (1883–1886). "Handbuch der geographischen und historischen Pathologie" (C. Creighton, transl.), 3 Vols. New Sydenham, London.

Loomis, W. F. (1967). Skin pigment regulation of vitamin D biosynthesis in man. *Science* **157,** 501–506.

Lyon, M. F. (1961). Gene action in the X-chromosome of the mouse (*Mus musculus L*). *Nature (London)* **190,** 372–373.

Motulsky, A. G. (1960). Metabolic polymorphisms and the role of infectious diseases in human evolution. *Hum. Biol.* **32,** 28–62.

Pattengale, P. K., Smith, R. W., and Gerber, P. (1974). B-cell characteristics of human peripheral and cord blood lymphocytes transformed by Epstein–Barr virus. *J. Natl. Cancer Inst.* **52,** 1081–1086.

Rymo, L., Lindahl, T., and Adams, A. (1979). Sites of sequence variability in Epstein–Barr virus DNA from different sources. *Proc. Natl. Acad. Sci. U.S.A.* **76,** 2794–2798.

Shanmugaratnam, K. (1977). Variations in nasopharyngeal cancer incidence among specific Chinese communities (dialect groups) in Singapore. *IARC Sci Publ.* **20,** 191–198.

Tosato, G., Magrath, I., Koski, I., Dooley, N., and Blaese, M. (1979). Activation of suppressor T-cells during Epstein–Barr-virus-induced infectious mononucleosis. *N. Engl. J. Med.* **301,** 1133–1137.

zur Hausen, H., Schulte-Holthausen H., Klein, G., Henle, W., Clifford, P., and Santesson, L. (1970). EBV DNA in biopsies of Burkitt tumors and anaplastic carcinomas of the nasopharynx. *Nature (London)* **228,** 1056–1058.

II
Populations and Disease

8

Diseases of North American Indians

MAURICE L. SIEVERS and JEFFREY R. FISHER

I. ORIGIN OF THE AMERICAN INDIAN

The Americas have been populated by immigrants. Even the aboriginal ancestors of the American Indian migrated to the western hemisphere from Siberia, 10,000–40,000 years before Columbus discovered the New World. These early

191

BIOCULTURAL ASPECTS OF DISEASE

Americans probably arrived during the last stage of the Pleistocene Ice Age, the Wisconsin glaciation, when ice sheets sequestered vast amounts of water, and caused the sea level to fall. Where the Bering Strait now exists, a broad land bridge connected Siberia with Alaska, and extended some 1000 miles in width when the glacial ice was at its maximum (Willey, 1966). Although the precise time of man's arrival in the New World is not established, Campbell (1963) presents compelling evidence that the optimum time for man to have crossed this land mass would probably have been after the final Wisconsin glacial advance, between 18,000 and 20,000 years ago. During that period, the land bridge was maximally exposed. Massive sheets of ice caused the forests to retreat, and with the subsequent spread of tundra vegetation, large herds of foraging game animals proliferated. Furthermore, the cold weather and glacial conditions facilitated traversing the otherwise wet and boggy terrain as man hunted the abundant herds of bison, caribou, mammoth, and musk-ox from Asia into the New World. When the ice melted and the sea level rose, the descendants of these early hunters were isolated from their Siberian origin by the narrowing and eventual disappearance of the land bridge more than 8000 years ago.

The American Indian, also referred to as "Amerind," entered the Western hemisphere at a time when neither human nor subhuman anthropoid forms existed in the New World. Whether the Amerind's subsequent evolution was from a single archaic *Homo sapiens* stock or from a mixture of *sapiens* types is debated (Jennings, 1974). In either case, the forebears of the American Indian resembled no modern racial group very closely. After the submersion of the Bering land bridge, the American Indian evolved in relative isolation from other members of the human family. With no competitive human population and in response to the wide variety of environmental zones, these paleo-Indian migrants developed phenotypic variation as they dispersed throughout the Americas. Geneotypic differentiation appeared in population isolates as the result of random mutation and natural selection. Genetic drift and the founder effect also contributed to many of the heritable differences that now exist among tribal groups. Variability in certain polymorphic genetic traits tends to obscure, but does not obliterate, the evidence of common ancestry and considerable racial homogeneity of the American Indian. We emphasize, however, that these observations apply only to the first migrants and their descendants, who, nonetheless, comprise most of the present tribes of North, South, and Meso-America. Excluded are the genetically distinct later arrivals of the past 6000 years—the Eskimo, Aleut, and Amerind of the Na-Déné language group, which includes the Athapascan-speaking Navajo and Apache of the southwestern United States.

II. MONGOLOID AFFINITY

The Asiatic origin of the American Indian is widely accepted. Contemporary Amerinds exhibit numerous phenotypic traits attesting to their Mongoloid origin.

They have oriental facial characteristics—high and broad cheek bones, moderate epicanthic folds, dark brown eyes, and coarse, straight, black hair. Facial and body hair is scanty, and hair follicles are characteristically absent on the middle phalanges of the hand (Danforth, 1921). The Indian men seldom show a receding hairline, and balding is unusual. Graying of the hair generally occurs only late in life. Skin pigmentation varies from light tan to dark brown. Among Amerind infants, the so-called Mongolian spot—a transitory, irregular, darkly pigmented area of skin over the lumbosacral area—occurs frequently. The teeth conform to the "Mongoloid master pattern" (Matis and Zwemer, 1971), which includes shovel-shaped maxillary incisors (Fig. 1), a low frequency of Carbelli's cusp (a pit, groove, ridge, or cusp on the lingual surface of the maxillary molars), a relatively high frequency of lingual exostoses or mandibular tori between the mandibular canines and molars at their apical level, and a low frequency of three-rooted mandibular first molars, similar to the dentition of several living Asian populations (Turner, 1971).

More subtle polymorphic traits characteristic of both Mongoloid and Amerind populations include relatively high prevalences of dry cerumen (Petrakis *et al.*, 1967) and typical cholinesterase alleles (Lubin *et al.*, 1971); the ability to inactivate the drug isoniazid (INH) rapidly (Scott *et al.*, 1969) and to taste phenylthiocarbamide (PTC) (Garn, 1971; Mourant *et al.*, 1976); and the capacity to secrete ABH substances in the saliva and to excrete β-aminoisobutyric acid (BAIB) in the urine (Garn, 1971; Mourant *et al.*, 1976). However, with regard to establishing Mongoloid affinity, none of these attributes alone discriminates meaningfully. Of greater utility are such factors as the Diego blood group (Di^a) and the atypical transferrin D$_{chi}$, which occur in Amerinds and Asiatics but are absent or rare in non-Mongoloids (Larisse, 1968).

Despite numerous similarities reflecting a common ancestry, the Amerind differ decidedly from contemporary Mongoloid populations. Indeed, having lived for millennia in geographic isolation from all other human populations, the

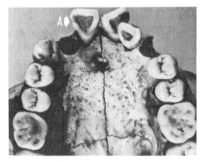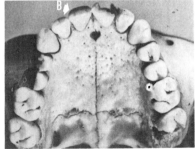

Fig. 1. Shovel-shaped incisors of an American Indian (arrow A) is one of several characteristic dental traits. Incisors of European origin (arrow B) lack shoveling. (Photographs by Christy G. Turner, II; reproduced by permission.)

American Indian is considered by many authorities to form a separate race. Amerind distinctiveness emerges on examination of composite genetic traits. Roychoudhury (1978) evaluated the gene frequencies of 14 blood groups and 12 protein loci in determining the genetic distance between the American Indian and three other races—Caucasoid, Negroid, and Mongoloid. This study and others, in which such factors as correspondence analysis of HLA-gene frequencies (Greenacre and Degos, 1977) and the characteristics of finger and palmar dermatoglyphics (Rife, 1968) were examined, support the concept of Amerind racial individuality with close Mongoloid affinity. In addition, certain hematologic traits present in other racial groups are not found in full-heritage American Indians. These traits include blood groups A_2, B, K, and Rh-factor negativity, as well as atypical alloimmunoglobulins and abnormal hemoglobins (Larisse, 1968; Garn, 1971; Mourant *et al.*, 1976; Gershowitz and Neel, 1978). When present, these findings indicate non-Indian admixture.

Despite considerable racial homogeneity, it should be stressed that somatic, biochemical, and hematologic variations do exist among, and even within, many Amerind tribes. For example, the serum albumin variant Naskapi is found primarily in the Algonquin and Athapascan language groups, whereas alloalbumin Mexico is noted predominantly in the more southern Uto-Aztecan-speaking tribes, but neither albumin type has been identified in the sera of non-Indians (Blumberg, 1969). American Indian populations clearly do not constitute a single gene pool. The extent, nature, and anthropological significance of this biologic heterogeneity have been reviewed elsewhere (Larisse, 1968; Garn, 1971; Mourant *et al.*, 1976), and will be considered in this chapter only as related to the variable expression of disease in different tribes. The preceding discussion of the origin and physical attributes of the American Indian provides a background for subsequent biomedical considerations.

III. MODERN INDIAN POPULATIONS

Where today is the Pequot? Where are the Narragansetts, the Mohawks, the Pokanowet. . . .?
(*Tecumseh*, Shawnee chief, 1765–1813)

In North America, more than 432 American Indian tribes have been identified, of which at least 391 reside within the United States (Swanton, 1952). The present U.S. population of Amerinds is slightly less than 1 million (U.S. Department of HEW, 1978a), which is fewer than the estimated number in that region about 500 years ago (Dobyn, 1966). After the early European contact, the American Indian population progressively decreased because of epidemic disease, famine, warfare, and hardship. It reached a nadir of about 250,000 in 1890 (Driver, 1969). The largest tribe, the Navajo, which now numbers about 150,000, was only about one-twentieth its present size 110 years ago (Dutton, 1976).

American Indians now reside throughout the United States but are located predominantly in 25 reservation states, ranging from Florida to Alaska (U.S. Department of HEW, 1978a). Oklahoma, Arizona, California, and New Mexico have the largest Amerind populations. Although many Indians have been assimilated to varying degrees into the non-Indian society, most live in their own Indian communities.

In the Southwest, Native Americans, who continue to reside mostly on isolated reservations, have retained a higher proportion of Indian heritage than in most other regions. However, both the genetic and the environmental conditions are changing. Although an estimated 94% of the southwestern Indians 15 years or older putatively have full heritage, only 80% of this population younger than 15 years are full-blooded. Differences between living conditions on- and off-reservation have rapidly narrowed. For example, as recently as 1959 at least 60% of the White Mountain Apache lived in wickiups, the traditional tribal dwelling (Tribal pamphlet, 1960), but now this type of housing is rare. In addition, contemporary Hopi Indians have substantially more lead, zinc, and copper and less strontium in their teeth than has been found in seventeenth century Hopis who lived in the same isolated geographic area (Kuhnlein and Calloway, 1977). Indeed, trace metal content in teeth is similar for Hopis of the post-industrial period and for California suburban residents.

IV. GENERAL HEALTH CONSIDERATIONS

A. Pre-Columbian and Early Historic Periods

The health status of prehistoric American Indians is largely conjectural. A frequently expressed opinion is that the absence of large and dense human populations in pre-Columbian North America spared the Amerind from the "crowd-dependent" epidemics that ravaged the Old World during that period (Hrdlička, 1932; Stewart, 1973). Furthermore, it has been postulated that the "cold screen" presented by the arctic route of man's entry into the New World effectively filtered many infectious agents, and that the subsequent isolation of the Americas limited the introduction of pathogenic micoorganisms before 1492 (Stewart, 1973). Indeed, Hrdlička (1932), the renowned Smithsonian anthropologist and physician, while categorizing the various diseases found in skeletal remains of paleo-Indians, concluded that in the pre-Columbian period the inhabitants of America were unusually healthy. This opinion was based largely on an examination of several thousand early Indian skeletons. We should stress, however, that the study of bones, even by currently available techniques, has major limitations for the discernment of most human diseases. Nevertheless, many reports by explorers and physicians who made early contact with the Indians of North America stressed the extraordinarily good health of the Native Americans.

The harsh environmental conditions endured by the early Amerind undoubtedly resulted in the natural selection of hardy people. Nonetheless, the otherwise sturdy descendants of these early Americans were decimated by certain viral diseases introduced by Europeans. The excessive morbidity and mortality experienced by American Indians during epidemics of smallpox, measles (rubeola), and influenza have been interpreted as being due to unusual racial vulnerability. However, the devastation caused by these epidemics was far more likely the result of inadequate medical care, overcrowded living conditions, and the susceptibility of every age-group because of the universal absence of acquired immunity from prior infection. Predictably, these viral diseases would have been especially severe in adults. Observations among nonimmunized populations of children have revealed that measles produces no more deleterious effects in Indians than among whites (Dale, 1949). Furthermore, the importance of medical and nursing care in the outcome of rubeola is supported by data from white populations in the United States. Early in this century the mortality from measles among U.S. whites exceeded 3%; within 50 years it declined to less than 0.1%. Most of this reduction antedated the availability of antibiotics and modern chemotherapy (Langmuir, 1962; Centerwall, 1968). Thus, the hypothesis of increased racial susceptibility of the Amerind to certain viral infections appears unsupported. In later sections of this chapter, the question of enhanced Amerind susceptibility to tuberculosis (Section V,M) and coccidioidomycosis (Section V,L) and to the effects of alcohol (Section V,H) will also be critically examined.

B. Contemporary Period

Recent health and vital statistics are consistent with the disproportionate numbers of Amerinds in the lower socioeconomic and educational categories. As a reflection of a high birthrate (almost twice the U.S. all-races rate) and decreased longevity (life expectancy at birth, 6 years less than for U.S. all-races), the Indian population of the 25 reservation states in 1970 had a median age of 19.4 years, in contrast to the 28.1 years for the U.S. general population (U.S. Department of HEW, 1978a). The Indian infant mortality has declined 70% between 1955 and 1975, from 61.2 to 18.1 infant deaths per 1000 live births. In 1975, the U.S. all-races infant death rate was 16.1 per 1000 live births. Table I presents comparative mortalities for Native Americans and U.S. all-races in 1975. The first six conditions listed accounted for almost two-thirds of the deaths among Indians and Alaska Natives. The other selected categories are presented because of unusual frequencies relative to the general population. The age-adjusted death rate for the Amerind was 1.3 times the U.S. all-races rate.

Health care for American Indians has been provided since 1955 by the Indian

TABLE I

Age-Adjusted Mortality Rates for Selected Causes of Death among Indians and Alaska Natives in Reservation States and the U.S. All-Races Populations, 1975[a]

Cause of death	Number of deaths	Indian and Alaska native (rate per 100,000 population)	U.S. all-races (rate per 100,000 population)	Ratio Indian to U.S. all-races
All causes	5774	824.8	638.3	1.3
Accidents	1256	170.5	44.8	3.8
Diseases of the heart	965	147.4	220.5	0.7
Malignant neoplasms	508	79.8	130.9	0.6
Cirrhosis of the liver	355	61.4	13.8	4.4
Cerebrovascular disease	291	43.5	54.5	0.8
Influenza and pneumonia	281	36.1	16.6	2.2
Homicide	185	26.5	10.5	2.5
Suicide	180	26.0	12.6	2.1
Diabetes mellitus	145	23.8	11.6	2.1
Tuberculosis, all forms	64	9.9	1.2	8.3
Bronchitis, emphysema, and asthma	27	3.7	8.6	0.4

[a] The first six categories listed were the leading causes of death among Native Americans in 1975 (U.S. Department of HEW, 1978a).

Health Service (IHS) of the U.S. Public Health Service, a responsibility originally assumed by the War Department in the early 1800s, and subsequently by the Department of Interior (Bureau of Indian Affairs) between 1849 and 1955 (U.S. Department of HEW, 1978b). Federal health services are based on treaties and laws enacted under authority specified within the Constitution. Most reservation Indians receive their medical care from the IHS, which has a system of 51 hospitals, 99 health centers, and more than 300 health stations and satellite field health clinics (US Department of HEW, 1978b). In 1900, the Indian Medical Service employed 83 physicians, including those giving part-time services. By 1978, there were more than 600 IHS physicians (U.S. Department of HEW, 1978b).

Despite widespread acceptance of Western medicine by contemporary American Indians, native healing practices continue to serve important therapeutic functions in many tribes. Traditionally, American Indians have regarded sickness to be a result of disharmony with nature or supernatural forces. Therefore, medicine and religion have been closely intertwined. The medicine man, or shaman, utilizing ritualistic practices and considerable knowledge of the curative properties of certain plants, has long treated illness, dressed wounds, and set broken bones. Native healing practices now generally complement rather than replace the services of physicians and other professional health workers. Indeed, the IHS has recognized the significance of the native healers, especially in the management of mental health problems, and, in recent years, has encouraged the training of Navajo medicine men, in a school that has been funded under a grant from the National Institute of Mental Health (Bergman, 1973).

V. AMERIND DISEASE PATTERNS

Generally, this section will be limited to diseases that occur more frequently or are less common in American Indians than in the general population, and it will examine the relative influences of heredity and environment on these conditions. Several disorders that occur frequently in some Native American groups (skeletal and dental fluorosis, trichinosis, echinococcus, plague, diphtheria, dysentery, bacterial pneumonia, and hepatitis) will not be discussed. These conditions result primarily from adverse environmental factors or inadequate health practices and do not appear to be associated with innate susceptibility. The scope of the material will usually be confined to the Amerind population of the United States, with emphasis on tribes of the Southwest, reflecting the authors' personal experiences. When appropriate, however, other Amerind and Mongoloid populations will also be included for comparisons.

A. Diabetes Mellitus and Obesity

1. Occurrence in Early and Contemporary Periods

Until the last 40 or 50 years, diabetes mellitus was conspicuously infrequent among North American Indians. West (1974), in reviewing the health reports of civilian and military physicians serving various Amerind groups between 1832 and 1939, discovered that diabetes was rarely encountered or, less likely, was not reported by those physicians. In 1937, Elliott Joslin, the eminent diabetologist, surveyed the morbidity among the Indians of Arizona. He discovered considerable differences in the prevalence of diabetes among various tribes, but he concluded that the overall frequency of the disease in those combined tribes was similar to the rate for the U.S. general population (Joslin, 1940). Later, Felsman (1955) reported no significant difference between the Amerind and the U.S. all-races rates for age-adjusted deaths from diabetes. By 1967, however, the diabetes-related death rate for U.S. Indians was reported to be 2.3 times as high as in the general population (Hill and Spector, 1971). In the past 20 years, diabetes has attained epidemic proportions in some tribes, although rates in other tribal groups have increased less markedly and are similar to the prevalence in the general population.

Because diagnostic criteria (West, 1975; Sievers, 1976a) and case-finding methods differ in the various studies, comparisons of reported rates for diabetes in Amerind populations have some limitations. Nonetheless, diabetes has become a major cause of morbidity and mortality in most North American native groups, with the exception of some Athapascan tribes and the Eskimo (West, 1974). The type of diabetes that occurs in the Amerind is almost exclusively noninsulin-dependent, ketosis-resistant (Sievers, 1966a; West, 1978; Savage *et al.*, 1979a), as it is in other Mongoloid populations.

Much of the subsequent discussion will summarize the results of recent prospective investigations among the Pima Indians living on the Gila River Reservation in southcentral Arizona. This geographically well-defined and relatively homogeneous tribe of almost 8000 persons has the highest recorded prevalence of diabetes in the world, and is ideally suited for examination of the genetics and natural history of diabetes. They have occupied this hot, arid, desert region for at least 2000 years. Almost 50% of the Pima aged 35 years and older are diabetic—10-15 times the overall U.S. rate. Obesity is also extremely prevalent among this tribe.

Diabetes in the Pima is primarily the maturity-onset (type II) variety, characterized by the infrequency of islet cell antibodies, resistance to ketosis, and lack of insulin dependence. It is strongly associated with the histocompatibility antigen HLA-A2 (Williams *et al.*, 1981), but not with the HLA types B8 or B15 that frequently accompany juvenile-onset (type I) diabetes mellitus (Knowler *et al.*, 1979). No association between chlorpropamide-alcohol-induced cutaneous flushing and type II diabetes has been observed in this tribe (M. Nagulesparan, 1980 personal communication). Evaluation of glucagon response to arginine infusion (Aronoff *et al.*, 1977a) and hepatic extraction of endogenously secreted insulin (Savage *et al.*, 1979b) have shown no significant differences between the Pimas and Caucasians. Furthermore, this tribe and other Amerind groups incur the usual vascular and other complications of diabetes (see "complications," Section V,A,4), thus supporting the probability that studies of diabetes in the Pimas are relevant to other Indian and non-Indian populations.

2. Possible Causative Factors

a. Heredity versus Environment. Heredity is clearly an important causative factor in diabetes, although the mechanism of inheritance remains undetermined and may differ between the juvenile-onset, insulin-dependent (type I) and the maturity-onset, insulin-independent (type II) forms of the disease (Rotter and Rimoin, 1981; Cudworth, 1979). Among the Pima, diabetes has strong familial aggregation. During a 6-year period the *incidence* of diabetes was 9% in the offspring of two diabetic parents, as compared with 1.6% in the children born to parents having normal glucose tolerance (Bennett *et al.*, 1976). Nonetheless, significant differences in the prevalence of carbohydrate intolerance are encountered that cannot be explained genetically.

The White Mountain and San Carlos Apache of Arizona reside on adjacent reservations. These two Athapascan tribes are similar genetically, but glucose intolerance occurs twice as often in the more obese San Carlos Apache as in the White Mountain Apache (Bennett, 1972). Both groups, however, have moderate rates of diabetes. By contrast, diabetes has become common in certain Athapascan tribes of Oklahoma (Ft. Sill Apache and Kiowa-Apache) (West, 1974). This spectrum of disease prevalence among related Athapascan tribes suggests that environmental factors, perhaps related to the development of obesity, contribute appreciably to the occurrence of diabetes in susceptible populations.

b. Relationship of Diabetes and Obesity. Congruent with the greatly increased prevalence of diabetes, obesity also has reached epidemic proportions in some Amerind groups within the past 40–50 years (Fig. 2). Study of photographs taken in the latter part of the nineteenth century reveals that Indians from most tribes were lean (Fig. 3). Early reports by physicians working with Indians (Hrdlička, 1908; Geare, 1915; Hancock, 1933) confirm the former infrequency

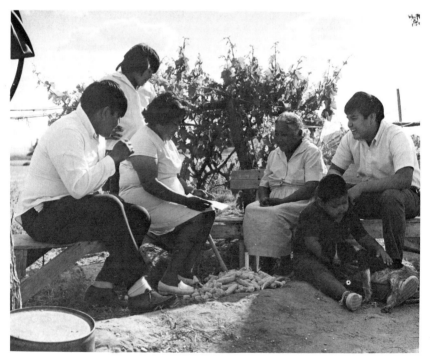

Fig. 2. A typical Pima family group, illustrating the early onset and generality of obesity.

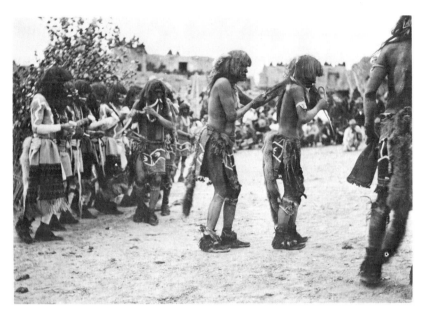

Fig. 3. Hopi snake dance at Oraibi, Arizona, August, 1900. The lean body habitus of the dancers contrasts with the obesity that is now prevalent among the Hopi and many other Indian tribes of North America. (Photograph by Summer W. Matteson; from the collection of the Milwaukee Public Museum, with permission.)

of obesity in North American Indians. As previously noted, considerable differences in prevalence of diabetes exist among various North American aboriginal groups, and, in general, tribes with the highest rates of diabetes have the greatest prevalence of obesity (West, 1974). Nonetheless, the extraordinary frequency of diabetes in the Pima cannot be attributed entirely to their obesity. Although the rate of diabetes is 2–3 times greater in obese (>125% of desirable weight) than in nonobese Pima men and women below 35 years of age, this relationship to body weight is not apparent in the older persons of this tribe (Bennett *et al.*, 1979a). These observations suggest that diabetes may emerge at an earlier age in extremely obese susceptible persons but that many elderly overweight members of the population do not have a genetic predisposition to the disease. Furthermore, in the less-obese persons with inherited susceptibility the onset of diabetes may be delayed until those persons become older.

Obesity and diabetes are clearly familial. Not yet established, however, is whether obesity is an independent variable that, if present for sufficient duration, produces diabetes in those with an inherited susceptibility or whether obesity is, itself, genetically linked to the diabetic trait. Genetic linkage of the two conditions is suggested by the observation that infants born to normal mothers and diabetic fathers have increased birth weights (Nilsson, 1962).

3. Hypothesis to Explain the Escalating Rates of Diabetes and Obesity in the Amerind

Diabetes and obesity, formerly uncommon, are now widespread among diverse Indian tribes of North America. Contemporary Amerinds undoubtedly ingest more calories and less fiber that did their ancestors. Nonetheless, the current diet of Pima Indians differs in only minor respects from that of the U.S. general population (Reid et al., 1971). The caloric expenditure has also probably decreased among American Indians, who formerly engaged regularly in strenuous physical activity but now are more sedentary.

The hypothesis of diabetes as a "thrifty" genotype rendered detrimental by "progress" was first proposed by Neel (1962). He reasoned that a people living for generations under conditions characterized by alternating periods of food scarcity and abundance might have evolved a particular propensity to expand adipose tissue during times of plenty and, therefore, have an enhanced ability to survive periods of famine. In the arid southwestern United States, tree-ring studies (Jennings, 1974) document the periodic occurrence of drought. The desert-dwelling Pima and Papago, who had relied for millennia on agriculture and food gathering for survival, now obtain most of their food from trading posts and markets. However, recent metabolic studies have not detected any significant difference between American Indians and Caucasians with regard to calorie requirements for maintenance or loss of body weight; obese persons of both races can be maintained on fewer calories than the nonobese (Hendrikx, 1979a,b). Perhaps these short-term observations may be too insensitive to detect the more subtle influences of a "thrifty" genotype producing weight gain over long periods.

A gene for "hyperinsulinemia," which promotes fat storage, would theoretically be advantageous in conditions of feast or famine, and would likely outweigh any disadvantages until food supplies became constant and plentiful. When such a change occurred, widespread obesity would supervene, especially if food supplies became abundant in a relatively short time, precluding genetic adaptation. Although hyperinsulinemia is associated with obesity in all races, nondiabetic Pima Indians have fasting and postglucose-load insulin levels that exceed those for age-matched similarly obese Caucasians (Fig. 4). The difference in insulin levels between Caucasians and Pimas is probably due to racial variation (Aronoff et al., 1977b). Nondiabetic Indians of the genetically distinct Navajo tribe also have been reported to have higher insulin levels after oral glucose administration than occurs in Caucasians of similar weight (Rimoin, 1969). Furthermore, fasting insulin levels in nondiabetic Pima children before the onset of obesity tend to be higher than in age-matched Caucasian children (Savage et al., 1976a). Nevertheless, further prospective studies are needed to determine whether hyperinsulinemia antedates and contributes to, or follows and

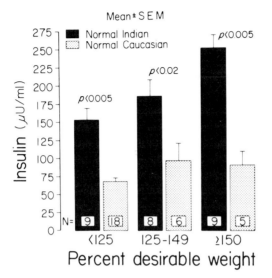

Fig. 4. Mean (± SEM) insulin responses 5 minutes after starting a rapid, 3-minute, 25-g intravenous glucose infusion in normal Pima Indians and normal Caucasians, according to percent desirable weight. (From Bennett *et al.*, 1976, with permission.)

results from, obesity. Other metabolic factors that may contribute to the high prevalence of obesity among the Pima are currently being investigated.

Obese Pima Indians with the recent onset of diabetes and fasting hyperglycemia have little or no additional insulin secretion in response to an oral glucose load. After a period of weight reduction, however, fasting glucose levels return to normal, and the response of insulin to oral glucose loading reverts to the elevated range seen in obese persons before the onset of glucose intolerance (Savage *et al.*, 1979c). Similar responses have been observed among non-Indians (Genuth, 1977). Before β-cell secretory failure appears in persons destined to develop adult-onset diabetes, a period of relatively rapid weight gain seems to occur, attended by increasing insulin levels and, later, by progressive carbohydrate intolerance with fasting hyperglycemia. Notably, the antilipolytic effects of insulin persist even when the hypoglycemic effects of the hormone are lost (Howard *et al.*, 1979). This retained activity may permit the continued deposition of fat and, thus, be an additional factor predisposing to obesity in maturity-onset diabetes mellitus.

4. Complications

American Indians with diabetes incur the usual vascular sequelae of the disease (West, 1974), but the prevalence of certain complications shows considera-

TABLE II

**Comparative Prevalence of Retinopathy and Proteinuria
in Three Racial Groups, among Persons with Diabetes of
10 or More Years in Duration**[a]

	Percent affected		
Condition	Pima	Japanese	Caucasian
Retinopathy	47	69	53
Proteinuria	43	69	<12

[a] From Bennett and Miller (1976).

ble racial variation. Table II compares the prevalence of retinopathy and proteinuria among diabetic Pima Indians, Japanese, and Caucasians. Among Pima
and Japanese, about one-half of all deaths from vascular causes in diabetics are
attributed to renal disease (diabetic nephropathy), as compared with only 11% in
the U.S. general population. On the other hand, three-fourths of vascular-
associated deaths in the diabetic general population are considered to have
cardiac causes, whereas the proportions for this cause in Pima and Japanese
diabetics are 31 and 16%, respectively (Bennett and Miller, 1976). Nonetheless,
the occurrence of diabetes does dramatically augment the otherwise low rate of
coronary heart disease in Indians (Sievers, 1967; Inglefinger *et al.*, 1976; Sievers
and Fisher, 1979a). Because diabetes in most tribes is complicated relatively
often by kidney failure, programs for the management of end-stage renal disease
should be assigned a high priority. Soft-tissue infection with nonclostridial gas-
producing organisms occurs unusually often in diabetic Indians (Fisher *et al.*,
1979), and amputation of gangrenous feet and legs is frequent (Sievers, 1976a).
In addition, diabetes is a major factor in fetal and neonatal loss and congenital
malformations among the Amerind (Bennett *et al.*, 1979b).

The age-adjusted mortality for diabetes in American Indians is 2.1 times the
U.S. all-races rate (U.S. Department of HEW, 1978a). Furthermore, Reinhard
and Greenwalt (1975), in a computerized evaluation of hospital utilization patterns among the Papago Indians, determined that diabetes produced a caseload
rate more than double that of nondiabetics. In addition, they noted that the
diabetic Indians had a greater frequency of illnesses unrelated to the well-
recognized complications of the disease than occurred among age-, sex-, and
geographically-matched nondiabetic Papagos.

Because of the epidemic proportions of diabetes among many Indian tribes of
North America and the likelihood that principles of disease management in this
racial group are applicable to other populations, Congress has appropriated special funds to the Indian Health Service to conduct a comprehensive diabetes

management program at five selected reservation hospitals and clinics. The project emphasizes the training of Indian people, who understand Native American diets, languages, and social customs, and will thus increase the number of allied health personnel for the management of diabetes mellitus. The model program is intended to determine the extent to which intensive application of conventional methods of treatment may improve the outcome of diabetes. New approaches with innovative techniques for patient education and motivation are clearly necessary to interrupt the increasing prevalence of this condition among North American Indians.

B. Biliary Disease

1. Prevalence

The Amerind have a remarkably high rate of biliary disease. Cholesterol gallstones, because of their pervasiveness, have been called the "American Indian's burden" (Sievers and Marquis, 1962a). Prevalence estimates for gallbladder disease, although collected by various methods, provide abundant evidence that cholelithiasis occurs at high rates in widely dispersed unrelated tribes throughout the United States. Indeed, at least 23 tribes have been reported to have clinical biliary disease significantly more often than does the U.S. white population (Table III). Undoubtedly, most, if not all, Indian tribes are similarly severely afflicted.

Comprehensive data, which are available for three population groups (Fig. 5), reveal that *symptomatic* gallbladder disease is much more frequent in the Pima of Arizona (Comess *et al.*, 1967) and the Chippewa of Minnesota (Thistle *et al.*, 1971) than among the white population of Framingham, Massachusetts (Friedman *et al.*, 1966). However, some patients with cholelithiasis may not seek

TABLE III

Tribes Reported to Have Significantly Higher Rates of Biliary Disease Than among the General U.S. Population[a]

Apache	Havasupai	Paiute	Ute
Arapaho	Hopi	Papago	Washoe
Chemehuevi	Hualapai	Pima	Yavapai
Chippewa	Maricopa	Quechan	Yuma
Choctaw	Mohave	Shoshone	Zuni
Cocopah	Navajo	Sioux	

[a] From Salsbury (1947); Lam (1954); Gilbert (1955); Hesse (1959, 1964); Sievers and Marquis (1962a); Kravetz (1964); Sievers (1966a); Reichenbach (1967); Comess *et al.* (1967); Brown and Christiansen (1967); Sampliner *et al.* (1970); Thistle *et al.* (1971); Nelson *et al.* (1971); Erickson (1972); Warren (1977); Morris *et al.* (1978).

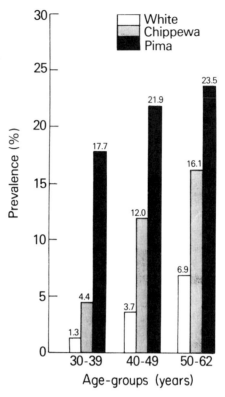

Fig. 5. Prevalence of clinical gallbladder disease among a white population (Framingham, Massachusetts) and in Chippewa (Cass Lake, Minnesota) and Pima Indians (Sacaton, Arizona), by age-groups (Friedman *et al.*, 1966; Comess *et al.*, 1967; Thistle *et al.*, 1971).

medical evaluation. Sampliner and co-workers (1970), therefore, systematically studied an age- and sex-stratified random sample of the Pima population on the Gila River Indian Reservation, and performed cholecystograms in persons having no clinically documented gallbladder disease (Table IV). Predictably, the prevalence of gallbladder disease was found to increase with age and to be greater in females than males. Remarkably, the frequency in Pima women 25 years of age or older was 75%. Autopsy and surgical findings have confirmed an extraordinarily high rate of cholesterol gallstones in southwestern Indians (Sievers and Marquis, 1962a; Kravetz, 1964; Reichenbach, 1967; Nelson *et al.*, 1971).

2. Lithogenicity

Gallstones are composed predominantly of cholesterol, whether they occur in the Amerind or in other ethnic groups of the United States (Bennion and Grundy,

TABLE IV

**Prevalence of Gallbladder Disease in Pima
Indians, by Age and Sex**[a]

Age-group (years)	Prevalence (%)	
	Males	Females
15–24	0	12.7
25–34	4.4	73.2
35–44	11.1	70.8
45–54	31.9	75.8
55–64	66.3	62.0
65+	67.8	89.5
All ages	31.7	65.4

[a] From Sampliner et al. (1970).

1978). In bile, the primary solubilizing agents for cholesterol are bile acids and lecithin. Stone formation, or lithogenesis, may occur when bile is supersaturated with cholesterol for prolonged periods, although a facilitative factor for nucleation may also be involved. The role of impaired gallbladder contraction in retaining microliths or in enhancing gallstone proliferation is uncertain (Bennion and Grundy, 1978). In Indians, lithogenic bile has been found (1) to be related to both enhanced cholesterol excretion in bile and inadequate amounts of bile acids (Grundy et al., 1972); (2) to occur in the healthy women more often than in the men, the former having significantly smaller bile acid pools than the latter (Bennion et al., 1978); (3) to increase abruptly during puberty, and to a greater measure in girls than in boys, although the degree of bile saturation in the prepubertal Pimas is no higher than for many normal white adults (Bennion et al., 1979); and (4) to be directly correlated with the extent of obesity and urinary estrogen level (Bennion and Grundy, 1975; Bennion et al., 1979). It has not been determined whether increased cholesterol synthesis by the liver in Indians may be attributed to high hepatic levels of 3-hydroxy-3-methylglutaryl-coenzyme A(HMG-CoA) reductase, which controls the production rate of this lipid (Bennion and Grundy, 1978).

3. Heredity versus Environment

The abundance of cholelithiasis in many broadly separated tribes suggests a widespread hereditary Indian trait. Nonetheless, this great lithogenic propensity does not extend to other Mongoloid populations. Indeed, gallstone formation is less frequent in Asiatics than in Europeans (Brett and Barker, 1976; Bennion and Grundy, 1978). Whether the paleo-Indians developed cholelithiasis is unknown, inasmuch as any cholesterol gallstones that may have existed would have decomposed in the burial sites. Early general reports of Indian diseases (Geare, 1915; Hancock, 1933) did not mention biliary disorders, suggesting an infrequency of either occurrence or diagnosis. Nonetheless, by 1937 (Salsbury, 1937), gallbladder disease was being detected almost as often as appendicitis in Navajo patients. Only 25 years later, however, cholecystectomy was being performed in southwestern Indians more than 3½ times as frequently as appendectomy (Sievers and Marquis, 1962a). This evidence suggests that some environmental influence, such as the changed diet of contemporary Indians, may have contributed to the emergence of latent lithogenic tendencies.

Although dietary influence may be contributory (Inglefinger, 1979), a hereditary propensity appears to be pre-eminent in the pathogenesis of cholelithiasis in the Amerind. Bennion et al. (1979) attribute the development of lithogenic bile by most Pima Indians to racial predisposition, and they conclude that the sharp postpubertal rise in bile saturation is related to the increasing obesity and estrogen production at that stage of maturation. Other causes considered for gallstone formation in Indians include the change from traditional foods to diets with more calories and less fiber (Reid et al., 1971), and an apparently rapid intestinal transit time (Goldman et al., 1972), which might contribute to chronic depletion of the bile acid pool.

In many Indian tribes adiposity is extremely common (Sievers, 1966a; Sievers and Hendrikx, 1972). Bennion and Grundy (1975) found an increased lithogenicity of bile in obesity, both among southwestern Indians and in white subjects. In Pima epidemiological studies, however, the mean percentage of desirable weight did not differ significantly between Indians with or without gallbladder disease (Sampliner et al., 1970). This inability to demonstrate a difference may be related to an extremely high rate of obesity and a paucity of Pimas with normal body weight for comparison. In addition, neither diabetes nor parity were significantly related to biliary disease. Indeed, diabetic Pimas were shown to have greater cholesterol synthesis but expanded bile acid pools and less lithogenic bile during uncontrolled hyperglycemia than during relative euglycemia with insulin administration (Bennion and Grundy, 1977).

4. Complications and Cholesterol

In the Indians, significant complications accompany the high rate of cholelithiasis. Biliary-enteric fistulas are relatively frequent (Zwemer et al., 1979), and acute pancreatitis occurs occasionally but, perhaps, less often than expected. In addition, biliary carcinoma is one of the more frequent malignant neoplasms in the Amerind (Sievers, 1976b; see also sections on cancer, p. 227). As compared with the U.S. white population, the Indians have at least three times the expected rate of cancer of the gallbladder (Creagan and Fraumeni, 1972).

Despite their increased production of cholesterol (Grundy et al., 1972), southwestern American Indians have significantly lower serum cholesterol levels than the white population (Sievers, 1968a). Among southwestern Indians, cholesterol precipitates in the gallbladder extremely often, but it is deposited in the walls of arteries relatively infrequently (Sievers, 1968a). However, no consistent difference in serum cholesterol levels has been found between the Pimas with and without gallbladder disease (Sampliner *et al.*, 1970). Further discussion of the occurrence of atherosclerosis and coronary heart disease in the Amerind is included in Section V,C.

C. Coronary Heart Disease

Coronary heart disease (CHD) is uncommon among full-heritage southwestern American Indians (Sievers, 1967; Inglefinger *et al.*, 1976; U.S. Department of HEW, 1978a; Sievers and Fisher, 1979a), although most of these tribes have high rates of diabetes mellitus and obesity (see Section V,A on diabetes), as well as a moderate but increasing prevalence of hypertension (Sievers, 1977b), factors associated with an increased risk of CHD. Acute myocardial infarction (AMI) occurs only about one-fifth as often in these Indians as in the U.S. general population (Sievers and Fisher, 1979a). The age- and sex-adjusted mortality (per 100,000) for AMI is much lower for southwestern Indians (14.7) than for U.S. all-Indians (135.0) or U.S. all-races (152.4) (U.S. Department of HEW, 1978a). This remarkably higher rate for U.S. all-Indians than for southwestern tribes reflects the greater frequency of CHD in nonsouthwestern tribes having considerable non-Indian admixture.

Several factors may be related to the relative infrequency of CHD in southwestern Indians.

1. Plasma cholesterol levels are significantly lower in these tribes than in whites (Sievers, 1968a; Savage *et al.*, 1976b), and the concentration rises little with advancing age.

2. A higher ratio of high-density lipoprotein (HDL) to low-density lipoprotein (LDL) cholesterol has been found among the Indians than in Caucasian controls (Garnick *et al.*, 1979).

3. Heavy cigarette smoking is rare among southwestern Indians (Sievers, 1966a, 1968b).

4. Interpersonal competitiveness is relatively infrequent in these tribes.

5. Blood group O, which occurs in more than 80% of southwestern Indians, may be associated with a reduced risk of CHD (Medalie *et al.*, 1971).

Ischemic heart disease apparently has become more prevalent in southwestern Indians during the past 15–20 years (Sievers and Fisher, 1979a), at a time when mortality from CHD in U.S. whites, blacks, and Chicanos has been declining (Stern, 1979). During this period, obesity, diabetes mellitus, and hypertension have also become more frequent in many tribes (West, 1974; Sievers, 1976a,

1977b). Tribal increases in rates of acute myocardial infarction generally have paralleled the extent of rise in rates of diabetes and hypertension. As shown in Fig. 6, this augmentation has been greater for the Athapascans (Apache and Navajo), who were traditionally nomadic hunters, than for the less aggressive agrarian Pimans (Pima and Papago). The Hopi Tribe, which had 19% of the population in the "other southwestern" category, experienced a disproportionate 35% of the infarctions for that group. Duodenal ulcer has exhibited a similar tribal pattern of increase (see Section V,D).

A vastly changing lifestyle of southwestern Indians has accompanied the recent increased frequency of acute myocardial infarction. Abrupt social changes and modernization have occurred, with substantial cultural disruption and an apparent decrease of physical activity but increased in psychological stress. Exist-

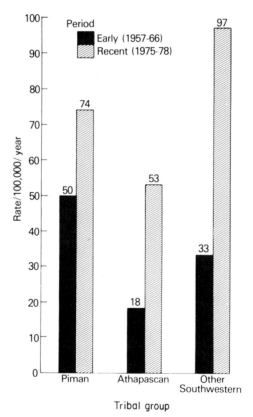

Fig. 6. Comparative rates, by tribe (age ≥ 30 years), for acute myocardial infarction during early (1957–1966) and recent (1975–1978) study periods. (From Sievers and Fisher, 1979a, with permission.)

ing evidence supports the probability that genetic factors relate to the relatively low levels of coronary artery disease among southwestern Indians. Despite their decreased vulnerability, however, they have the same predisposing risk factors as other ethnic groups. Thus, either the accentuation of adverse environmental conditions (e.g., heavy cigarette smoking) or the advent of significant non-Indian admixture would be expected to augment the frequency of acute myocardial infarction in the American Indians.

D. Peptic Ulcer Disease

Peptic ulcer disease is much less common in native Americans of the Southwest than in the U.S. white population (Sievers and Marquis, 1962b; Muggia, 1971; Sievers, 1973; Sievers and Fisher, 1979b). Observations among southwestern tribes that have been made at the Phoenix Indian Medical Center (PIMC) for the 23-year period 1956–1978 are shown in Table V. Overall, gastric carcinoma and pernicious anemia approximated expected numbers, based on comparison with rates for the general population, but there were distinct deficits in gastric ulcer and duodenal ulcer among the Indians. The number of person-years for the first 12 years (1956–1967) and last 11 years (1968–1978) are about equal. During the two periods, the rates for gastric carcinoma and pernicious anemia were similar, but both gastric and duodenal ulcer were almost twice as frequent in the recent as in the earlier interval.

More than 90% of all adult admissions to the PIMC were full-heritage southwestern Indians. This distribution was approximated by the patients with gastric carcinoma (95%) and pernicious anemia (92%), but only 55% (47/86) with

TABLE V

Comparative Frequency of Gastric Carcinoma, Pernicious Anemia, Gastric Ulcer, and Duodenal Ulcer at Phoenix Indian Medical Center during 1956—1967 and 1968—1978[a]

Disease category	Study period		Total	
	1956–1967	1968–1978	Observed	Expected[b]
Gastric carcinoma	42	40	82	71
Pernicious anemia	11	13	24	22
Gastric ulcer	18	34	52	346
Duodenal ulcer	12	22	34	1382
TOTALS	83	109	192	1821

[a] From Sievers and Fisher (1979b).
[b] Expected number based on rates for U.S. whites (Sievers, 1973; Sievers et al., 1973). Estimated Indian study population (mean) for 1956–1967=49,500 and for 1968–1978=55,000.

peptic ulcer were full-blooded southwestern Indians. Remarkably, *duodenal* ulcer was detected in only one *full-heritage* southwestern Indian during the first 12 years, but was noted in 8 during the last 11 years ($p < 0.025$). That this increase is only an artifact related to improved detection is unlikely, because the frequency of gastric carcinoma and pernicious anemia did not change appreciably. Significantly, 6 of the 9 full-blooded southwestern Indians with duodenal ulcer were Athapascans, but none was Piman (distribution of PIMC admissions was 43% Piman, 30% Athapascan). By contrast, gastric carcinoma had a relative excess for the Pimans (53/82, 65%) and a deficit for the Athapascans (13/82, 16%) ($p < 0.001$).

This increased frequency of duodenal ulcer has accompanied rapid social changes and a vastly altered life-style with concomitant cultural disruption and psychological stress. Contrasts between living conditions on- and off-reservation have abruptly narrowed. Nonetheless, many attributes of southwestern Indians have a negative correlation with duodenal ulcer: lower socioeconomic status, rural reservation residence, relative noncompetitiveness, phenythiocarbamide taste sensitivity, salivary secretion of ABH, a great prevalence of diabetes mellitus and cholelithiasis, a low rate of coronary artery disease, and infrequent cigarette smoking (Sievers, 1966a,b, 1973, 1976c).

Capper *et al.* (1967) showed that patients with gallstones have gastric acid hyposecretion more often than control subjects. Malhorta (1968) observed an inverse association between cholelithiasis and peptic ulcer in India. All southeastern American Indian tribes have much higher rates of gallstones (see Section V,B) and lower frequencies of peptic ulcer than have the U.S. whites. Significant tribal differences exist in the prevalence of each condition, but the rate of cholelithiasis maintains a direct relationship to the frequency of gastric carcinoma and pernicious anemia, and an inverse association with peptic ulcer (Sievers, 1973).

Achlorhydria has been found significantly more often in southwestern Indians than among American whites or blacks (Sievers, 1966b). Serum gastrin levels, however, did not differ significantly between Indian and white subjects in a limited evaluation (Sievers, 1973). Further detailed studies of gastric secretory function in the Amerind are in progress.

Peptic ulcer disease is noted disproportionately more often in off- than on-reservation Indians. In addition, the extent of non-Indian admixture is also directly related to the frequency of duodenal ulcer (Shore and Stone, 1973; Sievers, 1973; Thompson and Ackerstein, 1975). Thus, both heredity and environment appear to influence the rate of peptic ulcer in the Amerind.

Interestingly, during recent years the frequency of duodenal ulcer has been decreasing in the general population, at a time when this disease has become less rare among southwestern Indians (Elashoff and Grossman, 1980; Vogt and Johnson, 1980).

E. Inflammatory Bowel Disease

Both graunlomatous colitis (regional enteritis; Crohn's disease) and chronic idiopathic ulcerative colitis are less frequent in American Indians than among whites (Bebchuk *et al.*, 1961; Mendeloff, 1976). Furthermore, in the United States, the Japanese and Chinese appear to be at lower risk than the whites for developing these chronic inflammatory bowel diseases (Mendeloff, 1976). Some investigators have found that the HLA antigen B27 has a high association with chronic colitis, as well as with ankylosing spondylitis (Morris *et al.*, 1974; Mendeloff, 1976). This antigen and ankylosing spondylitis are common in some Amerind groups (see Section V,K), despite the infrequency of inflammatory bowel disease.

F. Lactose Intolerance

Abundant lactase activity in the small intestine is present at birth in human beings; but, except for the whites of northern and western European origin, most ethnic groups have a rapid decline in this disaccharide enzyme early in childhood (Newcomer *et al.*, 1977a). Lactose (milk sugar) malabsorption occurs in at least 90% of full-heritage North American Indian adults, but appears much less often among Indians with partial European ancestry (Duncan and Scott, 1972; Newcomer *et al.*, 1977a; Johnson *et al.*, 1978; Welsh *et al.*, 1978). Eskimo and Oriental adults also have high rates of lactose intolerance (Duncan and Scott, 1972). The studies of Newcomer *et al.* (1977b) among Chippewa Indians suggest that this trait has an autosomal-recessive pattern of inheritance. Because almost all full-heritage American Indians become intolerant to lactose after childhood, many adult Amerinds need some restriction of milk consumption to avoid diarrhea and intestinal cramping due to disaccharide malabsorption. However, most Native Americans are able to consume *small* amounts (1–1½ glasses) of milk and of other lactose-rich products without symptoms (Newcomer *et al.*, 1978).

G. Congenital Abnormalities

1. General Considerations

The overall rate of serious congenital malformations in most populations, including the American Indian, is about 2% of all births (Holmes, 1974; Niswander *et al.*, 1975), but the occurrence of specific anatomic defects varies considerably among the races. Racial contrasts are more pronounced for single defects, whereas multiple abnormalities are more often the result of sporadic, nongenetic factors (Erickson, 1976). The difficulties associated with comparing malformation rates among diverse populations have been reviewed elsewhere (Chung and

Myrianthopoulos, 1968; Lilienfield, 1970; Erickson, 1976). This presentation will focus on single major structural abnormalities of North American Indians found at birth. Chromosomal abnormalities, multiple birth defects, and inborn errors of metabolism (with the exception of albinism) do not appear in Amerinds with unusual frequency or distribution (Niswander *et al.*, 1975; McConnell *et al.*, 1976), and they will not be discussed here.

Niswander and colleagues (1975) reviewed the overall malformation rate and frequency of certain anomalies occurring in the Amerind during a 5-year period, 1964-1969. Among 43,711 live-born infants, 803 (1.8%) had one or more major defects. The study included 348 twin pairs. Monozygotic twin rates show little racial variation (about 3 or 4 pairs per 1000 births), whereas the frequency (per 1000 births) of dizygotic twins varies considerably among the races, being highest for blacks (11.0), intermediate for whites (7.0) and Indians (4.7), and lowest for Japanese (2.5) and other Mongoloid groups (Cavalli-Sforza and Bodmer, 1971; K. Morgan, 1979 personal communication). However, because the frequency of major malformations does not appear to differ between single and multiple births (Neel, 1958), this factor does not confound inter-racial comparisons.

2. Birth Defects With High or Unusual Frequencies

a. Polydactyly.   Polydactyly is the most prevalent major birth defect in the Amerind (Niswander *et al.*, 1975). This condition probably was also frequent in the prehistoric period, as ancient North American rock art depicted hands and feet with extra digits (Wellmann, 1972). The overall rate of this anomaly (per 1000 births) for Indians (2.4) is greater than that among Japanese (0.9) or whites (1.4), but only one-fifth as frequent as in blacks (12.8) (Neel 1958; Chung and Myrianthopoulos, 1968). Although American Indians are not ethnically homogeneous, no significant differences in the incidence of polydactyly have been found among the five major linguistic groups (Niswander *et al.*, 1975). Some of the racial differences in rates of polydactyly can be attributed to an increased frequency of specific types of this malformation, which have variable modes of inheritance (Bingle and Niswander, 1975). Existing evidence suggests that polydactyly is largely genetically determined.

b. Oral-Facial Clefts.   Mongoloid populations, in general, have a relatively high incidence of oral-facial clefts. Niswander and Adams (1967) found a rate of cleft lip, with or without cleft palate (CL ± P) in American Indians of 1.4 per 1000 births. Lowry and Trimble (1977), however, noted a higher rate (per 1000 births) of CL ± P in a large number of unrelated Indian tribes of British Columbia (3.7), which approximated the rate of Japanese (3.4) and exceeded the rate for whites (2.0) of that Canadian province.

The complex genetic, embryologic, and epidemiologic relationships that exist among the various types of oral-facial clefts have been extensively reviewed by

Shapiro (1976). He and others (Jaffe and DeBlanc, 1970) noted that the frequency of isolated cleft palate shows little racial variation. However, they report that cleft uvula, a microform of facial cleft, differs considerably in frequency among races, but shows a strong Mongoloid association—Amerind 13.9%, Japanese 9.8%, Chinese 6.8%, whites 1.5%, and blacks 0.3%. Most oral–facial clefts in human populations appear to result from the additive effects of several minor gene abnormalities. The role of exogenous or environmental factors in cleft anomalies is not discernible.

c. Congenital Hip Disease. Congenital dislocation of the hip has been found in the skeletal remains of prehistoric Indians (Clabeaux, 1977), and it is relatively common in several contemporary tribes of North America. The reported prevalence of dislocation and dysplasia (the latter characterized by a shallow deformed acetabulum, and by late development of the proximal femoral epiphysis) in population isolates of White Mountain Apache, Navajo, and Cree-Ojibwa Indians is 3.1, 3.8, and 6.0% respectively (Kraus and Schwartzmann, 1957; Rabin *et al.*, 1965; Walker, 1977). Neonatal examination has disclosed congenital hip dislocation less frequently (0–0.15%) in other populations of the United States (Mellin, 1963).

Not all hip dislocations are identified at birth, but most cases can be detected by physical examination within the first few days of life (Barlow, 1962). Congenital hip dysplasia, on the other hand, is a radiographic diagnosis. Dysplasia may represent a recovery stage from dislocation that frequently proceeds spontaneously to complete recovery.

The considerable variability in observed rates of congenital hip disease in various populations (Wynne-Davies, 1972) is due, in part, to differing diagnostic measures (physical examination versus radiographic study), methods of ascertainment (neonatal examination versus population surveys), and specificity of reporting (some published studies do and others do not differentiate between dysplasia and dislocation). Familial clustering of cases and twin studies suggest the probability that genetic factors are often involved, but it is also likely that nongenetic factors (such as breech presentation and a primiparous uterus) are important in the pathogenesis of congenital hip disease (Wynne-Davies, 1972).

More controversial is the relationship of infant swaddling to the development of hip dislocation. Epidemiologic studies have noted that children from populations with a high prevalence of congenital hip disease are tightly swaddled for several months after birth (Wynne-Davies, 1972). By contrast, congenital hip dislocation and dysplasia are rare in the native population of Hong Kong and in the Bantu of South Africa, societies that carry their young children with the infants' hip flexed and abducted (Clabeaux, 1977). The cradleboard (Fig. 7), which has been used for centuries by various Amerind groups (Wolman, 1970), has been implicated as a factor in preventing neonatal hip dislocations from correcting themselves (Coleman, 1968). However, reports of spontaneous im-

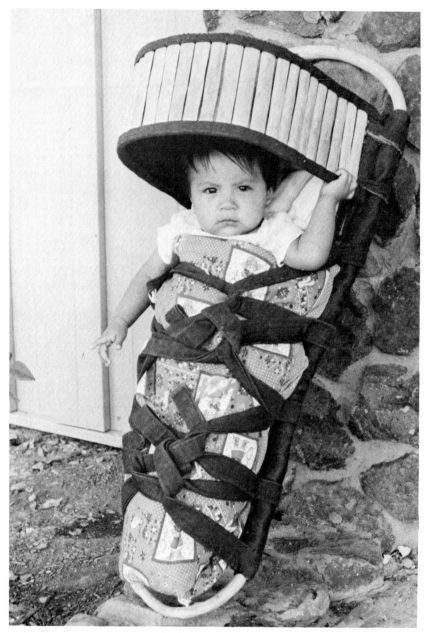

Fig. 7. Apache cradleboard. Cradleboards are still used, but traditional plant fiber fillers have been replaced by diapers, which limit extension of the infant's hip joints and may have reduced the incidence of hip dislocation.

provement of dysplasia despite continued cradleboard use (Rabin *et al.*, 1965), as well as the occurrence of hip dislocations in the early neonatal period, militate against swaddling as the primary cause. Although cradleboard use may retard normal hip development, other factors shared by populations with a high prevalence of congenital hip disease (isolation, small genetic pool, and consanguinity) are probably of greater importance.

d. Albinism. Generalized oculocutaneous albinism, an autosomal recessive trait, occurs with remarkable frequency in the Hopi, Zuni, and Jemez tribes of the southwestern United States, and in the Cuna Indians of Central America—about 1 in 200, as compared with an overall frequency of 1 in 20,000 among European populations (Woolf, 1965; Woolf and Dukepoo, 1969). With increasing age, the Zuni albinos develop some pigmentation of their hair and eyes, and nystagmus and photophobia decrease. They have the tyrosinase-positive form of albinism, which is also present in the Cuna and is believed to occur in the Hopi and Jemez tribes (Witkop *et al.*, 1972). Fascinating accounts of the social and cultural aspects of this condition among the Hopi, accompanied by unique photographs taken at the turn of the century, can be found elsewhere (Woolf and Grant, 1962; Woolf and Dukepoo, 1969). One such photograph is shown in Fig. 8.

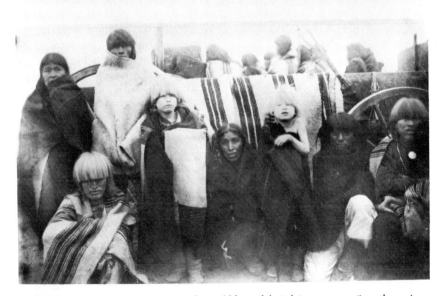

Fig. 8. Three Hopi albinos on the Second Mesa of their Arizona reservation, shown in an 1885 photograph. Albinos are active in the religious and social life of the tribe, and they have perpetuated the recessive trait among this Pueblo group. (From Smithsonian Institution, negative #48, 429-C, with permission.)

3. Other Abnormalities

The presence of teeth in newborn infants (natal teeth) is unexpectedly frequent in the Amerind (Gordon and Langley, 1970). Unconjugated hyperbilirubinemia is noted during the first few days of life significantly more often among Indians and other Mongoloid groups than among whites. This unexplained abnormality occurs in the absence of sepsis, respiratory distress, hemolytic disease, and hepatotoxic drugs, and it is observed in both breast- and bottle-fed babies (Saland *et al.*, 1974).

Hereditary methemoglobinemia due to a deficiency of the red blood cell enzyme DPNH-methemoglobin reductase has been found in the Navajo of the Southwest and in the Athapascan Indians and Eskimos of Alaska (Balsamo *et al.*, 1964). Inherited as an autosomal recessive trait, this disorder, in the homozygous state, produces cyanosis without other recognized pathophysiologic consequences. In the affected Alaskan natives, the serum level of methemoglobin exhibits seasonal variation. It is likely that a lower methemoglobin concentration in the autumn is related to the ingestion of wild berries rich in vitamin C, inasmuch as ascorbic acid reduces methemoglobin to hemoglobin.

Cystic fibrosis, which is assumed to be inherited as an autosomal recessive trait, is apparently rare in American Indian and Mongoloid populations (Harris and Riley, 1968). Phenylketonuria also seems to be rare in the Amerind (Wagner and Littman, 1967). Niswander and associates (1975) found the relative frequency of congenital heart defects to parallel the total malformation rate by linguistic group (Table VI). Anderson (1977) noted that, similar to Asiatic populations, Amerind children rarely had valvular aortic stenosis or coarctation of the aorta, but atrial septal defect was common. In addition, both left and right

TABLE VI

Frequency of Major Birth Defects (Total and for Five Selected Conditions) among 41,172 Single Live Births in American Indians and Alaskan Natives, by Linguistic Group (Cases per 1000) [a]

	Birth defects					
Linguistic group	All major malformations	Congenital heart disease	Cleft lip ± palate	Clubfoot	CNS[b] defects	Polydactyly
Aleut-Eskimo	26.3	5.2	1.8	3.6	—	1.6
Athapascan	20.6	3.6	2.1	1.5	1.4	2.8
Algonquian	17.2	3.4	0.8	3.2	0.5	3.4
Siouan	14.0	4.0	1.6	1.7	1.0	1.4
Uto-Aztecan	13.1	1.8	1.6	1.3	0.9	1.3

[a] From Niswander *et al.* (1975).
[b] CNS, central nervous system.

electrocardiographic axis deviation occur significantly more often among healthy young Navajo and Apache reservation students than among Tucson school children (Ewy *et al.*, 1979). Perhaps this difference reflects a normal hereditary variant in the two related Athapascan tribes.

4. Conclusions

The incidence of major birth defects in American Indians, including both multiple and single anomalies (18.4 per 1000 births), is similar to the frequency reported for other populations. However, among Amerind subgroups, based on linguistic affiliation, striking differences appear both in the overall rate of malformation and for specific anatomic defects (Table VI). Compared with whites, Indians have a higher rate of cleft lip ± palate and of polydactyly, but a lower frequency of clubfoot and central nervous system (CNS) abnormalities. These findings are similar to other Mongoloid populations. The Uto-Aztecan groups have the lowest incidence of birth defects (13.1 per 1000 births) but the highest incidence of diabetes mellitus. Both maternal diabetes and alcohol abuse are potentially teratogenic (Clarren and Smith, 1978; Bennett *et al.*, 1979b), and both conditions are prevalent in the Amerind (see Section V,A and Section V,H). The low frequency of CNS defects observed among American Indians is unexpected, in view of the reported association of neural tube defects with maternal alcohol abuse (Clarren, 1979). Apparently, the adverse effects of maternal diabetes and alcohol consumption are either counterbalanced by favorable genetic or environmental factors, or the results are not reflected in the overall frequency of congenital deformities reported by Niswander and associates (1975). Nonetheless, maternal diabetes mellitus clearly has a deleterious effect on the rate of birth defects in the Uto-Aztecan-speaking Pima Indians (Bennett *et al.*, 1979b). It is possible that the high rate of congenital anomalies observed by Niswander and co-workers (1975) in the more northern linguistic groups (Table VI) results from frequent consanguineous matings in these isolated populations (Scott, 1973).

H. Alcoholism and Alcohol-Related Diseases

Alcohol is a deadly companion to many North American Indians. The alcohol-related death rate for the Amerind population is 5–6 times the U.S. all-races rate (U.S. Department of HEW, 1978a). About 60% of the Indian deaths related to alcohol are attributed to Laennec's cirrhosis. Fatality from cirrhosis of the liver is disproportionately frequent among young Native Americans. For the age-group 25–34 years, the 1973–1975 Indian mortality for cirrhosis (60.8/100,000) was, tragically, 14.5 times the U.S. all-races rate (4.2/100,000). Other serious complications of chronic alcohol abuse, such as esophageal varices, erosive gastritis, hepatic encephalopathy, and alcohol withdrawal syndromes, occur frequently in Indians. However, in most tribes pancreatitis is relatively uncommon, despite the high prevalence of both alcoholism and cholelithiasis. In addition, alcoholic cardiomyopathy appears to develop less often than anticipated (Brandfonbrener et al., 1970).

Alcoholism is also a major contributor to the high rate of accidental death among Indian people—for 1973-1975, that rate being 3.2 times the U.S. all-races rate (U.S. Department of HEW, 1978a). In 1975, motor vehicle accidents accounted for 56% of all Indian accidental deaths. Furthermore, alcoholism is often closely associated with suicide (see Section V,I) and homicide, two violent events that occur more than twice as frequently in Indians as among the general population.

There is evidence that some tribes made a fermented drink from maize long before the arrival of white men. Nonetheless, the consumption of beverages with a *high* ethanol content was apparently unknown among the pre-Columbian Amerind of North America (Sievers, 1968b). Since the introduction of alcohol to the New World by the Europeans, a major controversy has existed as to whether Native Americans are more susceptible than the whites to alcohol intoxication and whether a racial predisposition contributes to excessive drinking. Indeed, the sale of alcoholic beverages to Indians was prohibited for many years by local, state, and federal laws. Not until 1953 did Congress give Indians the same rights as non-Indians to purchase liquor off reservations (Garbarino, 1976). Later, the selling of alcoholic beverages on some reservations was legalized by tribal government actions. From the observations and interpretations of early pioneers emerged the concept that "firewater" produced unusually severe intoxication with prolonged action in the Amerind. Since then, the opinions of laymen, legal and medical observers, anthropologists, sociologists, and psychologists have fluctuated in supporting or denying the existence in Indians of an inherent, genetically determined susceptibility to the effects of ethyl alcohol (Sievers, 1968b).

The racial vulnerability concept gained some support from the findings of Fenna and co-workers (1971) that, after the intravenous infusion of 10% ethanol, the blood alcohol concentration declined at a slower rate in western Canadian Indians than in whites. By contrast, Farris and Jones (1978) noted that, with the oral administration of ethyl alcohol, an Oklahoma Amerind group had a more rapid rate of absorption and a higher peak blood alcohol level but a faster rate of ethanol metabolism than occurred in the white controls. Furthermore, the Ojibwa (or Chippewa) Indians of Canada (Reed et al., 1976) and the Tarahumara Indians of Mexico (Zeiner et al., 1976) were found to metabolize ethanol more rapidly than Caucasians. Completing this spectrum of results, Bennion and Li (1976) reported no difference in rates of ethyl alcohol metabolism between southwestern Indians and white subjects. Perhaps of greater significance, their studies revealed no racial difference between the whites and Indians for the *in vitro* activity of alcohol dehydrogenase, the hepatic enzyme principally responsible for catalyzing the oxidation of ethanol to acetaldehyde. Several electrophoretically distinct forms (isoenzymes) of alcohol dehydrogenase are present in human liver, each having specific catalytic properties. Bennion and Li, however, found no difference in the isoenzyme pattern between the two racial groups. Those authors concluded that it is "unlikely that alleged racial differences in response to alcohol can be explained on the basis of racial differences in the rate of alcohol metabolism." They noted, however, as did Fenna and co-workers (1971), that ethanol is also metabolized by a less-specific hepatic microsomal system, which, unlike that of alcohol dehydrogenase, is activated by alcohol consumption. Both groups of investigators found that persons who chronically ingest alcohol had an increased rate of ethanol metabolism, the gain being greater in Indians than in whites. Lieber (1972) postulated that the high rate of alcoholism among Indians may be linked to augmented microsomal adaptation. At this time, however, no experimental data regarding this hypothesis are available.

The apparent discrepancies in reported rates of ethanol metabolism by the Amerind may be related, in part, to variations in study design, subject selection, and methods of determining blood alcohol levels (Lieber, 1972; Gilbert and Schaefer, 1977). On the other hand, differences in the rate of alcohol metabolism might, indeed, exist as a result of genetic heterogeneity among various tribal groups. If the Amerind tribes have a spectrum in the rate of alcohol metabolism, however, it has produced no discernable gradation in the prevalence of alcoholism among the North American Indians.

Interestingly, in some Mongoloid populations the prevalence of alcoholism is apparently lower than in Caucasoid groups. For this reason, Wolff (1972) compared cutaneous vasomotor response to alcohol drinking among Caucasoid, Japanese, Taiwanese, and Korean subjects. The Mongoloids who were studied responded with an early onset of severe facial flushing, which was infrequent and far less intense in the Caucasoids. This prompt vasomotor response to alcohol ingestion presumably is genetically determined because the racial differences were found not only in adults but also in *newborn infants,* for whom acquired influences were highly unlikely. Wolff suggests that the pronounced autonomic vascular reaction to ethanol and the associated unpleasant subjective symptoms "experienced by Mongoloids may well prevent many of them from consuming even moderate quantities of alcohol." Amerinds, despite a Mongoloid affinity, obviously have not been similarly deterred. Their vasomotor response to alcohol may be variable. For example, Wolff (1973) observed that Cree Indians approximated the Mongoloids' high incidence and intensity of facial flushing in response to oral alcohol. By contrast, in experiments among the Tarahumara tribe of Mexico (who are closely related to the Pima and Papago of Arizona), Zeiner and co-workers (1976) found less autonomic vasomotor responsiveness to ethanol among those Indians than in Caucasians.

Alcoholism is a serious problem of Indians residing on reservations (Brod,

1975), but it is even more devastating to Native Americans trying to adapt to urban living (Littman, 1970). It is widely accepted that in every ethnic group numerous social, cultural, economic, and other environmental factors closely relate to the development and progression of alcoholism. Nonetheless, this awareness has provided the basis for only limited success in programs to prevent and treat this devastating condition. Underlying factors in alcoholism among Amerinds likely include their prolonged catastrophic social and cultural disruption and economic deprivation. Whether genetic influences are also contributory remains unresolved, but the preponderance of evidence does not support that possibility.

I. Suicide

Native Americans commit suicide about twice as often as U.S. whites (U.S. Department of HEW, 1978a). Tribes vary considerably, however, in the extent of self-destructive behavior. Among the Apache, suicide occurs at four to five times the U.S. all-races rate, but the frequency varies among the Apache Reservations (Resnik and Dismang, 1971). In addition, the average rate for Pueblo Indians is low, although some New Mexico Pueblo reservations have high rates. Local factors appear to be major influences. On reservations where suicide is frequent, alcoholism, homicides, and insidious self-destructive behavior are also common. Suicide appears to be an even greater problem among urban than reservation Indians (Conrad and Kahn, 1974). Indian women make more suicide attempts than the men, but the completed suicide rate is much higher for the males (Sievers *et al.*, 1975). Trauma (inflicted by firearms, hanging, or self-incineration) is used more often by Indian men in suicide attempts, but ingestion of toxic substances is the preponderant method for the women.

In contrast to the U.S. non-Indian population, where the trend for suicide increases steadily with advancing age, the bulk of native American suicides is concentrated in the population 35 years or younger (U.S. Department of HEW, 1978a). During adolescence and early adulthood American Indians are often beset with unusually disruptive conditions, stresses of acculturation, and ambivalence about the culture bestowed at birth (Resnik and Dismang, 1971). These frustrations are likely to be greater for tribes that were once nomadic hunters, such as the Apache and Sioux, than for traditionally less mobile agrarian tribes, such as the Pima and Pueblo groups. The aggressiveness of the former tribes now appears to be exhibited by accentuated self-destructive behavior.

A loss of self-esteem by many Native Americans has been devastating. Early in life, the Amerind is confronted with an enormous struggle for identity and control of personal destiny. Hopefully, however, with "commitment to a perpetuation of the heritage of his people, the young Indian may well be able to perform and achieve . . . without being burdened by thoughts of his eventual dissolution" (Hammerschlag, 1970).

J. Cancer

1. Prevalence

American Indians are considered to be a low-risk population for cancer. In 1975, the age-adjusted mortality for malignant neoplasm was 39% lower for Indians that for the U.S. general population (U.S. Department of HEW, 1978a). Data from the National Cancer Institute (U.S. Department of HEW, 1976) indicate that the national age-adjusted mortality (per 100,000) for cancer was lower for the Amerind (100.7) than for the white (174.0), black (189.4), Chinese (189.7), or Japanese (158.3) populations of the United States.

However, among Indians, the relative frequency of cancer differs widely for various anatomic sites. Published studies regarding the frequency of malignant neoplasm in Indians have evaluated, either separately or in combination, clinical records, histological findings, autopsy reports, and mortality data (Smith et al., 1956; Smith, 1957; Sievers and Cohen, 1961; Sievers and Marquis, 1962a; Sievers, 1966a, 1976b; Hesse, 1964; Reichenbach, 1967; Muggia, 1971; Creagan and Fraumeni, 1972; Dunham et al., 1973; Bordin et al., 1977). Despite variability in methods, the studies agree substantially regarding comparative cancer prevalence among native Americans and the U.S. white population. Only mortality data will be analyzed statistically here, but morbidity studies and clinical findings confirm these results.

Table VII presents recent standardized mortality ratios (SMRs) by sex for

TABLE VII

Numbers and Standardized Mortality Ratios (SMRs) for the 10 Leading Cancer Sites among the Amerind of the 26 Reservation States, 1974–1976[a]

Site	Male SMR	Female SMR	Total Observed (No.)	Total Expected (No.)	Total SMR
Lung	39	66	153	352.1	43
Colon	51	47	89	181.8	49
Breast	—	53	78	148.0	53
Stomach	89	113	76	78.1	103
Pancreas	71	98	74	90.9	81
Cervix	—	229	66	28.8	229
Gallbladder	444	432	54	12.4	435
Prostate	57	—	53	93.5	57
Kidney and renal pelvis	145	171	52	33.8	154
Liver	101	138	29	25.3	115
All cancer deaths	55	89	1202	1736.9	69

[a] Items listed in order of frequency. Data from Indian Health Service (supplied by Mr. Mozart I. Spector, Director, Office of Program Statistics). SMR=(observed/expected) × 100.

cancer of the ten leading sites among the Amerind. The SMR is the proportionate relationship of observed to expected deaths, based on the standardized national rates in whites (a ratio of 100 = equality; > 100 = excess; < 100 = deficit). Because of the limited number of Indian cases (1,202) only SMRs that vary substantially from 100 indicate significant differences. These comparative findings agree generally with the conclusions of published studies cited above. Significant ($p < 0.05$) deficits occur among Indians for cancer of the lung, colon, breast, and prostate, and excesses are noted for malignancies of the cervix, gallbladder, and kidney. Not listed in Table VII, because of their low prevalences, are carcinoma of the bladder (SMR 25), rectum (SMR 50), brain (SMR 52), and ovary (SMR 56), as well as Hodgkin's disease (SMR 28), each of which has a significant deficit.

Interestingly, in the Amerind populations having substantial non-Indian ancestry *and* living off-reservation (e.g., tribes of Oklahoma), the cancer mortalities for most sites are intermediate between the national frequency and the rates for the tribes residing on reservations and having a high extent of Indian heritage (e.g., tribes of the southwestern states). Similarly, among Chicanos, most of whom have partial Indian heritage, cancer morbidities are intermediate between

TABLE VIII

Numbers and Standardized Mortality Ratios (SMRs) for Cancer of the Lung, Colon, and Gallbladder, 1974—1976, Compared by Sex, for the Tribes of the Southwest and of Oklahoma[a]

Site	Southwest			Oklahoma		
	Observed (No.)	Expected (No.)	SMR	Observed (No.)	Expected (No.)	SMR
Lung						
Male	5	105.8	5	47	55.1	85
Female	6	21.2	29	12	11.0	109
TOTAL	11	127.0	9	59	66.1	89
Colon						
Male	7	34.0	21	15	17.7	85
Female	4	31.4	13	9	16.3	55
TOTAL	11	65.4	17	24	34.0	71
Gallbladder						
Male	8	1.2	667	2	0.6	333
Female	20	3.2	625	3	1.6	188
TOTAL	28	4.4	636	5	2.2	227

[a] From Indian Health Service (IHS) data supplied by Mr. Mozart I. Spector, Director, Office of Program Statistics. The 1975 IHS Indian population base for the Southwest (Arizona, California, Colorado, Nevada, New Mexico, and Utah) = 223,437; for Oklahoma = 116,394; and for all 25 reservation states = 524,559 (U.S. Department of HEW, 1978a).

the national prevalence and the Amerind rates (Bordin *et al.*, 1977). Table VIII compares tribes of the Southwest and of Oklahoma in regard to cancer SMRs, by sex, for three selected sites. Overall, lung cancer mortality is lower in Indians (SMR 43) than in the general population, but the southwestern tribes have a much lower SMR (9) than do the Oklahoma Indians (89) ($p < 0.0001$). Similarly, death from colon cancer is relatively infrequent in the Amerind (SMR 49), but the frequency is much lower ($p < 0.001$) in the Southwest (SMR 17) than in Oklahoma (SMR 71). By contrast, the mortality for gallbladder cancer is strikingly augmented for Native Americans (SMR 435), the increase being significantly ($p < 0.05$) higher for tribes of the Southwest (SMR 636) than for Indians of Oklahoma (SMR 227).

2. Special Considerations for Cancer of Selected Sites

a. Low Prevalence

i. Lung.   Squamous cell bronchogenic carcinoma, the leading fatal malignant neoplasm in the United States (Robbins, 1974; American Cancer Society, 1979), is rare in southwestern Indians. However, these tribes approximate expected frequencies for the less common alveolar cell carcinoma and adenocarcinoma of the lung. The prevalence of both of these less-frequent malignant lesions in the general population is similar for each sex, but squamous cell carcinoma has a strong male preponderance. Significantly, in southwestern Indians, who rarely develop squamous cell carcinoma of the lung, the mean annual rate of lung cancer is about equal for men and women (Table IX).

Heavy cigarette smoking is associated with the occurrence of squamous cell bronchogenic carcinoma, but not with the other types of lung cancer (Robbins, 1974). Southwestern Indians seldom smoke extensively (Sievers, 1968b). By contrast, both cigarette smoking and lung cancer mortality among Oklahoma Indians more nearly approximate the national white experience (Table IX). The mean annual lung cancer mortality is nine times greater in Oklahoma tribes than in southwestern Indians (Table IX). In addition, unlike southwestern tribes, the Oklahoma Indians have a much higher average annual lung cancer mortality (per 100,000) for males (27.4) than for females (7.2). Amerinds do not have genetic immunity from bronchogenic carcinoma, because this lesion does occur occasionally among the few full-heritage southwestern Indians who smoke heavily. Furthermore, in Oklahoma tribes, where cigarette smoking is common, the rate of squamous cell lung cancer differs little from the national frequency. In addition, Navajo uranium miners have accentuated rates of lung cancer, mostly small-cell, undifferentiated, bronchogenic carcinoma (Archer *et al.*, 1976).

ii. Colon.   Comparable with the sex ratio in the general population (American Cancer Society, 1979), Indian males have a somewhat greater colon cancer mortality (5.8/100,000) than do the females (4.8/100,000). The colon cancer

TABLE IX

American Indian Mean Annual Cancer Mortality Rates[a] for Three Low-Prevalence Sites, 1974–1976, Compared by Sex for the Southwest, Oklahoma, and All 25 Reservation States[b]

	Indian areas		
Anatomic site[c]	Southwest	Oklahoma	All 25 states
Lung			
Male	1.7	27.4	13.9
Female	2.0	7.2	4.6
TOTAL	1.8	16.9	9.1
Colon			
Male	2.1	8.9	5.8
Female	1.0	5.0	4.8
TOTAL	1.6	6.9	5.4
Breast			
Female	2.7	6.3	4.7

[a] Deaths per 100,000 population.

[b] From Indian Health Service (IHS) data, supplied by Mr. Mozart I. Spector, Director, Office of Program Statistics.

[c] Statistical significance of differences between Indians of the Southwest and of Oklahoma: lung, $p < 0.001$; colon, $p < 0.001$; breast, $p < 0.05$.

SMR is much higher for Oklahoma tribes (71) than for the southwestern Indian population (17) (Table VIII). The possibility of a genetic influence is suggested by the significant non-Indian admixture of many Oklahoma Indians, but some regional cultural differences are equally likely to be contributory.

Burkitt and associates (1974) have noted that populations with high residue diets have rapid intestinal transit time, and seldom develop appendicitis, diverticular disease of the colon, or cancer of the colon and rectum. The southwestern Indians have relatively low rates of all three of these conditions, and they also may have a shortened intestinal transit time (Sievers, 1966a, 1976b; Goldman *et al.,* 1972). Pima Indians have a considerably greater intake of legumes (mostly beans), and, consequently, of dietary fiber than the U.S. mean (Reid *et al.,* 1971). Most other southwestern tribes also consume large amounts of beans much more frequently than do the Oklahoma Indians (Mayberry and Lindemann, 1963). Comparative studies of the intestinal transit time for southwestern and Oklahoma Indians, however, have not been performed. Nonetheless, environmental (dietary) factors likely contribute to the differing rates of colon cancer for these two regional Indian groups.

iii. Breast.   A relative deficit of breast cancer in Indians has been recognized for many years (Smith *et al.,* 1956; Smith, 1957). Pregnancy, multiparity, and lower socioeconomic status are more frequent in most tribes than among the whites, and these factors have been considered to be associated with a decreased incidence of breast cancer (Sievers, 1966a; Robbins, 1974). During the last 25 years, however, each of these conditions has decreased in many Indian populations, whereas the reported rate of breast cancer has increased modestly. It is unknown whether this small increment relates to improved discernment or to an augmented incidence associated with a change in diet (Hankin and Rawlings, 1978) or other altered environmental factors.

Oklahoma Indian women, who generally have substantial non-Indian heritage, have a much higher ($p < 0.05$) mortality for breast cancer (6.3/100,000) than occurs in southwestern tribes (2.7/100,000) (Table IX). Petrakis (1971) has reported an association between wet (or sticky) type of cerumen (earwax) and breast cancer. He noted that in western Europe and the United States, where breast cancer is a leading malignant neoplams of women, most of the white and black populations have wet cerumen. Mongloid groups, in whom dry cerumen predominates, have low mortalities for breast cancer. Most Amerinds have dry cerumen. Petrakis suggests that the association of breast cancer with wet cerumen may be plausible because the ceruminous and mammary glands are histologically of the same apocrine type, and both have biochemically similar secretions.

b. High Prevalence

i. Gallbladder.   An excess of biliary carcinoma in the Amerind is generally attributed to their high rate of cholelithiasis (Sievers, 1976b; Black *et al.,* 1977) (see above, p. 205). Lithogenic bile in Indians probably has a genetic basis, as discussed previously. However, it is unknown whether an irritant effect of gallstones is carcinogenic or whether some factor that accompanies gallstone formation may also influence cholecystic malignant neoplasia.

ii. Cervix.   Cervical carcinoma usually has been reported to be significantly more prevalent in Indians than in non-Indians, although there are exceptions (Bivens and Fleetwood, 1968; Jordan *et al.,* 1969). Lower socioeconomic status, early frequent sexual activity, and multiple pregnancies have been found to be associated with elevated rates of cervical cancer in various ethnic groups (Robbins, 1974). Each of these factors is applicable to most Indian populations. There is no substantial evidence that the Amerind have a genetic predisposition to carcinoma of the cervix.

3. Conclusions

Clearly, the same environmental factors that contribute to carcinogenesis in other populations have similar adverse effects in American Indians. However, the possibility of a genetic influence is suggested by the observation that the frequency of cancer of many sites in populations with partial Indian heritage is intermediate between the white and Indian rates. Overall, the occurrence and anatomic distribution of cancer in American Indians appear to be more influenced by cultural conditions and environmental factors than by any inherited resistance or innate predisposition to malignant neoplasia.

K. Arthritis

1. Ankylosing Spondylitis

The prevalence of sacroiliitis in four North American Indian communities is higher than that reported in any other population. Using the stringent New York criteria for radiographic diagnosis, Gofton and co-workers (1972) found evidence of definite (grades 3 and 4) sacroiliitis in 9.5% of Haida, 9.2% of Bella Bella, 5.2% of Bella Coola, and 4.5% of Pima men more than 25 years old (compared with an estimated rate of 0.5–1.0% in white and Japanese men). Those investigators considered the radiographic abnormalities to be manifestations of idiopathic ankylosing spondylitis, because the patients also had clinical evidence and complications characteristic of this condition. Furthermore, other chronic diseases associated with similar X-ray changes in the sacroiliac joints— ulcerative colitis, regional enteritis, Behçet's syndrome, psoriasis, and Reiter's syndrome—were rare or not encountered. Recently, however, a high frequency of Reiter's syndrome has been found among Navajo Indians, perhaps associated with a high prevalence of endemic shigellosis and of the histocompatibility antigen HLA B27 (36%) in this tribe (Morse et al., 1980). Indeed, the majority of male patients in this Athapascan group with symptomatic sacroiliitis and peripheral arthritis appear to have Reiter's syndrome and not ankylosing spondylitis.

An association between HLA B27 and ankylosing spondylitis is well documented (Schlosstein et al., 1973). The prevalence of the B27 antigen phenotype in Caucasian, Haida, and Bella Coola men with ankylosing spondylitis exceeds 90% (Gofton et al., 1975), but this relationship is less striking in other ethnic groups of men: Japanese 60%, Pima Indians 57%, blacks 50% (Calin et al., 1977; Khan et al., 1977). Despite a great difference in the frequency of HLA B27 in Haida (50%) and Caucasian (5–7%) populations, the risk for ankylosing spondylitis in persons with this antigen is about 20% in both groups (Gofton et al., 1975). Pima men, one-fifth of whom are B27 positive, also have a high risk of developing spondylitis, but B27 *negative* Pimas are much more likely to develop ankylosing spondylitis than B27 *negative* Caucasians (Calin et al., 1977). Thus, the frequency of this antigen does not entirely explain the prevalence of the disease in a population. The similar risk for ankylosing spondylitis in HLA B27-positive Haida and Caucasian men suggests that genetic influences related to the B27 locus predominate over environmental factors. Although inheritance is known to be important in predisposing to Reiter's syndrome and the "reactive arthropathies" (Moll et al., 1974), there is also evidence that certain microorganisms (Shigella, Salmonella, and Yersinia) may initiate these diseases. Direct evidence of an environmental factor associated with the development of idiopathic ankylosing spondylitis is lacking, but recent findings that associate the presence of Klebsiella pneumoniae in the gastrointestinal or genitourinary tract with active ankylosing spondylitis (Ebringer et al., 1978) are intriguing. In addition, the reported discordance for ankylosing spondylitis in three monozygotic twin pairs more than 45 years of age (Eastmond and Woodrow, 1977) suggests the probability that environmental influences contribute greatly to the pathogenesis of this disease in susceptible persons.

2. Rheumatoid Arthritis

Diagnostic evidence of peripheral rheumatoid arthritis has not been found in the skeletal remains of pre-Columbian man in either Europe or the western hemisphere (Short, 1974), suggesting that the origin of this condition may be recent and associated with some unidentified environmental change. In contrast to the sex incidence for ankylosing spondylitis, rheumatoid arthritis afflicts women more often than men. In most adult populations that have been studied, including several groups of native Americans (Gofton et al., 1964; O'Brien et al., 1967; Beasley et al., 1973a), the prevalence of definite rheumatoid arthritis (as defined by the New York and Rome criteria) for women ranges between 0.4 and 1.4% (Lawrence, 1961). Comparisons among the various studies, however, are complicated by differences in patient selection, diagnostic criteria, and the age range and structure of the populations studied. The geographic variation in the prevalence of definite rheumatoid arthritis appears to be less than in the combined probable plus definite cases, the latter being the category most often quoted (Beasley et al., 1973b; Henrard et al., 1976).

A survey among Yakima Indian women in central Washington state revealed definite rheumatoid arthritis in 3.4% (Beasley et al., 1973b), as compared with 1.4% among women of similar age in the general U.S. population (Engle et al., 1966). Interestingly, a high incidence of systemic lupus erythematosis has been recorded for three tribes (Crow, Arapahoe, and Sioux) living in the northern United States, contiguous to the area inhabited by the Yakima (Morton et al., 1976). The course and complications of rheumatoid disease in the Yakima and other Amerind groups are similar to those in non-Indian populations, except for a probable increased occurrence of untoward reactions to gold therapy in the Yakima (Willkens et al., 1976) and a low frequency of cervical spine involvement in the Pima (Lawrence, 1976).

Striking familial clustering of patients has been found in Yakima, Blackfeet, and Pima Indians, as well as in other ethnic groups (Bennett and Burch, 1968a,b;

Willkens *et al.*, 1976), but this aggregation of cases in close relatives was attributed to environmental influences that affected some families excessively, and not to hereditary factors. However, these conclusions were made before the association of the HLA antigen Dw4 with rheumatoid arthritis was recognized. The Dw4 antigen occurs in up to 54% of Caucasians with rheumatoid arthritis (Panayi *et al.*, 1978), suggesting that immunogenetic as well as environmental factors are operative in this disease. The prevalence of the Dw4 antigen and its association with rheumatoid disease in Amerind populations are currently being investigated.

3. Degenerative Joint Disease

Little is known about the racial or geographic distribution of osteoarthritis. Studies among the Blackfeet of Montana and Pima of Arizona, Indian tribes residing in the extremes of the U.S. climate range, failed to show any significant difference between the two groups in the age- and sex-adjusted prevalence rates for this degerative disease (Bennett and Burch, 1968c). Obesity is more frequent and the presence of rheumatoid factor more common in the Pima, whereas elevated serum uric acid levels are noted more often among the Blackfeet (Bennett and Burch, 1968a,d). These three factors are generally considered to correlate with an increased prevalence of osteoarthritis (Acheson and Collart, 1975), but their relative influence on the comparative prevalence of the disease in Blackfeet and Pima Indians is unknown.

Vertebral ankylosing *hyperostosis* (Forestier's disease) was originally considered to be an exaggerated form of spinal osteoarthritis. However, studies among the Pima (Spagnola *et al.*, 1978), where the condition is found in 48% of men and 12% of women more than 55 years of age, suggest that it is distinct from osteoarthritis. Also, contrary to reports from other ethnic groups, the condition was not associated with HLA B27, obesity, or diabetes in Pimas. The relative contributions of environment and heredity to the occurrence and progression of the degenerative types of arthritis remain unresolved.

L. Coccidioidomycosis

For many centuries, American Indian tribes have inhabited areas that are endemic for coccidioidomycosis. The non-Indians have lived only about 125 years in the Lower Sonoran Life Zone of the southwestern United States, where the soil is variably infested by *Coccidioides immitis*. Despite this difference in duration that their forebears had in exposure to *C. immitis*, the Amerind (and other nonwhite races) have generally been considered to be more vulnerable than whites to serious coccidioidal infection (Fiese, 1958; Pappagianis, 1972; Flynn *et al.*, 1979).

Indeed, relatively high rates of acute disease and of dissemination occur among populations of some reservations (Sievers, 1964, 1974, 1977a). As compared with whites, the Indians within the endemic region have disseminated coccidiodomycosis morbidity 3.6 times greater and mortality 5.1 times higher (Sievers, 1977a). These ratios, as well as even more augmented ones for blacks and other ethnic groups, have been the basis for the prevailing concept of nonwhite susceptibility to coccidioidomycosis.

Recently, however, the validity of evidence for this concept has been questioned (Sievers, 1977a, 1979, 1980; Huppert, 1978). Racial vulnerability infers a difference between whites and other races in the outcome of coccidioidal infection. Therefore, the only appropriate denominator for calculating dissemination rates is the number of infected persons for each race (as assessed by coccidioidin skin test results, for example). By contrast, almost all studies have used either the total regional population or the cases of acute pulmonary coccidioidomycosis for each race for computation of rates. Neither figure is appropriate. Inasmuch as dissemination occurs only among infected persons, the total population is not at risk for this event. The number of cases of acute coccidioidal disease diagnosed is also an imprecise basis for calculating dissemination rates because of variation in clinical discernment. Indeed, when infected populations (as determined from coccidioidin skin test results) were used as denominators, the disseminated disease rate was found to be similar (about 1:500) for southwestern Indians and whites (Sievers, 1977a). Nonetheless, various reservations within the endemic region had a fourfold variation (1:250 to 1:1000) in the rate that infection eventuated in dissemination. These differences probably relate directly to the density of the infecting inoculum, which reflects the magnitude of soil infestation by *C. immitis*.

Extensive observations among southwestern Indians indicate that some nonracial conditions unfavorably influence the extent of morbidity and mortality in coccidioidomycosis (Sievers, 1964, 1974, 1977a, 1979). These factors include high rates of coccidioidal infection, great density of infecting inoculum, younger ($\leq$ 5 years) or older ($\geq$ 50 years) age at infection or dissemination, intercurrent conditions that impair cell-mediated immune responses, and, probably, adverse socioeconomic conditions.

Epidemiological studies have limited potential for resolving the problem of whether race influences the rate of dissemination and survival in coccidioidomycosis and other granulomatous diseases. For meaningful comparisons, epidemiologists must use the appropriate denominator (the infected population) for each race and must consider other significant nonracial influences. Recovery from coccidioidal infection depends on cell-medicated immune responses. A spectrum in this activity exists, but whether the racial variation in the competency of this mechanism is significant is unknown. At this time, there is no substantial evidence that the Amerind are unusually vulnerable to coccidioidomycosis.

M. Tuberculosis

"Repeated studies show that certain races, such as the American Indian and Negro, have tendencies to develop the acute, grave types of tuberculosis. Other races, such as the Semites, seem particularly resistant. . . ." (Goldberg, 1944). This view, once widely espoused, merits critical examination. The hypothesis that Indians have enhanced susceptibility to tuberculosis is based on the disproportionately high prevalence of advanced disease in North American Indians. It also presumes that tuberculosis was introduced into the New World by European explorers after the fifteenth century, and, therefore, that an immunologically unprepared Native American population was exposed to the ravages of a disease new to them.

Contemporary Amerinds continue to have a high prevalence of tuberculosis. Indeed, in 1976 the case rate among Native Americans was 4.6 times the U.S. all-races rate (U.S. Department of HEW, 1978a). However, as discussed above for coccidioidomycosis, enhanced susceptibility to tuberculosis implies a more adverse outcome of *infection* (greater frequency and extent of clinical disease, poorer response to therapy, and higher mortality) in the Amerind than in whites. For such considerations, the appropriate denominator (the *number infected*) must be selected to compute meaningful comparative rates. The entire regional population of a race (as has usually been used) is a meaningless base in assessing relative racial vulnerability, because the risk to be considered does not involve the uninfected group. Clinical disease develops and progresses only among some portion of the persons infected with *Myobacterium tuberculosis* (as evidenced by skin reactivity to tuberculin). A further confounding factor is the latent interval between infection and clinical disease, which is common in tuberculosis but rare in coccidioidomycosis. This variable hiatus between the time of infection and the appearance of active disease, combined with the considerable difficulty in identifying racial populations with comparable socioeconomic conditions and known rates of tuberculin reactivity, explains why the question of enhanced racial susceptibility to tuberculosis remains unresolved.

In this regard, for many years the White Mountain Apache have had a much higher annual rate of tuberculosis than the San Carlos Apache. This great difference in disease prevalence between two genetically similar tribes living on adjacent reservations suggests that unfavorable environmental factors predominate over genetic influences. In addition, it has been noted that southwestern American Indians and some Amerind groups in South America (Nutels, 1968), when compared with other ethnic populations, have similar clinical manifestations of tuberculosis and responsiveness to chemotherapy.

Several years ago, Morse (1961, 1967) concluded that the available evidence regarding the possible presence of tuberculosis in prehistoric America was equivocal because (1) the hunchbacked caricatures (Fig. 9) found in pre-

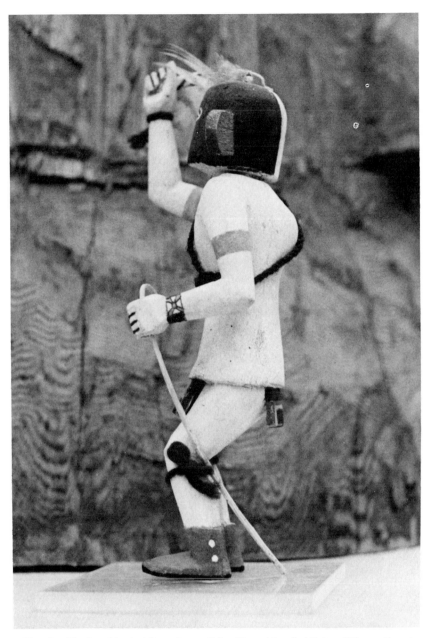

Fig. 9. The hunchbacked figure in pre-Columbian art is called Kokopelli by southwestern American Indians. Although thought by some to represent the gibbous deformity of spinal tuberculosis, the hump may have a purely symbolic meaning. In legend, Kokopelli is an energetic mischievous Don Juan, behavior not expected from a cripple. (From the collection of the Heard Museum, Phoenix, Arizona.)

Columbian art (Wellmann, 1979) and often presumed to depict Pott's disease may, in fact, represent at least 13 other conditions that could have caused spinal deformities; (2) the bony lesions discovered in ancient Amerind skeletons and attributed to tuberculosis lack pathologic specificity; and (3) if tuberculosis had existed in the New World during the pre-Columbian period, typical spinal lesions probably would have occurred more frequently than such findings have been discovered in skeletal remains of paleo-Indians. More recently, however, the dilemma seems to have been resolved by Allison and associates (1973), who reported definitive evidence of tuberculosis (miliary tubercles with acid-fast bacilli) in a Peruvian mummy, dated about 700 AD by carbon-14 studies and from estimates based on the associated pottery. In addition, recent skeletal findings in North America (Perzigian and Widmer, 1979), though not conclusive, make it likely that tuberculosis did exist in at least some of the pre-Columbian Indians. Thus, neither the archeologic nor the biomedical evidence appears to substantiate the hypothesis of an enhanced susceptibility to tuberculosis among the Amerind.

N. Chronic Obstructive Pulmonary Disease

The southwestern Indians rarely have chronic obstructive pulmonary disease (COPD/emphysema) (Muggia, 1971; Goldman et al., 1972; Samet et al., 1980). Heavy or even moderate cigarette smoking is unusual in these tribes (Sievers, 1968b). Significantly, COPD occurs occasionally among Oklahoma Indians, in whom both cigarette smoking and partial non-Indian heritage are more frequent than in the tribes of the Southwest (Sievers, 1966a, 1968b). A large proportion of Canadian Eskimos have impaired ventilatory function (Beaudry, 1968). In that population, cigarette smoking is frequent, and the ventilatory impairment is greater in the smokers than in the nonsmokers.

The low-to-moderate rate of COPD found in North American Indians is compatible with general observations that this disease is less common in rural than in urban populations, and in nonsmokers than in cigarette smokers, but not with the higher frequency reported for lower socioeconomic groups (Enterline, 1967; Mitchell, 1974). In recent years, cigarette smoking is increasing somewhat among the southwestern Indians, especially in the younger age-groups and in persons living off-reservation. Future trends for COPD in these tribes may indicate whether apparently favorable hereditary factors may be counterbalanced by the adverse environmental influences of cigarette smoking and air pollution.

O. Asthma and Allergies

Allergic (extrinsic) asthma and other atopic diseases occur less often in Native Americans than in whites (Salsbury, 1937; Kraus, 1954; Herxheimer, 1964; Sievers, 1966a; Slocum and Thompson, 1975; Gerrard et al., 1976, 1977). This racial difference appears to be largely genetically determined. Indeed, among southwestern tribes, more than 80% of the population less than 18 years of age have complete Indian heritage, but only 39% of the young asthmatics are fullblooded Indians ($p < 0.001$) (C. R. Westley and S. Nick, 1979 personal communication). However, environmental influences also seem to contribute, inasmuch as allergies are noted more frequently in off- than in on-reservation Indians, and asthma is more prevalent among tribes extensively engaged in farming (e.g., the Colorado River Reservation) than among tribes less involved with agriculture (e.g., the Papago Reservation).

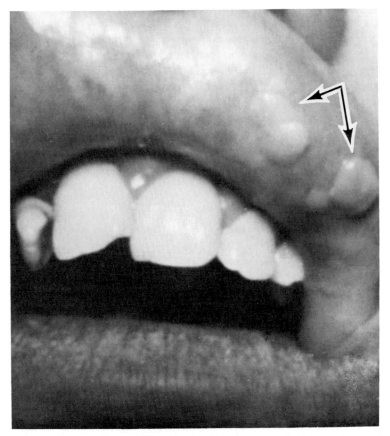

Fig. 10. Heck's disease, a wartlike disorder of the mouth, is probably contagious and shows a predilection for Native American groups. Among American Indians, the condition occurs most often in children, on the labial mucosa (shown here), whereas most of the lesions in Eskimos are found in adults, on the tongue. (Photograph by John W. Heck, D.D.S., reproduced with permission.)

P. Unusual Mucocutaneous Findings

Focal epithelial hyperplasia (Heck's disease), an apparently benign papular eruption of the tongue and oral mucosa (Fig. 10) associated with a papillomavirus infection has been observed predominantly in American Indians and Eskimos (Archard *et al.*, 1965; Praetorius-Clausen, 1973; Stiefler *et al.*, 1979). This distribution implies a high frequency of infection or an unusual vulnerability with more pronounced reactivity of the oral epithelium in native Americans than in other populations. The mode of transmission and natural history of this condition remain unknown. It is of interest that conjunctival papillomas, also related to papillomavirus infection, have been reported to occur with increased frequency among Canadian natives (Pearce *et al.*, 1975).

A distinctive photodermatitis of the polymorphic light eruption type (Fig. 11) occurs in diverse, broadly dispersed groups of American Indians and often produces severe actinic cheilitis (Birt and Hogg, 1979). The pathogenesis of this condition is unknown, but the presence of a dense perivascular lymphocytic infiltration in the cutaneous lesions suggests a cell-mediated immune mechanism. Birt and Davis (1975) found the condition to be transmitted as an autosomal dominant trait with incomplete penetrance. They found no abnormal

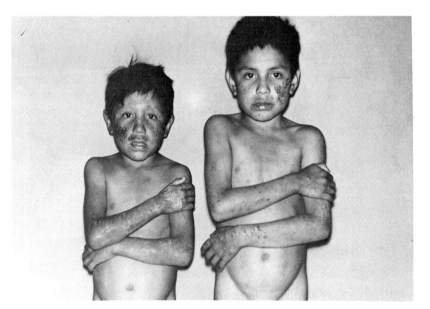

Fig. 11. Photodermatitis in Cree Indian brothers, demonstrating the characteristic skin eruption on sunexposed areas of the face, arms, and hands. (From Birt and Davis, 1975, with permission.)

porphyrins in the urine, feces, erythrocytes, or skin of those affected. Nonetheless, oral β-carotene treatment is as effective in controlling this condition as it is in erythropoietic protoporphyria (Fusaro and Johnson, 1980).

A deep diagonal ear-lobe crease has been considered to be associated with coronary heart disease (CHD) in other ethnic groups. Nonetheless, southwestern American Indians, who have a low rate of CHD, have about twice the frequency of diagonal ear-lobe creases reported for whites (Fisher and Sievers, 1980). Large pendulous ear lobes, a prominent physical attribute of the American Indian, especially the men, appear to develop creases with advancing age, independently from underlying pathologic conditions.

Q. Purulent Otitis Media

Otitis media is much more frequent in many native American groups than in the U.S. white population (Zonis, 1968a, 1970; Manning et al., 1974; Rowe, 1975; Wiet, 1979). New cases of middle-ear infections exceed all other notifiable diseases within the Indian Health Service (U.S. Department of HEW, 1978a). An estimated 50% of children in some areas of the Navajo Reservation have chronically perforated eardrums (Mortimer, 1973).

Middle-ear infections are often considered to occur more frequently in cold climates, but Zonis (1968a, 1970) found no significant difference in the prevalence of otitis media among children of the adjacent San Carlos and White Mountain Apache Reservations, although the former is a warm arid desert region, and the latter is a cold mountainous area. Early observations suggested that a deficiency of one or more immunoglobulins (especially secretory IgA) might be related to the high rates of chronic otitis media in Indians (Zonis, 1968b), but more recent studies have failed to find such an association (Zonis, 1970; Berg et al., 1971). Changing life-style with infrequent breast-feeding of infants has also been suggested as a contributing factor in the augmented prevalence of purulent otitis media in several Amerind tribes (Schaefer, 1972; Manning et al., 1974). The role of allergy in the cause of middle-ear disease among native Americans is uncertain (Zonis, 1970), but allergic diseases are less common in Indians than in whites (see Section V,O).

Cambron and co-workers (1965) noted that the preponderance of American Indians with middle-ear disease were from poor socioeconomic conditions. However, reservation-born Apache children who were adopted at an early age into middle-class non-Appache off-reservation homes had no significant difference in the number of episodes of otitis media during the first 2 years of life from the frequency among the reservation children (Spivey and Hirschhorn, 1977). The rate of middle-ear disease was also much higher for the Apache than for the non-Apache children in the adoptive households. Furthermore, Shaw et al. (1981), in extensive prospective observations, found no significant relationship between environmental factors (climate, housing, and sanitation) and the occurrence of otitis media among reservation Indian children of the Southwest.

Adenoid hypertrophy is considered an insignificant problem in Indians (Zonis, 1970). Recently, Beery *et al.* (1980) found lower resistance of the eustachian tube in Apaches than in whites, and suggested that a low tubal resistance might allow secretions (and infectious agents) to enter the middle ear more readily in Indians than in Caucasians. Furthermore, Klein (1979) cited evidence that the American blacks, whites, and Indians differ significantly in the length, width, and angle of the bony eustachian tube. These findings infer that anatomic factors may relate to racial differences in susceptibility to otitis media (which appears to be greatest in the Amerind, intermediate in American whites, and lowest in American blacks) (Griffith, 1979). In addition, genetic predisposition to middle-ear infection is suggested by observations that Boston children who had otitis media were more likely to have siblings with histories of middle-ear infections than were children who had no episodes of otitis media (Teele and Klein, 1978). Influences other than climate, sanitation, socioeconomic conditions, and immunologic competency appear to contribute to the high rate and severity of otitis media in the Amerind. Anatomic and genetic factors may predispose Native Americans to middle-ear infections.

R. Eye Diseases

Trachoma with its cicatrizing blinding complications was a frequent, serious ophthalmological problem of the American Indian until recently (Hoshiwara, 1971; Bettman, 1973). Since 1966, however, when an intensive trachoma control project was begun by the Indian Health Service, this infectious disease has been reduced from its epidemic proportions (1712 cases/100,000 population) to sporadic occurrences (1976 rate: 303/100,000), primarily in southwestern Indian children (Szuter and Hoshiwara, 1976; U.S. Department of HEW, 1978a).

Trauma is the most frequent cause of uniocular blindness in the Amerind, and diabetic retinopathy is the leading cause of binocular blindness in many southwestern tribes (Bettman, 1972; I. Hoshiwara, 1979 personal communication). Primary open-angle glaucoma, the most common cause of blindness in white adults, is infrequent in the Zuni (Kass *et al.*, 1978) and Chippewa (Thompson and Harper, 1974), but occurs at about expected rates in the Navajo and other southwestern Indians (Bettman, 1972). This tribal variability of rates suggests a genetic influence. An unusually high degree of astigmatism has been noted in the adolescents of some tribes (Hoshiwara, 1971; Mohindra and Nagaraj, 1977), but the relative contribution of genetic and environmental factors is unclear. Color-vision defects are rare among Native Americans (Garth, 1933; Adam, 1973), and strabismus (esotropia) is infrequent (Hoshiwara, 1971; Bettman, 1972).

In many tribes, congenital melanosis oculi has a high prevalence (Hoshiwara,

1971; Bettman, 1972). Retinoblastoma seems to occur unusually often in Indians, but ocular malignant melanoma is rare (Bettman, 1972; I. Hoshiwara, 1979 personal communication).

Vogt-Koyanagi-Harada syndrome, a rare inflammatory disorder characterized by ophthalmologic, neurologic, and dermatologic abnormalities, occurs most often in young adults. Many of the reported cases have been Orientals, and the condition appears to occur with greater than expected frequency among Native Americans, perhaps a reflection of their Mongoloid heritage (I. Hoshiwara and F. Jones, 1980 personal communication).

The Native Americans had what the world has lost. They have it now. It is the ancient reverence and passion for the human spirit, and for the earth and its web of life. *John Collier, Commisioner of Indian Affairs 1933–1945*

VI. CONCLUSIONS

After millennia of genetic adaptation to the varied ecologies of the New World, American Indians have experienced abrupt social and environmental changes in the last century. Increasing interaction with the prevailing Western culture has been accompanied by considerable alteration in the frequency of several disorders among Native Americans. This changing pattern of disease prevalence suggests that the Amerind are vulnerable to the same risk factors for disease that adversely affect other ethnic groups. Nonetheless, they appear to have genetically determined characteristics that enhance their propensity to some conditions (e.g., diabetes mellitus and cholesterol gallstones), but blunt their tendencies to develop others (e.g., duodenal ulcer and coronary heart disease).

Perhaps the high prevalence of obesity observed in contemporary North American Indians is the result of a "thrifty genotype" that permits maintenance of body weight with reduced caloric intake—advantageous in times of famine, but detrimental with constant food abundance. The burden of gallstones and escalating rates of diabetes mellitus and coronary artery disease in this ethnic group may be, in part, a manifestation of dietary alteration and of the widespread obesity. In addition, cholelithiasis appears to contribute to gastric hyposecretion and may be related to the low rate of peptic ulceration in Amerind groups. Multiple factors, however, probably contribute to the high prevalence of biliary disease and to the low rate of peptic ulcer. It is of interest that adoption of the Western diet and customs by another Mongoloid group, the Japanese, also has resulted in increased rates of diabetes (Kawate *et al.,* 1979), cholesterol gallstones (Nagase *et al.,* 1978), obesity, and coronary heart disease (Robertson *et al.,* 1977).

Native Americans have undergone drastic cultural disruption with concomitant decreased physical activity, increased psychological stress, and severe dietary alterations. Clearly, some modification of their current life-style is desirable to achieve an appropriate blend of the traditional Indian and Western cultures.

ACKNOWLEDGMENTS

We acknowledge the valuable assistance of Rebekah Hinton, administrative librarian (Phoenix Indian Medical Center), who obtained much of the reference material; Gwyneth Roske (Tucson Veterans Administration Medical Center), Eddie Deuel, Leon R. Doiron, Art Swieca, and Diana M. Zielinski (Phoenix Veterans Administration Medical Center), who prepared the illustrations; and Jennie Baldwin (Phoenix Area Indian Health Service) and Rose Mendoza (Phoenix Indian Medical Center), who patiently and meticulously prepared the manuscript.

REFERENCES

Acheson, R. M., and Collart, A. B. (1975). New Haven survey of joint diseases. Relationship between some systemic characteristics and osteoarthritis in a general population. *Ann. Rheum. Dis.* **34**, 379-387.

Adam, A. (1973). Colorblindness and gene flow in Alaskans. *Am. J. Hum. Genet.* **25**, 564-566.

Allison, M. J., Mendoza, D., and Pezzia, A. (1973). Documentation of a case of tuberculosis in pre-Columbian America. *Am. Rev. Respir. Dis.* **197**, 985-991.

American Cancer Society (1979). "Cancer Facts and Figures." Am. Cancer Soc., New York.

Anderson, R. C. (1977). Congenital heart malformations in North American Indian children. *Pediatrics* **59**, 121-123.

Archard, H. O., Heck, J. W., and Stanley, A. R. (1965). Focal epithelial hyperplasia: an unusual mucosal lesion found in Indian children. *Oral Surg.* **20**, 201-212.

Archer, V. E., Gilliam, J. D., and Wagoner, J. K. (1976). Respiratory disease mortality among uranium miners. *Ann. N.Y. Acad. Sci.* **271**, 280-293.

Aronoff, S. L., Bennett, P. H., and Unger, R. H. (1977a). Immunoreactive glucagon responses to intravenous glucose in prediabetes and diabetes among Pima Indians and normal Caucasians. *J. Clin. Endrocrinol. Metab.* **44**, 968-972.

Aronoff, S. L., Bennett, P. H., Gorden, P., Rushforth, N., and Miller, M. (1977b). Unexplained hyperinsulinemia in normal and "prediabetic" Pima Indians compared with normal Caucasians: an example of racial differences in insulin secretion. *Diabetes* **26**, 827-840.

Balsamo, P., Hardy, W. R., and Scott, E. M. (1964). Hereditary methemoglobinemia due to diaphorase deficiency in Navajo Indians. *J. Pediatr.* **65**, 928-931.

Barlow, T. G. (1962). Early diagnosis and treatment of congenital dislocation of the hip. *J. Bone Jt. Surg. Br. Vol.* **44**, 292-301.

Beasley, R. P., Retailliau, H., and Healey, L. A. (1973a). Prevalence of rheumatoid arthritis in Alaskan Eskimos. *Arthritis Rheum.* **16**, 737-742.

Beasley, R. P., Willkens, R. F., and Bennett, P. H. (1973b). High prevalence of rheumatoid arthritis in Yakima Indians. *Arthritis Rheum.* **16**, 743-748.

Beaudry, P. H. (1968). Pulmonary function survey of the Canadian Eastern Arctic Eskimo. *Arch. Environ. Health* **17**, 524-528.

Bebchuk, W., Rogers, A. G., and Downey, J. L. (1961). Chronic ulcerative colitis in a North American Indian. *Gastroenterology* **40**, 138-140.

Beery, Q. C., Doyle, W. J., Cantekin, E. I., Bluestone, C. D., and Weit, R. J. (1980). Eustachian tube function in an American Indian population. *Ann. Otol., Rhinol., Laryngol.* **89**, Suppl. 68, 28-33.

Bennett, P. H. (1972). Panel in Diabetes. *In* "Epidemiologic Studies and Clinical Trials in Chronic Diseases," Sci. Publ. No. 257, pp. 31-38. Pan Am. Health Organ., Washington, D.C.

Bennett, P. H., and Burch, T. A. (1968a). The distribution of rheumatoid factor and rheumatoid arthritis in the families of Blackfeet and Pima Indians. *Arthritis Rheum.* **11**, 546-553.

Bennett, P. H., and Burch, T. A. (1968b). The epidemiology of rheumatoid arthritis. *Med. Clin. North Am.* **52**, 479-491.

Bennett, P. H., and Burch, T. A. (1968c). Osteoarthrosis in the Blackfeet and Pima Indians. *In* "Population Studies of Rheumatic Diseases" (P. H. Bennett and P. H. N. Wood, eds.), pp. 407-412. Excerpta Med. Found., Amsterdam.

Bennett, P. H., and Burch, T. A. (1968d). Serum uric acid and gout in Blackfeet and Pima Indians. *In* "Population Studies of Rheumatic Diseases" (P. H. Bennett and P. H. N. Wood, eds.), pp. 358-362. Excerpta Med. Found., Amsterdam.

Bennett, P. H., and Miller, M. (1976). Vascular complications of diabetes in American Indians, Japanese, and Caucasians. *In* "Diabetes Mellitus in Asia" (S. Baba, Y. Goto, and I. Fykui, eds.), pp. 202-207. Excerpta Med. Found., Amsterdam.

Bennett, P. H., Rushforth, N. B., Miller, M., and LeCompte, P. M. (1976). Epidemiologic studies of diabetes in the Pima Indians. *Recent Prog. Horm. Res.* **32**, 333-376.

Bennett, P. H., Knowler, W. C., Rushforth, N. B., Hamman, R. F., and Savage, P. J. (1979a). The role of obesity in the development of diabetes in Pima Indians. *In* "Diabetes and Obesity" (J. Vague, P. H. Vague, and F. J. G. Ebling, eds.), pp. 117-126. Excerpta Med. Found., Amsterdam.

Bennett, P. H., Webner, C., and Miller, M. (1979b). Congenital anomalies and the diabetic and prediabetic pregnancy. *In* "Pregnancy Metabolism, Diabetes and the Fetus" (K. Elliott and M. O'Connor, eds.), pp. 207-225. Excerpta Med. Found., Amsterdam.

Bennion, L. J., and Grundy, S. M. (1975). Effects of obesity and caloric intake on biliary metabolism in man. *J. Clin. Invest.* **56**, 996-1011.

Bennion, L. J., and Grundy, S. M. (1977). Effects of diabetes mellitus on cholesterol metabolism in man. *N. Engl. J. Med.* **296**, 1365-1371.

Bennion, L. J., and Grundy, S. M. (1978). Risk factors for the development of cholelithiasis in man. *N. Engl. J. Med.* **299**, 1161-1167, 1221-1227.

Bennion, L. J., and Li, T.-K. (1976) Alcohol metabolism in American Indians and whites: lack of racial differences in metabolic rate and liver alcohol dehydrogenase. *N. Engl. J. Med.* **294**, 9-13.

Bennion, L. J., Drobny, E., Knowler, W. C., Ginsberg, R. L., Garnick, M. B., Adler, R. D., and Duane, W. C. (1978). Sex differences in the size of bile pools. *Metab., Clin. Exp.* **27**, 961-969.

Bennion, L. J., Knowler, W. C., Mott, D. M., Spagnola, A. M., and Bennett, P. H. (1979). Development of lithogenic bile during puberty in Pima Indians. *N. Engl. J. Med.* **300**, 873-876.

Berg, D. E., Larsen, A. E., and Yarington, C. T., Jr. (1971). Association between serum and secretory immunoglobulins and chronic otitis media in Indian children. *Ann. Otol., Rhinol., Laryngol.* **80**, 766-772.

Bergman, R. L. (1973). A school for medicine men. *Am. J. Psychiatry* **130**, 663-666.

Bettman, J. W., Jr. (1972). Eye disease among American Indians of the Southwest. I. Overall analysis. *Arch. Ophthalmol.* (*Chicago*) **88**, 263-268.

Bettman, J. W., Jr. (1973). Eye disease among American Indians of the Southwest. II. Trachoma. *Arch. Ophthalmol.* (*Chicago*) **90**, 440-446.

Bingle, G. J., and Niswander, J. D. (1975). Polydactyly in the American Indian. *Am. J. Hum. Genet.* **27**, 91-99.

Birt, A. R., and Davis, R. A. (1975). Hereditary polymorphic light eruption of American Indians. *Int. J. Dermatol.* **14,** 105–111.

Birt, A. R., and Hogg, G. R. (1979). The actinic cheilitis of hereditary polymorphic light eruption. *Arch. Dermatol.* **115,** 699–702.

Bivens, M. D., and Fleetwood, H. O. (1968). A 10-year survey of cervical carcinoma in Indians of the Southwest. *Obstet. Gynecol.* **32,** 11–16.

Black, W. C., Key, C. R., Carmany, T. B., and Herman, D. (1977). Carcinoma of the gallbladder in a population of southwestern American Indians. *Cancer (Philadelphia)* **39,** 1267–1279.

Blumberg, B. S. (1969). The epidemiology of alloalbuminemia. *Arch. Environ. Health* **18,** 1–3.

Bordin, G. M., Key, C. R., McQuade, C. E., Kutvirt, D. M., Hughes, W. B., and Brylinski, D. A. (1977). Multiple primary cancers: relative risk in New Mexico's triethnic population. *Cancer (Philadelphia)* **30,** 1793–1800.

Brandfonbrener, M., Lovekin, W. S., and Leack, J. K. (1970). Cardiomyopathy in the southwest American Indians. *Br. Heart J.* **32,** 491–496.

Brett, M., and Barker, D. J. P. (1976). The world distribution of gallstones. *Int. J. Epidemiol.* **5,** 335–341.

Brod, T. M. (1975). Alcoholism as a mental health problem of Native Americans. *Arch. Gen. Psychiatry* **32,** 1385–1391.

Brown, J. E., and Christensen, C. (1967). Biliary tract disease among Navajos. *J. Am. Med. Assoc.* **202,** 1050–1052.

Burkitt, D. P., Walker, A. R. P., and Painter, N. S. (1974). Dietary fiber and disease *J. Am. Med. Assoc.* **229,** 1068–1074.

Calin, A., Bennett, P. H., Jupiter, J., and Terasaki, P. I. (1977). HLA 27 and sacroiliitis in Pima Indians—association in males only. *J. Rheumatol.* **4,** Suppl. 3, 44–48.

Cambron, K., Galbraith, J. D., and Kong, G. (1965). Middle ear disease in Indians of the Mount Currie Reservation, British Columbia. *Can. Med. Assoc. J.* **93,** 1301–1305.

Campbell, J. M. (1963). Ancient Alaska and paleolithic Europe. *Anthropol. Pap. Univ. Alaska* **10**(2), 29–49.

Capper, W. M., Butler, T. J., Kilby, J. O., and Gibson, J. J. (1967). Gallstones, gastric secretion, and flatulent dyspepsia. *Lancet* **1,** 413–415.

Cavalli-Sforza, L. L., and Bodmer, W. F. (1971). "The Genetics of Human Populations." Freeman, San Francisco, California.

Centerwall, W. R. (1968). A recent experience with measles in a "virgin-soil" population. *In* "Biomedical Challenges Presented by the American Indian" (J. V. Neel, ed.), pp. 77–80. World Health Organ., Washington, D.C.

Chung, C. S., and Myrianthopoulos, N. C. (1968). Racial and prenatal factors in major congenital malformations. *Am. J. Hum. Genet.* **20,** 44–60.

Clabeaux, M. S. (1977). Congenital dislocation of the hip in the prehistoric Northeast. *Bull. N.Y. Acad. Med.* **53,** 338–346.

Clarren, S. K. (1979). Neural tube defects and fetal alcohol syndrome. *Pediatrics* **95,** 328.

Clarren, S. K., and Smith, D. W. (1978). Fetal alcohol syndrome. *N. Engl. J. Med.* **298,** 1063–1067.

Coleman, S. S. (1968). Congenital dysplasia of the hip in the Navajo infant. *Clin. Orthrop. Relat. Res.* No. 56, 179–193.

Comess, L. J., Bennett, P. H., and Burth, T. A. (1967). Clinical gallbladder disease in Pima Indians: its high prevalence in contrast to Framingham, Massachusetts. *N. Engl. J. Med.* **277,** 894–898.

Conrad, R. D., and Kahn, M. W. (1974). An epidemiological study of suicide and attempted suicide among the Papago Indians. *Am. J. Psychiatry* **131,** 69–72.

Creagan, E. T., and Fraumeni, J. F. (1972). Cancer mortality among American Indians 1950–1967. *J. Natl. Cancer Inst.* **49,** 959–967.

Cudworth, A. G. (1979). Type 2 (insulin-independent) diabetes-fibre and flushers. *Diabetologia* **17,** 67–69.

Dale, E. D. (1949). "The Indians of the Southwest." Univ. of Oklahoma Press, Norman.

Danforth, C. H. (1921). Distribution of hair on the digits of man. *Am. J. Phys. Anthropol.* **4,** 189–204.

Dobyn, H. F. (1966). Estimating aboriginal American population. An appraisal of techniques with a new hemispheric estimate. *Curr. Anthropol.* **7,** 395–416.

Driver, H. E. (1969). "Indians of North America." Univ. of Chicago Press, Chicago, Illinois.

Duncan, I. W., and Scott, E. M. (1972). Lactose intolerance in Alaskan Indians and Eskimos. *Am. J. Clin. Nutr.* **25,** 867–868.

Dunham, L. J., Bailar, M. C., and Laquer, G. L. (1973). Histologically diagnosed cancers in 693 Indians of the United States, 1950–1965. *J. Natl. Cancer Inst.* **50,** 1119–1127.

Dutton, B. P. (1976). "Navajos and Apaches: The Athabascan Peoples." Prentice-Hall, Englewood Cliffs, New Jersey.

Eastmond, C. J., and Woodrow, J. C. (1977). Discordance for ankylosing spondylitis in monozygotic twins. *Ann. Rheum. Dis.* **36,** 360–364.

Ebringer, R. W., Caldwell, D. R., Cowling, P., and Ebringer, A. (1978). Sequential studies in ankylosing spondylitis. Association of *Klebsiella pneumoniae* with active disease. *Ann. Rheum. Dis.* **37,** 146–151.

Elashoff, J. D., and Grossman, M. I. (1980). Trends in hospital admissions and death rates for peptic ulcer in the United States from 1970 to 1978. *Gastroenterology* **78,** 280–285.

Engle, A., Robert, J., and Burch, T. A. (1966). "Rheumatoid Arthritis in Adults," DHEW, Natl. Cent. Health Stat., Publ. 1000, Ser. 11, No. 17. U.S. Gov. Print. Off., Washington, D.C.

Enterline, P. E. (1967). The effects of occupation on chronic respiratory disease. *Arch. Environ. Health* **14,** 189–200.

Erickson, J. D. (1976). Racial variations in the incidence of congenital malformations. *Ann. Hum. Genet.* **39,** 315–320.

Erickson, W. (1972). Cholecystectomy and the American Indian: a ten-year comparative study. *Rocky Mt. Med. J.* **69,** 33–35.

Ewy, G. A., Okada, R. D., Marcus, F. I., Goldberg, S. J., and Phibbs, B. P. (1979). Electrocardiographic axis deviation in Navajo and Apache Indians. *Chest* **75,** 54–58.

Farris, J. J., and Jones, B. M. (1978). Ethanol metabolism in male American Indians and whites. *Alcoholism* **2,** 77–81.

Felsman, F. W. (1955). "Health Status Report on Diabetes Mellitus." Div Indian Health, USPHS, Rockville, Maryland.

Fenna, D., Mix, L., Schaefer, O., and Gilbert, J. A. L. (1971). Ethanol metabolism in various racial groups. *Can. Med. Assoc. J.* **105,** 472–475.

Fiese, M. J. (1958). "Coccidioidomycosis." Thomas, Springfield, Illinois.

Fisher, J. R., and Sievers, M. L. (1980). Ear-lobe crease in American Indians. *Ann. Intern. Med.* **93,** 512.

Fisher, J. R., Conway, M. J., Takeshita, R. T., and Sandoval, M. R. (1979). Necrotizing fasciitis. Importance of radiographic studies for soft-tissue gas. *J. Am. Med. Assoc.* **241,** 803–806.

Flynn, N. M., Hoeprich, P. D., Kawachi, M. M., Lee, K. K., Lawrence, R. M., Kundargi, R. S., and Wong, G. A. (1979). An unusual outbreak of windborne coccidioidomycosis. *N. Engl. J. Med.* **301,** 358–361.

Friedman, G. D., Kannel, W. B., and Dawber, T. R. (1966). The epidemiology of gallbladder disease: observations in the Framingham study. *J. Chronic Dis.* **19,** 273–292.

Fusaro, R. M., and Johnson, J. A. (1980). Treatment of photosensitive American Indians with oral beta carotene. *J. Am. Med. Assoc.* **243**, 231.

Garbarino, M. S. (1976). "Native American Heritage." Little, Brown, Boston, Massachusetts.

Garn, S. M. (1971). "Human Races." Thomas, Springfield, Illinois.

Garnick, M. B., Bennett, P. H., and Langer, T. (1979). Low density lipoprotein metabolism and lipoprotein cholesterol content in southwestern American Indians. *J. Lipid Res.* **20**, 31–39.

Garth, T. R. (1933). The incidence of color blindness among races. *Science* **77**, 333–334.

Geare, R. I. (1915). Some diseases prevalent among Indians of the Southwest and their treatment. *Med. World* **33**, 305–310.

Genuth, S. M. (1977). Insulin secretion in obesity and diabetes: an illustrative case. *Ann. Intern. Med.* **87**, 714–716.

Gerrard, J. W., Geddes, C. A., Reggin, P. L., Gerrard, C. D., and Horne, S. (1976). Serum IgE levels in white and metis communities in Saskatchewan. *Ann. Allergy* **37**, 91–100.

Gerrard, J. W., Ko, C. G., Dalgleish, R., and Tan, L. K. T. (1977). Immunoglobulin levels in white and metis communities in Saskatchewan. *Clin. Exp. Immunol.* **29**, 447–456.

Gershowitz, H., and Neel, J. V. (1978). The immunoglobulin allotypes (Gm and Km) of 12 Indian tribes of Central and South America. *Am. J. Phys. Anthropol.* **49**, 289–302.

Gilbert, J. (1955). Absence of coronary thrombosis in Navajo Indians. *Calif. Med.* **82**, 114–115.

Gilbert, J. A. L., and Schaefer, O. (1977). Metabolism of ethanol in different racial groups. *Can. Med. Assoc. J.* **116**, 476.

Gofton, J. P., Robinson, H. S., and Price, G. E. (1964). A study of rheumatic disease in a Canadian Indian population. *Ann. Rheum. Dis.* **23**, 364–371.

Gofton, J. P., Bennett, P. H., Smythe, H. A., and Decker, J. L. (1972). Sacroiliitis and ankylosing spondylitis in North American Indians. *Ann. Rheum. Dis.* **31**, 474–481.

Gofton, J. P., Chalmers, A., Price, G. E., and Reeve, C. E. (1975). HLA B27 and ankylosing spondylitis in B.C. Indians. *J. Rheumatol.* **2**, 314–318.

Goldberg, B. (1944). "Clinical Tuberculosis." Davis, Philadelphia, Pennsylvania.

Goldman, S. M., Sievers, M. L., Carlile, W. K., and Cohen, S. L. (1972). Roentgen manifestations of diseases in southwestern Indians. *Radiology* **103**, 303–306.

Gordon, R. C., and Langley, R. N. (1970). Natal teeth in American Indian children. *J. Pediatr.* **76**, 613–614.

Greenacre, M. J., and Degos, L. (1977). Correspondence analysis of HLA gene frequency data from 124 population samples. *Am. J. Hum. Genet.* **29**, 60–75.

Griffith, T. E. (1979). Epidemiology of otitis media—an interracial study. *Laryngoscope* **89**, 22–30.

Grundy, S. M., Metzger, A. L., and Adler, R. D. (1972). Mechanisms of lithogenic bile formation in American Indian women with cholesterol gallstones. *J. Clin. Invest.* **51**, 3026–3043.

Hammerschlag, C. A. (1970). Pride, powerlessness and rebellion: the red and the black. *J. Hum. Relat.* **18**, 656–669.

Hancock, J. C. (1933). Diseases among the Indians. *Southwest. Med.* **17**, 126–129.

Hankin, J. H., and Rawlings, V. (1978). Diet and breast cancer: a review. *Am. J. Clin. Nutr.* **31**, 2005–2016.

Harris, R. L., and Riley, H. D. (1968). Cystic fibrosis in the American Indian. *Pediatrics* **41**, 733–738.

Hendrikx, M. E. (1979a). Measurement of caloric needs for weight maintenance in southwestern Indian and Caucasian diabetic and nondiabetic patients. *Proc. USPHS Prof. Assoc., Commissioned Officers Assoc., Washington, D.C.* pp. 30–31.

Hendrikx, M. E. (1979b). Adaptive response to caloric deprivation in southwestern Indians and Caucasians. *Proc. USPHS Prof. Assoc., Commissioned Officers Assoc., Washington, D.C.* p. 31.

Henrard, J., Bennett, P. H., and Burch, T. A. (1976). Rheumatoid arthritis in the Pima Indians of

Arizona: an assessment of the clinical components of the New York criteria. *Int. J. Epidemiol.* **4**, 119–126.

Herxheimer, H. (1964). Asthma in American Indians. *N. Engl. J. Med.* **270**, 1128–1129.

Hesse, F. G. (1959). Incidence of cholecystitis and other diseases among Pima Indians of southern Arizona. *J. Am. Med. Assoc.* **170**, 1789–1790.

Hesse, F. G. (1964). Incidence of disease in the Navajo Indians: a necropsy study of coronary and aortic atherosclerosis, cholelithiasis, and neoplastic disease. *Arch. Pathol.* **77**, 553–557.

Hill, C. A., Jr., and Spector, M. I. (1971). Natality and mortality of American Indians compared with U.S. whites and nonwhites. *HSMHA Health Rep.* **86**, 229–246.

Holmes, L. B. (1974). Inborn errors of morphogenesis. A review of localized hereditary malformations. *N. Engl. J. Med.* **291**, 763–773.

Hoshiwara, I. (1971). Ophthalmological care for American Indians. *Arch. Ophthalmol.* (*Chicago*) **86**, 368.

Howard, B. V., Savage, P. J., Nagulesparan, M., Bennion, L. J., Unger, R. H., and Bennett, P. H. (1979). Evidence for marked sensitivity to the antilipolytic action of insulin in obese maturity-onset diabetics. *Metab., Clin. Exp.* **28**, 744–750.

Hrdlička, A. (1908). "Physiological and Medical Observations among the Indians of Southwestern United States and Mexico," Bull. No. 34. Smithsonian Inst., Bur. Am. Ethnol., Washington, D.C.

Hrdlička, A. (1932). Disease, medicine, and surgery among American aborigenes. *J. Am. Med. Assoc.* **99**, 1661–1666.

Huppert, M. (1978). Racism in coccidioidomycosis? *Am. Rev. Respir. Dis.* **118**, 797–798.

Inglefinger, F. J. (1979). The chemistry of the American Indian's burden. *N. Engl. J. Med.* **300**, 917–918.

Inglefinger, J. A., Bennett, P. H., Liebow, I. M., and Miller, M. (1976). Coronary heart disease in Pima Indians. *Diabetes* **25**, 561–565.

Jaffe, B. F., and DeBlanc, G. B. (1970). Cleft palate, cleft lip, and cleft uvula in Navajo Indians: incidence, and otorhinolaryngologic problems. *Cleft Palate J.* **7**, 300–305.

Jennings, J. D. (1974). "Prehistory of North America." McGraw-Hill, New York.

Johnson, J. D., Simoons, F. J., Hurwitz, R., Grange, A., Sinatra, F. R., Sunshine, P., Robertson, W. V., Bennett, P. H., and Kretchmer, N. (1978). Lactose malabsorption among adult Indians of the Great Basin and American Southwest. *Am. J. Clin. Nutr.* **31**, 381–387.

Jordan, S. W., Munsick, R. A., and Stone, R. S. (1969). Carcinoma of the cervix in American Indian women. *Cancer* (*Philadelphia*) **23**, 1227–1232.

Joslin, E. P. (1940). The universality of diabetes. A survey of diabetic morbidity in Arizona. *J. Am. Med. Assoc.* **115**, 2033–2038.

Kass, M. A., Zimmerman, T. J., Alton, E., Lemon, L., and Becker, R. (1978). Intraocular pressure and glaucoma in the Zuni Indians. *Arch. Ophthalmol.* (*Chicago*) **96**, 2212–2213.

Kawate, R., Yamakido, M., Nishimoto, Y., Bennett, P. H., Hamman, R. F., and Knowler, W. D. (1979). Diabetes mellitus and its vascular complications in Japanese migrants on the islands of Hawaii. *Diabetes Care* **2**, 161–170.

Khan, M. A., Kushner, I., Braun, W. E., Schacter, B. Z., and Steinberg, A. G. (1977). HLA-B27 and ankylosing spondylitis in American blacks. *N. Engl. J. Med.* **297**, 513.

Klein, J. O. (1979). Epidemiology of otitis media. *Proceedings Natl. Conf. Otitis Media, 2nd, Ross Lab., Columbus, Ohio* pp. 18–20.

Knowler, W. C., Bennett, P. H., Bottazzo, G. F., and Doniach, D. (1979). Islet cell antibodies and diabetes mellitus in Pima Indians. *Diabetologia* **17**, 161–164.

Kraus, B. S. (1954). "Indian Health in Arizona." Univ. of Arizona, Tucson.

Kraus, G., and Schwartzmann, J. (1957). Congenital dislocation of the hip in Fort Apache Indians. *J. Bone Jt. Surg., Am. Vol.* **39**, 448–449.

Kravetz, R. E. (1964). Etiology of biliary tract disease in southwestern American Indians. *Gastroenterology* **48**, 392-398.

Kuhnlein, H. V., and Calloway, D. H. (1977). Minerals in human teeth: differences between preindustrial and contemporary Hopi Indians. *Am. J. Clin. Nutr.* **30**, 883-886.

Lam, R. C. (1954). Gallbladder disease among the American Indians. *J.-Lancet* **74**, 305-309.

Langmuir, A. D. (1962). Medical importance of measles. *Am. J. Dis. Child.* **103**, 224-246.

Larisse, M. (1968). Biological subdivisions of the Indian on the basis of genetic traits. *In* "Biomedical Challenges Presented by the American Indian" (J. V. Neel, ed.), pp. 35-46. World Health Organ., Washington, D.C.

Lawrence, J. S. (1961). Prevalence of rheumatoid arthritis. *Ann. Rheum. Dis.* **20**, 11-17.

Lawrence, J. S. (1976). Radiological cervical arthritis in populations. *Ann. Rheum. Dis.* **35**, 365-371.

Lieber, S. (1972). Metabolism of ethanol and alcoholism: racial and acquired factors. *Ann. Intern. Med.* **76**, 326-327.

Lilienfield, A. M. (1970). Population differences in frequency of malformations at birth. *In* "Congenital Malformations: Proceedings of the Third International Conference" (F. C. Fraser and V. A. McKusick, eds.), pp. 251-263. Excerpta Med. Found., Amsterdam.

Littman, G. (1970). Alcoholism, illness, and social pathology among American Indians in transition. *Am. J. Public Health* **60**, 1769-1787.

Lowry, R. B., and Trimble, B. K. (1977). Incidence rates for cleft lip and palate in British Columbia 1952-71 for North American Indians, Japanese, Chinese, and total populations: secular trends over twenty years. *Teratology* **16**, 277-283.

Lubin, A. H., Garry, P. J., and Owen, G. M. (1971). Sex and population differences in the incidence of a plasma cholinesterase variant. *Science* **172**, 161-164.

McConnell, T. S., Foreman, R. E., and Bergren, N. K. (1976). Chromosome abnormalities in southwest American Indian patients. *Am. J. Hum. Genet.* **10**, 398-445.

Malhorta, S. L. (1968). Epidemiological study of cholelithiasis among railroad workers in India with special reference to causation. *Gut* **9**, 290-295.

Manning, P., Avery, M. E., and Ross, A. (1974). Purulent otitis media: differences between populations in different environments. *Pediatrics* **53**, 135-136.

Matis, J. A., and Zwemer, T. J. (1971). Odontognathic discrimination of United States Indian and Eskimo groups. *J. Dent. Res.* **50**, 1245-1248.

Mayberry, R. H., and Lindemann, R. D. (1963). A survey of chronic disease and diet in Seminole Indians in Oklahoma. *Am. J. Clin. Nutr.* **13**, 127-134.

Medalie, J. H., Lavene, C., Papier, C., Goldbourt, U., Dreyfuss, F., Oron, D., Neufeld, H., and Riss, E. (1971). Blood groups, myocardial infarction and angina pectoris among 10,000 adult males. *N. Engl. J. Med.* **285**, 1348-1352.

Mellin, G. W. (1963). The frequency of birth defects. *In* "Birth Defects" (M. Fishbein, ed.), pp. 7-17. Lippincott, Philadelphia, Pennsylvania.

Mendeloff, A. I. (1976). Epidemiological aspects of inflammatory bowel disease. *In* "The Small Intestine and Colon" (H. L. Bockus, J. E. Berk, W. S. Hanbrick, M. Kalser, J. L. Roth, and F. Vilardell, eds.), Gastroenterology, Vol. 2, pp. 540-549. Saunders, Philadelphia, Pennsylvania.

Mitchell, R. S. (1974). Chronic airway obstruction. *In* "Textbook of Pulmonary Diseases" (G. L. Baum, ed.), pp. 579-600. Little, Brown, Boston, Massachusetts.

Mohindra, I., and Nagaraj, S. (1977). Astigmatism in Zuni and Navajo Indians. *Am. J. Optom. Physiol. Opt.* **4**, 121-124.

Moll, J. M. H., Haslock, I., Macrae, I. F., and Wright, V. (1974). Associations between ankylosing spondylitis, psoriatic arthritis, Reiter's disease, the intestinal arthropathies, and Behçet's Syndrome. *Medicine (Baltimore)* **53**, 343-364.

Morris, D. L., Buechley, R. W., Key, C. R., and Morgan, M. W. (1978). Gallbladder disease and gallbladder cancer among American Indians in tricultural New Mexico. *Cancer (Philadelphia)* **42**, 2472-2477.

Morris, R. I., Metzger, A. L., Bluestone, R., and Terasaki, P. I. (1974). HLA-W-27-a useful discriminator in the arthropathies of inflammatory bowel disease. *N. Engl. J. Med.* **290**, 1117-1119.

Morse, D. (1961). Prehistoric tuberculosis in America. *Am. Rev. Respir. Dis.* **83**, 489-504.

Morse, D. (1967). Tuberculosis. *In* "Diseases in Antiquity" (D. Brothwell and A. T. Sandison, eds.), pp. 249-271. Thomas, Springfield, Illinois.

Morse, H. G., Rate, R. G., Bonnell, M. D., and Kuberski, T. (1980). High frequency of HLA-B27 and Reiter's syndrome in Navajo Indians. *J. Rheumatol.* **7**, 900-902.

Mortimer, E. A. (1973). Indian Health: an unmet problem. *Pediatrics* **51**, 1065-1066.

Morton, R. O., Gershwin, M. E., Brady, C., and Steinberg, A. D. (1976). The incidence of systemic lupus erythematosis in North American Indians. *J. Rheumatol.* **3**, 186-190.

Mourant, A. E., Kopec, A. C., and Domaniewska-Sobczak, K. (1976). "The Distribution of the Human Blood Groups and Other Polymorphisms." Oxford Univ. Press, London and New York.

Muggia, A. L. (1971). Diseases among the Navajo Indians. *Rocky Mt. Med. J.* **68**(9), 39-49.

Nagase, M., Tanimura, H., Setoyama, M., and Hikasas, Y. (1978). Present features of gallstones in Japan: a collective review of 2,144 cases. *Am. J. Surg.* **135**, 788-790.

Neel, J. V. (1958). A study of major congenital defects in Japanese infants. *Am. J. Hum. Genet.* **10**, 398-445.

Neel, J. V. (1962). Diabetes mellitus: A "thrifty" genotype rendered detrimental by "progress?" *Am. J. Hum. Genet.* **14**, 353-362.

Nelson, B. D., Porvaznik, J., and Bernfield, J. R. (1971). Gallbladder disease in southwestern American Indians. *Arch. Surg.* **103**, 41-43.

Newcomer, A. D., Thomas, P. J. McGill, D. B., and Hofman, A. F. (1977a). Lactase deficiency: a common genetic trait of the American Indian. *Gastroenterology* **72**, 234-237.

Newcomer, A. D., Gordon, H., Thomas, P. J., and McGill, D. B. (1977b). Family studies of lactase deficiency in the American Indian. *Gastroenterology* **73**, 985-988.

Newcomer, A. D., McGill, D. B., Thomas, P., and Hofman, A. F. (1978). Tolerance to lactose among lactase-deficient American Indians. *Gastroenterology* **74**, 44-46.

Nilsson, S. E. (1962). Genetic and constitutional aspects of diabetes mellitus. *Acta Med. Scand.*, Suppl. No. 375, 1-96.

Niswander, J. D., and Adams, M. S. (1967). Oral clefts in the American Indian. *Public Health Rep.* **82**, 807-812.

Niswander, J. D., Barrow, M. V., and Bingle, F. J. (1975). Congenital malformations in the American Indian. *Soc. Biol.* **22**, 203-215.

Nutels, N. (1968). Medical problems of newly contacted Indian groups *In* "Biomedical Challenges Presented by the American Indians" (J. V. Neel, ed.), pp. 68-76. World Health Organ., Washington, D.C.

O'Brien, W. M., Bennett, P. H., Burch, T. A., and Bunim, J. J. (1967). A genetic study of rheumatoid arthritis and rheumatoid factor in Blackfeet and Pima Indians. *Arthritis Rheum.* **10**, 163-179.

Panayi, G. S., Wooley, P., and Batchelor, J. R. (1978). Genetic basis of rheumatoid disease: HLA antigens, disease manifestations, and toxic reaction to drugs. *Br. Med. J.* **ii**, 1326-1328.

Pappagianis, D. (1972). Coccidioidomycosis. *In* "Infectious Diseases" (P. D. Hoeprich, ed.), pp. 405-416. Harper, New York.

Pearce, W. G., Nigam, S., Mielke, B., and Wyatt, H. T. (1975). Conjunctival papillomas in Northern Canadian Natives. *Can. Med. Assoc. J.* **112**, 1423-1427.

Perzigian, A. J., and Widmer, L. (1979). Evidence for tuberculosis in a prehistoric population. *J. Am. Med. Assoc.* **241**, 2643-2646.

Petrakis, N. L. (1971). Cerumen genetics and human breast cancer. *Science* **173**, 347-349.

Petrakis, N. L., Molohon, K. T., and Tepper, D. J. (1967). Cerumen in American Indians: Genetic implications of sticky and dry types. *Science* **158**, 1192-1193.

Praetorius-Clausen, F. (1973). Geographic aspects of oral focal epithelial hyperplasia. *Pathol. Microbiol.* **39**, 204-213.

Rabin, D. L., Barnett, C. R., Arnold, W. D., Freiberger, R. H., and Brooks, G. (1965). Untreated congenital hip disease. A study of the epidemiology, natural history and social aspects of the disease in a Navajo population. *Am. J. Public Health* **55**, 1-44.

Reed, T. E., Kalant, H., Gibbins, R. J., Kapur, B. M., and Rankin, J. G. (1976). Alcohol and acetaldehyde metabolism in Caucasians, Chinese, and Amerinds. *Can. Med. Assoc. J.* **115**, 851-855.

Reichenbach, D. D. (1967). Autopsy incidence of diseases among southwestern American Indians. *Arch. Pathol.* **84**, 81-86.

Reid, J. M., Fullmer, S. D., Pettigrew, K. D., Burch, T. A., Bennett, P. H., Miller, M., and Whedon, G. D. (1971). Nutrient intake of Pima Indian women: relationships to diabetes mellitus and gallbladder disease. *Am. J. Clin. Nutr.* **24**, 1281-1289.

Reinhard, K. R., and Greenwalt, N. I. (1975). Epidemiological definition of the cohort of diseases associated with diabetes in southwestern American Indians. *Med. Care* **13**, 160-173.

Resnik, H. L. P., and Dismang, L. H. (1971). Observations on suicidal behavior among American Indians. *Am. J. Psychiatry* **127**, 58-64.

Rife, D. C. (1968). Finger and palmar dermatoglyphics in Seminole Indians of Florida. *Am. J. Phys. Anthropol.* **28**, 119-126.

Rimoin, D. L. (1969). Ethnic variability in glucose tolerance and insulin secretion. *Arch. Intern. Med.* **124**, 659-700.

Robbins, S. L. (1974). ''Pathogenic Basis of Disease.'' Saunders, Philadelphia, Pennsylvania.

Robertson, T. L., Kato, H., Gordon, T., Kagan, A., Rhoads, G. G., Land, C. E., Worth, R. M., Belsky, J. L., Dock, D. S., Miyanishi, M., and Kawamoto, S. (1977). Epidemiologic studies of coronary heart disease and stroke in Japanese men living in Japan, Hawaii and California. *Am. J. Cardiol.* **39**, 244-249.

Rotter, J. I., and Rimoin, D. L. (1981). The genetics of the glucose intolerance disorder. *Am. J. Med.* **70**, 116-126.

Rowe, D. S. (1975). Acute suppurative otitis media. *Pediatrics* **51**, 285-294.

Roychoudhury, A. K. (1978). Genetic distance between the American Indians and the three major races of man. *Hum. Hered.* **28**, 380-385.

Saland, J., McNamara, H., and Cohen, M. I. (1974). Navajo jaundice: a variant of neonatal hyperbilirubinemia associated with breast feeding. *J. Pediatr.* **85**, 271-275.

Salsbury, C. G. (1937). Disease incidence among the Navajos. *Southwest. Med.* **21**, 230-233.

Salsbury, C. G. (1947). Incidence of certain diseases among the Navajos. *Ariz. Med.* **4**, 29-31.

Samet, J. M., Key, C. R., Kutvirt, D. M., and Wiggins, C. L. (1980). Respiratory disease mortality in New Mexico's American Indians and Hispanics. *Am. J. Public Health* **70**, 492-497.

Sampliner, R. E., Bennett, P. H., Comess, L. J., Rose, F. A., and Burch, T. A. (1970). Gallbladder disease in Pima Indians: demonstration of high prevalence and early onset by cholecystography. *N. Engl. J. Med.* **283**, 1358-1364.

Savage, P. J., Flock, E. V., Zahnhiser, L., and Bennett, P. H. (1976a). Hyperinsulinism and its age of onset in Pima Indians. *Diabetes* **25**, Suppl. 1, p. 384.

Savage, P. J., Hamman, R. F., Bartha, G., Dippe, S. E., Miller, M., and Bennett, P. H. (1976b). Serum cholesterol levels in American (Pima) Indian children and adolescents. *Pediatrics* **58**, 274-282.

Savage, P. J., Bennett, P. H., Senter, R. G., and Miller, M. (1979a). High prevalence of diabetes in young Pima Indians: evidence of phenotypic variation in a genetically isolated population. *Diabetes* **28**, 937-942.

Savage, P. J., Flock, E. V., Mako, M. E., Blix, P. M., Rubenstein, A. H., and Bennett, P. H. (1979b). C-peptide and insulin secretion in Pima Indians and Caucasians: constant fractional hepatic extraction over a wide range of insulin concentrations and in obesity. *J. Clin. Endocrinol. Metab.* **48**, 594-598.

Savage, P. J., Bennion, L. J., Flock, E. V., Nagulesparan, M., Mott, D., Roth, J., Unger, R. H., and Bennett, P. H. (1979c). Diet-induced improvement of abnormalities in insulin and glucagon secretion and in insulin receptor binding in diabetes mellitus. *J. Clin. Endocrinol. Metab.* **48**, 999-1007.

Schaefer, O. (1972). Otitis media and bottle-feeding: an epidemiological study of infant feeding habits and incidence of recurrent and chronic middle ear disease in Canadian Eskimos. *Can. J. Public Health* **62**, 478-489.

Schlosstein, L., Terasaki, P. I., Bluestone, R., and Pearson, C. M. (1973). High association of an HL-A antigen, W27, with ankylosing spondylitis. *N. Engl. J. Med.* **288**, 704-706.

Scott, E. M. (1973). Genetic disorders in isolated populations. *Arch. Environ. Health* **26**, 32-35.

Scott, E. M., Wright, R. C., and Weaver, D. D. (1969). The discrimination of phenotypes for rate of disappearance of isonicotinoyl hydrazide from serum. *J. Clin. Invest.* **48**, 1173-1176.

Shapiro, B. L. (1976). The genetics of cleft lip and palate. *In* "Oral Facial Genetics" (R. E. Stewart and G. H. Prescott, eds.), pp. 473-499. Mosby, St. Louis, Missouri.

Shaw, J. R., Todd, N. W., Goodwin, M. H., Jr., and Feldman, C. M. (1981). Observations on the relation of environmental and behavioral factors to occurrence of otitis media among Indian children. *Public Health Rep.* **96**, 342-349.

Shore, J. H., and Stone, D. L. (1973). Duodenal ulcer among Northwest Coastal Indian women. *Am. J. Psychiatry* **130**, 774-777.

Short, C. L. (1974). The antiquity of rheumatoid arthritis. *Arthritis Rheum.* **17**, 193-205.

Sievers, M. L. (1964). Coccidioidomycosis among southwestern American Indians. *Am. Rev. Respir. Dis.* **90**, 920-926.

Sievers, M. L. (1966a). Disease patterns among southwestern Indians. *Public Health Rep.* **81**, 1075-1083.

Sievers, M. L. (1966b). A study of achlorhydria among southwestern Indians. *Am. J. Gastroenterol.* **45**, 99-108.

Sievers, M. L. (1967). Myocardial infarction among southwestern American Indians. *Ann. Intern. Med.* **67**, 800-807.

Sievers, M. L. (1968a). Serum cholesterol levels in southwestern American Indians. *J. Chronic Dis.* **21**, 107-115.

Sievers, M. L. (1968b). Cigarette and alcohol usage by southwestern American Indians. *Am. J. Public Health* **58**, 71-82.

Sievers, M. L. (1973). Unusual comparative frequency of gastric carcinoma, pernicious anemia, and peptic ulcer in southwestern American Indians. *Gastroenterology* **65**, 867-876.

Sievers, M. L. (1974). Disseminated coccidioidomycosis among southwestern American Indians. *Am. Rev. Respir. Dis.* **109**, 602-612.

Sievers, M. L. (1976a). Diabetes mellitus in American Indians—standards for diagnosis and management. *Diabetes* **25**, 528-531.

Sievers, M. L. (1976b). Cancer of the digestive system among American Indians. *Ariz. Med.* **33**, 15-20.

Sievers, M. L. (1976c). Peptic-ulcer factors in American Indians. *Ann. Intern. Med.* **84**, 755-756.

Sievers, M. L. (1977a). Prognostic factors in disseminated coccidioidomycosis among southwestern

Indians. *In* "Coccidioidomycosis. Current Clinical and Diagnostic Status" (L. Ajello, ed.), pp. 239–252. Symposia Specialists, Miami, Florida.

Sievers, M. L. (1977b). Historical overview of hypertension among American Indians and Alaskan Natives. *Ariz. Med.* **34,** 607–610.

Sievers, M. L. (1979). Coccidioidomycosis and race. *Am. Rev. Respir. Dis.* **119,** 830.

Sievers, M. L. (1980). Racial susceptibility to coccidioidomycosis. *N. Engl. J. Med.* **302,** 58–59.

Sievers, M. L., and Cohen, S. L. (1961). Lung cancer among Indians of the southwestern United States. *Ann. Intern. Med.* **54,** 912–915.

Sievers, M. L., and Fisher, J. R. (1979a). Increasing rate of acute myocardial infarction in southwestern American Indians. *Ariz. Med.* **36,** 739–742.

Sievers, M. L., and Fisher, J. R. (1979b). Peptic ulcer in southwestern Indians. *Gastroenterology* **77,** 423–424.

Sievers, M. L., and Hendrikx, M. E. (1972). Long-term results: two weight reduction programs among southwestern Indians. *Health Serv. Rep.* **87,** 530–536.

Sievers, M. L., and Marquis, J. R. (1962a). The southwestern American Indian's burden: biliary disease. *J. Am. Med. Assoc.* **182,** 172–174.

Sievers, M. L., and Marquis, J. R. (1962b). Duodenal ulcer among southwestern American Indians. *Gastroenterology* **42,** 566–569.

Sievers, M. L., Metzger, A. L., Goldberg, L. S., and Fudenberg, H. H. (1973). Pernicious anemia in southwestern American Indians. *Blood* **41,** 309–317.

Sievers, M. L., Cynamon, M. H., and Bittker, T. E. (1975). Intentional isoniazid overdose among southwestern American Indians. *Am. J. Psychiatry* **132,** 662–665.

Slocum, R., and Thompson, F. (1975). Rarity of asthma among Cheyene Indians. *Ann. Allergy* **34,** 201.

Smith, R. L. (1957). Recorded and expected mortality among the Indians of the United States with special reference to cancer. *J. Natl. Cancer Inst.* **18,** 385–396.

Smith, R. L., Salsbury, C. G., and Gilliam, A. G. (1956). Recorded and expected mortality among the Navajo with special reference to cancer. *J. Natl. Cancer Inst.* **17,** 77–89.

Spagnola, A. M., Bennett, P. H., and Terasaki, P. I. (1978). Vertebral ankylosing hyperostosis (Foreister's disease) and HLA antigens in Pima Indians. *Arthritis Rheum.* **21,** 467–472.

Spivey, G. H., and Hirschhorn, N. (1977). A migrant study of adopted Apache children. *Johns Hopkins Med. J.* **140,** 43–46.

Stern, M. P. (1979). The recent decline in ischemic heart disease mortality. *Ann. Intern. Med.* **91,** 630–640.

Stewart, T. D. (1973). "The People of America." Scribner's, New York.

Stiefler, R. S., Solomon, M. P., and Shalita, A. R. (1979). Heck's disease (focal epithelial hyperplasia). *J. Am. Acad. Dermatol.* **1,** 499–502.

Swanton, J. R. (1952). "The Indian Tribes of North America." Smithsonian Inst. Press, Washington, D.C.

Szuter, C., and Hoshiwara, I. (1976). Trachoma, a vanishing disease. *Proc. USPHS Prof. Assoc., Commissioned Officers Assoc., Washington, D.C.* p. 15.

Telle, D. W., and Klein, J. O. (1978). Greater Boston collaborative otitis media program: epidemiology of otitis media during first two years of life. *Pediatr. Res.* **12,** 428.

Thistle, J. L., Eckhart, K. L., Nensen, R. E., Nobrega, F. T., Poehling, G. G., Reimer, M., and Schoenfield, L. J. (1971). Prevalence of gallbladder disease among Chippewa Indians. *Mayo Clin. Proc.* **46,** 603–608.

Thompson, J. R., and Harper, I. H. (1974). The low incidence of chronic primary open angle glaucoma in the Chippewa (Ojibwa) Indians of Minnesota. *Minn. Med.* **57,** 975–976.

Thompson, W. M., and Ackerstein, H. (1975). Peptic ulcer disease in the Alaska Natives: a four-year retrospective study. *Alaska Med.* **17**(3), 43–44.

Tribal Pamphlet (1960). "The White Mountain Apache Indians." White Mountain Apache Tribe, Whiteriver, Arizona.

Turner, C. G. (1971). Three-rooted mandibular first permanent molars and the question of American Indian origins. *Am. J. Physical Anthropol.* **34**, 229-242.

U.S. Department of Health, Education, and Welfare (1976). "Atlas of Cancer Mortality among U.S. Nonwhites: 1950-1969." U.S. Gov. Print. Off., Washington, D.C.

U.S. Department of Health, Education, and Welfare (1978a). "Indian Health Trends and Services." U.S. Gov. Print. Off., Washington, D.C.

U.S. Department of Health, Education, and Welfare (1978b). "The Indian Health Program of the U.S. Public Health Service." U.S. Gov. Print. Off., Washington, D.C.

Vogt, T. M., and Johnson, R. E. (1980). Recent changes in the incidence of duodenal and gastric ulcer. *Am. J. Epidemiol.* **111**, 713-720.

Wagner, M. G., and Littman, B. (1967). Phenylketonuria in the American Indian. *Pediatrics* **39**, 108-110.

Walker, J. M. (1977). Congenital hip disease in a Cree-Ojibwa population—a retrospective study. *Can. Med. Assoc. J.* **116**, 501-504.

Warren, D. L. (1977). Gallbladder disease in the Mississippi Choctaw Indian. *Proc. USPHS Prof. Assoc., Annu. Meet., 12th, USPHS Commissioned Officers Assoc., Washington, D.C.* p. 4.

Wellmann, K. F. (1972). New Mexico's mutilated hand: finger mutilation and polydactylism in North American Indian rock art. *J. Am. Med. Assoc.* **219**, 1609-1610.

Wellmann, K. F, (1979). North American Indian rock art. Medical connotations. *N.Y. State J. Med.* **79**, 1094-1105.

Welsh, J. D., Poley, J. R., Bhatia, M., and Stevenson, D. E. (1978). Intestinal disaccharide activities in relation to age, race, and mucosal damage. *Gastroenterology* **75**, 847-855.

West, K. M. (1974). Diabetes in American Indians and other native populations of the New World. *Diabetes* **23**, 841-855.

West, K. M. (1975). Substantial differences in diagnostic criteria used by diabetic experts. *Diabetes* **24**, 641-644.

West, K. M. (1978). "Epidemiology of Diabetes and Its Vascular Lesions." Elsevier, Amsterdam.

Wiet, R. J. (1979). Patterns of ear disease in southwestern American Indians. *Arch. Otolaryngol.* **105**, 381-385.

Willey, G. R. (1966). "An Introduction to American Archeology. Vol. 1: North and Middle America." Prentice-Hall, Englewood Cliffs, New Jersey.

Williams, R. C., Knowler, W. C., Butler, W. J., Pettitt, D. L., Lisse, J. R., Bennett, P. H., Mann, D. L., Johnson, A. H., and Terasaki, P. I. (1981). HLA-A2 and type II diabetes in Pima Indians: an association and decrease in allele frequency with age. *Diabetologia* (to be published).

Willkens, R. F., Blandau, R. L., Aoyama, D. T., and Beasley, R. P. (1976). Studies of rheumatoid arthritis among a tribe of northwest Indians. *J. Rheumatol.* **3**, 9-14.

Witkop, C. J., Niswander, J. D., Bergsma, D. R., Workman, P. L., and White, J. G. (1972). Tyrosinase positive oculocutaneous albinism among the Zuni and the Brandywine triracial isolate: biochemical and clinical characteristic and fertility. *Am. J. Phys. Anthropol.* **36**, 397-405.

Wolff, P. H. (1972). Ethnic differences in alcohol sensitivity. *Science* **175**, 449-450.

Wolff, P. H. (1973). Vasomotor sensitivity to alcohol in diverse Mongoloid populations. *Am. J. Hum. Genet.* **25**, 193-199.

Wolman, C. (1970). The cradleboard of the Western Indians: a baby-tending device of cultural importance. *Clin. Pediatr.* **9**, 306-308.

Woolf, C. M. (1965). Albinism among Indians in Arizona and New Mexico. *Am. J. Hum. Genet.* **17**, 23-35.

Woolf, C. M., and Dukepoo, F. C. (1969). Hopi Indians, inbreeding, and albinism. *Science* **164**, 30–37.

Woolf, C. M., and Grant, R. B. (1962). Albinism among the Hopi Indians in Arizona. *Am. J. Hum. Genet.* **14**, 391–400.

Wynne-Davies, R. (1972). The epidemiology of congenital dislocation of the hip. *Dev. Med. Child. Neurol.* **14**, 515–517.

Zeiner, A. R., Parades, A., and Cowden, L. (1976). Physiologic responses to ethanol among the Tarahumara Indians. *Ann. N.Y. Acad. Sci.* **273**, 151–158.

Zonis, R. D. (1968a). Chronic otitis media in the southwestern American Indian: I. Prevalence. *Arch. Otol.* **88**, 40–45.

Zonis, R. D. (1968b). Chronic otitis media in the southwestern American Indians: II. Immunologic factors. *Arch. Otol.* **88**, 46–49.

Zonis, R. D. (1970). Chronic otitis media in the Arizona Indian. *Ariz. Med.* **27**(6), 1–6.

Zwemer, F., Kwart, V., and Conway, M. (1979). Biliary-enteric fistulas. Management of 47 cases in Native Americans. *Am. J. Surg.* **138**, 301–304.

9
Diseases of Latin America

ANTHONY B. WAY

I. INTRODUCTION

This chapter provides an overview of the pattern of human diseases in Latin America. Because they are of general interest to the student of human evolution and epidemiology, certain diseases and disease patterns have been selected. My intent is to discuss disease from an evolutionary point of view. No attempt was made to be comprehensive; for that purpose, the reader is referred to publications on tropical medicine (Hunter et al., 1976; Maegraith, 1976; Wilcocks and Manson-Bahr, 1972), epidemiology (Puffer and Serrano, 1973; Rodenwalt and Jusatz, 1952, 1956, 1961), zoonoses (Hubbert et al., 1975), geographic medicine (Ackerknect, 1965; Henschen, 1966; Howe, 1977), medical history (Crosby, 1972; McNeill, 1976), paleopathology (Brothwell and Sandison, 1967; Janssens, 1970), medical and biological anthropology (Ciba Foundation, 1977; Logan and Hunt, 1978; Pan American Health Organization, 1968; Wood, 1979), mortality statistics (Preston, 1976; Preston et al., 1972; Puffer and Griffith,

BIOCULTURAL ASPECTS OF DISEASE
Copyright © 1981 by Academic Press, Inc.
ISBN 0-12-598720-X

1967; United Nations, 1978; World Health Organization, 1978), and various case studies (e.g., Buck *et al.*, 1968; Shattuck, 1933, 1938). The reader should appreciate the size and diversity of Latin America (Fig. 1). It consists of all the land area south of the United States of America, that is, South America, the Caribbean, Central America, and Mexico. Its climate varies from tropical to temperate, and its ecology from rain forests to arid deserts. The land ranges from flat lowlands to mountains habitable above 4000 m, and from maritime regions to the continental interior. The 1977 estimate of the number of persons living in its 43 nations and colonies was 342 million (U.S. Bureau of the Census, 1978). The four major genetic groups are Europeans, American Indians, Africans, and Mestizos (primarily European and American Indian hybrids). The principal languages are Spanish, Portuguese, and several American Indian ones. The economy encompasses the range from modern industry to subsistence agriculture to hunting and gathering. Economically, however, Latin America can be generally characterized as a developing area.

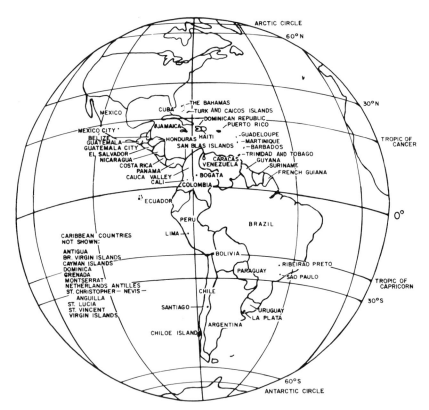

Fig. 1. Geopolitical map of Latin America.

II. THEORETICAL ASSUMPTIONS

A brief statement of the theoretical assumptions made in this chapter may assist the reader to understand the point of view being used in this chapter. In discussing disease from an evolutionary perspective, genetic evolution is considered to result from differences in fertility and mortality of individuals (Crow, 1958; Neel and Chagnon, 1968) and disease is considered to be any biological abnormality that causes either an actual or a potential reduction of the ability of individuals to function (i.e., both symptomatic and presymptomatic states are included). A major assumption in this chapter is that, in any population, the pattern of diseases results from the interaction of persons with each other and with their biological and physical environments, both now and in the past. Thus, by looking at disease not only as the cause of mortality and morbidity, but also as the effect of various factors, one can infer generalizations about humans and their societies.

Another major assumption here is that an understanding of biological evolution can do much to help in obtaining this type of information from the pattern of diseases. One conclusion from evolution is that every disease, except senility, evolves toward its own extinction. This conclusion follows from the logical observation that a population will evolve complete resistance to any disease if (1) there is any genetically based variation in resistance/susceptibility and (2) such genetic variation has any effect on the contribution to subsequent generations of reproducing descendants. Since there is no theoretical reason why both conditions cannot obtain in any population for any disease, natural selection should eventually eliminate virtually all disease. Even postreproductive diseases can, for human beings, also act as their own agents of negative natural selection, since the health and survival of postreproductive parents can, in human societies, influence the survival and reproductive success of their children and possibly even their grandchildren. For infectious diseases, this evolutionary process is speeded by the tendency of living pathogens to evolve to a nonpathogenic state (Cockburn, 1963, 1967a,b, 1971; Dubos, 1965a,b). The evolution of the parasite itself is the result of the impediments to continued transmission of the parasite if it causes death or illness in its host.

Recognizing that the family of bipedal, tool-using hominids has existed for about 200,000 generations (4 million years), and the genus *Homo* for about 75,000 generations (1.5 million years), and the species *Homo sapiens* for about 12,500 generations (250,000 years), one can appreciate that there has been sufficient time for even a low level of natural selection to have a large cumulative effect in eliminating diseases. Thus, the existence of even a minor disease requires explanation in terms of some evolutionarily recent change that has resulted in the temporary appearance of that disease. Such change could be either genetic or environmental. A genetic change may reflect either a random mutation or a side effect of some genetic adaptation (perhaps to another disease). Environmental changes relevant to noninfectious diseases are physical, nutritional, behavioral, and social. For infectious diseases these same environmental changes may allow a formerly nonpathogenic parasite of humans to become a pathogen. In addition, a change in the biological environment may expose people to new organisms capable of becoming human parasites. The most likely source of new parasites is another closely related host organism such as other human populations, other primates, domesticated animals, household scavengers or hunted animals.

The last major assumption underlying this chapter is that disease is one of the most important agents of natural selection for human beings. Similar opinions have been expressed by Charles Darwin (cited in Montalenti, 1965) and J. B. S. Haldane (1956–1957; also cited in Dubos, 1965b). This sweeping generalization derives from the recognition that all deaths must be due to disease as defined, and thus a major portion of natural selection must be due to disease.

III. FACTORS INFLUENCING THE PATTERN OF DISEASES

Two major groups of factors help explain the specific pattern of diseases found in Latin America. One group comprises those factors that arose in the past but whose influences can be seen today or in the resurrectable past. The second group comprises those factors that continue to operate today.

A. Past Events

1. Plate Tectonics

Until about 65 million to 135 million years ago, in the Mesozoic period, South America was part of a continuous land mass with Africa (Dietz and Holden, 1970; Hurley, 1968). This fact suggests that some common organisms should be capable of becoming human parasites in both South America and in Africa and Eurasia. Examples are the trypanosomes and the leishmanias found in both the Old and New World, human pathogens in both places. A relationship that is due' to past geographical connections should be distinguished from the current ubiquity of some infectious diseases produced by human transportation. Examples of the latter include malaria and measles.

On the other hand, 65 million to 135 million years of geographic isolation should have resulted in much evolutionary divergence of the fauna (both micro- and macro-) in South America and the Old World. The separation of South America from Africa occurred about the time of the evolution of the prosimian primates but before the development of the monkeys. Thus, the South American monkeys genetically relate more distantly to humans than do the Old World monkeys. The hominoids (apes and humans) evolved even later, only in Africa. For that reason, parasites that could potentially become human pathogens should have been fewer in South America than in the Old World. The long separation of the Old and New World, therefore, should have meant that when humans first migrated to the New World 30,000 to 40,000 years ago (Jennings, 1978), they found an environment relatively free of infectious disease.

2. Human Migrations

The first human invasion of the New World began about 30,000–40,000 years ago and probably continued for tens of thousands of years (Jennings, 1978). We can probably ignore the genetic contribution of trans-Pacific and trans-Atlantic wayfarers. Morison's (1971) recounting of the repeated failure of more recent European colonizers in the New World shows the difficulty of establishing viable colonies in an unfamiliar environment without close logistic support. The bulk of the first migrants to the New World surely came by land, directly from eastern Eurasia by way of Beringia, the broad land mass that made Siberia continuous with Alaska when the sea level was lowered during the Ice Ages. During that time, the expansion of *Homo sapiens* in the Old World came to include the contiguous New World. It is likely that various populations of eastern Eurasia spread into the New World during the long or repeated existence of Beringia. Nevertheless, the different people indigenous to the New World can all be considered to be an extension of Asian people. This relationship means that we should not expect to find European or African or Australian genetic diseases in the American Indians, except as the result of more recent gene flow.

In 1960, Stewart proposed that an arctic route to the New World should have filtered out many Old World pathogens. Cockburn (1963, 1967b) makes a similar argument. Thus, we can expect that Old World infectious agents that require nonarctic vectors (such as yellow fever), intermediate hosts (such as schistosomiasis), or external environments (such as ascariasis) would be absent in the New World. In addition, Crosby (1972) may be right in suggesting that the rigors of an arctic climate might tend to eliminate more human carriers of illness than would less hostile environments. However, the large numbers of persons who had time to spread into the New World make this latter effect of questionable importance.

On the other hand, one must not give this arctic filter undue credit. For instance, the dearth of infections requiring dense human populations (the "crowd" infections) in the New World, as compared with such infections in the Old World, should be attributed in part to the small population supportable in the arctic and not to the arctic cold itself (Newman, 1976; St. Hoyme, 1969; Wood, 1979). More importantly, when the bulk of the first migrants spread into the New World, no dense human population existed anywhere in the world. In other words, the crowd infections had not yet evolved. When they developed in the Old World, the waters of the Bering Strait, combined with the primitiveness of the local transportation, would serve as a better filter than the arctic cold. The second major human migration to the New World began about 500 years ago and has been decreasing only recently. Most of the migrants came from Europe and Africa. One effect of this migration was the introduction of European and African genetic diseases to Latin America. In addition, the ability by that time to move large numbers (hundreds) of persons quickly (weeks) across the Atlantic Ocean permitted the introduction of the European and African crowd infections to Latin America. Table I lists some diseases that have been proposed as exotic to the New World. The similarity of climates in Latin America and Africa even enabled some insect vectors of crowd infections (e.g., those of malaria and yellow fever) to be introduced to the New World.

TABLE I

Some Infectious Diseases That Have Been Proposed as Being Introduced to the New World by European or African Migrants

Disease	Reference
Viral	
Influenza	Wood (1979, p. 163)
Measles	Ball (1977); Henschen (1966, p. 138); Newman (1976); Wood (1979, pp. 159–160)
Mumps	Wood (1979, pp. 159–160)
Poliomyelitis	Newman (1976)
Smallpox	Wood (1979, pp. 159–160)
Yellow fever (Z)[a]	Ackerknecht (1965, p. 53); Neel (1971); Newman (1976); Wood (1979, pp. 159–160)
Bacterial	
Cholera	Cockburn (1967b); Newman (1976); Wood (1979, p. 163)
Diphtheria	Newman (1976); Wood (1979, p. 163)
Plague (Z)	Ackerknecht (1965, p. 21); Newman (1976); Wood (1979, pp. 159–160)
Protozoal	
Malaria (Z)	Ackerknecht (1965, p. 88); Henschen (1966, pp. 59, 138, 142); Neel (1971); Newman (1976); Wood (1979, pp. 159–160)
Metazoal	
Ascariasis (Z)	Cockburn (1967c, 1977)
Onchocerciasis (Z)	Newman (1976)
Schistosomiasis (Z)	Maegraith (1976, p. 368)

[a] Z, human zoonoses.

3. Development of Agriculture

The development of agriculture has enabled human populations to become both large and dense. Such crowding enables a new pathogen (possibly from a domesticated animal) that produces acquired immunity to persist in a population until more susceptible persons are born. Previously such infections would die out when most of the population had developed immunity. Without a reservoir, they could not be reintroduced (Armelagos and McArdle, 1975; Cockburn, 1963, 1967b, 1977; Haldane, 1956–1957; Polgar, 1964). Black (1975) and Black and colleagues (1977) evaluated the viral disease pattern in relatively isolated American Indians in Latin America. They found that herpes simplex, chickenpox and herpes zoster, infectious mononucleosis, hepatitis B, and cytomegalovirus infections, as indicated by antibodies, were common. This finding corresponds with our knowledge of persistent viral infections and demonstrates that such infections are not crowd dependent. On the other hand, measles, mumps, rubella, influenza, parainfluenza, and polio infections all appeared to be sporadic one-time epidemic diseases. Niederman and co-workers (1967) made similar observations in some other Latin American populations. These latter are clearly crowd infections.

Confirming that 500 years ago the crowd infections in the New World were fewer than those in the Old World is difficult (Crosby, 1972; McNeill, 1976). However, the relative absence of serious disease threats for Europeans in the New World as compared with those in Asia and Africa suggests that this was the case (Newman, 1976; St. Hoyme, 1969; Wood, 1979). Nonetheless, this dearth of crowd infections in the New World is not well explained. Perhaps the few

TABLE II

Human Zoonoses With a Geographically Localized (Not Worldwide) Distribution[a]

Continent	Continental area $\times 10^6$ km²	Continental population $\times 10^6$	No. of zoonoses found in two or more continents (*proportion*)	No. of zoonoses unique to one continent (*proportion*)
Eurasia	53.5	3223	41 (0.28)	14 (0.26)
Africa	29.8	431	34 (0.24)	12 (0.22)
North America	24.2	304	24 (0.17)	6 (0.11)
Central and South America	18.4	249	40 (0.28)	20 (0.37)
Australia	7.7	14	5 (0.03)	2 (0.04)
			Total 144 (1.00)	54 (1.00)

[a] From Hubbert *et al.* (1975).

TABLE III

Infectious Diseases in Latin America Restricted to, or Originating in, the New World

Agent	Disease
Viruses	
Arbovirus Group A (Z)[a]	Eastern equine encephalomyelitis
	Western equine encephalomyelitis
	Venezuelan equine encephalitis
	Mayaro infection[b]
	Mucambo infection
Arbovirus Group B (Z)	St. Louis encephalitis
	Ilheus infection[b]
	Bussuquara infection
Arbovirus Group C (Z)	Apeu infection[b]
	Caraparu infection[b]
	Itaqui infection[b]
	Madrid infection[b]
	Marituba infection[b]
	Muratuca infection[b]
	Oriboca infection[b]
	Ossa infection
	Restan infection
Arbovirus Group Bunyamwera (Z)	Guaroa infection[b]
	Wyeomyia infection[b]
Arbovirus Group Changuinola (Z)	Changuinola fever
Arbovirus Group Guama (Z)	Cata infection[b]
	Guama infection[b]
Arbovirus Group Phlebotomus (Z)	Candiru infection
	Chagres infection
	Puntu Toro infection
Arbovirus Group Simbu (Z)	Oropouche infection[b]
Arbovirus Group VSV (Z)	Indiana vesicular stomatitis[b]
	Piry vesicular stomatitis[b]
Junin Virus (Z)	Argentine hemorrhagic fever[b]
Machupo virus (Z)	Bolivian hemorrhagic fever[b]
Bacteria	
Rickettsia rickettsi (Z)	Rocky Mountain spotted fever
Bartonella bacilliformis	Bartonellosis (Carrion's disease, Oroya fever, verruga peruana)
Treponema carateum	Pinta (carate)
Fungi	
Coccidioides immitis	Coccidioidomycosis
Parococcidioides brasiliensis	South American blastomycosis
Protozoa	
Leishmania brasiliensis (Z)	American leishmaniasis[b] (chiclero ulcer, espundia, pian-bois, uta)
Tryponosoma cruzi (Z)	American trypanosomiasis (Chagas' disease)

(*continued*)

TABLE III (Cont.)

Agent	Disease
Metazoa	
Echinococcus oligarthrus (Z)	Polycystic hydatidosis[b]
Mansonella ozzardi	Mansonelliasis
	(filariasis ozzardi)
Trichuris trichuria	Trichuriasis
Ixodes and *Ornithodorus* Ticks (Z)	Local necrosis
Tunga penetrans (Z)	Tunga infection
(Chigoe flea)	

[a] (Z), human zoonoses.
[b] The 20 zoonoses unique to Central and South America counted in Table II. [From Cockburn (1967c), Crosby (1972), Hubbert *et al.* (1975), Hunter *et al.* (1976), and Newman (1976).]

domesticated animals (Newman, 1976; St. Hoyme, 1969; Wood, 1979) or the absence of closely related primates (Cockburn, 1977) in the New World resulted in fewer zoonoses becoming crowd infections. Perhaps the arid climate of some of the Latin American pre-Columbian civilizations protected them (Bruce-Chwatt, 1965). Perhaps the fact that fewer agricultural societies developed in the New World than in the Old World, and developed later, limited the opportunity for different crowd infections to evolve in different places. Likely, however, a combination of these and other unknown factors kept the New World relatively free of crowd infections. Today, virtually all of the crowd diseases can be traced to importation from Europe and Africa (Table I).

B. Current Conditions

1. Tropical Environment

Although Latin America is climatically diverse, it is bisected by the equator (Fig. 1) and thus has a predominately tropical climate. Because the tropics support a diversity of fauna, including biting insects as vectors, that zoonotic infections of humans are common in Latin America is not surprising. Table II, derived from "Diseases Transmitted from Animals to Man" by Hubbert and colleagues (1975) compares the number of zoonoses in the five inhabited continents, restricting attention to those diseases that are not ubiquitous. Although the area and population of Central and South America combined are smaller than those of any other inhabited continent except Australia, they have more (20) unique zoonoses than any other continent and almost as many (40) shared zoonoses as Eurasia. Table III is a partial list of infections of Latin America that are either unique to, or probably originated in, the New World, including North America. All except 6 of the 42 diseases are zoonoses. Note especially the plethora of arthropod-borne viruses in Table III. These are human zoonoses from the tropical fauna. For example, Niederman and co-workers (1967) have shown that the zoonotic arboviruses cause ten times as many infections in Brazil as they do in the United States. Six exotic diseases noted in Table I—yellow fever, plague, some malarias, ascariasis, onchocerciasis, and schistosomiasis—are also zoonoses.

2. Geography and Geology

The form and composition of the land in Latin America have direct and indirect impacts on the disease pattern there. The mountains of the Andes have created temperate zones within the tropics, altering the distribution of animals that act either as reservoirs for, or vectors of, infectious diseases. Examples of such diseases discussed later in this chapter are arboviruses, malaria, trypanosomiasis, leishmaniasis, and bartonellosis. In addition to the indirect effects, geography and geology have direct effects, such as iodide deficiency and mountain sickness.

a. **Iodide Deficiency.** Iodide deficiency is generally manifested by thyroid enlargement (goiter) and by disruption of normal growth and development in childhood (cretinism). Except for the Chilean nitrate deposits, iodide is not common in the New World (Barzelatto and Covarrubias, 1968). This lack is probably enhanced by soil leaching in the high rainfall areas of Latin America. As a result, human iodide deficiency is common throughout Latin America (Fig. 2), particularly in the mountainous regions of Mexico, Central America, and South America (Barzelatto and Covarrubias, 1968; Fierro-Benitez *et al.*, 1969; Henschen, 1966; May, 1977; Neel, 1971; Scrimshaw, 1960; Stanbury and Kevany, 1970). The proportion of the local population affected can be substantial in some regions, i.e., 54–80% with goiter and 6% with cretinism (Barzelatto and Covarrubias, 1968; Fierro-Benitez *et al.*, 1969; Greene, 1977; May, 1977).

The soil content of iodide is not, however, the only factor influencing iodide deficiency in Latin America. In the Cauca Valley of Colombia (Fig. 1), iodide deficiency is endemic despite an apparently adequate iodide availability (Fierro-Benitez *et al.*, 1974). The problem has been traced to a naturally occurring goitrogen in the ground water (Gaitan, 1973; Gaitan *et al.*, 1969). This thiourea-like substance is probably derived from local organic sedimentary rocks. Barzelatto and Covarrubias (1968) point out that the pinon nuts consumed in Chile are also goitrogenic.

Because the effects of iodide deficiency are deleterious to survival and repro-duction, and because iodide deficiency should have been present since the first

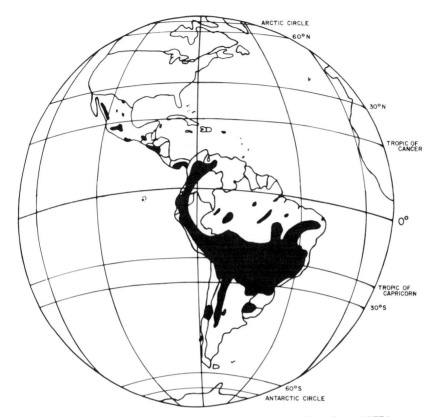

Fig. 2.   Distribution of endemic goiter in Latin America. (From Giggs, 1977.)

migrants arrived as much as 40,000 years ago, it is reasonable to enquire whether any genetic adaptation to this stress has occurred (Neel, 1968, 1971). Some evidence suggests that the ability to taste phenylthiocarbamide (PTC) may be protective in Latin America (Barzellato and Covarrubias, 1968; Greene, 1974). The genetic ability to taste thiourea-like molecules may enable some Latin American people to reduce their consumption of goitrogenic foods. In regions where the iodide supply is marginal, this protective trait may be important.

b. Mountain Sickness.   This disease is another that is a correlate of geography (Houston, 1976; Hurtado, 1942; Monge-M., 1937, 1948; Monge-M. and Monge-C., 1966). Mountain sickness may occur anyplace in the world, usually at altitudes at or above 3000 m (Fig. 3). Because extensive portions of the Andes—from Ecuador through Peru to Bolivia, northern Argentina, and Chile—support millions of people at high altitude, mountain sickness is a problem in Latin America. The illness results from maladaptation to hypoxia and has

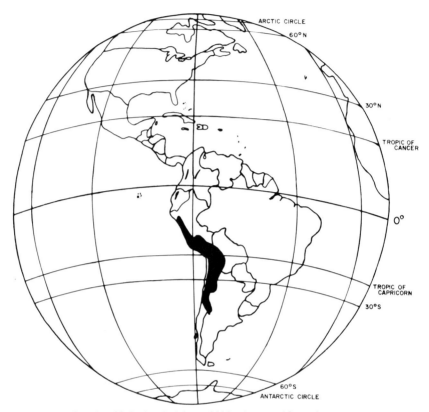

Fig. 3. High altitude (above 3000 m) areas of Latin America.

both acute and chronic forms. Persons who have recently arrived at an altitude above 3000 m frequently experience the malaise of acute mountain sickness, and occasionally also have pulmonary and cerebral edema. Long-term residents sometimes develop chronic mountain sickness, possibly as a result of other pulmonary cardiovascular disease (Buck *et al.*, 1968; Monge-M. and Monge-C., 1966). Whether there has been any genetic adaptation to hypoxia and mountain sickness among the American Indians of the Andes remains unclear (Monge-M., 1948; Monge-M. and Monge-C., 1966).

3. Current Agriculture

Most of the people in Latin America depend on agriculture. For this reason, agriculture plays a major role in the diseases there. One effect is the fostering of certain infectious diseases by the concentration in one place of large numbers of human hosts, pathogens, and vector insects (Cockburn, 1971). Malaria and schistosomiasis are examples of such agriculture-dependent infections in Latin America.

Agriculture also tends to influence the nutritional diseases. As Dubos (1965b) points out, persons who depend on agriculture for their livelihoods tend to maximize their calories from carbohydrates at the expense of dietary balance. The result is often nutritional deficiency (St. Hoyme, 1969). One might expect pellagra (niacin deficiency) in the maize culture of Mexico and Central America, kwashiorkor (protein deficiency) in the manioc culture of South America, and beri-beri (thiamine deficiency) in the rice culture developing throughout Latin America (May, 1977). Actually, one sees mixed deficiencies of calories, proteins, vitamins, and minerals throughout Latin America, largely due to the local dependence on a few crops. In many cases, potential deficiencies are avoided either by mixing appropriate agricultural staples, such as beans with corn or rice (May, 1977), or by appropriate preparation of a staple food, such as lime-water treatment of corn, which makes more tryptophane, niacin, and calcium available (Behar, 1968; May, 1977).

4. Economy

All of Latin America is considered to be a developing region (U.S. Bureau of the Census, 1978). This fact accounts for many of the nutritional problems seen in both the agricultural and urban areas of Latin America. As people move from a self-subsistent to a wage economy, one may expect that their diet would suffer. On the one hand, money can be saved by reducing the variety and quantity of food; on the other, ignorance of what to buy or the unavailability of traditional foods may result in a deficient diet. Malnutrition may be a predisposing factor to the infectious diseases. Another effect of a developing economy may be a rise in those degenerative diseases that are more prevalent in the industrialized world.

IV. SPECIFIC DISEASES AND PATTERNS

In section III, diseases were discussed as being the effects of various determining factors. If that perception is proper, diseases can also be used to draw conclusions about those factors. This section reviews various specific diseases, and the general pattern of diseases, with an emphasis on shedding light on the determining factors.

A. General Pattern of Diseases

Lacking data on living persons, and thus information about nonlethal morbidity, one can estimate the general pattern of diseases in a population from mortality statistics. Such data are available from most countries, although their

TABLE IV

Cause-Specific Age-Standardized Death Rates, Population per Physician, and Gross National Product per Capita for Countries of Latin America, the United States, and the United Kingdom in Early 1960s[a]

Cause of death	Sex	Guatemala (GU)	El Salvador (ES)	Chile (CH)	Colombia (CO)	Mexico (ME)	Trinidad and Tobago (TT)	Costa Rica (CR)	Venezuela (VE)	Panama (PA)	Puerto Rico (PR)	Latin America (mean)	United States (US)	England and Wales (UK)
All causes	M	1927	1744	1618	1397	1303	1409	1154	1162	1118	1018	1385	1148	1133
	F	1840	1592	1196	1188	1152	996	982	932	913	737	1153	713	693
All other causes and unknown causes (residual) O-U	M	621	714	293	424	429	256	285	383	339	166	391	107	91
	F	618	744	223	374	412	171	237	332	290	137	354	64	67
Cardiovascular diseases (330-4,400-68) CVD	M	121	90	384	281	150	624	264	289	312	340	286	613	543
	F	124	79	311	247	149	436	238	225	261	273	234	383	347
Malignant and benign neoplasms (140-239) NEO	M	52	35	187	117	66	120	189	121	115	148	115	180	225
	F	82	58	175	132	90	131	165	132	97	109	117	129	140
Influenza, pneumonia, bronchitis (480-502) PNE	M	293	122	208	106	157	95	69	44	63	46	120	42	148
	F	292	114	168	104	145	61	81	42	50	35	109	24	62
Other infectious and parasitic diseases (010-138) INF	M	318	231	45	80	65	31	46	48	50	16	93	7	5
	F	305	235	43	71	63	15	41	36	45	12	87	4	3
Diarrhea, gastritis, enteritis (543,571,572) DIA	M	222	244	47	71	85	32	75	31	32	32	87	4	4
	F	231	219	44	66	85	30	76	29	29	28	84	4	5
Other accidents, violence (E800-2,E840-999) VIO	M	89	176	143	127	124	73	75	80	74	77	104	66	38
	F	17	21	33	29	27	24	20	23	29	22	25	26	24
Certain disease of infancy (760-776) DOI	M	109	38	102	71	84	56	60	44	29	65	66	35	26
	F	84	30	86	56	68	42	42	32	25	43	51	26	19
Certain degenerative diseases (260,540-1, 581,590-4) DEG	M	41	44	120	62	92	84	51	58	40	68	66	48	25
	F	27	29	57	53	69	66	52	41	39	48	48	34	16
Respiratory tuberculosis (001-8) TBC	M	46	49	78	35	38	21	25	26	43	32	39	6	7
	F	36	38	37	26	23	8	14	22	27	20	25	2	2
Motor vehicle accidents (E810-35) MOV	M	16	3	11	23	14	18	16	39	20	28	19	38	23
	F	3	2	2	6	4	3	2	8	7	7	4	14	7
Complication of pregnancy (640-89) MAT	M	0	0	0	0	0	0	0	0	.	0	0	0	0
	F	20	22	17	22	17	9	14	10	14	0	15	2	1
Population per physician		3600	6000	2100	2270	1810	2550	2560	1300	2260	1310	2576	700	830
Gross national product per capita (U.S. dollars)		299	238	324	266	386	653	370	768	472	982	476	3166	1603

[a] Death rates per 100,000 population. Abbreviations indicate causes of death that are comparable with Table V and are same as Figs. 4–6. Year for death rates: ES 1950, TT 1963, remainder 1964. Year for population per physician: ES 1952; ME 1966; PA, PR, UK, 1964; remainder 1963. Year for

accuracy may vary. Preston and colleagues (1972) (Table IV) and Puffer and Griffith (1967) (Table V) have assembled reliable, and comparable, cause-specific mortality statistics from countries and cities, respectively, of Latin America in the early 1960s. They removed the effect of population age structure on mortality by standardizing the data for age. Their values are not comparable between each other, however, because each used a different standardization and different age ranges. I have rank-ordered their statistics for this chapter and included data from the United States and United Kingdom for comparison.

The relative reliability of the data can be judged from the frequency of "other-unknown" as the cause of death (Tables IV and V). In Latin America (Figs. 4, 5, and 6), "other-unknown" is often the most common diagnosis, accounting for 6-47% (mean = 29%) of all deaths as compared with 5-10% in the United States or United Kingdom. The general heterogeneity of Latin America is reflected in the variation in each cause of death.

The high mortality from "all causes" in Latin America as compared with the United States and United Kingdom mortalities is consistent with the developing economies in that region (Preston, 1976). One should note, however, that this total mortality is lower in some places in Latin America than in the United States and the United Kingdom (Figs. 5 and 6; Tables IV and V). The relationships between overall mortality and such indicators of economic development (Tables IV and V) as the number of persons per physician and per capita gross national product are as expected. Mortality declines as the population per physician declines and as the gross national product per capita increases. Correlations are statistically significant, or nearly so, for the country, but not for the city data. Better correlations for the city data might result from indicators of the local rather than the national economy. The effect of economics and technology on specific cause of death are apparent in Figs. 4-6. The incidence of other infectious diseases, diarrhea, and tuberculosis are generally more frequent in Latin America than in the United States or the United Kingdom, whereas motor vehicle deaths are often less frequent.

The above observations may support my earlier thesis that the general pattern of diseases in Latin America will reflect the fact that it is an economically developing area. Other infections, diarrhea, tuberculosis, and infant and maternal deaths are much affected by hygiene (especially public), nutrition, education, and medical care (and probably in that order). The number of motor vehicle-caused deaths clearly is contingent on the number of automobiles available.

A common belief is that cardiovascular and neoplastic diseases result from a modern technological life-style. For this reason, I find it interesting that the range of Latin American death rates for these diseases causes overlaps those for the United States and the United Kingdom (Figs. 4-6). Even the country data (Fig. 5) follow this pattern, if we accept Preston's (1976) conclusion that excess "other-unknown" causes of death usually conceal cardiovascular deaths. Car-

Cause of death	Sex	Santiago Chile SA-CH	Bogota Colombia BO-CO	Ribeirao Preto Brazil RP-BR	Mexico City Mexico MC-ME	Gu Gu C
All causes	M	981	684	794	727	
All	F	536	634	492	501	
Cardiovascular diseases	M	210	223	245	162	
(330-4,400-68) CVD	F	148	232	189	141	
Malignant and benign	M	129	117	143	64	
neoplasms (140-205,	F	123	131	90	98	
210-39) NEO						
Certain degenerative	M	189	62	44	175	
diseases (260,540-1,	F	66	62	40	90	
581,590) DEG						
All other and unknown	M	75	39	58	64	
causes (600-36,780-95, and	F	35	38	34	35	
remainder) O-U						
Other accidents and	M	107	82	54	87	
violence (E800-2,840-62,	F	24	28	21	20	
963-5,970-9,980-99) VIO						
Tuberculosis, all forms	M	93	32	35	35	
(001-019) TBC	F	26	21	14	17	
Respiratory diseases	M	83	46	38	52	
(470-527) PNE	F	33	47	18	28	
Other disease of digestive	M	33	24	19	32	
system (remainder	F	36	37	14	31	
of 530-87) DIA						
Other infective and parasitic	M	14	16	132	18	
diseases (020-138)	F	8.4	13	64	11	
INF						
Motor vehicle accidents	M	50	43	26	38	
(E810-35) MOV	F	8.2	8.3	2.6	9.3	
Deliveries and complica-	M	0	0	0	0	
tions of childbirth,	F	30	17	6.5	21	
and the puerperium						
(640-89) MAT						
Population per		2100	2270	2290	1810	
physician						
Gross national		324	266	268	386	
product per capita						
(U.S. dollars)						

[a] Death rates per 100,000 population. Abbreviations indicate causes of death that are compara population per physician: AR 1962; ME 1966; BR, PE, UK 1964; remainder 1963. Year for gross (Puffer and Griffith, 1967; United Nations, 1965, 1966, 1968, 1970).

	Lima Peru LI-PE	Sao Paulo Brazil SP-BR	Caracas Venezuela CR-VE	La Plata Argentina LP-AR	Latin America Mean	San Francisco United States SF-US	Bristol United Kingdom BR-UK
ia /)	645	621	633	687	609	724	630
	459	427	397	340	470	398	319
	195	256	213	247	204	282	273
	117	191	130	114	151	127	127
	115	105	131	184	119	129	157
	140	98	118	106	114	102	98
	57	51	56	50	78	99	17
	38	32	36	25	46	59	9.6
	50	42	46	61	64	37	33
	35	27	31	29	42	28	23
	50	45	91	43	77	87	28
	12	15	18	15	19	46	18
	87	28	14	12	43	10	5.7
	50	9.7	9.1	5.9	23	4.1	2.1
	30	43	19	31	39	28	78
	16	19	11	6.5	21	7.4	23
	20	17	17	18	23	11	8.5
	21	14	17	20	25	10	6.6
	12	15	25	11	28	7.4	3.8
	7.6	10	10	4.3	15	2.1	0.8
	29	19	20	32	34	34	27
	7.2	4.3	6.7	6.3	6.6	12	9.1
	0	0	0	0	0	0	0
	17	7.5	12	7.4	16	0.5	1.1
	2230	2290	1300	680	2084	700	830
	236	268	768	564	365	3166	1603

own in Table IV and are same as Figs. 4–6. Year for death rates: 1962–1964. Year for per capita: 1963. International Classification of Diseases code numbers in parentheses.

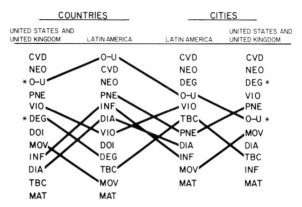

Fig. 4. Rank order of cause of death means in countries and cities (ages 15–74 years) of Latin America and the United States and the United Kingdom in early 1960s, males and females combined. O-U, all other and unknown causes; CVD, cardiovascular diseases; NEO, malignant and benign neoplasms; PNE, influenza, pneumonia, bronchitis; INF, other infectious and parasitic diseases; DIA, diarrhea, gastritis, enteritis; VIO, other accidents and violence; DOI, certain diseases of infancy; DEG, certain degenerative diseases; TBC, tuberculosis; MOV, motor vehicle accidents; MAT, complications of pregnancy; *, major difference between countries and cities of United States and the United Kingdom, i.e., first and last columns. Only differences of more than one rank are indicated. See Tables IV and V for values (Preston *et al.*, 1972; Puffer and Griffith, 1967).

diovascular or neoplastic disease is often the most common specific cause of death in Latin America (Figs. 4-6). Together the two diseases account for an average of 30-49% of all deaths (Tables IV and V).

I conclude from these observations that cardiovascular and neoplastic diseases are not merely diseases of a modern Western society. Economic and technological development may aggravate these problems, but the data from Latin America suggest that they may be inherent diseases of all humans who can live long enough.

It is true that cardiovascular and neoplastic mortality are much lower in Latin America than in the more-developed countries of the world (Howe *et al.*, 1977; World Health Organization, 1978) if one does not adjust for the population differences in the proportion of young and old persons. The age-adjusted statistics presented suggest, however, that economic and technological development will do as much to uncover, as to create, cardiovascular and neoplastic diseases in Latin America.

B. Some Infectious Diseases Introduced to Latin America

When the Europeans migrated to the New World, they brought with them much more than just their culture. They were able to dominate the New World

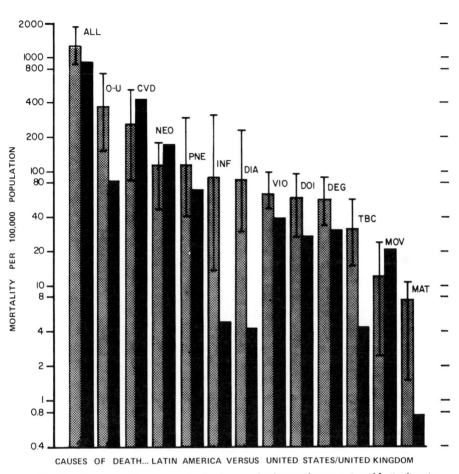

CAUSES OF DEATH...LATIN AMERICA VERSUS UNITED STATES/UNITED KINGDOM

Fig. 5. Cause-specific, age-standardized mean death rates for countries of Latin America and the United States and the United Kingdom in early 1960s, males and females combined. Latin American on left (stippled), United States and the United Kingdom on right (solid). Ranges also shown for Latin America. Logarithmic (proportional) scale used. ALL, all causes. See Fig. 4 for other abbreviations. See Table IV for values. (Preston *et al.*, 1972.)

largely because they and their African slaves introduced new infections to the American Indians (Brown, 1977; Hunter *et al.*, 1976). Virtually the entire indigenous population of the New World apparently was susceptible to such diseases as measles and smallpox (Dubos, 1965a; Wood, 1979). The consequence was that the bulk of the American Indians were exterminated often even without seeing the new invaders (Nutels, 1968). One reason the Europeans preferred African to American Indian slaves was the major difference in susceptibility to these Old World infections. This difference in susceptibility to the crowd dis-

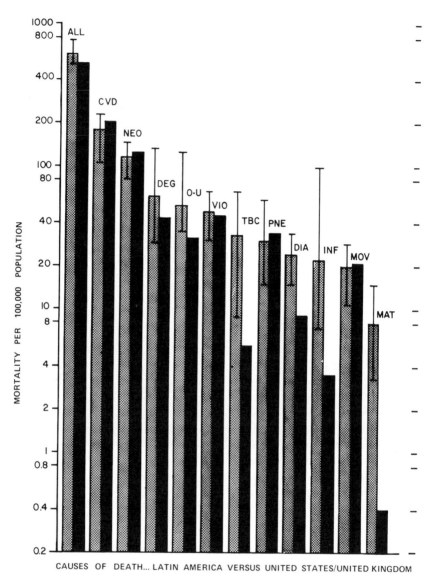

CAUSES OF DEATH... LATIN AMERICA VERSUS UNITED STATES/UNITED KINGDOM

Fig. 6. Cause-specific, age-standardized mean death rates for cities of Latin America and the United States and the United Kingdom in early 1960s, males and females combined, ages 15–74 years. Latin America on left (stippled), United States and the United Kingdom on right (solid). Ranges also shown for Latin America. Logarithmic (proportional) scale used. ALL, all causes. See Fig. 4 for other abbreviations. See Table V for values. (Puffer and Griffith, 1967.)

eases became even more important when malaria and yellow fever were introduced (Goodyear, 1978; Wood, 1979). One important question that should be
addressed is whether this susceptibility of the American Indians can be ascribed
to genetic factors. Malaria and measles provide good grounds for discussing this
question.

1. Malaria

The best example that students of human evolution have of genetic adaptation
to an infectious disease is malaria (Allison, 1964; Livingstone, 1958; Wiesenfeld,
1967). Human malaria probably evolved in Africa when the environmental and
demographic alterations produced by agriculture enabled a nonhuman primate
zoonosis to establish itself in, and become adapted to, people (Ackerknecht,
1965; Cockburn, 1977; Dunn, 1965). The major effect of agriculture is to bring
large enough numbers of both mosquito vectors and human hosts together so that
one mosquito is likely to bite two persons, the first already infected and second
not yet infected. Nonagricultural, hunting and gathering people neither will
disrupt the environment sufficiently to become the major target of the malaria-
bearing mosquitos, nor will they provide a sufficiently dense population for
malaria to be transmitted among humans.

Malaria is not only a recent human disease [i.e., since the development of
agriculture (Wiesenfeld, 1967)], it is also rather devastating. The infection tends
to be chronic, having a severe effect on both mortality and fertility (Allison,
1964; Black, 1975; Conly, 1972; Giglioli, 1968, 1972; Livingstone, 1958;
Montalenti, 1965). These conditions suggest that some genetic adaptations
should have arisen among those populations that have been exposed the longest.
Likely contenders for such adaptations are various abnormalities in hemoglobin
(e.g., hemoglobin S and C, and thalassemia), red blood cell enzymes (e.g.,
glucose-6-phosphate dehydrogenase deficiency), and the red blood cell surface
membrane (e.g., Duffy-negative blood type). Most of these genetic abnormalities occur in Africans, the population in which malaria may have arisen.
Calculations by Livingstone (1976) show that the 175 generations (3500 years)
since the last likely development of agriculture in Africa is sufficient time for
these traits to achieve their current high levels. Investigators have known for
some time that hemoglobin S provides genetic protection from falciparum
malaria (Allison, 1964; Livingstone, 1958; Montalenti, 1965; Wiesenfeld,
1967). Furthermore, in Latin America the absence of the Duffy substance from
red blood cell membranes was recently shown also to protect persons from vivax
malaria (Miller *et al.*, 1975; Spencer *et al.*, 1978).

Although malaria may have been indigenous to the New World (Learmonth,
1977), the bulk of the evidence is that it was introduced from the Old World,
probably by Africans [see Bruce-Chwatt (1965) for another pre-Columbian alter-
native] only a few hundred years ago (Ackerknecht, 1965; Dunn, 1965;

Henschen, 1966). Malaria is now well established in Latin America (Fig. 7; Giglioli, 1968), although it has been brought under control in many areas (Learmonth, 1977). Despite this prevalence of malaria, no genetic characteristic that has been implicated as an adaptation to malaria has been found in the American Indian population (Dunn, 1965; Saldanha et al., 1976).

Although protective traits do exist in Latin America, they can all be traced to the more recent Old World migrants, usually from Africa (Arends, 1971). Studies in Latin America have consistently shown that the Africans there are resistant to vivax malaria and tolerant to falciparum malaria, in contrast with the American Indians (Giglioli, 1968) and Europeans there (Spencer et al., 1978). This resistance to vivax malaria has been shown in Honduras to be due to the Duffy-negative red blood cell trait from Africa (Spencer et al., 1978).

Malaria provides good examples of the relationship of a disease to the human and nonhuman environment. Conditions in Latin America are well suited for the

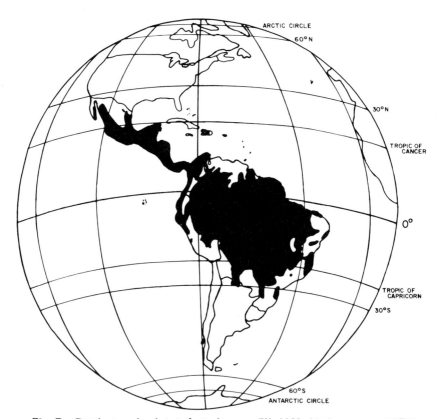

Fig. 7.   Distribution of malaria in Latin America. (World Health Organization, 1979.)

maintenance of malaria. The climate supports the necessary vector; the economy supports the necessary dense (human) host population; and the agricultural technology both fosters the vector and host populations and brings them together. Likely, these conditions existed before the introduction of malaria and have only been enhanced since the recent Old World migrations. Genetic adaptations to malaria in Latin America all derive from the Old World. Apparently 20 generations (400 years) of severe disease stress is insufficient time for even the molecularly simple adaptations to malaria to develop (Section IV,D,1,a). This observation reinforces the belief that malaria has only recently been introduced to the New World.

2. Measles

The devastation wrought in the New World by the acute, infectious, viral diseases such as measles and smallpox has raised a suspicion of genetic susceptibility in the American Indians (Crosby, 1972). Although American Indians clearly lack genetic resistance to malaria (as do most Europeans also), recent evidence from Latin America suggests that they do not lack such resistance to measles.

Measles is a good example of an infection that could only have arisen since the development of dense human population (i.e., since agriculture developed). It probably arose from the closely related, but different, distemper of dogs or rinderpest of cattle (Ball, 1977; Cockburn, 1977). This viral infection produces a permanent and complete immunity in all infected normal people. Its infectivity is so high that virtually the only people who will be susceptible after an epidemic are those who were born after the epidemic. Because no reservoir for measles exists other than humans, it will become extinct in any small population. This phenomenon has been observed worldwide, including Latin America (Black, 1975; Niederman et al., 1967). Based on epidemiological evidence, an estimated population of 200,000 to 1.25 million is needed to maintain measles (Black et al., 1977; Cockburn, 1967b, 1977). In a population of that size, the birthrate can keep pace with the circulation of the disease. For these reasons, diseases such as measles could not become established in human populations until after the development of agriculture, which enabled such large populations to exist in reasonably circumscribed geographical areas.

Clearly measles was introduced into the New World by the European and/or African migrants (Ball, 1977; Newman, 1976; Wood, 1979). Ordinarily, without modern medical care, measles can have a 10% mortality (Grossman and Jawetz, 1979). However, shortly after the Old World migrations the American Indians experienced a much higher mortality (Crosby, 1972). Although a genetic susceptibility (or lack of genetic resistance) has been suspected, recent observations in unexposed American Indian populations in Latin America support an alternative explanation.

Black and co-workers (1977) studied the effect of measles vaccine (an attenuated live measles virus) on three tribes of American Indians in Brazil that were totally susceptible to measles. Neel and colleagues (1970) actually observed a measles epidemic in another totally susceptible Venezuelan–Brazilian tribe. Both sets of investigators concluded that the bulk of the excess mortality was due to the social disorganization brought about by the epidemic (Neel, 1977). When an entire population is susceptible to an infection, no one is well enough during an epidemic to provide food, water, and other basic care to the sick (Crosby, 1972). This situation does not obtain, however, when an infection recurs in a population more than once in the lifetime of the average person and leaves a pool of survivors resistant to the disease. Newman (1976) also points out that effective folk medicine responses, which may include basic nursing, may be abandoned because of apparent failure in the face of a novel infection. I conclude from this evidence that if American Indians have a genetic susceptibility to measles, the difference between them and the Old World populations is small.

C. Some Infectious Diseases Indigenous to Latin America

Although the long isolation of the New World fauna from humans and the arctic filter may have reduced the variety of diseases facing people in Latin America, one must not imagine that this was a disease-free paradise. Undoubtedly, many viral, bacterial, fungal, protozoal, and metazoal diseases of pre-agricultural humans are well adapted for transportation through the arctic. In addition, there was sufficient variety among the New World animals so that many of their infections are transmissible to humans (Table III). Thus, even though the Europeans may not have encountered disease barriers in the New World tropics comparable with those in the Old World tropics (Newman, 1976), the pre-Columbian American Indians had their share of misery.

Earlier, it was pointed out that the natural co-evolution of a parasite and its host is from a pathological, poorly infectious disease to a nonpathological, highly infectious coexistence. Just such a pattern can be detected among the indigenous diseases of Latin America.

1. American Trypanosomiasis and Leishmaniasis

The most likely origin of a new infectious disease of humans is other animals. A characteristic of such a new infection should be that, although it is highly pathological, it is not easily transmitted among humans. American leishmaniasis and trypanosomiasis are examples of two such diseases. Both leishmaniasis (Ackerknecht, 1965; Cockburn, 1977; Garnham, 1971; Lainson and Shaw, 1978; Newman, 1976) and trypanosomiasis (Cockburn, 1977; Henschen, 1966; Lambrecht, 1964, 1967; Newman, 1976) are interesting because they have independently become human infections in both the Old World and the New World. Both of these related protozoal diseases are serious problems in Latin America (Guerra, 1970; Lainson and Shaw, 1978; Figs. 8 and 9). Although some leishmanial infections can be transmitted among humans in the Old World (e.g., kala-azar), American leishmaniasis is not transmitted among humans (Biagi, 1976; Lainson and Shaw, 1978). That is, American leishmaniasis has not evolved beyond being a zoonosis. Some types of trypanosomiasis, however, have evolved in both the Old and New World to become transmissible among humans, although no trypanosome is restricted to humans in the New World as it is in the Old World (Arean, 1976; Lambrecht, 1964, 1967; Maegraith, 1976). Both of these infections depend on human technology for their maintenance in Latin America. American leishmaniasis is a zoonosis that affects humans when they invade, but have not yet eliminated, the forest (Garnham, 1971; Herrer and Christensen, 1976). American trypanosomiasis is often maintained as a human

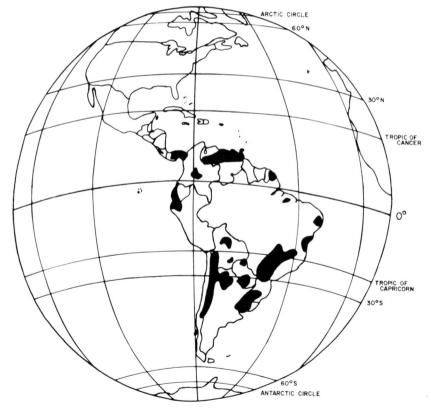

Fig. 8. Distribution of American trypanosomiasis in Latin America. (From Wilcocks and Manson-Bahr, 1972, p. 109.)

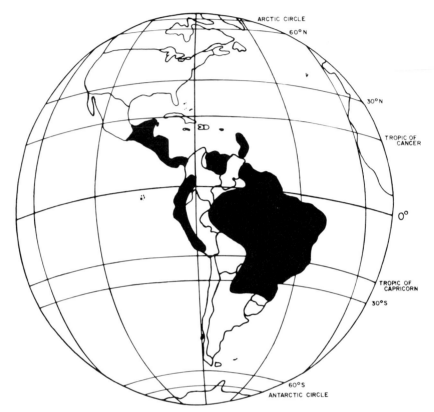

Fig. 9. Distribution of American leishmaniasis in Latin America. (From Biagi, 1976, p. 412.)

infection when thatched roofing provides a shelter for the vector near humans (Whitlaw and Chaniotis, 1978; Wilcocks and Manson-Bahr, 1972).

2. Bartonellosis

Bartonellosis (Herrer, 1976; Maegraith, 1976; Wilcocks and Manson-Bahr, 1972) is an example of a disease that developed in South America and has probably become restricted to humans. Bartonellosis (Carrion's disease) is a bacterial infection having two manifestations: Oroya fever and verruga peruana. This disease is limited by the distribution of phlebotomine sandflies to the Andes between 2° N and 13° S, and from 800 m to 3000 m in altitude; that is the region bordering the high altitude area shown in Fig. 3. *Bartonella* must have originally been derived from a zoonosis. However, although wild rodents can be infected, humans are the only known reservoir. The disease is maintained because of the large number of asymptomatic carriers. The possibility that American Indians of the area have evolved some tolerance to the parasite is raised by the observation that severe disease is more common among nonresidents (usually Europeans). This pattern may, of course, be accounted for by the lack of acquired immunity during childhood among the intrusive people. In summary, bartonellosis appears to be a Latin American example of a parasite that has evolved, perhaps with its host, from a zoonosis to a human-restricted disease of moderate-to-severe pathology and prolonged infectivity.

3. Pinta

Pinta is a treponemal infection found only in tropical Latin America (Fig. 10). It is probably a good example of a disease that is evolving an even more advantageous relationship with its host. Four closely related treponematoses are known: pinta, yaws, nonvenereal (endemic) syphilis, and venereal syphilis. The treponemal infections of humans are probably related to those of Old World primates (Cockburn, 1967d, 1977; Willcox, 1977). The evolution and relationship of the human treponematoses have been the subject of extensive speculation

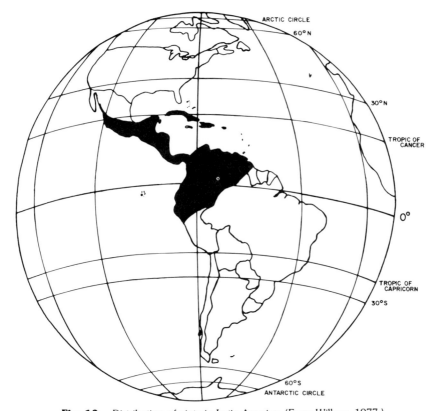

Fig. 10.   Distribution of pinta in Latin America. (From Willcox, 1977.)

(Hackett, 1963; Hudson, 1963, 1965a,b; Willcox, 1972), as has been the apparent emergence of venereal syphilis after Columbus' discovery of the New World (Crosby, 1972; Hudson, 1968). Because there is no known treponematosis of nonhuman New World primates (Lee *et al.*, 1978), and because human treponemal infections were known in the pre-Columbian New World (Crosby, 1972; El-Najjar, 1979), some treponemal organisms must have been brought there by the Asian migrants sometime during the last 40,000 years. Since pinta is probably not found outside of the New World (Brubaker, 1976; Wilcocks and Manson-Bahr, 1972; Willcox, 1977), it must have evolved in Latin America, possibly from that treponeme carried across Beringia.

Pinta does, in fact, behave like a disease that has had time to evolve a less pathological, but more infectious, relationship with its host. Of all the treponematoses, pinta produces the fewest pathological manifestations. Its lesions are probably limited to the skin, and may not involve deeper structures (Brubaker, 1976; Maegraith, 1976; Wilcocks and Manson-Bahr, 1972) as do the other treponematoses. Black (1975) and Lee and co-workers (1978) have recently found evidence of a possibly asymptomatic, unknown, treponemal infection in some isolated American Indians of South America. I raise the possibility that this infection may represent a further evolution of pinta. Unlike the other treponematoses, pinta remains infectious for many years (Wilcocks and Manson-Bahr, 1972). All of the evidence suggests that pinta is a treponemal infection that is following the expected pattern of evolution. Whether American Indians are also evolving tolerance is unknown. However, Hopkins and Florez (1977) noted that, in Colombia, pinta is most common in American Indians and their descendents, whereas yaws is more frequent in Africans living there, and venereal syphilis is most frequent in the European-dominated urban areas (but is also found in Africans and American Indians).

4. Mansonelliasis

Mansonelliasis (de Paola, 1971; Hubbert *et al.*, 1975; Hunter *et al.*, 1976; Maegraith, 1976; Wilcocks and Manson-Bahr, 1972) is an example of an indigenous New World infection that has evolved to a virtually nonpathogenic state. The helminthic parasite *Mansonella ozzardi*, also known as Ozzard's filaria, is only found in tropical Latin America (Fig. 11). Similar, but different, microfilaria have been detected in the local fauna, but humans are the only known host. In endemic areas, most people are infected. If any symptoms or lesions are produced from this infection, they are mild. Possibly this parasite, which originally must have been a zoonosis, was never pathological for humans. However, a consideration of the usually highly pathological response of humans to other filarial infections suggests that it too may have passed through a pathological state. That the life requirements of a host and a parasite will be sufficiently matched for either not to be pathological to the other without some

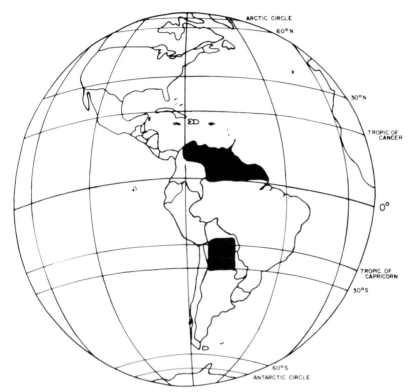

Fig. 11. Distribution of mansonelliasis in Latin America (Gelman, 1976; Wilcocks and Manson-Bahr, 1972, p. 193).

genetic evolution is unlikely. More probably mansonelliasis is an example of host-parasite coevolution to the point of host tolerance to prolonged parasite infection.

D. Genetic Diseases

By genetic disease, I mean genetic traits that produce morbidity independent of the effect of the environment. Thus, susceptibility and resistance to nutritional, infectious, or other environmentally derived diseases are not considered here. Private genes are distinguished from public genes or genetic disease.

By a private gene I mean a genetic characteristic that is unique to one small group of persons and for which no evolutionary advantage is known. Private genes may be considered to have arisen by a single mutation that seldom recurs in a population. Their frequencies in a population have probably risen to noticeable levels merely because of chance phenomena such as population growth, inbreeding, or genetic drift. Private genes are considered transient traits that will shortly disappear.

On the other hand, public genes are more long-lasting, often widespread, characteristics of populations. They may arise because of a high mutation rate at a particular chromosomal locus, or they may be side effects of more important genetic adaptations. These genetic adaptations may themselves be evolutionary responses to infectious or other disease. Although these public genetic diseases will eventually be selected out of the population, such extinction will not occur as rapidly as for a private gene.

1. Some Genetic Diseases Introduced to Latin America

The large number of migrants in the last 500 years ensures that many of the genetic diseases of Europe and Africa are also found in Latin America. Examples of both public and private Old World genetic diseases are palatolabial defects (Arce-Gomes *et al.*, 1970; Salzano and Freire-Maia, 1970), hemoglobins S, C, D, A $'_2$ (B $_2$), thalassemia, glucose-6-phosphate dehydrogenase deficiency (Arends, 1971), Portugese-type familial amyloid polyneuropathy (Juliao *et al.*, 1974), color blindness (Mueller and Weiss, 1979), familial chondrocalcinosis (Reginato *et al.*, 1975), osteopetrosis, hemophilias A and B (Salzano and Freire-Maia, 1970), and the X-linked muscular dystrophies (Zatz *et al.*, 1976, 1977). Panchaszadeh (1979) lists at least 51 additional genetic disorders found in Venezuela alone.

a. Hemoglobin S. Typical of the public genetic diseases introduced to Latin America is hemoglobin S homozygosity. Hemoglobin S arose in Africa as a response to falciparum malaria (Allison, 1964; Livingstone, 1958; Wiesenfeld, 1967), as was discussed earlier. Hemoglobin S is the result of a mutation of normal hemoglobin A, a single nucleotide change that results in a single amino acid difference on the beta protein chain of hemoglobin. This change interferes with the growth of the parasite and thus reduces its pathological effects. Although hemoglobin S is protective against falciparum malaria in the heterozygous AS state, it is lethal in the homozygous SS state because of the destructive effect of pure hemoglobin S on the red blood cell (sickle cell anemia). From the strong selective pressure of malaria and its recent onset, a simple genetic adaptation has resulted that for homozygous AA persons necessarily leaves them unprotected and for homozygous SS persons is lethal. Apparently, the short time since the beginning of human malaria (no more than 500 generations or 10,000 years, since the beginning of agriculture) has not been long enough for a better adaptation to evolve.

Hemoglobin S was introduced to the New World by migrants from Africa. Arends (1971) extensively surveyed the literature which shows that hemoglobin

S (as well as other probable adaptations to malaria) is never found in pure American Indians. Among Latin American Africans, the frequency of hemoglobin AS heterozygotes ranges from 3 to 23%. Among other Latin American populations, the presence of this gene relates directly to the admixture with African genes. One may presume that for the immediate future the frequency of this genetic disease in Latin America will depend jointly on gene flow from Latin American Africans to Latin American Indians and Europeans and on the effect (both positive and negative) of human culture on malaria.

b. Familial Chondrocalcinosis. Familial (or articular) chondrocalcinosis (Reginato *et al.*, 1975) is an example of a private genetic disease introduced to Latin America from Europe. Probably due to an autosomal gene, either dominant or recessive, it is found in the descendents of the European settlers of the Chiloe Islands of Chile (Fig. 1). Because this disease has been reported in Europe, and because three affected families can be traced back almost to the original European migrants in the 1500s without American Indian admixture, apparently familial chondrocalcinosis was not indigenous to the New World. Reginato and colleagues surmised that it was introduced by one of the migrants from Portugal or Spain. As the Chiloe islanders are reported to be a small population with little gene flow with other groups, I propose that the high frequency of this genetic disease is the combined result of genetic drift, inbreeding, and cultural protection of the affected persons.

2. Some Genetic Diseases Indigenous to Latin America

Unlike the Old World, the New World has few indigenous genetic diseases that can be pointed to (Salzano, 1972). Neel (1971) detected a high incidence of major congenital defects and of chromosomal abnormalities in some isolated American Indians in Latin America. (Whether the congenital defects reflect inbreeding, and the chromosomal abnormalities reflect technical problems, remains to be answered.) In a review of the genetic basis for many diseases among the populations of the world, Damon (1969) lists no clearly genetic diseases among the American Indians and only a few diseases that are possibly genetic. This dearth of genetic diseases may be accounted for by the relative lack of in tensive study of the indigenous New World populations, as compared with Old World populations. Because many Old World genetic diseases are probably the side effects of adaptations to Old World crowd diseases, and because such crowd diseases had not developed as much in the pre-Columbian New World, perhaps American Indians do have fewer genetic diseases. Nevertheless, the following genetic diseases can be listed as indigenous to Latin America: hereditary polymorphic light eruption (Birt and Davis, 1975), focal epithelial hyperplasia (possibly viral) (Borghelli *et al.*, 1975; Praetorius-Clausen and Emmertsen, 1973), and albinism (Keeler, 1970; Witkop *et al.*, 1978) for the American

Indians, and Parana hard-skin syndrome (probably genetic) (Cat *et al.*, 1974), and acheiropodia (Freire-Maia, 1975; Freire-Maia *et al.*, 1975a,b) for the Latin American Europeans.

a. Albinism. The occulocutaneous albinism of the Tele Cuna Indians of the San Blas Islands (Fig. 1) in Panama (Keeler, 1970; Witkop *et al.*, 1978) is an example of a public (at least within that group) genetic disease. This tyrosine-positive albinism is produced by an autosomal, partially codominant, gene. Among this population of 24,800 persons are 61–67 albinos per 10,000. Only the Jemez Indians and the Brandywine isolate in North America have higher frequencies of albinism.

Albinism has been known to be present among the Cuna for at least 17 generations (340 years). The reason for the presence of this gene is not clear. The gene is deleterious in the homozygous state. Albinos have slower growth, poorer health, worse vision, and higher mortality than nonalbinos. At least among the males, fertility is reduced. Nevertheless, the frequency of albinos did not decline between 1925 and 1970, and was probably not higher in 1681. A high mutation rate is possible, but more likely is some advantage for the heterozygotes. Keeler (1970) does in fact point out that heterozygotes are often lighter in color than normal homozygotes, and that light-colored skin is preferred in that society. These conditions could give the heterozygotes a reproductive advantage that compensates for the disadvantage of the albino homozygotes.

b. Acheiropodia. A genetic disease that has arisen among the European (Portuguese) population of Latin America (Brazil) (Freire-Maia, 1975; Freire-Maia *et al.*, 1975a,b), acheiropodia is a condition of congenitally absent hands and feet. The afflicted persons have a genetic fitness 1% of normal. The disease results from an autosomal recessive gene that has complete penetrance. The gene frequency is about 9/10,000. The disadvantage that the homozygotes suffer is expected to eliminate this recessive gene from the population within 2300 generations (46,000 years). Investigators estimate that some 25,000 acheiropodia genes have arisen in the Brazillian population in less than 400 years. However, they doubt that this gene increase is a case of recurrent mutation. Since population growth alone is insufficient to account for this relatively high frequency, they hypothesize, and I agree, that genetic drift must have played a role initially.

V. CONCLUSION

This chapter reviews diseases found in the populations of Latin America. The enormity of this region, the diversity of its population, and the range of its environment, however, preclude an encyclopedic treatment. (A computer search of *Index Medicus* for publications from 1966 to 1979 about diseases in Latin America produced more than 2000 citations). Rather than being comprehensive, I have chosen to discuss some selected diseases or disease patterns that demonstrate an evolutionary principle or a biocultural interaction.

In general, two basic patterns emerge from a consideration of Latin American diseases. The first is that the evolution of diseases had not progressed as far in the pre-Columbian New World as in the Old World. Humans arrived late there, and agriculture arose later and less frequently than in the Old World. As a result, most, but not all, of the diseases unique to Latin America are still zoonoses and are not well adapted to humans. I believe that this fact reflects both the absence of closely related animal reservoirs for new diseases and the late development of dense populations. Even a relative lack of genetic diseases among the American Indians may be accounted for by the dearth of indigenous crowd diseases of recent (10,000 years) origin. The bulk of the crowd diseases in Latin America can be traced to the European and African migrations.

The other pattern is that Latin America has a disease pattern that might be expected for an economically developing region. Nutritional deficiency and infectious diseases are major and interacting causes of morbidity and mortality. Contrariwise, cardiovascular and neoplastic diseases are not as common as in the developed world. Surprising is the observation that despite this fact, cardiovascular and neoplastic diseases are still the most common causes of death in Latin America when differences in population age structure between developed and developing countries are allowed for. These findings suggest that a human susceptibility to cardiovascular and neoplastic diseases may merely be enhanced, rather than caused, by modern civilization.

In conclusion, I reaffirm my original thesis that the maximum amount of information can be extracted from the knowledge of diseases in populations if they are viewed as resulting from novel interactions among peoples and between persons and their environment. Diseases are more than randomly occurring events. The existence of any disease is the expression of a transient evolutionary process that ought to be explainable.

REFERENCES

Ackerknecht, E. H. (1965). "History and Geography of the Most Important Diseases." Hafner, New York.

Allison, A. C. (1964). Polymorphism and natural selection in human populations. *Cold Spring Harbor Symp. Quant. Biol.* **29**, 137–149.

Arce-Gomes, B., Azevedo, J. B. C., Chautard, E. A., and Freire-Maia, N. (1970). A genetic study of palatolabial defects. *Hum. Hered.* **20**, 580–589.

Arean, V. M. (1976). American trypanosomiasis. *In* "Tropical Medicine" (G. W. Hunter, J. C. Swartzwelder, and D. F. Clyde, eds.), 5th ed., pp. 440–450. Saunders, Philadelphia, Pennsylvania.

Arends, T. (1971). Hemoglobinopathies and enzyme deficiencies in Latin American populations. *In* "The Ongoing Evolution of Latin American Populations" (F. M. Salzano, ed.), pp. 509–559. Thomas, Springfield, Illinois.

Armelagos, G. J., and McArdle, A. (1975). Population, disease, and evolution. *In* "Population Studies in Archeology and Biological Anthropology: A Symposium" (A. C. Swedlund, ed.), Memoir of the Society for American Archeology, No. 30, pp. 1–10.

Ball, A. P. (1977). Measles. *In* "A World Geography of Human Diseases" (G. M. Howe, ed.), pp. 237–254. Academic Press, New York.

Barzelatto, J., and Covarrubias, E. (1968). Study of endemic goiter in the American Indian. *In* "Biomedical Challenges Presented by the American Indian," Sci. Publ. No. 165, pp. 124–132. Pan Am. Health Organ., Washington, D.C.

Behar, M. (1968). Food and nutrition of the Maya before the conquest and at the present time. *In* "Biomedical Challenges Presented by the American Indian," Sci. Pub. No. 165, pp. 114–119. Pan Am. Health Organ., Washington, D.C.

Biagi, F. (1976). Leishmaniasis—Introduction. Kala-azar. Cutaneous and mucocutaneous leishmaniasis. *In* "Tropical Medicine" (G. W. Hunter, J. C. Swartzwelder, and D. F. Clyde, eds.), 5th ed. pp. 411–414, 415–422, 423–429. Saunders, Philadelphia, Pennsylvania.

Birt, A. R., and Davis, R. A. (1975). Hereditary polymorphic light eruption of American Indians. *Int. J. Dermatol.* **14**, 105–111.

Black, F. L. (1975). Infectious diseases in primitive societies: many common diseases are not maintained in primitive society and probably did not affect human evolution. *Science* **187**, 515–518.

Black, F. L., Pinheiro, F. de P., Hierholzer, W. J., and Lee, R. V. (1977). Epidemiology of infectious disease: the example of measles. *In* "Health and Disease in Tribal Societies," Ciba Foundation Symposium, No. 49, pp. 115–130. Elsevier, Amsterdam.

Borghelli, R. V., Stirparo, M. A., Paroni, H. C., Barros, R. E., and Dominquez, F. V. (1975). Focal epithelial hyperplasia; report of five new cases from Argentina. *Oral Surg.* **40**, 107–112.

Brothwell, D., and Sandison, A. T., eds. (1967) "Diseases in Antiquity: A Survey of the Diseases, Injuries and Surgery of Early Populations." Thomas, Springfield, Illinois.

Brown, A. W. A. (1977). Yellow fever, dengue, and dengue haemorrhagic fever. *In* "A World Geography of Human Diseases" (G. M. Howe, ed.), pp. 271–317. Academic Press, New York.

Brubaker, M. L. (1976). Pinta. *In* "Tropical Medicine" (G. W. Hunter, J. C. Swartzwelder, and D. F. Clyde, eds.), 5th ed., pp. 162–164. Saunders, Philadelphia, Pennsylvania.

Bruce-Chwatt, L. J. (1965). Paleogenesis and paleo-epidemiology of primate malaria. *Bull W. H. O.* **32**, 363–387.

Buck, A. A., Sasaki, T. T., and Anderson, R. I. (1968). "Health and Disease in Four Peruvian Villages: Contrasts in Epidemiology." Johns Hopkins Press, Baltimore, Maryland.

Cat, I., Magdalena, N. I. R., Marinoni, L. P., Wong, M. P., Freitas, O. T., Malfi, A., Costa, O., Esteves, L., Giraldi, D. J., and Opitz, J. M. (1974). Parana hard-skin syndrome: study of seven families. *Lancet* **1**, 215–216.

Ciba Foundation (1977). "Health and Disease in Tribal Societies," Symposium No. 49. Elsevier, Amsterdam.

Cockburn, T. A. (1963). "The Evolution and Eradication of Infectious Diseases." Johns Hopkins Press, Baltimore, Maryland.

Cockburn, (T.) A. (1967a). Parasitism. *In* "Infectious Diseases: Their Evolution and Eradication" ((T.) A. Cockburn, ed.), pp. 22–37. Thomas, Springfield, Illinois.

Cockburn, (T.) A. (1967b). The evolution of human infectious diseases. *In* "Infectious Diseases: Their Evolution and Eradication" ((T.) A. Cockburn, ed.), pp. 84–107. Thomas, Springfield, Illinois.

Cockburn, (T.) A. (1967c). Paleoepidemiology. *In* "Infectious Diseases: Their Evolution and Eradication" ((T.) A. Cockburn, ed.), pp. 50-65. Thomas, Springfield, Illinois.

Cockburn, (T.) A. (1967d). Infections of the order primates. *In* "Infectious Diseases: Their Evolution and Eradication" ((T.) A. Cockburn, ed.), pp. 38-49. Thomas, Springfield, Illinois.

Cockburn, (T.) A. (1971). Infectious diseases in ancient populations. *Curr. Anthropol.* **12**, 45-62.

Cockburn, (T.) A. (1977). Where did our infectious diseases come from? The evolution of infectious disease. *In* "Health and Disease in Tribal Societies," Ciba Foundation Symposium, No. 49, pp. 103-112. Elsevier, Amsterdam.

Conly, G. N. (1972). The impact of malaria on economic development: a case study. *Am. J. Trop. Med. Hyg.* **21**, 668-674.

Crosby, A. W., Jr. (1972). "The Columbian Exchange: Biological and Cultural Consequences of 1492," Contributions in American Studies, No. 2. Greenwood Press, Westport, Connecticut.

Crow, J. F. (1958). Some possibilities for measuring selection intensities in man. *Hum. Biol.* **30**, 1-13.

Damon, A. (1969). Race, ethnic group, and disease. *Soc. Biol.* **16**, 69-80.

de Paola, D. (1971). Mansonelliasis (mansonelliasis ozzardi, ozzard's filariasis). *In* "Pathology of Protozoal and Helminthic Diseases: with Clinical Correlation" (R. A. Marcial-Rojas, ed.), pp. 955-959. Williams & Wilkins, Baltimore, Maryland.

Dietz, R. S., and Holden, J. C. (1970). The breakup of Pangaea. *Sci. Am.* **223**(4), 30-41.

Dubos, R. J. (1965a). The evolution of microbial diseases. *In* "Bacterial and Mycotic Infections of Man" (R. J. Dubos and J. G. Hirsch, eds.), 4th ed, pp. 20-36. Lippincott, Philadelphia, Pennsylvania.

Dubos, R. (J.) (1965b). "Man Adapting." Yale Univ. Press, New Haven, Connecticut.

Dunn, F. L. (1965). On the antiquity of malaria in the Western Hemisphere. *Hum. Biol.* **37**, 385-393.

El-Najjar, M. Y. (1979). Human treponematosis and tuberculosis: evidence from the New World. *Am. J. Phys. Anthropol.* **51**, 599-618.

Fierro-Benitez, R., Penafiel, W. DeGroot, L. J., and Ramirez, I. (1969). Endemic goiter and endemic cretinism in the Adean region. *N. Engl. J. Med.* **280**, 296-302.

Fierro-Benitez, R., Ramirez, I., Garces, J., Jaramillo, C., Moncayo, F., and Stanbury, J. B. (1974). The clinical pattern of cretinism as seen in highland Ecuador. *Am. J. Clin. Nutr.* **27**, 531-543.

Freire-Maia, A. (1975). Genetics of acheiropodia (the handless footless families of Brazil), VIII. Penetrance and expressivity. *Clin. Genet.* **7**, 98-102.

Freire-Maia, A. Freire-Maia, N., Morton, N. E., Azevedo, E. S., and Quelce-Salgado, A. (1975a). Genetics of acheiropodia (the handless and footless families of Brazil), VI. Formal genetic analysis. *Am. J. Hum. Genet.* **27**, 521-527.

Freire-Maia, A., Li, W. H., and Maruyama, T. (1975b). Genetics of acheiropodia (the handless and footless families of Brazil), VII. Population dynamics. *Am. J. Hum. Genet.* **27**, 665-675.

Gaitan, E. (1973). Water-borne goitrogens and their role in the etiology of endemic goiter. *World Rev. Nutr. Diet.* **17**, 53-90.

Gaitan, E., Island, D. P., and Liddle, G. W. (1969). Identification of a naturally occurring goitrogen in water. *Trans. Assoc. Am. Physicians* **82**, 141-152.

Garnham, P. C. C. (1971). American leishmaniasis. *Bull. W. H. O.* **44**, 521-527.

Gelman, A. C. (1976). Distribution of selected communicable diseases in the tropical and subtropical areas of the world. *In* "Tropical Medicine" (G. W. Hunter, J. C. Swartzwelder, and D. F. Clyde, eds.), 5th ed., pp. 843-869. Saunders, Philadelphia, Pennsylvania.

Giggs, J. A. (1977). Mental disorders and mental subnormality. *In* "A World Geography of Human Diseases" (G. M. Howe, ed.), pp. 477-506. Academic Press, New York.

Giglioli, G. G. (1968). Malaria in the American Indian. *In* "Biomedical Challenges Presented by the

American Indian,'' Sci. Pub. No. 165, pp. 104-113. Pan Am. Health Organ., Washington, D.C.

Giglioli, G. (1972). Changes in the pattern of mortality following the eradication of hyperendemic malaria from a highly susceptible community. *Bull. W. H. O.* **46**, 181-202.

Goodyear, J. D. (1978). The sugar connection: a new perspective on the history of yellow fever. *Bull. Hist. Med.* **52**, 5-21.

Greene, L. S. (1974). Physical growth and development, neurological maturation, and behavioral functioning in two Ecuadorian Andean communities in which goiter is endemic: II PTC taste sensitivity and neurological maturation. *Am. J. Phys. Anthropol.* **41**, 139-151.

Greene, L. S. (1977). Goiter and social organization in Eucador. *In* "Malnutrition, Behavior, and Social Organization" (L. S. Greene, ed.), pp. 55-94. Academic Press, New York.

Grossman, M., and Jawetz, E. (1979). Infectious diseases: viral and rickettsial. *In* "Current Medical Diagnosis and Treatment" (M. A. Krupp and M. J. Chatton, eds.), 18th ed., pp. 823-846. Lange Med. Pub., Los Altos, California.

Guerra, F. (1970). American trypanosomiasis: an historical and a human lesson. *J. Trop. Med. Hyg.* **73**, 83-118.

Hackett, C. J. (1963). On the origin of the human treponematoses: pinta, yaws, endemic syphilis and venereal syphilis. *Bull. W. H. O.* **29**, 7-41.

Haldane, J. B. S. (1956-1957). Natural selection in man. *Acta Genet. Stat. Med.* **6**, 321-332.

Henschen, F. (1966). "The History and Geography of Diseases." Delacorte Press, New York.

Herrer, A. (1976). Bartonellosis. *In* "Tropical Medicine" (G. W. Hunter, J. C. Swartzwelder, and D. F. Clyde, eds.), 5th ed., pp. 256-259. Saunders, Philadelphia, Pennsylvania.

Herrer, A., and Christensen, H. A. (1976). Epidemiological patterns of cutaneous leishmaniasis in Panama. *Ann. Trop. Med. Parasitol.* **70**, 59-65.

Hopkins, D. R., and Florez, D. (1977). Pinta, yaws, and venereal syphilis in Colombia. *Int. J. Epidemiol.* **6**, 349-355.

Houston, C. S. (1976). High altitude illness: disease with protean manifestations. *J. Am. Med. Assoc.* **236**, 2193-2195.

Howe, G. M., ed. (1977). "A World Geography of Human Diseases." Academic Press, New York.

Howe, G. M., Burgess, L., and Gatenby, P. (1977). Cardiovascular disease. *In* "A World Geography of Human Diseases" (G. M. Howe, ed.), pp. 431-476. Academic Press, New York.

Hubbert, W. T., McCulloch, W. F., and Schnurrenberger, P. R., eds. (1975). "Diseases Transmitted from Animals to Man," 6th ed. Thomas, Springfield, Illinois.

Hudson, E. H. (1963). Treponematosis and anthropology. *Ann. Intern. Med.* **58**, 1037-1048.

Hudson, E. H. (1965a). Treponematosis in perspective. *Bull. W. H. O.* **32**, 735-750.

Hudson, E. H. (1965b). Treponematosis and man's social evolution. *Am. Anthropol.* **67**, 885-901.

Hudson, E. H. (1968). Christopher Columbus and the history of syphilis. *Acta Trop.* **25**, 1-16.

Hunter, G. W., Swartzwelder, J. C., and Clyde, D. F. (1976). "Tropical Medicine," 5th ed. Saunders, Philadelphia, Pennsylvania.

Hurley, P. M. (1968). The confirmation of continental drift. *Sci. Am.* **218**, 52-64.

Hurtado, A. (1942). Chronic mountain sickness. *J. Am. Med. Assoc.* **120**, 1278-1282.

Janssens, P. A. (1970). "Paleopathology: Diseases and Injuries of Prehistoric Man." Baker, London.

Jennings, J. D. (1978). Origins. *In* "Ancient Native Americans" (J. D. Jennings, ed.), pp. 1-41. Freeman, San Francisco, California.

Juliao, O. F. Querioz, L. S., and Lopes de Faria, J. L. (1974). Portuguese type of familial amyloid polyneuropathy: anatomo-clinical study of a Brazilian family. *Eur. Neurol.* **11**, 180-195.

Keeler, C. (1970). Cuna moon-child albinism, 1950-1970. *J. Hered.* **61**, 273-278.

Lainson, R., and Shaw, J. J. (1978). Epidemiology and ecology of leishmaniasis in Latin America. *Nature (London)* **273**, 595-600.

Lambrecht, F. L. (1964). Aspects of evolution and ecology of tsetse flies and trypanosomiasis in prehistoric African environment. *J. Afr. Hist.* **5**, 1-24.

Lambrecht, F. L. (1967). Trypanosomiasis in prehistoric and later human populations: a tentative reconstruction. *In* "Diseases in Antiquity" (D. Brothwell and A. T. Sandison, eds.), pp. 132-151. Thomas, Springfield, Illinois.

Learmonth, A. T. A. (1977). Malaria. *In* "A World Geography of Human Diseases" (G. M. Howe, ed.), pp. 61-108. Academic Press, New York.

Lee, R. V., Black, F. L., Hierholzer, W. R., Jr., and West, B. L. (1978). A novel pattern of treponemal antibody distribution in isolated South American Indian populations. *Am. J. Epidemiol.* **107**, 46-53.

Livingstone, F. (1958). Anthropological implications of sickle-cell gene in West Africa. *Am. Anthropol.* **60**, 533-562.

Livingstone, F. B. (1976). Hemoglobin history in West Africa. *Hum. Biol.* **48**, 487-500.

Logan, M. H., and Hunt, E. E., Jr. (1978). "Health and the Human Condition: Perspectives on Medical Anthropology." Duxbury Press, North Scituate, Massachusetts.

McNeill, W. H. (1976) "Plagues and Peoples." Anchor Press/Doubleday, Garden City, New York.

Maegraith, B. G. (1976). "Adams and Maegraith: Clinical Tropical Diseases," 6th ed. Blackwell, Oxford.

May, J. M. (1977). Deficiency diseases. *In* "A World Geography of Human Diseases" (G. M. Howe, ed.), pp. 535-575. Academic Press, New York.

Miller, L. H., Mason, S. J., Dvorak, J. A., McGinnis, M. H., and Rothman, I. K. (1975). Erythrocyte receptors for (Plasmodia knowlesi) malaria: Duffy blood group determinants. *Science* **189**, 561-563.

Monge-M., C. (1937). High altitude disease. *Arch. Intern. Med.* **59**, 32-37.

Monge-M., C. (1948). "Acclimatization in the Andes: Historical Confirmation of 'Climatic Aggression' in the Development of Andean Man." Johns Hopkins Press, Baltimore, Maryland.

Monge-M., C., and Monge-C., C. (1966). "High Altitude Diseases: Mechanism and Management." Thomas, Springfield, Illinois.

Montalenti, G. (1965). Infectious diseases as selective agents. *In* "Biological Aspects of Social Problems" (J. E. Meade and A. S. Parkes, eds.), pp. 135-151. Oliver & Boyd, Edinburgh.

Morison, S. E. (1971). "The European Discovery of America: The Northern Voyages, AD 500-1600." Oxford Univ. Press, London and New York.

Mueller, W. H., and Weiss, K. M. (1979). Color blindness in Colombia. *Ann. Hum. Biol.* **6**, 137-145.

Neel, J. V. (1968). The American Indian in the International Biological Program. *In* "Biomedical Challenges Presented by the American Indian," Sci. Pub. No. 165, pp. 47-54. Pan Am. Health Organ., Washington, D.C.

Neel, J. V. (1971). Genetic Aspects of the ecology of disease in the American Indian. *In* "The Ongoing Evolution of Latin American Populations" (F. M. Salzano, ed.), pp. 561-590. Thomas, Springfield, Illinois.

Neel, J. V. (1977). Health and disease in unacculturated Amerindian populations. *In* "Health and Disease in Tribal Societies," Ciba Foundation Symposium, No. 49, pp. 155-168. Elsevier, Amsterdam.

Neel, J. V., and Chagnon, N. A. (1968). The demography of two tribes of primitive, relatively unacculturated American Indians. *Proc. Natl. Acad. Sci. U.S.A.* **59**, 680-689.

Neel, J. V., Centerwall, W. R., Chagnon, N. A., and Casey, H. L. (1970). Notes on the effect of measles and measles vaccine in a virgin-soil population of South American Indians. *Am. J. Epidemiol.* **91**, 418-429.

Newman, M. T. (1976). Aboriginal new world epidemiology and medical care, and the impact of old world disease imports. *Am. J. Phys. Anthropol.* **45**, 667-672.

Niederman, J. C., Henderson, J. R., Opton, E. M., Black, F. L., and Skvrnova, K. (1967). A nationwide serum survey of Brazilian military recruits, 1964 II: antibody patterns with arboviruses, polioviruses, measles and mumps. *Am. J. Epidemiol.* **86,** 319-329.

Nutels, N. (1968). Medical problems of newly contacted Indian groups. *In* "Biomedical Challenges Presented by the American Indian," Sci. Pub. No. 165, pp. 68-76. Pan Am. Health Organ., Washington, D.C.

Pan American Health Organization (1968). "Biomedical Challenges Presented by the American Indian," Sci. Pub. No. 165. Washington, D.C.

Panchaszadeh, V. B. (1979). Frequency and characteristic of birth defect admissions to a pediatric hospital in Venezuela. *Am. J. Med. Genet.* **3,** 359-369.

Polgar, S. (1964). Evolution and the ills of mankind. *In* "Horizons of Anthropology" (S. Tax, ed.), pp. 200-211. Aldine, Chicago, Illinois.

Praetorius-Clausen, F., and Emmertsen, M. (1973). Occurrence of focal epithelial hyperplasia among Amerindians in Ecuador. *Int. J. Oral Surg.* **2,** 45-53.

Preston, S. H. (1976). "Mortality Patterns in National Populations: With Special Reference to Recorded Causes of Death." Academic Press, New York.

Preston, S. H., Keyfitz, N., and Schoen, R. (1972). "Causes of Death; Life Tables for National Populations." Seminar Press, New York.

Puffer, R. R., and Griffith, G. W. (1967). "Patterns of Urban Mortality; Report of the Inter-American Investigation of Mortality," Sci. Pub. No. 151. Pan Am. Health Organ., Washington, D.C.

Puffer, R. R., and Serrano, C. V. (1973). "Patterns of Mortality in Childhood," Sci. Pub. No. 262. Pan Am. Health Organ., Washington, D.C.

Reginato, A. J., Hollander, J. L., Martinez, V., Valenzuela, F., Schiapachasse, V., Covarrubias, E., Jocabelli, S., Arinoviche, R., Silcox, D., and Ruis, F. (1975). Familial chondrocalcinosis in the Chiloe Islands, Chile. *Ann. Rheum. Dis.* **34,** 260-268.

Rodenwaldt, E., and Jusatz, H. J., eds. (1952, 1956, 1961). "World Atlas of Epidemic Diseases," Parts 1, 2, and 3. Falk-Verlag, Hamburg.

St. Hoyme, L. E. (1969). On the origins of New World paleopathology. *Am. J. Phys. Anthropol.* **31,** 295-302.

Saldanha, P. H., Lebensztajn, B., and Itskan, S. B. (1976). Activity of glucose-6-phosphate dehydrogenase among Indians living in a malarial region of Mato Grosso and its implication to the Indian mixed populations in Brazil. *Hum. Hered.* **26,** 241-251.

Salzano, F. M. (1972). Visual accuity and color blindness among Brazilian Cayapo Indians. *Hum. Hered.* **22,** 72-79.

Salzano, F. M., and Freire-Maia, N. (1970). "Problems in Human Biology: A Study of Brazilian Populations." Wayne State Univ. Press, Detroit, Michigan.

Scrimshaw, N. S. (1960). Endemic goiter in Latin America. *Public Health Rep.* **75,** 731-737.

Shattuck, G. C., ed. (1933). "The Peninsula of Yucatan, Medical, Biological, Meteorological and Sociological Studies," Carnegie Institution of Washington, Pub. No. 431. Washington, D.C.

Shattuck, G. C., ed. (1938). "A Medical Survey of the Republic of Guatemala," Carnegie Institution of Washington, Pub. No. 499. Washington, D.C.

Spencer, H. C., Miller, L. H., Collins, W. E., Knud-Hansen, C., McGinnis, M. H., Shiroishi, T., Lobas, R. A., and Feldman, R. A. (1978). The Duffy blood group and resistance to Plasmodium vivax in Honduras. *Am. J. Trop. Med. Hyg.* **27,** 664-670.

Stanbury, J. B., and Kevany, J. P. (1970). Iodine and thyroid disease in Latin America. *Environ. Res.* **3,** 353-363.

Stewart, T. D. (1960). A physical anthropologists' view of the peopling of the New World. *Southwest. J. Anthropol.* **16,** 259-273.

United Nations (1955, 1965, 1966, 1967, 1968, 1970, 1978). "Statistical Yearbook." Stat. Off. UN, New York.

U.S. Bureau of the Census (1978). "World Population: 1977-Recent Demographic Estimates for the Countries and Regions of the World." U.S. Dep. Commer., Bur. Census, Washington, D.C.

Whitlaw, J. T., Jr., and Chaniotis, B. N. (1978). Palm trees and Chagas' disease in Panama. *Am. J. Trop. Med. Hyg.* **27**, 873–881.

Wiesenfeld, S. L. (1967). Sickle-cell trait in human biological and cultural evolution. *Science* **157**, 1134–1140.

Wilcocks, C., and Manson-Bahr, P. E. C. (1972). "Manson's Tropical Diseases," 17th ed. Williams & Wilkins, Baltimore, Maryland.

Willcox, R. R. (1972). The treponemal evolution. *Trans. St. John Hosp. Dermatol. Soc.* **58**, 21–37.

Willcox, R. R. (1977). Venereal diseases. *In* "A World Geography of Human Diseases" (G. M. Howe, ed.), pp. 201–235. Academic Press, New York.

Witkop, C. J., Jr., Quevedo, W. C., Jr., and Fitzpatrick, T. B. (1978). Albinism. *In* "The Metabolic Basis of Inherited Disease" (J. B. Stanbury, J. B. Wyngaarden, and D. S. Fredrickson, eds.), 4th ed., pp. 283–316. McGraw-Hill, New York.

Wood, C. S. (1979). "Human Sickness and Health: A Biocultural View." Mayfield, Palo Alto, California.

World Health Organization (1978). "World Health Statistics Annual 1978. Vol. 1: "Vital Statistics and Causes of Death." WHO, Geneva.

World Health Organization (1979). Epidemiological assessment of status of malaria, December 1977. *Wkly. Epidemiol. Rec.* **54**, 172.

Zatz, M., Froto-Pessoa, O., Levy, J. A., and Peres, C. A. (1976). Creatine-phosphokinase (CPK) activity in relatives of patients with X-linked muscular dystrophies: a Brazilian study. *J. Genet. Hum.* **24**, 153–168.

Zatz, M., Lange, K., and Spence, M. A. (1977). Frequency of Duchenne muscular dystrophy carriers. *Lancet* **1**, 759.

10
Diseases of the Japanese

KOJI OHKURA

293

BIOCULTURAL ASPECTS OF DISEASE
Copyright © 1981 by Academic Press, Inc.
All rights of reproduction in any form reserved.
ISBN 0-12-598720-X

I. INTRODUCTION

During the three centuries before the *Meiji* Restoration about a century ago, the Japanese were, with a few exceptions, isolated from other countries. Since that time, when Dutch and German scientists and physicians introduced Western medicine to Japan, knowledge of the cause of the diseases, of methods of diagnosis and treatment, and of transmission of diseases and abnormalities have accumulated rapidly.

Treatment of infectious and communicable diseases steadily improved—up to the mid-1960s, efforts in clinical medicine and public health for preventing tuberculosis and other diseases were exhaustive. As treatment effectiveness has increased, constitutional diseases and congenital and hereditary abnormalities have become more important. Today, in all developed countries, efforts are increasing to investigate the pathogenesis of genetic conditions; consequently, ethnic differences in disease patterns have become a primary focus of studying these diseases. In Japan, however, the study of genetic and constitutional diseases is rather recent, and academic support and social acceptance for conducting epidemiological, particularly genetic, research have been minimal. Unfortunately, also, few statistical or epidemiological data are available comparing ethnic differences of diseases patterns among Korean, Chinese, and other Asian populations with other groups.

As general hygiene and public health have improved during the past generation, morbidity and mortality from infectious or communicable diseases have decreased. Industrialization coincidentally has grown rapidly during this period, introducing different diseases—particularly in industrial centers and their environs. A notorious example, Minamata disease, is caused by organic mercury.

II. HISTORICAL INSIGHTS

Almost all bases of Japanese culture—philosophy, religion, literature, fine arts, and medicine—were introduced from China to Japan since about the sixth century AD. In each of these cases, Japanese and Chinese medical thought were identical.

Instead of a belief in an all-powerful creator, the Japanese conceived of creation as accomplished by *Ko* (*Tao* in Chinese), an impersonal spiritual force that requires simply that one live in accord with the laws of nature. Elaborated by Chinese philosophers, the concept of Tao became an ethical superstructure providing for all eventualities and for the foundation of personal relationships. A guide for society, Tao lets each man be the chief guardian and judge of his own behavior. This concept became an important dogma in Confucianism, which also supported the Chinese partriarchal system through insistence on filial piety.

The Tao philosophy arose as early as the fourth century BC and included the concept of *Mien,* the face. We often use such expressions as "to lose face" and "to save face" and other variations. In China, Mien involves social or public supervision of personal conduct and significantly influences the behavior pattern of the Chinese. In some persons, however, it produces extreme sensitivity. For example, if a student fails an examination, he and sometimes his family believe that he and they lose face. Such disappointments have led to serious consequences, including acute psychosis and suicide.

In a broad sense, Tao, filial piety, and the Mien were the psychological foundations of the traditional Chinese personality. As evident from the above mentioned cultural concepts, the Chinese people do not clearly separate mind and matter, soul and body.

One cause of mental disorder or deviation is the belief that a person's soul may be stolen. The theft is thought to occur during sleep, when the soul is occupied with a dream and can be lured away very easily. The powerful spirit *Tengu,* for example, is believed to possess victims and force them to madness. Regarded as a mountain demon in Japan, it is *Tienku* in China (meaning celestial dog and originally imagined to be a dog-faced comet). In time, Tengu became incorporated into Buddhism. The spirit was presumed to fulfill the role of the ghosts of dead priests or of the secret messenger of the devil. The spirit powers are considered infinite and dangerous to all.

Specific forces are also held to cause disease. Any component of the vegetable, mineral, and animal classifications is recognized as a potential dwelling for malign spirits. This animism, persisting from early Chinese religion, was never abandoned completely, although with historical change it became transformed in Japanese folklore.

As a vestige of animism in Japan, "fox possession" (*kitsune tsuki*) remains the most apparent and specified folk belief. The fox is regarded as the messenger in *Inari,* the rice goddess, who believed herself to have a vulpine shape. On the other hand, the fox is also believed to be an animal of the darkness. Evil, in the form of the fox, enters a human being, assuming the shape of man, and bewitching, possessing, and diminishing his or her light-spirit. The person's original or ordinary character is lost and becomes empty, and the emptiness itself becomes possessed only of the spirit of the darkness. Bad demons have easy access in that dark emptiness. Besides the fox, such animals as the dog, badger, fowl, snake, and toad also have been included in the animal-possession belief. That belief is not unique to the Chinese or Japanese; it has been described in historical documents and in folklore of several cultures, including the Amerindian, Eskimo, and some Siberian ethnic groups. For many centuries in Europe, the possession has been described as lycanthropy, that is, taking on the characteristics of a wolf.

The history of psychiatry in East Asia has never been studied systematically. Only recently have studies on folk or folkloristic psychiatry begun. For modern medicine, the study of fox possession began at the end of the nineteenth century. Later, animal possession was included among the autosuggestive psychoses that appear as acute or subacute mental derangements including change in personality and resulting from fear, anticipative impressions or incantations, and prayer. In general, the female who is mentally retarded, or one who is susceptible to suggestions, is believed to be more frequently affected. The mental derangement is paroxysmal and hysteric. The person "possessed by a fox" behaves with a foxlike movement or cries like a fox, and also speaks in nonsense. Recently, Takaesu *et al.* (1976) suggested that the meaning of the possession was based on both self-punishment and self-relief.

III. DISEASES HAVING GREATER THAN NORMAL PREVALENCE IN JAPAN

As in most developed countries, the leading cause of death in Japan is circulatory system disease, especially cerebrovascular disease and ischemic heart disease.

A. Congenital Heart Disease (CHD)

Available information on the overall incidence of cardiovascular anomalies does not show critical ethnic difference among Caucasians (Mitchel *et al.*, 1971; Hoffman, 1968), American blacks (Mitchel *et al.*, 1971), and Japanese (Neel, 1958). However, Maron *et al.* (1973) found blacks and Caucasians differed significantly from the Japanese in the incidence of particular cardiac anomalies.

Advances in heart surgery have enabled a classification of anatomical types of congenital heart defects. Recently, Ando *et al.* (1977) compared the frequencies of anatomically different types and subtypes of cardiac defects among Japanese and compared types and frequencies of cardiac abnormalities found in the survey of school children among Japanese (Ando, 1975) and among Caucasians in Liverpool, England (Hay, 1966) (Table I). In Japanese higher frequencies are found for ventricular septal defect (VSD), tetralogy of Fallot (TOF), and auricular septal defect (ASD). On the other hand, incidences of pulmonary stenosis, aortic stenosis (AS), and coarctation of the aorta are significantly higher in Caucasians.

TABLE I

Prevalence of Cardiac Anomalies at School Age

Anomaly	Japanese (%)[a]	Liverpool (%)[b]
Ventricular septal defect	44.0	28.1
Auricular septal defect	22.0	15.1
Patent ductus arteriosus	11.6	14.1
Pulmonary stenosis	5.7	17.5
Tetralogy of Fallot	5.6	3.8
Aortic stenosis	—	11.7
Coarctation of aorta	—	2.5
Other CHD	10.7	7.2

[a] Based on 1,282 patients found in 533,829 Japanese school children (Ando, 1975).
[b] Based on 291 patients found in a survey of 130,936 school children (Hay, 1966).

According to Nora and Nora (1979), the proportion of CHD that is due to the single mutant gene is only 3% of all cases, 5% are due to chromosomal aberration, and less than 2% are believed to be due primarily to environmental factors. The remaining 90% of CHD may be explained by a genetic–environmental interaction or multifactorial inheritance.

B. Ventricular Septal Defect (VSD)

Simple VSDs are classified according to the defect's anatomical location. The ventricular septum anatomically or developmentally comprises the infundibular, membranous, and muscular sinus septa. The muscular sinus septum has two parts: inflow smooth septum and apical trabeculated septum. The ventricular defect occurs in each septal component and also at their junction.

Table II compares Ando and associates' (1977) data of 146 defects in 145 Japanese specimens with Goor and co-workers' (1970) data of 269 defects in 251 American specimens. The frequency of infundibular VSD in Japanese (59.6%) is about twice that in Americans (30.1%), and distal conus septum defect is especially preponderant in Japanese (23.3% in Japanese, 1.5% in Americans). For membranous canal type VSD, Japanese and American incidences do not differ. Contrariwise, muscular VSD is much more frequent in Americans (45.0%) than in Japanese (15.7%). Thus, remarkable ethnic differences exist. Ando and Takao (1975) compared the frequency of several anatomical effects of coarctation or interruption type of VSD. They found subpulmonary VSD is twice as frequent in Caucasians (82% of 32 cases) as in Japanese (44% of 36 cases).

TABLE II

Frequencies of Subtypes of Simple Ventricular Septal Defect

VSD Type	Japanese (%)[a]	American (%)[b]
Infundibular	87 (59.6)	81 (30.1)
Membranous canal	36 (24.7)	67 (24.9)
Muscular	23 (15.7)	121 (45.0)
Total	146 (100.0)	269 (100.0)

[a] From Ando et al. (1977).
[b] From Goor et al. (1970).

C. Tetralogy of Fallot

Two morphological types of tetralogy of Fallot have been described: one, the classical type, and the other, subpulmonary VSD with pulmonary stenosis. The latter is not rare in Japanese but is extremely rare in Caucasians (Ando, 1974; Rao and Edwards, 1974). In their surgical series, Ando et al. (1977) found 30 cases (9.6%) with subpulmonary VSD and pulmonary stenosis among 312 cases of clinical tetralogy. Of 1050 autopsy specimens, 131 had clinical evidence of tetralogy. Of these, 22 (16.8%) were subpulmonary VSD involving pulmonary stenosis, compared with only 2 cases out of 111 (1.8%) with clinical tetralogy among 1500 autopsies at the Boston Children's Hospital.

D. Cerebrovascular "Moyamoya" Disease (Occlusion of the Circle of Willis)

An unusual form of cerebrovascular occlusive disease was first reported in 1955 as hypoplasia of bilateral internal carotid arteries by Shimizu and Takeuchi as the Fifteenth annual meeting of the Japanese Society of Brain and Neurosurgery. Although it has many symptoms, it is most commonly referred to as Moyamoya disease or occlusion of the circle of Willis.

A study group of the Ministry of Health and Welfare in 1979 presented a guide for diagnosis (Goto, 1979) (Table III). According to a nationwide survey (1976–1977), Yamaguchi et al. (1979) estimated the average annual incidence of the disease as 0.15/100,000, with a range between 0.11 and 0.20 by districts.

E. Malignant Neoplasms

The second leading cause of death in Japan is cancer, the most common form being cancer of the stomach. The mortality due to breast cancer (Table IV) is low among Japanese women when compared with women of other developed coun-

TABLE III

Guide for Diagnosis of Cerebrovascular "Moyamoya" Disease[a]

Clinical Feature	Description
Age of onset	Bimodal distribution (0–5 years and 30–39 years) but may occur at any age.
Sex ratio	Male:female = 2:3.
Major symptoms	Infants: cerebral ischemia, hemiplegia, monoplegia, sensory abnormalities, involuntary movements, headaches, recurrent spasms and paroxysms (sometimes from side to side), occasional mental retardation. Adults: sudden onset, cranial hemorrhage.
Course	Varies from asymptomatic to severe, from transient to chronic neurological symptoms.
Diagnosis	Cerebral angiography: stenosis or obliteration of terminal parts of internal carotid arteries, proximal parts of anterior and midcerebral arteries. Abnormal bilateral vascular anastomoses.
Cause	Unknown.

[a] From Goto (1979).

tries. Table IV compares mortality by site of neoplasm and by sex for Japan, the United States (whites only), and England and Wales (Health and Welfare Statistics Assoc., Japan, 1978). The data show that the general mortality from neoplasm is much lower in Japan than in the other countries.

Compared with neoplasm sites in white Americans, the following were more frequent in Japanese: stomach (6.56 times in males, 6.39 times in females), liver (2.97 and 2.23 times), esophagus (1.85 and 1.69 times), and gallbladder and bile ducts (2.0 and 1.46 times). In contrast, the Japanese had lower mortality for all other sites, particularly breast cancer in females (only 17.6% that in American whites) and prostate cancer in males (only 12.1%). Mortality for other neoplasms ranged between 25 and 50% of the rates in American whites.

Recently, Yanai et al. (1978) analyzed the change in mortality by site of neoplasm based on records obtained between 1958 and 1971. They divided the data into three periods (T_1, 1958–1962; T_2, 1962–1967; T_3, 1968–1971) and estimated the correlations of the geographical distributions of 20 sites of neoplasm between each two of three periods. Although their statistical procedure is complicated, the comparable correlation coefficients obtained from the analysis are clear. For example, for stomach cancer the correlation coefficients between T_1 and T_2 (0.916 in males, 0.932 in females), T_2 and T_3 (0.946 and 0.882), and T_1 and T_3 (0.916 and 0.937) are stable. Esophageal cancer shows almost the same high correlation. Inaba et al. (1979), analyzing the same basic data by other procedures, concluded that the geographical distribution of mortality in general had not changed over time. However, they suggested that geographical

TABLE IV

Comparative Mortality[a] from Malignant Neoplasms by Sex and Site[b]

	Mortality (per 100,000)					
	Male			Female		
Cause of Death	Japan	United States	England and Wales	Japan	United States	England and Wales
Malignant neoplasm[c]	138.5	188.7	271.0	104.5	152.2	218.7
Buccal cavity and pharynx	1.5	5.3	3.9	0.8	2.0	2.4
Digestive organs and peritoneum	85.7	50.7	84.2	57.3	43.3	75.9
Esophagus	7.4	4.0	7.5	2.2	1.3	5.7
Stomach	57.7	8.8	29.7	36.4	5.7	20.1
Intestine (except rectum)	4.7	18.4	18.1	5.1	19.9	24.5
Rectum	5.6	5.9	13.3	4.6	4.4	11.0
Liver	11.9	4.0	1.4	6.7	3.0	0.8
Gallbladder and bile ducts	3.2	1.6	1.7	4.1	2.8	2.8
Pancreas	5.6	10.1	11.6	3.9	7.8	10.1
Respiratory system	20.8	61.5	112.7	8.1	15.5	25.7
Larynx	1.4	2.6	2.5	0.2	0.4	0.6
Trachea, bronchus and lung	17.5	58.0	108.8	6.5	14.6	24.3
Bone	0.9	1.1	1.2	0.6	0.8	0.9
Skin	0.8	2.9	2.2	0.6	2.1	2.2
Breast	0.1	0.3	0.3	5.4	30.6	45.2
Uterus	—	—	—	11.0	10.7	15.1
Ovary	—	—	—	2.5	10.0	13.6
Male genital organs	2.6	18.3	19.2	—	—	—
Prostate	2.1	17.3	17.7	—	—	—
Urinary organs	3.5	11.0	15.9	1.8	4.9	7.3
Bladder	2.3	6.6	11.7	1.1	2.5	4.7
Kidney	1.0	4.3	4.1	0.6	2.3	2.5
Lymphatic and hemato-poietic tissue	7.8	19.4	16.0	5.4	15.0	12.8
Leukemia	4.1	8.5	7.1	3.1	6.2	5.3

[a] For 1973 for Japan, England, and Wales, 1972 Americans (white only).

[b] From Vital Statistics 1973. Vital Statistics of the United States 1972. Volume II, Mortality, Part A and Statistical Review of England and Wales, 1973, Part I, Tables, Medical (Health and Welfare Statistics Association, Tokyo, 1978, by permission).

[c] Secondary (197.7) and unspecified (197.8) neoplasms of liver are not included in England and Wales.

differences between periods were observed for bone, breast, and bladder cancers and for leukemia among both sexes; in prostate and kidney cancers among males; and in rectum, skin, uterus, ovary, and lymphatic tissue cancers among females.

Dunham and Bailer (1970) plotted mortality of 18 sites of neoplasm for about 100 geographical areas worldwide. They again emphasized the extremely high mortality of gastric cancer in Nara prefecture and some other districts of Japan. Among these prefectures, mortality is more than twice that of the lowest prefectures (Segi and Kurihara, 1972). Many other scientists have reported geographical variations of mortality for specific neoplasms. However, no study has revealed any factors related to the cause of neoplasm. Hirayama (1975) attributed the decline to the change of diet in Japan since 1949, since which time there has been a general dietary improvement, specifically an increase in consumption of milk and milk products.

F. Myopia

Japan has an extremely high frequency of myopia. According to the School Health Statistics, 1976 (Ministry of Education, 1977), that frequency, including pseudomyopia, was 12.20% among primary school children (boys, 10.34% and girls 14.11%), 29.17% among junior high school students (25.29% and 33.17%), and 45.8% among senior high school students (44.04% and 47.74%). These frequencies have been going up gradually since 1950; in about a quarter of a century, they have increased nearly threefold. The cause remains unclear. However, an environmental factor is suggested as one cause, because the frequencies differ between rural and urban populations; the vision of children and students residing in a rural area is much better than that of children in an urban area.

G. Behçet's Disease

Since the first report of Behçet (1937) in Turkey, this condition has been reported in many countries of Europe and the Middle East, but few reports have come from the American continent. Since World War II, a considerable increase in the incidence of the condition has been reported in Japan according to Eietti and Bruna (1966). The disease's prevalence in Japan is greater than that of any other country.

Major clinical manifestations are as follows: (1) aphthous lesions (ulceration) of mucous membranes of the mouth and genitalia; (2) skin erythema (multiforme, bullosum, or nodosum); (3) gradual loss of vision, with occasional complete blindness; (4) arthritis; and (5) neurological involvement and intestinal disease. The disease, which occurs in adults, predominantly in females, is chronic, and complete remission is rare.

In Japan, the disease is an important cause of blindness, and, as a result, a study group on origin, treatment, and prevention of the disease (Behçet's Disease Research Committee of Japan, Ministry of Health and Welfare) was established in 1959. In 1972, the group, along with others, carried out an epidemiological survey on eight selected diseases, and the total number of patients with the disease was estimated to be 7000–8500 with a prevalence of 8.5/100,000 population (Yamamoto et al., 1974). In general, the prevalence rate was higher in the northern districts and lower in the southern districts. From 1957 to 1971 the incidence of the disease increased every year (Ohno et al., 1975). In 1959 about 100 new cases were found, and by 1971 the number was more than 400.

Two surveys have been done among Japanese immigrants and their descendants residing in Hawaii or the West Coast of the United States. In Hawaii, 258 physicians reported that they had never seen a patient with Behçet's disease during the 5 years from 1969 to 1973 (Kuratsune et al., 1975). Ohno and Sugiura (1976) found only 17 cases among American whites and two cases among Mexicans, but none for Japanese among 5400 medical records (1947–1975) at the Uveitis Survey Clinic, University of California, San Francisco, California.

H. Subacute Myelo-Optico Neuropathy (SMON)

Subacute myelo-optico neuropathy (SMON) is a disease that first appeared in medical literature during the latter half of the 1950s, particularly in Japan. The total of persons affected has been estimated at about 11,000. The early symptoms—diarrhea, constipation, and abdominal pain—progress to sensory and motor nerve disorders. In serious cases, the disease causes visual disturbances and may eventually cause death.

Because there are no appropriate diagnostic laboratory tests, the diagnosis is based on clinical signs and symptoms. Table V shows the guide to clinical diagnosis of SMON adopted by the clinical group of the SMON Research Commission (1970). Pathologically the disease is characterized by the presence of symmetrical degeneration in peripheral nerves, long tracts of the spinal cord, particularly the posterior column and corticospinal tract, and, in many cases, the optic nerve and tract. Takasu et al. (1970) noticed that the tongues of some patients were colored green, and Igata et al. (1970) found that some patients excrete greenish urine. Subsequently Yoshioka and Tamura (1970) isolated green pigment from the green urine and feces of SMON patients and identified the pigment as the iron (III) chelate of 5-chloro-7-iodo-8-hydroxyquinoline (clioquinol, chinoform). They also found that the green urine contained crystals of free clioquinol in large amounts.

SMON was thus found to be caused by ingestion of "chinoform" (clioquinol), an antiamebicidal and antibacterial drug prescribed by doctors to treat abdominal

TABLE V

Guide to Clinical Diagnosis of SMON

Cardinal Signs

1. Abdominal symptoms (abdominal pain, diarrhea, etc.) before onset of neurological symptoms
2. Acute or subacute onset of bilateral ascending paresthesia and dysesthesia of the lower extremities
3. Occasionally, one or more of the following: (A) bilateral impairment of vision; (B) disturbances of consciousness; convulsions, psychic symptoms, and other cerebral symptoms; (C) greenish discoloration of the tongue and feces; (D) sphincter disturbances
4. Protracted course with occasional relapses
5. No significant laboratory findings in the blood and cerebrospinal fluid
6. Rare occurrence in children

disturbances. Emafor, Entero-Vioform, and Medaform were the most frequently used preparations in Japan.

Besides the dosage and duration of usage, personal vulnerability or efficiency of detoxication seems to play a significant role in manifestation of the clinical disorder, since not all persons exposed to the drug were subjected to the disease.

Racial differences may play a role, because reported cases outside Japan have been relatively rare, although clioquinol is ingested in many other countries (Wadia, 1977).

I. Kawasaki Disease (Mucocutaneous Lymph Node Syndrome, MLNS)

In 1961, Kawasaki examined a boy aged 4 years 3 months who had a high fever and many unusual clinical features. After observing 50 more patients with similar conditions, Kawasaki (1967) reported the new syndrome as mucocutaneous lymph node syndrome. No confirmatory test exists to validate the diagnosis, which is made by the clinical manifestations. Today in Japan, more than 12,000 persons, including adolescents and adults, are recorded as having been afflicted with the syndrome. About 80% of patients are less than 4 years old, and boys have a higher incidence (1.5 male to 1 female).

In 1974, a group organized by the Japanese Ministry of Health and Welfare to study MLNS established six diagnostic criteria (Kawasaki, 1976) (Table VI). A patient with five of the six major symptoms is diagnosed as having Kawasaki disease.

Usually the illness lasts less than a month. Especially important are the cardiac complications, including coronary artery thrombosis and aneurysm, myocarditis,

TABLE VI

Kawasaki Disease Diagnostic Information[a]

Body part, organ systems, or specimen	Symptoms and signs
A. Major	
Whole body	High fever (about 39°C, 102°F), occurs without any prodromal signs; fever does not respond to antibiotics and usually persists for 5 days or more
Exanthema	Occurs without blister or crust, mostly as erythema with irregular form, frequently on the trunk
Extremities	In acute phase, indurative edema appears on the extremities and hot and dry areas appear on palms and soles. In convalescent phase, membranous desquamation of fingertips occurs
Conjunctiva	Conjunctivitis differs from usual because no exudation is evident; congestive papillary vessels are recognizable
Lips, oral cavity	Redness and fissuring of the lips, strawberry colored tongue, similar to that seen in scarlet fever
Lymph nodes	In acute phase, nonpurulent swelling of the cervical lymph nodes
B. Minor	
Cardiovascular	Carditis with prolongation of PQ and QT intervals, low-voltage, changes in ST and T, arrhythmia, and abnormal physical signs (e.g., murmur)
Gastrointestinal	Diarrhea (about 35%) and occasional vomiting and abdominal pain
Urine	Proteinuria (about 30%) and often increased number of leukocytes in the sediment
Blood	Leukocytosis may be seen, with immature leukocytes, slight anemia, increasing globulin, with or without increase of the ASO titer
Respiratory	Occasional cough and nasal discharge
Joints	Pain and swelling are common
Miscellani	Meningeal irritation, slight jaundice

[a] From Kawasaki (1976).

and pericarditis. From 1 to 2% of patients die of acute cardiac failure. Autopsy findings have shown coronary aneurysm and thrombus due to coronary arteritis. The cause of the disease is unknown. Viral, rickettsial, and bacterial (especially hemolytic streptococcus) infections were suggested as the cause of MLNS. Hamashima *et al.* (1973) described rickettsia-like bodies in the skin and lymph node biopsies in 12 of 23 subjects with acute MLNS. However, that cause has not yet been confirmed, nor has any other cause–effect relationship been found. Thus far, epidemiological studies have not shown detectable environmental factors (Shigematsu and Yanagawa, 1976; Hamashima, 1976).

First described in Japan and especially prevalent there, cases have also been reported from Korea, Hawaii (most had some Oriental heritage), Australia,

Greece, Sweden, the United States, and Holland. No basis for the ethnic differences in distribution has been postulated.

J. Ossification of Posterior Longitudinal Ligament (OPLL)

Since the first report by Tsukimoto in 1960, numerous orthopedic observations have been published in Japan on the specific clinical features of the spinal cord lesions of OPLL. Chief complaints include numbness of extremities, disturbance in walking, clumsiness of fingers, sensory abnormality, and muscular weakness. These are part of spinal paralytic symptoms or signs that appear after injury to the head and/or neck, gradually in some cases and suddenly in others. Neurological symptoms vary and correspond with the site and grade of the lesion of the spinal cord. Diagnosis is made from radiological examination of the cervical spine; lateral tomography is definitive.

The basic defect of this disease is the ossification or cartilaginification of the posterior longitudinal ligament. The defect develops gradually and depresses the spinal canal, which then narrows and depresses the spinal cord. The cause of the ossification or the cartilaginification is not known, but physical or mechanical and unidentified ossification factors are suspected. Although endocrinological, biochemical (especially calcium metabolism), and immunological studies have continued, no definite explanation has been found.

According to the report of the study group, supported by the Japanese Ministry of Health and Welfare (Tsuyama, 1976), ossification may be classified into four types (Fig. 1). The study group recommended this criterion for clinical diagnosis: the association of one of the above-mentioned radiographical findings with (1) pain in the nape of the neck, (2) limitation of the mobility of the spine, (3) numbness or pain on the extremities or the trunk, (4) sensory abnormality of the

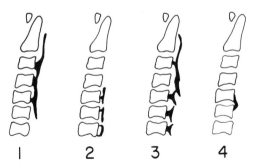

Fig. 1. Schematic illustration of ossification of posterior longitudinal ligament. (1) Consecutive type. (2) Segment type. (3) Mixed type. (4) Other type.

extremities or trunk, (5) reflex abnormalities of the extremities or trunk, or (6) bladder–rectum disturbance.

More than 2000 cases were registered in Japan in 1976. From an epidemiological survey by this study group, the incidence in Japan was estimated to be 19.8 per million. Recently, Yamaura *et al.* (1978) examined 332 lateral cervical X-ray films in Manila, and found four Filipinos and one Chinese with these abnormal findings. They estimated the hospital population incidence of this abnormality as 1.5%. Furthermore, they found 602 cases in 32,464 cervical X-ray films in a literature survey of the Japanese hospital population. They estimated the average incidence, based on 12 studies from nine institutions, as 1.8%, with the range between 0.9 and 2.8%.

In 1969, Minagi and Gronner reported two cases in American whites. Thereafter, 15 cases (among 12 whites, 1 black, 1 East Indian, and 1 Chinese) were reported. Yamauchi *et al.* (1977) examined 854 American whites at Mayo Clinic and found only two cases. This frequency, 0.2%, is extremely low.

K. Elastofibroma

In 1959, Järvi and Saxén observed four cases of elastofibroma involving the subscapular region, and in 1961 they described the condition as elastofibroma dorsi (Järvi and Saxén, 1961). The condition is a rare soft-tissue tumor. Recently, however, a number of patients were observed in Japan, particularly in the Okinawa islands.

According to a literature survey by Nagamine *et al.* (1978), of 222 cases reported, 144 were found in Okinawa (Ryukyu) and 23 in other places of Japan. Only 55 cases were reported from other countries. (Two cases in Hawaii involving Japanese persons were included in the 55 cases.) Of 144 cases found in Okinawa, 141 were observed by Nagamine and colleagues (1978, 1979); all patients, with one exception, were the inhabitants of Okinawa islands. Of 23 Japanese patients 13 were found in the Amami islands, northeast of Okinawa and in the same archipelago. The distribution of patients having this tumor is strikingly restricted to that area (Fig. 2).

Most patients are asymptomatic except for complaints referable to the tumor. A few patients complain of shoulder muscle stiffness, chest pain, and pain at the area of tumor. Nagamine *et al.* (1979) reported that in 116 cases the tumor was in the subscapular region, and in 21 cases the tumor occurred at the infraolecranon area. Multiple appearances of tumors were observed in three patients, one having a tumor on the infraolecranon bilaterally but not in the subscapular region.

Distribution differed between the sexes. Females predominated, with 132 cases, compared with only nine cases in males (Nagamine *et al.*, 1978). The reason for the disparity by sex is not yet known.

Since the first report of Järvi and Saxén (1961), belief that the tumor results

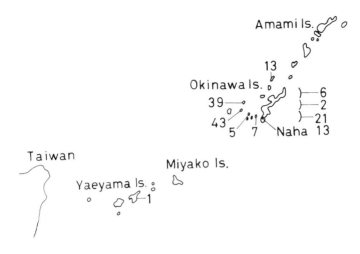

Fig. 2. Distribution of elastofibroma in Okinawa.

from mechanical action of the scapula against the ribs has been common. Later, the tumor was suggested to be a reactive hyperplasia and not a true tumor. Supporting the belief were the occupations of most of the patients—farmers or heavy laborers. However, Nagamine *et al.* (1979) recently pointed out the importance of intrinsic factors in the origin of the lesions. Of 141 patients, 88 were isolated cases and 53 (37.6%) had a positive family history. This observation might suggest a genetic factor as the cause. I rearranged their data and classified 15 families as ascertained (examined by Nagamine) and 15 unascertained (with hearsay evidence).

L. Pulseless Disease (Takayasu Disease, Martorell Syndrome, Aortic Arch Syndrome, Reversed Coarctation Syndrome)

One case of this disease was probably described in a medical book written in the 1830s in Japan. Nonetheless, Takayasu is credited with having described this disease, an arteritis of unknown cause that may involve the aorta, its branches, and the pulmonary arteries. Its characteristic feature is diminished or absent pulsation of arteries of the head, neck, and upper limbs (Jervell, 1954). Complaints of attacks of orthostatic syncope and dizziness are common. Epileptic seizures, facial atrophy, transient hemiplegia, intermittent claudication, transient blindness, or blurring of vision may also occur. Several other clinical signs or symptoms appear because of the diminished supply of blood to tissues or organs by arteria anonyma (truncus brachiocephalicus), carotis communis, subclavia, and vertebralis. Signs of hypertension due to stenosis of the aorta or renal artery have been observed.

The pathological feature is nonspecific inflammatory occlusive arteritis of the above-mentioned arteries. The histological findings are disorganization of the elastic membrane, adventitia, and tunica media of arteries, and the presence of giant cells. This disease is most prevalent in young women (female to male ratio is 8:1). Although the disease may occur from early childhood to old age, its peak incidence is between 5 and 25 years of age. Although worldwide in distribution, the disease most frequently affects the Japanese. Other types of occlusive vascular diseases (atherosclerosis and syphilis) are distinguishable by the histological features and narrowing of the aorta.

M. Vogt-Koyanagi-Harada's Disease (Harada's Disease, Uveitis-Vitiligo-Alopecia-Poliosis Syndrome)

The diseases originally described by Harada (1926) and by Vogt (1906) and Koyanagi (1929) were considered separate entities. However, Bruno and McPherson (1949) suggested that they are the same condition but with different manifestations. This concept is now widely accepted.

The disease usually occurs in young adults. Its course is chronic, often resulting in considerable loss of vision and hearing. Later, vision sometimes improves remarkably. Other ocular findings are as follows: white rashes, secondary glaucoma, bilateral uveitis, sympathetic ophthalmitis, exudative iridocyclitis, steamy cornea, many vitreous opacities, bilateral serous retinal detachment and edema (with spontaneous reattachment after weeks), depigmentation and patches of scattered pigment later on, acute diffuse exudative choroiditis bilaterally, occasional retinal hemorrhages, and papilledema.

Other clinical findings include alopecia and poliosis (frequent); vitiligo occurs in nearly 50% of cases; and headache, vomiting, meningeal irritation, and tinnitus are also commonly associated.

A viral cause has been suggested, but no supportive evidence has been found. The Japanese and Italians are affected more commonly than other ethnic groups.

IV. OTHER CONGENITAL ANOMALIES

A. Anencephalus and Spina Bifida

The cause and the distribution of anencephalus with or without spina bifida has been studied extensively. Recently, this condition became included among items to be checked in the monitoring of congenital abnormalities. Because of the striking nature of this defect, figures of its incidence are probably reliable. The extensive world literature on this defect was assembled by Penrose (1957); it was shown that the incidence of the defect varies widely from locality to locality. Among Japanese, the incidence of anencephalus and spina bifida based on the investigation of 49,645 newborn infants was estimated at 0.063 and 0.022%, respectively, by Mitani (1943). An epidemiological study by Neel (1958) showed an incidence of 0.063% for anencephalus and 0.020% for spina bifida, based on 63,796 births in Hiroshima and Nagasaki.

These figures have been compared with those of several other populations by Neel (1958). The incidence of anencephalus in Japanese is nearly half that of American and English populations. The incidence of spina bifida is one-fifth to one-tenth that of the Americans or the English.

B. Cleft Lip and Palate

Cleft lip and palate is the most common congenital malformation among the Japanese. The incidence is roughly twice that among Caucasians. According to one literature survey, the incidence of cleft lip and palate in Caucasians was estimated as 0.111%, an average based on 56 studies; the lowest incidence was 0.079% and the highest was 0.203% (Akasaka, 1970). Among American blacks, the estimate was 0.051%, an average based on 10 studies. In 15 studies among the Japanese, 1447 affected were found among 761,394 births, including stillbirths, and the incidence was estimated as 0.190%. Of those 15 studies, two include the Japanese residing in Hawaii or other places of the mainland of the United States. With those two studies omitted, the incidence becomes 0.193%. The highest incidence was 0.319% and the lowest, 0.131%. However, the most reliable and detailed large-scale epidemiological study has been done by the Atomic Bomb Casualty Commission at Hiroshima and Nagasaki. The observa-

TABLE VII

Comparative Data on Type of Clefts by Sex

Group	Lip		Lip and palate		Palate	
	Male	Female	Male	Female	Male	Female
Caucasian						
No.	2775	1652	5308	2806	2613	3490
ratio	1.68 to	1.00	1.89 to	1.00	0.75 to	1.00
Japanese						
No.	1568	1701	3046	1588	881	1436
ratio	0.92 to	1.00	1.92 to	1.00	0.61 to	1.00

tion was reported by Neel (1958) with an incidence of 0.268% among 63,796 livebirths and stillbirths. So, generally, the relative incidence is about four Japanese to two Caucasians to one American black.

Some investigators suggested that each type of cleft did not appear equally in both sexes. Using Akasaka's data and additional new data from Japan, I found differences in the distributions of these anomalies between Japanese and Caucasians (Table VII). A significant preponderance of cleft lip among male Caucasians was observed. In contrast, a significant excess of cleft palate was observed among Japanese females. On the other hand, for both cleft lip and palate, an excess was found in both Japanese and Caucasian males.

V. EFFECTS OF THE ATOMIC BOMB

Data collected on the Japanese A-bomb survivors of Hiroshima and Nagasaki at the end of World War II has enabled us to assess the risk of radiation-induced diseases. In both detonations, large amounts of γ-rays and neutrons were released. The doses received by those exposed depended on their distance from the hypocenter, presence of shielding, and like factors.

A. Cancer and Leukemia

An excessively high incidence of leukemia appeared within a few years, reached a peak at 5–7 years, and declined after 15 years postirradiation. Among Hiroshima victims, the incidence of leukemias clearly exceeds that of the control sample—even for the low-dose group, which received 20–49 rads. At Nagasaki, however, a different nuclear device was used, with the result that there 90% of the air dose was due to γ-rays, whereas at Hiroshima the dose was equally divided between γ-rays and neutrons. At Hiroshima there was a high risk of acute myeloid, acute lymphocytic, and chronic myeloid leukemias; at Nagasaki the excessive risk was primarily due to acute myeloid and acute lymphocytic leukemias. No evidence exists today to show that the incidence of chronic lymphocytic leukemia is affected by irradiation. In both cities, as always, males were more susceptible than females.

The data for Japanese A-bomb survivors show elevated incidences of myelofibrosis, multiple myeloma, lung cancer, breast cancer, and particularly thyroid cancer. No single tumor type has been observed in sufficient numbers to support a reliable estimate of the magnitude of the risk as a function of dose, except to indicate that such risk is plainly much lower than the leukemogenic effect.

B. Genetic Effects

The largest group of humans available for the study of the genetic hazards of radiation exposure are the descendants of the Japanese survivors from Hiroshima and Nagasaki. Significant differences were noted in the frequency of cells with radiation-induced chromosome aberrations in the peripheral blood between the exposed and control groups. Furthermore, among the exposed, the frequency of abnormal cells apparently generally increased proportionately with increasing dose (Awa et al., 1969). Although 20 years after the bombing the bone marrow of survivors showed some statistically significant differences in the appearance of plasma cells, most failed to show other significant differences when compared with controls (Kamada, 1969).

Extensive studies of offspring conceived after the exposure of their parents to the atomic bombs have revealed no increased frequency of stillbirths, neonatal deaths, or gross malformations (Neel, 1963). Furthermore, mortality in the next generation has not increased overall (Kato et al., 1966), and initial impressions of an alteration in the sex ratio have not been substantiated. Nor have any detectable cytogenetic effects been noted in the progeny of persons who survived exposure to the atomic bombs. However, the possibility of selection against chromosomally or genetically damaged germ cells cannot be ruled out (Awa et al., 1968). Evidence for a lack of hereditary defects caused by radiation remains inconclusive; insufficient time has passed for recessive mutations to show up, since several generations must elapse before they can be expressed.

Consanguineous marriages are encountered in relatively high rates in Japan (Komai, 1972). Schull and Neel (1965) estimated the first-cousin marriage rate to be about a 5–7%. This estimate is much higher than that for most European populations, where the corresponding rate is given as 0.1–2%. Schull and Neel stressed that the consanguinity rate is relatively high among present-day city people, even in large cities. This high rate may be attributed to the age-old Japanese custom that marriage in general is an affair of the family rather than of individuals, so that the initiative in matrimonial selection is customarily taken by some person other than the would-be mates. In Japan, much as in old European communities, each family has had a recognized social status, and a match between families of similar status has been preferred to one between those of different status. Moreover, most elders of the family are inclined to want to limit the dispersal of inherited property.

However, such social isolation has rapidly diminished. The rate of first cousin marriage is now reported as high as 2.315 on average (Imaizumi et al., 1975). This figure is still rated higher than other countries. To maintain this figure other social factors might be considered under the situation of urbanization.

VI. GENETIC DISEASES

A. Inborn Errors of Metabolism

Since 1960, Japan has screened infants for phenylketonuria (PKU) by means of the urine test. In 1966 and 1967, no one was found to be positive among 147,107 newborn babies. In Hyogo Prefecture between 1967 and 1972, only two positive cases were found among 382,892 babies; in Tokyo, during 1970–1973, only one PKU was found in 632,932 infants tested. Although more examinations were done by the local governments and some physicians' associations independently, no further positives were reported. After the experimental stage of screening, the Japanese Ministry of Health and Welfare in 1977 decided to expand the program to include such inborn errors of metabolism as galactosemia (by the Guthrie and the Beulher methods), histidinemia, homocystinemia, and maple syrup urine disease. Today, Japan is the only Far East country that screens for inborn errors of metabolism.

Between October 1977 and March 1979, the newborn infants screened numbered 1,871,906. In all, 266 cases of inborn errors of metabolism were reported. Because of ascertainment bias, the true incidence may be lower. Table VIII shows the incidence of each abnormality. That for PKU is exceptionally low when compared with the figure for Caucasians. Galactosemia is also rare in Japan, and its incidence is almost one-third that of Caucasians. In contrast, histidinemia is more frequently observed in Japan than among Caucasians. Use-

TABLE VIII

Incidence of Inborn Errors of Metabolism

Inborn error	No. affected	Incidence
Phenylketonuria	26	1/72,000
Maple syrup urine disease	5	1/374,400
Histidinemia	191	1/9,800
Homocystinemia	13[a]	1/144,000
Galactosemia	12	1/156,000
Others	19	1/98,500
Hypermethionemia	(9)	1/208,000
Hyperphenylalaninemia	(3)	1/624,000
Tyrosinosis	(5)	1/374,400
Citrullinemia	(1)	1/1,871,900
Lipid metabolism disorder	(1)	1/1,871,900
Total	266	1/7,000

[a] All of these 13 are believed to be the infants affected with liver diseases and other diseases. Therefore, they may not have had homocystinemia.

ful for comparing incidences among populations is the review by Thalhammer (1975).

B. Acatalasemia

This disease was discovered in 1946 by Takahara when he attempted to cleanse the site of an oral necrotic ulcer with diluted hydrogen peroxide after a radical operation. Surprisingly, no bubbling occurred and the surface of the lesion immediately turned brownish-black. Blood specimens from the patient's parents and six siblings were examined. Three siblings reacted to hydrogen peroxide in the same manner as the proband, whereas three others and the parents did not (Takahara and Miyamoto, 1949; Takahara, 1951; Ogata and Takahara, 1966).

Acatalasemia due to a rare autosomal recessive gene is the absence of catalase in both red and white blood cells (also apparently in other tissue cells as well, although the study on this observation has not yet been completed). However, by means of a manometric and permanganate titration procedure, 1/500–1/1000 of normal catalase activity is revealed. The nature of this residual activity is not yet clearly explained.

The red blood cells of the parents and some of siblings of the acatalasemics showed only a half of the normal catalase activity and were designated as hypocatalasemics (Nishimura *et al.*, 1959). A greater than 70% rate of parental consanguinity was observed (Ogura, 1965).

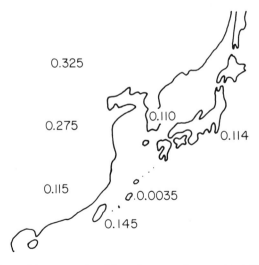

0.325

0.275

0.110

0.114

0.115

0.0.0035

0.145

Fig. 3. Distribution and frequency of acatalasemic gene and geographical cline in East Asia.

Up to the end of 1967, 39 Japanese families with 78 affected members were reported. In addition, 1 Korean family with 3 affected, 3 Swiss families with 11 affected, and 1 affected from Israel have been reported (Takahara *et al.*, 1969). In Japan, the distribution of the gene corresponding to acatalasemia seems to be limited. Since 1961 large-scale surveys on gene distribution have been done by Takahara and me jointly and independently.

Because the screening procedure of hypocatalasemia is simple, we have begun to screen for the distribution and frequency of the gene. So far, more than 130,000 blood specimens from many different populations in East Asia have been analyzed. As shown in Fig. 3, the gene is distributed in East Asian populations with different frequencies (Takahara, 1968; Takahara *et al.*, 1969; K. Ohkura *et al.*, unpublished data).

C. Isolated Lactase Deficiency (Lactose Intolerance) in Adults

Although infantile lactose intolerance in man is rare, a common condition among some Japanese adults is severe gastrointestinal disturbance after an intake of an amount of milk. The cause of the lactose intolerance was not clearly recognized until Auricchio *et al.* (1963) and later Haemmerli *et al.* (1965) found that the milk intolerance in adults is due to the deficiency of isolated intestinal lactase.

That the frequencies of milk intolerance vary greatly in adults of different ethnic groups has been reported. In general, Caucasians (non-Jews) in Europe, the United States, and Australia had low frequencies (10–20%). However, high frequencies (60–100%) were reported for Greeks, Jews, Palestinian Arabs, African and American Negroes, Thais, Eskimos, and Japanese.

Among Japanese, Shibuya *et al.* (1970) revealed changes of the ability to digest lactose according to age by applying the lactose-tolerance test. Lowered ability begins at age 1 year, nearly 70% of children cannot digest lactose at age 8 years, and progressively almost all of Japanese lose the ability.

The reason for this difference in frequency of primary lactose intolerance between ethnic groups is not known. Genetic adaptation (evolutionary) based on natural selection have been proposed.

D. Cystic Fibrosis of Pancreas (Mucoviscidosis)

A common belief is that cystic fibrosis of the pancreas is almost nonexistent or extremely rare in Oriental populations. However, since the 1950s, several cases with cystic fibrosis or meconium ileus have been reported in Japan. Wright and Morton (1968) reported that the incidence of cystic fibrosis in pure non-Caucasian infants in Hawaii is 1 in 90,000.

Komi *et al.* (1966; Komi, 1967) re-evaluated 21 cases reported as cystic fibrosis or meconium ileus. Most of the patients showed the clinical and pathological features, but only four were examined by means of the sweat metabolite test. Two of four patients showed abnormally high sweat electrolyte levels with a reasonable ratio of sodium to chloride. The diagnosis was based mostly on clinical manifestations of the disease and on the findings of fibrocystic changes of the pancreas. Komi and Seki (1967) found fibrocystic changes of the pancreas in 46 cases of 422 autopsy records in infants and children aged lower than 5 years. Although fibrocystic changes of the pancreas are not specific for cystic fibrosis, Komi (1967) found such pancreatic changes in a large number of autopsies of Japanese infants and children. However, after a strict check of the medical and autopsy records, no cystic fibrosis case was found in that series.

Komi and Kawasaki (1969) carried out a questionnaire survey and collected 46 records. The sweat test was included for 13 cases and abnormally high sweat electrolyte levels were reported in 7 cases. In that series, they found only one typical case with clinical, laboratory, and pathological data.

Komi *et al.* (1971) compared Japanese and Caucasian cases for differences in the presence of the Spock factor and of metachromasia in cultured fibroblasts. They concluded that the cystic fibrosis among Japanese is type II. The features of type II are a negative Spock factor and a metachromatic and severe clinical manifestations, and perhaps death. Therefore, finding the affected case from clinical observations alone is difficult.

E. Glucose-6-Phosphate Dehydrogenase (G6PD) Deficiency

The distribution of glucose-6-phosphate dehydrogenase (G6PD) deficiency, transmitted by an X-linked recessive gene, differs by region and ethnic group. Among Japanese, the Ministry of Health and Welfare organized and sponsored a population study of hemolytic anemia. According to the report of the group (Arakawa *et al.*, 1977; Miwa *et al.*, 1977; Takagi and Kawai, 1977; Fujioka *et al.*, 1977; Shibata *et al.*, 1977), 27,383 specimens obtained from six different areas in Japan were screened by the Beutler's fluorescent screening method and seven cases with G6PD deficiency were found. The overall frequency is estimated as 0.026% in Japanese males, which is low when compared with frequencies of other ethnic groups (see Chapter 4).

F. Abnormal Hemoglobins

For many years, the general belief was that no abnormal hemoglobin existed in Japan (Fukutake, 1953). Tamura *et al.* (1959) reported a large pedigree with peculiar cyanotic conditions. The blood of affected persons was blackish. They presented the condition under the name of hereditary black blood disease (Tamura and Takahashi's disease or nigremia hereditaria). Tamura and co-workers postulated that a hemoglobin with abnormal heme moiety was present in these patients. The hemoglobin was extremely prone to conversion into a hematin-like substance by oxidization. By means of electrophoresis, Shibata *et al.* (1960) demonstrated an abnormal band of hemoglobin and subsequently showed that it was a new variant of HbM, and the condition was established to be HbM Iwate (Shibata *et al.*, 1964). According to the family history and documents, the condition could be traced back to a probable affected ancestor who lived about 200 years ago (Tamura *et al.*, 1959). Another HbM found in Kurume (Kimura *et al.*, 1960) was identified as HbM Saskatoon (Shibata *et al.*, 1962).

Recently, S. Shibata (personal communication) reviewed and compiled the types of abnormal hemoglobins found in Japan. So far, 47 different substitutions by point mutation, one deletion, and one fusion gene have been reported by several investigators, though a frame shift and elongated chain have not been observed. Ratio of α-chain and β-chain abnormalities is 1:2. A γ-chain abnormality was observed, but its structure is not yet determined. HbS has been found in the offspring of Japanese–Negro parents.

According to Shibata's literature survey 55 persons with abnormal hemoglobins were found among about 305,000 specimens screened. The incidence is estimated as 1 in 5550. However, his own survey revealed an incidence of 1:4000 (40/160,000).

For a long time, thalassemia had been thought not occur in Japan. However, the first instance of a β-thalassemia heterozygote was reported in Tokyo in 1960 (Amaki *et al.*, 1960). Since then, nearly 30 sporadic cases of β-thalassemia carriers have been reported. One case of β-thalassemia major was reported by Kokuhu and Ishihara (1967) in Kagoshima.

VII. GENETIC DISEASES UNIQUE TO JAPAN

A. Dyschromatosis Symmetrica Hereditaria (Toyama)

This disease is characterized by bilateral small pigmented flecks and spots with depigmentation that occur on the extensor side of the fingers, hands, and feet (Toyama, 1924). The size, form, and grade of pigmentation varies, but the margin is distinct. Age of onset varies from 1 to 13 years, and the disease then progressively affects the forearms and legs, and sometimes the trunk. Usually flecks exist on the face. No difference in incidence by sex is observed. The only findings are histological: two locations on the basal stratum, one with and the other without melanin pigments.

This rare disorder has been reported only in Japanese. Of 29 sporadic cases of this disorder, seven of the patients were born to consanguineous parents. That finding suggested an autosomal recessive inheritance. Genetic heterogeneity may exist; other authors have suggested autosomal dominant transmission with a high degree of penetrance.

B. Lepromembranous Polycystic Osteodysplasia (LMPO)

This disease has been reported only in Japan and Scandinavia (Yagishita *et al.*, 1976). Skeletal symptoms usually begin at about age 20 years. Fractures in connection with minor accidents are the initial sign. Roentgenography shows large symmetric cystic cavities in the metaphyses of the long bones, in metatarsal bones, and in the phalanges of the toes. The ribs, cranium, spinal column, and pelvic bones are rarely affected. Psychiatric symptoms usually begin several years after the bone changes. In autopsied cases pathological changes of the brain are leukodystrophy of the sudanophilic type.

Light microscopy shows many peculiar undulating membranous structures in the adipose tissue. With the electron microscope the membrane seems to be composed of an accumulation of endoplasmic reticulum-like tubular profiles. They appear first within the mesenchymal cell, in close connection with fat droplets.

The disorder is probably due to an autosomal recessive gene.

C. Dyschromatosis Universalis Hereditaria (Toyama-Ichikawa-Hiraga)

This rare disorder, described only in the Japanese, has clinical features similar to dyschromatosis symmetrica hereditaria, although the relation to that condition is not clear. However, the pigmentation and depigmentation usually start on the trunk, then spread over the body. The mode of inheritance is probably autosomal dominant, although consanguinity occurred in each of four successive generations in the kindred reported by Suenaga (1952).

D. Oguchi's Disease

Since the initial observation by Oguchi in 1907, more than 80 cases have been observed in Japan. Although the disease is more frequent in Japan, François (1961) described a total of 26 cases among non-Japanese in his book. The disease is also called congenital stationary or static night blindness.

The characteristics of the disease are congenital, static hemeralopia and diffuse gray or golden coloration of the fundus in the light. Light adaptation is either slow or absent. The coloration returns to normal after a variable time (2–3 hr) in complete darkness and is called Mizuo-Nakamura's phenomenon. It is valuable for differentiating the condition from other types of hemeralopia. The central photopic visual acuity and the central color sense are both normal. Pathologically, the cones have abnormal structure and pigmented syncytium is present between the rods and pigment epithelium.

The disease itself is transmitted by an autosomal recessive gene. Essential hemeralopia or nyctalopia consists of night blindness without any degenerative ophthalmologic abnormality. The photopic visual functions, at least those concerning central visual acuity, visual fields, and color sense, are apparently normal, but the scotopic functions are severely affected. No defect is found in the retinal structure, and the rhodopsin concentration levels are normal. Physiological examinations suggest the cause of the hemeralopia to be due to a defect in neural transmission. Two types of genetically different hemeralopia are especially characterized by the association of high-grade myopia. One is transmitted by an autosomal recessive gene and the other by a sex-linked gene.

E. Nevus Fusco-Ceruleus Ophthalmo-Maxillaris (Ota)

First described by Ota (1939; Ota and Tanino, 1939), this abnormality is now commonly called the nevus of Ota. The condition is due to hyperplasia of melanocytes on the area innervated by the trigeminal (fifth) nerve (rarely by the third). Brownish-blue or bluish-black pigmentation appears during childhood or puberty. Usually it appears unilaterally, but sometimes it occurs bilaterally, either symmetrically or asymmetrically.

The symmetric type of the nevus often appears in the second or third decades of life. Pigmentation appears in the forehead, cheek, eyelids, nose, and earlobes. Besides involving the periorbital region, the nevus may extend to the pharynx and the ear. Scleral and conjunctival pigmentation mainly occurs in the palpebral region, particularly near the lid margins. Occasionally infantile glaucoma and optic disc pigmentation are noted. There is a female preponderance (4:1).

No evidence of hereditary transmission is demonstrated in either the unilateral type or the asymmetric type. The symmetric type is almost limited to females and is presumed to be autosomal dominant (Hidano, 1977), although that presumption remains to be proved.

F. Acropigmentatio Reticularis (Kitamura)

In this disorder many small polygonal-shaped pigmentations appear on the extensive side of the periphery of the extremities. The pigmentation becomes reticular when the flecks fuse. Onset usually occurs during childhood or puberty and sometimes in adulthood. The abnormality gradually develops with age.

This abnormality is found only in Japanese. The mode of inheritance is autosomal dominant, and penetrance is almost complete. However, its expression has been noted to vary within and between families. Selective pressure is also low.

G. Congenital Muscular Dystrophy (Fukuyama Type)

The congenital type of muscular dystrophy has been defined and classified as due to an autosomal recessive gene (Walton and Nattrass, 1954; World Federation of Neurology, 1968). Fukuyama *et al.* (1960) described a peculiar form of congenital progressive muscular dystrophy with clinical features as follows: (1) onset is early, (2) both sexes are affected equally, (3) muscular wasting is diffuse and extensive but predominantly proximal, (4) facial muscles are frequently involved, (5) contracture of joints is frequent, in some cases showing a clinical picture resembling arthrogryposis multiplex congenita, (6) in younger infants, hypotonia, hypokinesia, and myotonia congenita are observed, (7) almost invariably, mental deficiency and developmental speech disorders are associated. Febrile or nonfebrile recurrent convulsions were observed in about half of the cases.

Recently a detailed analysis has been done by Osawa (1978) (see Table IX).

VIII. GENETIC COUNSELING SYSTEM IN JAPAN

Despite the prevailing emphasis on health and medical education for all the people in general, many Japanese, not only those of the older generation but also those of the younger one as well, do not wish to have their genetic problems made known. The attitude is based completely on the traditional and emotional upbringing among the Japanese. The existence of such a disease in a family is

TABLE IX

Genetic Features of Congenital Muscular Dystrophy[a]

Feature	Description
Comparative frequency	With Duchenne type, estimated as 546:252 (2.2:1)
Consanguinity	Among parents of patients = 26.80% including 15% of first-cousin marriages
Mode of inheritance	Autosomal recessive type
Gene frequency	$5.2-9.7 \times 10^{-3}$
Theoretical frequency	6.9–11.9/100,000 (prevalence rate)

[a] From Osawa (1978).

thought to be shameful, not only for the person affected but for all members of the family, like "losing face" or "losing the family name."

In Japan, genetic counseling had been done voluntarily by a few physicians and human geneticists. With a few exceptions, no specific facility had been established or organized for the public. In 1972, the Japanese Society of Human Genetics established the Committee on Genetic Counseling Network and began to consider the practical and appropriate system for genetic counseling in Japan. Today the potential need of genetic counseling is estimated to involve 20,000 to 30,000 cases per year.

Secondarily, we pointed out the importance of collection, maintenance, and supply of information and references relating to genetic counseling and clinical genetics. In 1974, the committee began a short-term training course of genetic counseling for physicians and began to establish a systematic information service.

In 1977, the Ministry of Health and Welfare decided to establish a new project as "the family planning special counseling project" to increase the quantity and quality of the genetic counseling services and to improve their distribution. Under the name of the project, the Genetic Counseling Center was set up as an attached facility of the Japan Family Planning Association, Inc., in Tokyo. Their main projects are (1) training of genetic counselors, (2) providing an information service, and (3) staffing the genetic counseling service. Furthermore, they provide seminars for allied health professionals, particularly for public health nurses and midwives, and several other activities (Ohkura and Kon, 1978).

Since the project was established, a number of local (prefectural and municipal) governments have begun to deliver or to plan genetic counseling services. The systems differ because of local circumstances (Ohkura and Handa, 1978).

REFERENCES

Akasaka, Y. (1970). Statistical and cytogenetic study on the cleft lip, alveolus and/or plate (in Japanese). *Jinrui Idengaku Zasshi* **15**, 35–95.

Amaki, I., Serizawa, T., Harashima, S., Okada, F., Seino, H., Shoji, K., and Kawashima, T. (1960). A case of thalassemia-like anemia. *Jpn. J. Clin. Hematol.* **1**, 193–197.

Ando, M. (1974). Subpulmonary ventricular septal defects with pulmonary stenosis. (Letter to editor.) *Circulation* **50**, 412.

Ando, M. (1975). Epidemiology of congenital heart disease (in Japanese). *In* "Rinsho Junkankibyo Koza," Vol. 2, p. 83. Kanehara, Tokyo.

Ando, M., and Takao, A. (1975). Anatomic variabilities between races in some major cardiac anomalies. *Teratology* **12**, 194.

Ando, M., Takao, A., and Mori, K. (1977). Genetic and environmental factors in congenital heart disease. *In* "Gene-Environment Interaction in Common Diseases" (Medical Research Foundation, ed.), pp. 71–88. Univ. of Tokyo Press, Tokyo.

Arakawa, T., Narisawa, K., Ogasawara, Y., and Hayashi, K. (1977). Study on the fluorescent screening method for glucose 6 phosphate dehydrogenase deficiency (in Japanese). *In* "Report of Group Study on Hemolytic Anemia" (S. Miwa, ed.), pp. 203–206. Minis. Health Welfare, Tokyo.

Auricchio, S., Rubino, A., Landolt, M., Semenza, G., and Prader, A. (1963). Isolated intestinal lactase deficiency in the adult. *Lancet* **ii**, 324–326.

Awa, A., Bloom, A. D., Yoshida, M. C., Neriishi, S., and Archer, P. G. (1968). Cytogenetic study of the offspring of atom bomb survivors. *Nature (London)* **218**, 367–368.

Awa, A., Neriishi, S., Honda, T., Sofuni, M. C., Sofuni, T., Matsui, T., and Hamilton, H. B. (1969). Variation in chromosomes in human populations: I. chromosomal aberrations and karyotypic variants in normal and exposed human populations. *Jinrui Idengaku Zasshi* **14**, 225–227.

Behçet, H. (1937). Über rezidivierende, aphthöse, durch ein Virus verurachte Geshwure am Mund, am Auge und an den Genitalien. *Dermatol. Wochenschr.* **105**, 1152–1157.

Bruno, M. G., and McPherson, S. D. (1949). Harada's disease. *Am. J. Ophthamol.* **32**, 513–522.

Dunham, L. J., and Bailer, J. C. (1970). World maps of cancer rates and frequency rates, Part I. *Ind. Med.* **39**, 89–100.

Eietti, G. B., and Bruna, F. (1966). An ophthalmic report on Behçet's disease. *In* "International Symposium on Behçet's Disease," pp. 75–100. Karger, Basel.

François, J. (1961). "Heredity in Ophthalmology," p. 404. Mosby, St. Louis, Missouri.

Fujioka, S., Asai, T., and Ikeda, K. (1977). Screening for glucose-6-phosphate dehydrogenase deficiency in Chiba prefecture (in Japanese). *In* "Report of Study Group on Hemolytic Anemia" (S. Miwa, ed.), pp. 209–210. Minist. Health Welfare, Tokyo.

Fukutake, K. (1953). Clinical investigation of abnormal hemoglobins (Hb F and Hb S) (in Japanese). *Rinsho Byori* **1**, 164–174.

Fukuyama, Y., Kawazura, M., and Haruna, H. (1960). A peculiar form of congenital progressive muscular dystrophy. *Pediatr. Univ. Tokyo* **4**, 5–8.

Goor, D. A., Lillehei, C. W., Rees, R., and Edwards, J. E. (1970). Isolated ventricular septal defects: development bases for various types and presentation of classification. *Chest* **58**, 462–482.

Goto, F. (1979). Guide for diagnosis of occlusion of the circle of Willis (in Japanese). *In* "Report of the Study Group on Occlusion of the Circle of Willis, 1978" (F. Goto, ed.), p. 18. Minist. Health Welfare, Tokyo.

Haemmerli, U. P., Kistler, H., Ammann, R., Marthaler, T., Semenza, G., Aurrichio, S., and Prader, A. (1965). Acquired milk tolerance in the adult caused by lactose malabsorption due to a selective deficiency of intestinal lactase deficiency. *Am. J. Med.* **38**, 7–30.

Hamashima, Y. (1976). Etiology of Kawasaki disease (in Japanese). *In* "Advances in Study of Kawasaki Disease (MCLS)" (T. Kawasaki, S. Kusakawa, and I. Shigematsu, eds.), pp. 52–64. Kindai Shuppan, Tokyo.

Hamashima, Y., Kishi, K., and Tasaka, K. (1973). Rickettsia-like bodies in infantile acute febrile mucocutaneous lymph-node syndrome. *Lancet* **ii**, 42.

Harada, E. (1926). Clinical observations on non-purulental chorioiditis (acute diffuse chorioiditis) (in Japanese). *Nippon Ganka Gakkai Zasshi* **30**, 356–378.

Hay, J. D. (1966). Population and clinical studies of congenital heart disease in Liverpool. *Br. Med. J.* **ii**, 661–667.

Health and Welfare Statistics Association (1978). "Annual Statistical Report of National Health Condition, 1978" (in Japanese). Health Welfare Stat. Assoc., Tokyo.

Hidano, S. (1977). Skin tumor and nevus (in Japanese). *In* "Genetics of Skin and Urinary Disease" (O. Miura and K. Ochiai, ed.), pp. 138–166. Igaku Shoin, Tokyo.

Hirayama, T. (1975). Epidemiology of cancer of the stomach with special reference to its recent decrease in Japan. *Cancer Res.* **35**, 3460–3463.

Hoffman, J. E. (1968). Natural history of congenital heart disease, problems in its assessment with special reference to ventricular septal defects. *Circulation* **37**, 97.

Igata, A., Hasebe, M., and Tsuji, T. (1970). On the green pigment found in SMON patients: two cases excreting greenish urine. *Jpn. J. Med. Sci. Biol.* (No. 2421), **23**, 25-28.

Imaizumi, Y., Shinozaki, N., and Aoki, M. (1975). Inbreeding in Japan: Results of a nation-wide study. *Jinrui Idengaku Zasshi* **20**, 91-108.

Inaba, Y., Takagi, H., and Yanai, H. (1979). An epidemiological study on cancer mortality for selected sites in Japan by means of factor analysis (in Japanese). *Jpn. J. Public Health* **26**, 67-76.

Järvi, O. H., and Saxén, E. (1961). Elastofibroma dorsi. *Acta Pathol. Microbiol. Scand., Suppl.* No. 144, 83-84.

Jervell, A. (1954). Pulseless disease. *Am. Heart J.* **47**, 780-784.

Kamada, N. (1969). The effects of radiation on chromosomes of bone marrow cells: II. Studies on bone marrow chromosomes of atomic bomb survivors in Hiroshima. *Nippin Ketsueki Gakkai Zasshi* **32**, 236-248.

Kato, H., Schull, W. J., and Neel, J. V. (1966). A cohort-type study of survival in the children of parents exposed to atomic bombing. *Am. J. Hum. Genet.* **18**, 339-373.

Kawasaki, T. (1967). Febrile oculo-oro-cutaneo-acrodesquamatous syndrome with or without acute non-suppuration cervical lymphadenitis in infancy and childhood: clinical observations of 50 cases (in Japanese). *Jpn. J. Allergy* **16**, 178-222.

Kawasaki, T. (1976). Symptomatology of Kawasaki disease (in Japanese). *In* ''Advances in Study of Kawasaki Disease (MCLS)'' (T. Kawasaki, S. Kusakawa, and I. Shigematsu, eds.), pp. 18-28. Kindai Shuppan, Tokyo.

Kimura, N., Nishimoto, S., Nawata, Y., Mori, F., Kodama, S., and Nakakura, S. (1960). Hemoglobin disease (in Japanese). *Jpn. Heart J.* **1**, 456-465.

Kokuhu, H., and Ishihara, Y. (1967). A kindred of thalassemia major. *Nippon Ketsueki Gakkai Zasshi* **30**, 643.

Komai, T. (1972). Genetic studies on inbreeding in some Japanese populations: introductory remarks. *Jinrui Idengaku Zasshi* **17**, 87-113.

Komi, N. (1967). Fibrocystic changes of the pancreas in Japanese infants. *Recent Adv. Gastroenterol. Proc. World Congr. Gastroenterol., 3rd* **4**, 402-405.

Komi, N., and Kawasaki, S. (1969). Meconium ileus and cystic fibrosis in Japan: re-evaluation of 46 cases. *Bull. Tokyo Med. Dent. Univ.* **16**, 1-6.

Komi, N., and Seki, Y. (1967). An analysis of 46 autopsy cases of Japanese children, showing fibrocystic changes of the pancreas and one case of fibrocystic disease of the pancreas. *Bull. Tokyo Med. Dent. Univ.* **14**, 407-414.

Komi, N., Miyanaga, T., and Murakami, K. (1966). Meconium ileus and fibrocystic disease of the pancreas in Japan. *Bull. Tokyo Med. Dent. Univ.* **15**, 1-8.

Komi, N., Danes, B. S., and Ono, M. (1971). On the feature of cystic fibrosis (Meconium ileus) (in Japanese). *J. Jpn. Pediatr. Surg.* **7**, 199-202.

Koyanagi, Y. (1929). Dysacusis, Alopecia, und Poliosis bei schwerer Uveitis nicht traumatischen Ursprung. *Klin. Monatsbl. Augenheilkd.* **82**, 194.

Kuratsune, M., Jimi, S., Hirohata, T., and Nomura, A. (1975). Epidemiological survey of Behçet's disease in Hawaii: comparison of Japanese-American and Japanese (in Japanese). *In* ''Report of Studies on Etiology, Treatment and Prevention of Behçet's Disease, 1974'' (T. Shimizu, ed.), pp. 27-28. Minist. Health Welfare, Tokyo.

Maron, B. J., Applefield, J. M., and Krovetz, L. J. (1973). Racial frequencies in congenital heart disease. *Circulation* **47**, 359-361.

Minagi, H., and Gronner, A. T. (1969). Classification of the posterior longitudinal ligament: a cause of cervical myelopathy. *Am. J. Roentgenol.* **105**, 365-369.

Ministry of Education (1977). "The School Health Statistics, 1976." Minist. Educ., Tokyo.

Mitani, S. (1943). Malformations of newborns (in Japanese). *Sanka to Fujinka* **11**, 345–356.

Mitchell, S. C., Korones, S. B., and Berendes, H. W. (1971). Congenital heart disease in 56,109 births: incidence and natural history. *Circulation* **43**, 323–332.

Miwa, S., Nakashima, K., Matsumoto, N., and Fujii, H. (1977). Incidence of glucose-6-phosphate dehydrogenase (G6PD) deficiency in Yamaguchi prefecture. The second report (in Japanese). *In* "Report of Group Study on Hemolytic Anemia" (S. Miwa, ed.), pp. 213–214. Minist. Health Welfare, Tokyo.

Nagamine, N., Ito, E., and Nohara, Y. (1978). Summary of cases and geographical distribution of elastofibroma in Okinawa (in Japanese). *Ryukyu Univ. J. Health Sci. Med.* **1**, 269–295.

Nagamine, N., Nohara, Y., and Ito, E. (1979). Clinico-pathological study of extra-subscapular elastofibroma (in Japanese). *Rinsho Seikei Geka* **14**, 282–289.

Neel, J. V. (1958). A study of major congenital defects in Japanese infants. *Am. J. Hum. Genet.* **10**, 398–445.

Neel, J. V. (1963). "Changing Perspectives on the Genetic Effects of Radiation." Thomas, Springfield, Illinois.

Nishimura, E. T., Hamilton, H. B., Kobara, T. Y., Takahara, S., Ogura, Y., and Doi, H. H. (1959). Carrier states in human acatalsemia. *Science* **130**, 333–334.

Nora, J. J., and Nora, A. J. (1979). Genetics of cardiovascular diseases. *In* "Clinical Genetics: A Source Book for Physicians" (L. G. Jackson and R. N. Schimke, eds.), pp. 269–284. Wiley, New York.

Ogata, M., and Takahara, S. (1966). On minimal catalase activity in Japanese acatalasemic blood. *Proc. Jpn. Acad.* **42**, 828–832.

Ogura, Y. (1965). Families of acatalasemia (in Japanese). *Igaku no Ayumi* **54**, 307–339.

Ohkura, K., and Handa, Y., eds. (1978). "Regional Genetic Counseling Systems—Its Views and Methods" (in Japanese). Genet. Counsel. Cent. Jpn. Fam. Plann. Assoc., Tokyo.

Ohkura, K., and Kon, Y. (1978). Family planning special counseling project as a national project (in Japanese). *In* "Regional Genetic Counseling Systems—Its Views and Methods" (K. Ohkura and Y. Handa, eds.), pp. 127–132. Genet. Counsel. Cent. Jpn. Fam. Plann. Assoc., Tokyo.

Ohno, M., Yamamoto, S., Yanai, H., and Nakae, K. (1975). Addition of the result of nation-wide epidemiological study of Behçet's disease (in Japanese). *In* "Report of Studies on Etiology, Treatment and Prevention of Behçet's Disease, 1974" (T. Shimizu, ed.), pp. 9–12. Minist. Health Welfare, Tokyo.

Ohno, S., and Sugiura, S. (1976). Behçet's disease in the Department of Ophthalmology, University of California, San Francisco (in Japanese). *In* "Report of Studies on Etiology, Treatment and Prevention of Behçet's Disease, 1975" (T. Shimizu, ed.), pp. 15–17. Minist. Health Welfare, Tokyo.

Osawa, M. (1978). A genetical and epidemiological study on congenital progressive muscular dystrophy (Fukuyama type) (in Japanese). *Tokyo Joshi Ika Daigaku Zasshi* **48**, 204–241.

Ota, M. (1939). Naevus fusco-caeruleus ophthalmo-maxillaris. *Tokyo Iji Shinshi* **63**, 1243.

Ota, M., and Tanino, H. (1939). Über eine in Japan sehr häufig vorkommende Navus Form, Navus Fusco-caeruleus Ophtalmomaxillaris, und ihre Beziechungen zu der Augenmelanose. *Hifuka Hitsunyokika Zasshi* **45**, 119.

Penrose, L. S. (1957). Genetics of anencephaly. *J. Ment. Defic. Res.* **1**, 4–15.

Rao, B. N. S., and Edwards, J. E. (1974). Conditions simulating the tetralogy of Fallot. *Circulation* **49**, 173–178.

Schull, W. J., and Neel, J. V. (1965). "The Effects of Inbreeding on Japanese Children." Harper, New York.

Segi, M., and Kurihara, M. (1972). "Age-Adjusted Death Rates and Specific Death Rates of Cancer in Prefectures of Japan, 1958-1967'' (in Japanese), pp. 1-16. Segi Inst. Cancer Epidemiol. Sendai.

Shibata, S., Tamura, A., Iuchi, I., and Takahashi, H. (1960). Hemoglobin M_1: Demonstration of a new abnormal hemoglobin in hereditary nigremia. *Nippon Ketsueki Gakkai Zasshi* **23**, 46-105.

Shibata, S., Miyaji, T., Iuchi, I., Ueda, S., Takeda, I., Kimura, N., and Kodama, S. (1962). Hemoglobin M Kurume: its identity with hemoglobin M Saskatoon. *Nippon Ketsueki Gakkai Zasshi* **25**, 690-694.

Shibata, S., Tamura, A., Iuchi, I., and Miyaji, T. (1964). Hereditary nigremia and hemoglobin M. Iwate. *Proc. Jpn. Acad.* **40**, 220-225.

Shibata, S., Yawata, Y., Yamada, O., and Koresawa, S. (1977). Results of screening tests for detection of glucose-6-phosphate dehydrogenase deficiency in human red cells in Okayama-Kurashiki district in Japan: the report in the third year (in Japanese). *In* ''Report of Group Study on Hemolytic Anemia'' (S. Miwa, ed.), pp. 211-212. Minist. Health Welfare, Tokyo.

Shibuya, Y., Yamashita, F., Funatsu, T., and Funatsu, I. (1970). Ability of lactose digestion in Japanese—changes by age (in Japanese). *Igaku no Ayumi* **72**, 323-324.

Shigematsu, I., and Yanagawa, H. (1976). Epidemiology of Kawasaki disease (in Japanese). *In* ''Advances in Study of Kawasaki Disease (MCLS)'' (T. Kawasaki, S. Kusakawa, and I. Shigematsu, eds.), pp. 3-17. Kindai Shuppan, Tokyo.

SMON Research Commission (1970). Results of nation-wide survey of SMON patients. *Rep. SMON Res. Comm.*, No. 1, 4-38.

Suenaga, M. (1952). Genetical studies of skin-disease: VII. Dyschromatosis universalis hereditaria in five generations. *Tohoku J. Exp. Med.* **55**, 373-376.

Takaesu, Y., Sugano, K., Sato, S., Hiruta, G., and Handa, Y. (1976). Folk psychiatric consideration of animal possession (in Japanese). *Seishin Shinkeigaku Zasshi* **78**, 568.

Takagi, K., and Kawai, T. (1977). A result of mass screening for G6PD deficiency among Japanese male individuals (in Japanese). *In* ''Report of Study Group on Hemolytic Anemia'' (S. Miwa, ed.), pp. 207-208. Minist. Health Welfare, Tokyo.

Takahara, S. (1951). Acatalasemia (lack of catalase in blood) and or progressive gangrene. *Proc. Jpn. Acad.* **27**, 259-301.

Takahara, S. (1968). Acatalasemia in Japan. *In* ''Hereditary Disorders of Erythrocyte Metabolism'' (E. Beutler, ed.), p. 21. Grune & Stratton, New York.

Takahara. S., and Miyamoto, H. (1949). Clinical and experimental study of progressive necrotic gingivitis due to lack of catalase in the blood (in Japanese). *Jibi Inkoka Rinsho.* **21**, 53-56.

Takahara, S., Ogura, Y., Koyama, T., Kishimoto, H., Chiba, K., Sadamoto, M., Takehisa, T., Mitani, Y., Kuroda, Y., Kasai, H., and Ohkura, K. (1969). A report of field survey on acatalasemia and hypocatalasemia in 1966 and 1967 (in Japanese). *Okayama Igakkai Zasshi* **81**, 135-141.

Takasu, T., Igata, A., and Toyokura, Y. (1970). On the green tongue observed in SMON patients. *Igaku no Ayumi* **72**, 539-540.

Tamura, A., Takahashi, M., Ishii, H., and Akashi, S. (1959). A study on the hereditary black blood disease (Tamura and Takahashi's disease or nigremia hereditaria) (in Japanese). *Jinrui Idengaku Zasshi* **4**, 180-195.

Thalhammer, O. (1975). Frequency of inborn errors of metabolism, especially PKU, in some representative newborn screening centers around the world: A collaborative study. *Humangenetik* **30**, 273-286.

Toyama, G. (1924). Symmetrische Pigmentanomalie der Extremitaten. *Arch. Dermatol. Syph.* **147**, 389-393.

Tsukimoto, H. (1960). A case report—Autopsy of syndrome of compression of spinal cord owing to ossification within spinal canal of cervical spines (in Japanese). *Nihon Greka Hokan.* **29**, 1003-1007.

Tsuyama, N., ed. (1976). "Report of the Study Group on Ossification of Posterior Longitudinal Ligament" (in Japanese), p. 93. Minist. Health Welfare, Tokyo.

Vogt, A. (1906). Frühzeitiges Ergrauen der Silien und Bemerkungen über den sogenannten plötzlichen Eintritt dieser Erscheinung. *Klin. Monatsbl. Augenheilkd.* **44,** 228.

Wadia, N. H. (1977). Some observations on SMON from Bombay. *J. Neurol., Neurosurg. Psychiatry* **40,** 268–275.

Walton, J. N., and Nattrass, F. J. (1954). On the classification, natural history and treatment of the myopathies. *Brain* **77,** 169–231.

World Federation of Neurology, Research Group on Neuromuscular Disease (1968). Classification of the neuromuscular disorders. *J. Neurol. Sci.* **6,** 165–177.

Wright, S. W., and Morton, N. E. (1968). The incidence of cystic fibrosis in Hawaii. *Hawaii Med. J.* **27,** 229–232.

Yagishita, S., Ito, Y., and Ikezaki, R. (1976). Lipomembranous polycystic osteodysplasia. *Virchows Arch. A: Pathol. Anat. Histol.* **372,** 245–251.

Yamaguchi, T., Tashiro, M., Sugi, T., and Kitamura, K. (1979). A nationwide survey on the occlusion of the circle of Willis (in Japanese). *In* "Report of the Study Group on Occlusion of the Circle of Willis, 1978" (F. Goto, ed.), pp. 9–16. Minist. Health Welfare, Tokyo.

Yamamoto, S., Toyokawa, H., Matsubara, J., Yanai, H., Inaba, Y., Nakae, K., and Ono, M. (1974). A nation-wide survey of Behçet's disease in Japan: I. Epidemiological survey. *Jpn. J. Ophthalmol.* **18,** 282–290.

Yamauchi, H., Izawa, K., and Fujiwara, M. (1977). X-ray investigation of cervical spine for ossification of posterior longitudinal ligament in the States (in Japanese). *Seikei Geka.* **28,** 757–765.

Yamaura, I., Kamikozuru, M., Shinoyama, K., and Kaneda, A. (1978). X-ray investigation of ossification of posterior longitudinal ligament in Southeast Asia: Philippines (in Japanese). *Kanto Seisai Shi* **9,** 292–297.

Yanai, H., Inaba, Y., Takagi, H., Toyokawa, H., and Yamamoto, S. (1978). An epidemiological study on mortality rates of various cancer sites during 1958–1971 by means of factor analysis. *Behaviormetrika* **5,** 55–74.

Yoshioka, M., and Tamura, Z. (1970). On the nature of the green pigment found in SMON patients. *Igaku no Ayumi* **74,** 320–322.

11

Diseases of the Chinese

ROSALIND Y. TING

I. INTRODUCTION

Covering a territory of nearly 3.7 million square miles (9.6 million km²), China is slightly larger than the United States (3.6 million square miles). China's population, however, accounts for about one fourth of the whole of humankind. According to the latest statistics released by its government in 1979, the total population at the end of 1978 was estimated to be 958,030,000, not including the 17,200,000 Chinese residing on Taiwan and about 5,000,000 in Hong Kong. Ninety-five percent of China's total population is concentrated in the eastern 40% of the land. The remaining 60% is occupied by less than 6% of her people. Of China's 55 ethnic groups, the Han people are the overwhelming majority, accounting for 94% of the total population.

BIOCULTURAL ASPECTS OF DISEASE
Copyright © 1981 by Academic Press, Inc.
All rights of reproduction in any form reserved.
ISBN 0-12-598720-X

Of China's total population, 6% are minority ethnic groups, living scattered over some 50-60% of the northwestern and southwestern parts of the country. Traditionally they have lived their own life styles, segregated mostly because of geographic distances. Recently, efforts have been made on all fronts to integrate them more fully into the life of China as a whole. Even intermarriages, although still rare, are somewhat more frequent in recent times. All of these peoples have their distinctive genetic heritages, customs, diets, ways of making their living— factors that influence their disease patterns and their susceptibilities to various diseases. These complicating factors have further compounded the already complex picture of disease and medical history in China.

The largest minority group, the Zhuang, totals more than 8 million persons, most of them (about 90%) residing in the Guangxi Zhuang Autonomous Region. The remaining 10% have emigrated to the adjacent Yunnan Province and the Guangdong autonomous areas. In the days before the 1949 Liberation, the most common disease of the Zhuang in Guangxi was goiter, called, because of the obvious symptom of swelling under the chin, "Big Neck Blister Disease" (Chen, 1976). The prevalence of goiter resulted from the scarcity of iodized salt in that area. The disease has now become almost a thing of the past because of the improved supply of iodized salt to the area as well as to a better medical care and health delivery system.

The second largest minority group, the Uighur, numbering more than 5 million, lives in Xinjiang Uighur Autonomous Region, mostly in the oases of Tarim Basin and Dzungarian Basin. Turkic-speaking Muslims, their diet consists of wheat or corn flour, mutton, and dairy products, but not many vegetables. Uighur girls used to marry in their early teens, sometimes even as early as age 9 or 10 years. Before 1949 and the outreach of modern medical care, they relied on and believed in their witch doctors—without even the benefit of traditional herbal medicine, which was almost exclusively a Han heritage.

Throughout China, more than 4 million Hui people are spread over Ningxia, Gansu, Honan, Qinghai, Hobei, Shandong, Yunnan, Anhui, Xinjiang, Liaoning, Beijing, and Tianjin (Tan, 1976). The heaviest concentration of these Chinese Muslims, numbering more than 600,000, is in the Ningxia Hui Autonomous Region. The Hui people use Chinese mandarin as the common language, but they learn Arabic in their own special schools. They have their own customs and religion, Islam, with their mosques. They tend to live together among their own people, usually concentrated in certain districts, even within cities. Their clannishness leads to marriage among close relatives. Their diet adheres to Muslim traditions and restrictions.

More than 3 million Tibetans are scattered in Tibet, Qinghai, Sichuan, Gansu, and Yunnan (Tan, 1976). In 1979, there were 1.74 million persons in the Tibet Autonomous Regions, 120,000 of them recent Han Chinese settlers (Butterfield,

1979). For centuries, Tibetan Buddhism, or Lamaism, has greatly influenced the Tibetans, albeit the lamas themselves have dwindled from 110,000 in the 1950s to about 2000 in 1979. The Tibetan diet consists basically of barley flour, yak meat, mutton, wheat flour, butter, milk, and cheese. Tea and barley beer (chang) are their main beverages, the tea thickly mixed with salt and butter, consumed in even greater quantities than we drink coffee. Traditionally they have practiced monogamy, polygamy, and polyandry, though the latter two forms of marriage, while notorious, were never predominant.

In the old times, lamas were the medicine men of Tibet (Chen, 1937). Before the 1950s, public health services and medical facilities were unheard of. Fortunately, cold temperatures and cool dry air, year around, kept down epidemics, but infant mortality was extremely high (Tan, 1976) and pregnant women often gave birth while working in the fields. In the 1,221,700 km^2 of the "roof of the world" there was not a single school, or a hospital. Today Tibet has 10,000 miles of roads, 6300 schools (Butterfield, 1979), and many childcare centers and hospitals (Tan, 1976).

The most widely dispersed of China's minority groups is the Mongolian, a nomadic people. Most of the more than 2 million Mongolians live in the Inner Mongolian Autonomous Region, but small Mongolian and Mongolian-related groups are scattered from Xinjiang through Qinghai, and Gansu, and into the provinces of the northeast. Before 1949, infant mortality was as high as 98% in some areas. Since then, new hospitals, clinics, and health stations, along with anti-epidemic centers, have been set up throughout Inner Mongolia, giving the newborn a better chance of survival.

Besides the major minority groups described above, an additional 20–30 smaller minority ethnic groups reside in China. These include the Miao, Yi, Puyi, Tung, Pai, Tuchia, Hani, and Tai, living in the southwestern provinces of Yunnan, Guizhou, and Sichuan, and Hunan in south-central China. The Kazakhs and Kirghiz live in the border areas of northern Xinjiang. More than 1 million Koreans inhabit the three northeastern provinces, predominantly Jilin.

II. HEALTH CARE

The changes in health care in China since the Liberation in 1949 have been many and dramatic. Briefly, China, perhaps in its worst condition in its four millenia history, had a shortage of doctors and food and lacked adequate sanitation. Diseases, inflation, and corruption were rampant. In 1949, China had fewer than 20,000 modern-trained physicians, about one doctor for every 26,000 persons. Health care facilities—hospitals, clinics, medical colleges—were inadequate in quantity and quality and were concentrated in a few major cities. The whole countryside was practically without modern medical care facilities. The people depended on traditional Chinese herbal medicine provided by poorly trained Chinese traditional doctors.

Since 1949 the government has tried vigorously to mass produce intermediate level physicians, provided with shorter and less extensive training. Thus the number of doctors has increased from fewer than 20,000 in 1949 to 70,000 in 1957 and to about 150,000 in 1966. In the face of the continuing shortage of Western-trained physicians and the popular confidence in traditional Chinese medicine, the government decided to make use of this abundant resource. First, the traditional doctors, 486,700 in number, were registered. Confident that, to have survived thousands of years, the traditional herbal medicine had to be of some benefit, the government undertook to study it and to combine its techniques and therapeutic measures selectively with those of modern Western medicine, thereby creating what the Chinese call the "new medicine."

To further increase the supply of medical practitioners, the government has trained many secondary practitioners, or paraprofessionals. About 1 million of these dedicated "barefoot doctors" have been trained (U.S. DHEW, 1978). Mostly women, they are selected by their peasant peers to receive training in basic medical education and techniques. After completing this training, they are capable of treating most of the common illnesses, give immunizations, provide education, supervision, and counseling in health and sanitation, and refer patients with serious conditions to more highly trained medical practitioners.

As a result of this aggressive health care policy, China has the highest doctor-to-patient ratio in Asia. As former Senator Mike Mansfield observed in a 1974 report to the U.S. Senate:

> The misery of the Old China, where famines and pestilence were common and millions wandered aimlessly, is gone. . . . It is evident that the Chinese have made remarkable accomplishments in health care delivery, disease prevention and disease control during the past twenty-five years. They are using the contemporary Western medical concepts together with new techniques in traditional Chinese medicine. The combination is producing promising results, which could be of benefit to the entire world (Mansfield, 1977).

Now China's major medical problems are those she shares with the industrialized world—heart disease and cancer—and one she shares with the developing countries of the world—an enormous and still expanding population.

As noted, the latest census figure is staggering. China's 1949 population of 541,670,000 has nearly doubled. This continuous population increase greatly concerns the Chinese government. Since 1954, the government has been advocating a family planning program that since 1956 has been vigorously implemented by the Ministry of Public Health. Late marriage—25 or 26 years of age for women, 27 or 28 for men—as well as small families has been encouraged. Until 1978, the ideal family size was two children. To achieve this ideal, various contraceptive methods are freely provided, and for third pregnancies, abortion is easily obtained.

Currently the government has as its goal a further decrease in family size, and now vigorously promotes the one-child family by providing not only contraceptive methods but also positive incentives. The child of the one-child family is guaranteed an education. Single-child families are given special health care and medical attention, and provided with extra income. The effects of these policies are not yet apparent, but in the big cities young couples seem to have decided to have only one child and to claim the benefits to which their restraint entitles them.

The effect of these policies in the remote rural areas remains problematic. The people there generally resisted the previous campaigns for limited population, showing great reluctance to practice birth control. For them the old fear of having no children, or too few children, to care for them in old age proved a more powerful motivation than government policies. Minority nationalities too have been increasing their numbers dramatically. While the government works to achieve a zero population growth, the population of the Mongolian people has increased 3.27 times, and that of the Uighurs in Xinjiang by 42%.

Because of China's concern in providing basic health care to its people since the Liberation and the anti-intellectual atmosphere generated by the Cultural Revolution from 1965 to 1975, little attention has been paid to describing and investigating the unique and genetic diseases prevalent in China. Thus, the diseases discussed here should be considered in the perspective of the historical and political changes of the country. Because of the limited data available at present and with the new spirit of scientific inquiry now prevalent, this chapter hopefully will serve as the foundation for future reviews which will be able to be more specific about diseases of the Chinese.

III. INFANT MORTALITY AND GROWTH PATTERNS

A. Infant Mortality

Infant mortality may be a sensitive index to reflect national health status. Table I shows the dramatic decrease of total infant death rate in China, from 58.1/1000 in 1951 to 6.0/1000 in 1974–1976. Because of improved medical care, the diseases that in the past usually killed infants during their first year of life have been controlled or eliminated. These measures have shifted the pattern of problems. In 1951 the death rate from congenital heart disease was 1.5/1000; whereas by 1974 it had increased to 1.8/1000. At present, among the five major causes of infant mortality, congenital anomalies account for the greatest number of deaths

TABLE I

**Main Causes of Infant Death[a] in Beijing:
Comparison between 1951 and 1974–1976**

Cause of Death	1951	1974–1976
Diphtheria	0.1	0.0
Scarlet Fever	0.2	0.0
Measles	4.5	0.0
Tuberculosis	2.1	0.0
Congenital Syphilis	2.1	0.0
Epidemic Encephalitis	0.0	0.18
Tetanus	2.6	0.02
Prematurity	16.0	1.6
Pneumonia	16.0	2.3
Diarrhea	5.2	0.1
Malnutrition	7.8	0.0
Congenital Heart Disease	1.5	1.8
Total	58.1	6.0

[a] Deaths per thousand.

(23.4%). Of these, 90% were caused by congenital heart defects, brain malformations, severe gastrointestinal malformations, myelomeningocele, anencephaly, hydrocephalus, and multiple congenital anomalies (Liu, 1978).

B. Growth Patterns

Recently the Chinese Academy of Medical Sciences (1977) conducted a massive survey of Chinese children's growth characteristics. Nine cities and their rural areas were divided into three zones: (1) northern zone at latitude 34–36°, and included Harbin, Beijing, and Xian; (2) middle zone, at latitude 31–33°, and included Shanghai, Nanjing, Wuhan; and (3) southern zone, at latitude 23–26°, and included Guangzhou, Fuzhou, and Oumin. Of the 273,735 children surveyed, 140,229 were city residents and 133,506 were rural-farming residents. 139,130 were boys and 134,605 were girls. When the data were compared with 1976 U.S. figures, the measurements for the Chinese were similar until about age 12 months (Tables II and III). If anything, Chinese children appear to be slightly taller than U.S. children. A factor influencing the slightly higher average birth weights and lengths of Chinese children could be the lower incidence of premature infants born to Chinese women. A factor that may account for the slightly larger measurements up to age 6 months is the high incidence of breast-feeding in China. After 6 months of age, the quality of supplementary food probably be-

TABLE II

Comparison of Heights and Weights of U.S. and Chinese Boys

	Weight			Height		
Age	U.S.	Chinese urban	Chinese rural	U.S.	Chinese urban	Chinese rural
Newborn	3.27	3.27	3.22	50.5	50.6	50.2
6 Months	7.85	8.22	7.79	67.8	68.1	66.8
12 Months	10.15	9.66	8.97	76.1	75.6	73.7
18 Months	11.27	10.67	9.96	82.4	80.7	78.3
24 Months	12.59	11.95	11.28	87.6	86.5	83.6
36 Months	14.69	13.63	13.11	96.5	93.8	90.5
4 Years	16.69	15.26	14.61	102.9	100.8	97.1
5 Years	18.68	16.88	16.08	109.9	107.2	103.9
6 Years	20.69	19.25	18.11	116.1	114.7	109.8
7 Years	22.85	21.01	19.81	121.7	120.6	115.2
8 Years	25.30	23.08	21.77	127.0	125.3	120.3
9 Years	28.13	25.33	23.81	132.2	130.6	125.3
10 Years	31.44	27.15	25.95	137.5	134.4	129.7
11 Years	35.30	30.13	28.07	143.3	139.2	133.7
12 Years	39.78	33.05	30.84	149.7	144.2	138.6
13 Years	44.95	36.90	33.89	156.5	149.8	143.9
14 Years	50.77	42.03	38.54	163.1	156.5	150.3
15 Years	56.71	46.91	43.64	169.0	162.0	156.5
16 Years	62.10	50.90	47.93	173.5	165.6	161.0
17–18 Years	67.78	53.17	50.68	176.7	167.7	163.5

comes increasingly important and is demonstrated by the difference in birth weight and height between city children and rural children. Beginning at age 12 months, Chinese children fall steadily behind U.S. children in size. The distance widens from 8–9 years of age to age 18 years and is most striking in the weight of adolescent boys. Dietary patterns, cultural influences, and nutritional education, as well as heredity, may all play a part in causing these differences.

IV. DISEASES

During the past 25 years many diseases have been conquered through modern therapeutic and preventive medical techniques. Now that the Chinese have improved health and increased longevity, the problems common to industrialized countries have become more prevalent: hypertension, cardiovascular diseases, cerebrovascular diseases, and cancer.

Zhao and Wang (1978) reported mass surveys that were done in 1958, 1973,

TABLE III

Comparison of Heights and Weights of U.S. and Chinese Girls

Age	U.S.	Weight		Height	
		Chinese urban	Chinese rural	Chinese urban	Chinese rural
Newborn	3.23	3.17	3.15	49.9	50.0	49.7
6 Months	7.21	7.62	7.24	65.9	66.7	65.4
12 Months	9.53	9.04	8.43	74.3	74.1	72.3
18 Months	10.82	10.08	9.37	80.9	79.4	76.7
24 Months	11.90	11.37	10.66	86.5	85.3	82.2
36 Months	13.93	13.10	12.48	95.6	92.8	89.2
4 Years	15.96	14.89	14.15	101.6	100.1	95.9
5 Years	17.66	16.46	15.56	108.4	106.5	102.0
6 Years	19.52	18.67	17.53	114.6	113.9	109.0
7 Years	21.84	20.35	19.16	120.6	119.3	114.3
8 Years	24.84	22.43	21.08	126.4	124.6	119.6
9 Years	28.46	24.57	23.07	132.2	129.5	124.1
10 Years	32.55	27.05	25.35	138.3	134.8	129.2
11 Years	36.96	30.51	28.09	144.8	140.6	134.4
12 Years	41.53	34.74	31.86	151.5	146.6	140.4
13 Years	46.10	38.52	35.80	157.1	150.7	145.7
14 Years	50.28	42.26	39.73	160.4	153.7	150.1
15 Years	53.68	45.37	43.83	161.8	155.5	153.0
16 Years	55.89	47.43	46.40	162.4	156.8	154.3
17–18 Years	56.71	48.57	48.00	163.4	157.4	155.2

and 1977 (Table IV). The 1977 survey, covering more than 95% of the members of five factories and nine large farming communes, included manual laborers in urban and rural areas in and around Shanghai; the men were 60 years of age or less, the women 55 years of age or less (Zhao and Wang, 1978). Table IV shows the consistently higher prevalence of hypertension among urban residents. This high prevalence is most significant on the 1977 data ($p < 0.01$). Table V shows the prevalence of hypertension between 1973 and 1977 by age and residence. Clearly, for each age-group over 20 years, prevalence of hypertension is higher in urban areas. In the urban areas, prevalence rose sharply after age 30 years, and in rural areas, after age 40 years. Not only did the rise occur earlier, it also occurred more rapidly in the urban group than in the rural group. The prevalence among the 40- to 45-year-old group in rural areas was similar to that among the 20- to 25-year-olds in urban areas, a 20-year difference. Whereas the prevalence among those more than age 55 years was highest for both urban and rural groups, it was two-and-a-half times higher in the urban than in the rural group.

TABLE IV

The Percentage of Hypertension in Urban and Rural Area Residents

Year	Urban		Rural	
	Male	Female	Male	Female
1958	9.47	7.02	2.02	2.27
1973	9.99	7.01	4.55	3.52
1977	12.53		2.36	

The survey also showed that prevalence was highest among white-collar workers, next highest among urban manual laborers, and lowest among rural workers. However, more of the rural residents had diastolic pressures above 110 mm Hg. EKGs, done on 92% of the study group, showed significantly higher abnormalities, particularly left ventricular hypertrophy, among those in rural areas. These statistics suggest that, whereas the incidence of hypertension was higher in urban areas, its intensity was more severe among residents of rural areas.

TABLE V

A Comparison of the Frequency of Hypertension among Greater Shanghai Residents

Age (Years)	Urban				Rural			
	1973		1977		1973		1977	
	Number	(%)	Number	(%)	Number	(%)	Number	(%)
15	6,158	(1.3)	379	(1.1)	7,020	(1.1)	1,483	(1.5)
20	1,226	(4.2)	1,353	(2.4)	5,449	(2.0)	2,229	(1.7)
25	10,382	(3.6)	1,304	(4.1)	4,077	(2.1)	1,796	(1.6)
30	8,405	(4.9)	1,086	(7.0)	3,050	(1.8)	1,061	(1.1)
35	14,054	(6.6)	900	(13.2)	2,724	(2.4)	680	(1.3)
40	19,982	(9.2)	1,587	(13.3)	3,002	(3.5)	534	(3.6)
45	15,813	(13.7)	1,732	(19.2)	2,950	(4.5)	704	(4.7)
50	8,577	(18.2)	977	(26.4)	2,329	(6.4)	680	(5.7)
55	4,614	(25.7)	599	(26.4)	1,580	(10.0)	618	(10.0)

A. Cardiovascular Diseases

Table VI, based on data collected by the Beijing Fu Wai Hospital on persons aged 40 years and more, shows specific regional variations in the prevalence of coronary artery disease. The data suggest that the different cultural life-styles and dietary habits in different geographic locations influence the incidence of coronary artery disease. Most notable is the low prevalence among the fishermen living on the Zhoushan archipelago and the group in Guangdong whose major source of protein is fish, in contrast to the high prevalence among the nomads of Xinjiang Province, whose protein source is the large amount of animal meat and fat they consume. Both availability and distribution limit the kind of food people consume, and these limitations may be reflected in the varied incidences of artery disease.

Recently Li (1979) reported the causes of death for persons aged more than 30 years in Beijing, a city with a population of 228,017 (Table VII). During the 3-year period from 1975 to 1977, cardiovascular diseases were listed as the number one cause of death. This survey showed a reversal of the trend reported in 1972 from Shanghai (Lamm and Sidel, 1974), where cancer was the number one killer (25.3%), followed by cerebrovascular diseases (19.3%), and cardiovascular diseases (12.1%). Whether these two surveys represent a national trend or geographical and ethnic differences is not clear, but the changing pattern is worth noting.

A survey of serum lipids of 954 herdsmen of Sizuwang Banner, Inner

TABLE VI

Prevalence of Coronary Artery Disease—Regional Differences[a]

		Male		Female		Total	
Year	Region	Number	(%)	Number	(%)	Number	(%)
1960	Beijing	2726	(2.2)	641	(3.6)	3367	(2.5)
1960	Shanghai	5473	(3.2)	1806	(3.2)	7279	(3.2)
1965	Kansu	1129	(1.9)	155	(9.0)	1284	(2.7)
1965	Beijing (factory workers)	500	(4.4)			500	(4.4)
1965	Sichuan	217	(7.4)	66	(8.5)	283	(7.8)
1965	Zhoushan (fisherman)	1625	(0.6)			1625	(0.6)
1965	Xinjiang (administrators)	195	(2.5)				
	Xinjiang (nomad)	81	(19.8)				
	Xinjiang (total)	276	(7.6)			276	(7.6)
1971	Shanghai (factory workers)	1747	(6.9)			1747	(6.9)
1971	Quangdong	912	(1.5)	181	(4.4)	1093	(2.0)

[a] Courtesy of Dr. Y. K. Wu, Fu Wai Hospital, Beijing.

TABLE VII

Major Cause of Death

Year	Cardiovascular disease	Cerebrovascular disease	Coronary disease	Malignancy	Accidents	Mortality from all causes
1975	662	342	104	215	37	11.4
1976	656	348	125	255	50	11.2
1977	670	396	139	272	30	12.3
1975–1977	1988	1085	368	742	117	11.7
Percent of all deaths (1975–1977)	46.2%	25.2%	8.6%	17.3%	2.7%	

Mongolia, was done by Hsia and co-workers (1977). Of these, 740 (77.6%) were Mongolians (384 males, 356 females), and 214 (22.4%) were Han (160 males, 54 females). The Han who were included in the survey had lived in the pastoral area more than 10 years. Mean cholesterol levels were 197.1 ± 32.8 mg/dl, which is higher than levels reported from other parts of China. Mean triglyceride values were 78.9 ± 30.1 mg/dl, lower than in other areas. When the data were broken down by ethnic group, Mongolian males showed higher cholesterol levels than did Han males, whereas triglyceride levels shown in both sexes were higher among the Han than among Mongols ($p < 0.01$). Both cholesterol and triglyceride levels were significantly higher among the 17.4% males who were overweight ($p < 0.001$), but the levels were not higher among the 32.1% overweight females ($p < 0.05$). Smokers of both sexes had higher levels of serum lipids; drinkers had higher levels of triglycerides than did nondrinkers ($p < 0.01$). The 158 persons with coronary artery disease, the 144 with hypertension, and the 142 showing arteriosclerosis of ocular fundi, all had serum cholesterol and triglyceride levels higher than did the healthy subjects surveyed ($p < 0.001$).

In 1957–1958, the leading form of cardiovascular diseases was rheumatic heart disease (about 50%). By 1973, coronary heart disease, hypertensive heart disease, pulmonary heart disease, and congenital heart disease had steadily increased in incidence. Data collected by Fu Wai Hospital in Beijing in 1960 showed that coronary artery disease was more prevalent among females than among males. The prevalence among women more than 50 years of age was twice that among men. However, the sample surveyed was relatively small and nonrandomized and, therefore, may not represent the total population.

B. Schistosomiasis

Because of its devastating effects on patients, the most important parasitic disease of China is schistosomiasis. *Schistosoma japonicum* eggs were found in an unearthed female corpse buried between 195 and 188 BC. Historically, this disease entity was first established in China in 1905 in Hunan Province, 1 year after the discovery of the parasite *S. japonicum* in Japan.

From 1905 to 1924, sporadic cases of schistosomiasis were seen, mostly by missionary doctors in central and southern China. Faust and Meleney (1924) reported as the endemic area nine provinces: Jiangsu, Zhejiang, Anhuei, Jiangsi, Hubei, Hunan, and Sichuan in Central China; Fujian and Guangdong in South China.

In 1932, a severely affected endemic area was reported (Kan and Yao, 1932). Chih Huai Pan, Kaihua Xian, Zhejiang Province, a fertile area of 600 acres, had been reduced to only 65 persons, because of the severity of the disease. The land had been taken over by a thriving population of *Oncomelania* (snails) and weeds. By 1977, the endemic area had expanded to include Yunnan, Guangxi, Fujian, Taiwan, and Shanghai, a total of 13 provinces, municipalities, and autonomous territories, spreading over an area of about 8–10 million m^2 (Chai, 1977). About 6–10 million persons were infected, and the population at risk numbered about 100 million.

The magnitude of the devastation from schistosomiasis may be appreciated by the numerous samples of epidemiologic evidence gathered (Chung, 1977). Nienzieun Village, in Guiji County, Anhui Province, had 120 households a century ago. By 1949, when the People's Republic of China was established, 119 had been wiped out, and three of the four members of the one remaining family were infected.

Also a century ago, Qianjiazhuang Village (literally, the village of 1000 families), in Zhujian County, Guangdong Province, had more than 800 households with more than 3000 inhabitants. By 1949, only nine families with 15 members were left; each of them had schistosomiasis and four were in late stages of the disease.

Since the establishment of the People's Republic of China in 1949, great efforts have been made to eradicate parasitic diseases. In 1956, control and eradication of schistosomiasis were included in the National Program for Agricultural Development by the Central Committee of the Chinese Communist Party (Chung, 1977). Through the combined measures of snail destruction, medical treatment, excreta control, water management, and individual protection in accordance with the epidemiological characteristics of schistosomiasis and the peculiarities of the specific geographic environments, the endemic areas were cleaned up, one after another. Since the early 1970s, the *Oncomelania* snail has been eliminated from 5000 million m^2 of once snail-infested land and 3–5 million patients have been cured. The *People's Daily* in Beijing reported recently that the disease has now been eradicated from 204 counties in China, although it remains in more than 140 others. According to Dr. Mao Shoubai, the Director of the Institute of Parasitology in Shanghai (Sullivan, 1979), the disease remains entrenched in some low-lying coastal areas and around such great inland lakes as Dongting Hu in Hunan Province and Poyang Hu in Jiangxi Province. It also occurs in relatively inaccessible mountain areas where crops are cultivated on terraces, the snails having been found as high as 10,000 feet above sea level.

C. Nasopharyngeal Carcinoma

Nasopharyngeal carcinoma (NPC) has attracted worldwide interest because patients with this tumor were found to contain high titers of antibodies to Epstein-Barr virus (EBV) (DeSchryver *et al.*, 1969; Henle *et al.*, 1970; Klein *et al.,* 1970; Ho, 1972). As noted in Chapter 7, EBV has been associated with this tumor and Burkitt's lymphoma and has been shown to cause infectious mononucleosis.

Rare in other parts of the world, NPC is one of the most important and highly prevalent cancers in China. Of all biopsy-diagnosed malignant tumors in China, the incidence of NPC is remarkably high, particularly among males. Table VIII shows the occurrence and distribution of malignancies for males and females, based on data from the 1958 Shanghai tumor registry (personal communication).

During 1970–1972, a tumor survey of 436,786 persons of a population of 447,006 persons more than 10 years of age was conducted in three counties and one city in Guangdong. The total prevalence of NPC was 39.8/100,000; all were histopathologically confirmed. Of the total, 56.8/100,000 were male and 22.5/100,000 were female. NPC comprised 44% of all male malignancies and 18.6% of all female malignancies.

Another notable feature of NPC in Guangdong was the early age of onset. NPC occurred two decades earlier than most other epithelial cancers and two decades earlier than among residents of Sweden (Doll *et al.,* 1970) and Great Britain (Lederman, 1961), where the incidence of NPC is extremely low.

In Singapore, a multiracial community, the age-adjusted incidence for NPC during a 15-year period from 1950 to 1964 was highest among the Chinese, next among Malays, and lowest among East Indians. The prevalence rates expressed per 100,000 population were: 20.3 for Chinese males, 9.0 for Chinese females,

TABLE VIII

Distribution of Malignancies in Shanghai[a]

Area	Percentage
Male	
Stomach	17.1
Esophagus	14.9
Liver	10.4
Lung	10.1
NPC	9.6
Colon	6.5
Blood	4.2
Female	
Cervix	46.2
Breast	15.1
Stomach	6.2
Colon	4.0
Ovary	2.6
NPC	2.4
Liver	2.4

5.8 for Malay males, 2.0 for Malay females, 0.2 for Indian males, and 0.0 for Indian females (Muir and Shanmugaratnam, 1967). The authors suggested that an ethnic factor, rather than the geographic locality, determines the risk. However, one must remember that even when multiracial groups live in the same geographic area, they tend to remain culturally and dietarily distinct. Furthermore, Buell's (1974) data showed that rates of NPC for U.S.-born Chinese are consistently lower than for China-born Chinese, which suggests that environmental factors are at least one of the responsible agents of the disease.

Data collected by Ho (1972) illustrate a striking difference in the relative frequency of NPC in China by geographic distribution. Some overlapping occurs between North and Central China, but the difference between them when compared with South China is striking, the frequency of NPC being much higher in South China than in North China (Table IX). In Guangdong Province, for exam-

TABLE IX

A Geographical Comparison of Nasopharyngeal Carcinoma in China[a]

Locality	All cancers	NPC (%)	
North China			
Beijing	5,137	206	(4.0)
Tientsin (male only)	1,562	123	(7.9)
Jinan	2,738	140	(5.1)
		Average	(5.4)
Central China			
Xian	879	59	(6.7)
Hunan			
Changsha	5,805	476	(9.7)
Sichuan	3,696	292	(8.2)
Chengdu	3,714	259	(7.0)
Shanghai			
Tumor Hospital 1949–1958	8,049	1,008	(12.5)
Tumor Registration 1958	9,612	523	(5.4)
Male only	8,332	Average	(8.1)
South China			
Guangxi, Nanning			
Total	1,484	273	(18.4)
Male only	672	210	(31.4)
Guangdong, Guangzhow	11,087	2,794	(25.2)
Zhongshan Medical College, 1961	16,417	5,068	(30.9)
Population survey 1970–1972	557	174	(31.2)
Male only	577	122	(44.0)
		Average	(33.7)

[a] Adapted and modified from Wen (1974).

ple, NPC accounted for 56.9% of 3010 malignancies in males and 17.4% of 4026 malignancies in females.

The frequencies of NPC among Taiwan residents who had been born south and north of the Yangtse River have been reported to be 100/100,000 and 3/100,000, respectively, whereas corresponding figures for other cancers were 107 and 28. Among those born south of the Yangtse River, the increase in NPC was ninefold (Ku and Liu, 1959).

A mass survey done by the Shanghai researchers (Chungshan Medical College, 1978) divided persons aged 10 years and above into two groups: (1) 20,000 persons who moved to Guangdong (in the high prevalence South China) from Central and North China and had resided in Guangdong longer than 5 years (5–15 years), (2) 257,700 persons who had moved to Shanghai from Guangdong Province. Table X shows that lung cancer and liver cancer were the first and second leading causes of cancer deaths in both groups. NPC, the third highest cause of

TABLE X

**Comparison of Cancer Mortality
between Guangdong Natives
and Immigrants to Guangdong**

Cancer Site	per 100,000
Native Residents	
Lung	22.6
Liver	18.4
NPC	10.9
Stomach	10.2
Esophagus	6.3
Uterus	5.6
Breast	2.9
Leukemia	2.6
Other	12.3
Total	97.7
Immigrant Residents	
Lung	29.1
Liver	19.1
Stomach	11.8
Esophagus	6.4
Intestine (Colon)	5.5
Uterus	4.6
NPC	3.6
Breast	3.6
Leukemia	2.7
Other	6.4
Total	92.8

cancer deaths among the Tungshan natives, was three times greater among them than among the immigrants. The mortality due to NPC was 13.0/100,000 for native inhabitants of Guangdong and 3.6/100,000 for immigrants to this province. In Shanghai, the mortality for immigrants from Guangdong was 4.76/100,000 and for Shanghai natives 1.99/100,000, a ratio of 2.39:1. Of note is that the death rate for those Guangdong people who resided continuously in their native area (13.01/100,000) was 2.75 higher than that for those who had emigrated to Shanghai. Because NPC is highly malignant and usually diagnosed rather late in its course, one may reasonably assume that the death rate is equivalent to the incidence of the disease. If these incidences represent the true difference, then the data may be interpreted as follows:

1. The Guangdong people had much higher incidence of NPC than did immigrants to Guangdong.
2. The Guangdong people who were permanent residents of Guangdong had a higher incidence of NPC than did their contemporaries who emigrated to Shanghai.
3. The Guangdong people who immigrated north and resided in Shanghai for 5–15 years still had a higher incidence of NPC than did the native Shanghai residents.

Therefore, a genetic factor and an environmental factor besides the EBV may have contributed to the high prevalence of NPC among Guangdong people.

D. Concave Fingernail Syndrome

Concave fingernail syndrome (Lai, 1960; Wu et al., 1978) is a disability most prevalent in persons who live at high altitudes and do manual labor that requires prolonged or frequent immersion of the hands in water. The degree of involvement varies from mild, irregular ridges of the fingernails to thickened, rough, and dull-grey nails with peripheral detachment, pain, bleeding, and partial loss of nails.

Mild morphologic manifestation of the syndrome consists of flattening of the fingernails, appearance of longitudinal marks and grooves that produce a wrinkled look, and almost normal color and luster. When moderately affected, the distal part of the nail is flattened and sunken, whereas the middle part is elevated to resemble a duck's beak. The longitudinal marks remain and multiple small dents interspersed with small ridges give the nails an irregular surface, and luster of the nails is decreased. Severely affected nails show thickening, loss of luster, rough, dull-grey surfaces, and brittleness. The concavity becomes spoon-shaped or saddlelike with some nail detachment around the edges of the nail bed. Symptoms include bleeding, pain, and loss of part of the fingernail. The right hand is more frequently affected than the left; the thumb and index and middle fingers are affected more often than ring and small fingers. A small number of

TABLE XI

**Prevalence of Concave Fingernail Syndrome,
According to Altitude**

Altitude (m)	Number examined	Number positive (%)
2231–2500	1487	258 (17.4)
2900–3200	5968	1752 (29.4)
3750–4888	887	268 (30.1)
Total	8342	2278 (27.3)

patients also show minimal changes on their toes. This syndrome was first reported from Changdu City in 1955. Wu *et al.* (1978), in reviewing the syndrome, examined the records of 8342 persons for the years 1960 to 1975. The syndrome is most prevalent in such high-altitude areas (Table XI) as Tibet and Qinghai Provinces. In Qinghai Province, where the altitude varies from 2200 m to 4900 m, the prevalence of the syndrome for the total population can be as high as 30%. The incidence for similar groups living at sea level is only 3.4% ($p <$ 0.01). Prevalence also varies with age and sex, primarily as associated with occupation. Prevalence is extremely high (83.2%) among 20- to 40-year olds, more frequent in Han Chinese men (30.8%) than women (13.8%) but more frequent in Tibetan women (24.8%) than men (22.0%). The comparative frequency among 20- to 40-year-old Chinese men and Tibetan women is probably related to the degree of physical labor they do that requires excessive use of hands and prolonged immersion of the hands in water, e.g., transporting water and milking. Table XII, correlating relative incidence to occupation, shows that dishwashers have the highest incidence.

TABLE XII

**Prevalence of Concave Fingernail Syndrome,
According to Occupation**

Occupation	Number examined	Number positive (%)
Washer	198	139 (70.2)
Cook	85	53 (62.4)
Mason	750	275 (36.7)
Housewife	576	196 (34.0)
Peasant	2953	874 (29.6)
Other laborer	1634	378 (23.1)
Soldier	1454	278 (19.1)
Office worker	692	85 (12.3)
Total	8342	2278 (27.3)

No significant difference can be seen in the incidence between native residents of these high altitudes and migrant residents. (For native residents the incidence is 24.4%; for migrant residents, 29.1%). Natives begin to show the syndrome in their twenties, migrants after 6 months to 1 year's residence. No obvious seasonal variation has appeared, nor does nutritional status seem to affect the incidence of the syndrome. Further, no relationship between appearance of the syndrome and maladjustment to high altitude can be found. For all but 4.7% of those affected and 5.3% of those unaffected, the hemoglobin values were within normal range for residents of high altitudes.

Because the survey showed that physiologic maladjustment to high altitude is not a contributing cause and the relative iron deficiency anemia of high altitudes is not related to this phenomenon, the most likely explanation for the development of the concave fingernail syndrome is that the low oxygen saturation at high altitude leads to lowered arterial oxygen saturation, the distal tissues being especially vulnerable. This lowered oxygen supply interferes with normal metabolism of the fingernails. Generally the body adjusts to high altitudes by redistributing the blood supply, increasing it to the brain and heart by dilation of cerebral and coronary arteries, decreasing it to the skin and distal extremities by vasoconstriction. Overexertion of the extremities and fingers increases the demand for oxygen on an already decreased blood supply. That such overexertion is the probable cause of the condition is indicated by worse conditions on right hands and on thumbs, index fingers, and middle fingers. Natural water temperature at high altitudes is lower. Constant contact with water causes distal capillary spasm that could also be a predisposing factor.

So far treatment has been palliation and prevention. Using vitamins B_1, and C, iron, or calcium remedies for 1–6 months produced no improvement. Cutting down the contact with water by wearing gloves improved the condition in differing degrees, sometimes resulting in total cure.

E. Kaschin-Beck Disease

A chronic disease of the bones and joints, prevalent in the farmland of Northeast, North, and Northwest China, Kaschin-Beck disease has also been reported in Japan, Korea, and Siberia (Chu and Tsui, 1978). Incidence is higher among school children and young adults. Rarely is the disease found in children less than 3 years of age. Its cause is unknown, but generally it is considered to be related to the mineral content in local soil and water, as deficiencies or as excesses. Some postulate a lack of magnesium and sulfates, excessive strontium and iron or other trace elements. Others believe the disease relates to increased content of acid in water when rain is washed through the humus soil and the water is contaminated by organic acids that convert magnesium and calcium ions into nonsoluble salts. Still others believe that the disease relates to decreased salivation. Certain diseases have also been considered predisposing factors.

The disease is usually ushered in by lethargy, with occasional muscle spasm of the extremities. Movements of the extremities become sluggish and awkward, especially in extension of fingers. Patients often awaken with pain in the extremities and difficulty with motion that improves with movement. As the condition progresses, the joints become symmetrically enlarged, and flexion and extension become more difficult and are accompanied by a grating sound. The consequent restricted movements leads to muscle atrophy and joint deformity. With early growth arrest of tubular bones, shortening, contracture deformity, and short stature result. The appearance then is that of a midget with a waddling gait. The disease progresses slowly. In severe cases, patients can be crippled by middle age.

Diagnosis is by endemic history and symptomatology. The disease affects the whole articular system. X rays show early union of the epiphyseal plate and deformity of bone ends. The films may show three stages of changes. In the first stage, epiphyseal cartilage and metaphysis become irregular. There are concavity and sclerosis at the central part and small areas of bone destruction at the edges of the epiphysis. The temporary calcification zone is irregular and has a different density. The second stage is characterized by bony union of the epiphysis and diaphysis. Some scleroses of the epiphyseal nucleus are evident. In the third stage epiphyseal plate cartilage is gradually absorbed, separated, and ossified, causing bony union and arrest of longitudinal growth of the long bones. Due to the different timing of bone union, the lengths of the different tubular bones may vary. Bone ends are thickened and deformed. Decreased density of the bones as well as irregularities and narrowing of the joint spaces may cause subluxation. At the same time, periarticular soft tissue is swollen. The described changes are usually symmetrical, which is pathognomonic for diagnosis. No laboratory abnormalities have been reported. Pathological findings show degeneration and necrosis of the cartilage, absorption and proliferation of the cartilage and bony tissues, and various manifestations accompanying connective tissue repair.

These degenerative changes are nonspecific. The appearance of fibrils is the result of refractive changes caused by disturbance of colloid structure of the cementing matter. "Asbestos degeneration" with necrosis may be a late manifestation. Irregular lamination and alignment of chondrocytes and degeneration and necrosis of epiphyseal cartilage often result in abnormal endochondral ossification of the epiphyseal plate and premature, irregular intrusion of primordial marrow into necrotic epiphyseal plate cartilage. With the active chondroclastic process, the epiphyseal plate cartilage is gradually absorbed, separated, and ossified, causing bony union and arrest of longbone growth.

Zonal necrosis below the articular cartilage is the direct cause of ulceration of the articular surface, subchondral bone plate absorption, and repair. Cartilage destruction due to absorption is much more severe and is an important cause of early union of the epiphyseal plate and deformity of bone ends. The severity of the cartilage destruction relates to severe metabolic disturbance of the cartilage. Mosaic structure formation of bone trabeculae mainly involves epiphyses and metaphyses but not the cortical bone and spongy bone distal to the epiphyseal plate. Such selective involvement cannot be explained as a general metabolic change of the bone. Destructive bone absorption appears on X ray as cystic change.

F. Keshan Disease

An endemic idiopathic cardiomyopathy, Keshan disease was first identified in Keshan, Heilongjiang Province in 1935 (Heilongjiang Institute, 1959). It is characterized by its intermittent endemic pattern in mountainous or hilly areas and in the villages of Heilongjiang, Jilin, Liaoning, Shansi, Kansu, Shandong, Shanxi, Hebei, Henan, Hubei, Sichuan, Yunnan, and Tibet. It does not appear in major cities and coastal areas. The incidence of Keshan disease shows a seasonal variation: in North China it is higher in severe winter seasons, whereas in Southwest China it is more prevalent in the hot summer season. In North China, the disease most frequently affects persons between 20 and 50 years of age, the highest incidence being among women of childbearing age. In the southwest region, it is more frequently seen among children between 2 and 7 years of age. During major endemics, several members in a family may be affected.

Studies have searched for the causes of the disease without success. Toxicity, nutritional deficiency, and infection have all been considered.

Pathologic changes usually seen include globular cardiac enlargement not accompanied by thickening. In severe cases, the heart wall becomes thin. The most serious pathologic change is in the myocardium especially the left ventricle with flattening of the papillary muscles. In subacute cases, however, the right ventricle may be equally or more seriously affected. Mural thrombus formation occurs in 25% of the cases. In acute cases, the striated muscle may be affected, usually not as severely damaged as the myocardium. Histologically, the myocardial fibers may show focal necrotic lesions, diffuse degeneration and patchy fibrosis.

Depending on the severity of the disease, the clinical picture varies. The acute type manifesting as shock or acute heart failure is most commonly seen among young adults and in children more than 7 years of age. The subacute type manifesting as fatigability and chronic wasting accompanied by gastrointestinal complaints and circulatory disturbances is more commonly seen in children between 2 and 6 years of age. Onset of the chronic type is insidious with patients usually having a previous history of acute attack. The prominent feature is chronic cardiac failure. The chronic form of Keshan disease can be exacerbated to the acute state by upper respiratory infection, physical overexertion, and emotional disturbance. All three types of the disease can be accompanied by pulmonary or cerebral embolism and their sequelae. Diagnosis is usually based on the endemic characteristics, history, X-ray findings, and EKG.

Treatment is symptomatic and depends on the severity of manifestations. In acute types, large doses of intravenous vitamin C in glucose solution may enhance therapeutic efforts (Lu, 1978). Because the cause of the disease is unclear, preventive measures rely on improvement of nutritional status and of environmental sanitation, e.g., eliminating insect–rodent vectors, decreasing air pollution, improving quality of drinking water, and ensuring proper grain storage. With the advent of these measures, morbidity and mortality have shown noticeable reduction.

G. Hemolytic Diseases

Hemolysis has not been a common disorder among Chinese. At present more than 20 different kinds of abnormal Hb have been identified in China (Zhu *et al.*, 1980). In Guangxi Province (Cheng *et al.*, 1978), six different abnormal Hb have been identified. In the United States about 15% of whites and 7% of blacks are Rh negative. Among Chinese in the United States Rh-negative incidence is estimated at about 1%. In Shanghai, the result of testing 50,000 Han descendants revealed the incidence for Rh negative to be 0.34% (Peking Children's Hospital, 1975). Among the minorities, the incidence was 4.9%.

During the 12-year period from 1960 to 1972, there were 487 cases of hemolytic disease of newborns reported in Shanghai. Of these, 29.4% were due to Rh incompatibility and 69.8% to ABO incompatibility. Thirty percent of Chinese have type O blood. The ABO incompatibility is divided into 41.0% anti-A and 28.8% anti-B. Of the 487 reported cases, 34.3% of the total reported in the 12-year period occurred during 1971 and 1972. This sudden increase in incidence is caused primarily by the increased awareness of the problem, one that is certainly not as rare as had been believed.

Of 91 patients admitted to Shanghai Children's Hospital (X.-Y. Liu, personal communication) during 1977 for hemolytic anemia 10 had Rh incompatibility and 81 had ABO incompatibility. Of the 81 ABO incompatible cases, 75.8% of the mothers were type O with the infants' blood type equally distributed between groups A and B.

Because 62 of the infants had to be transferred from rural farming areas, admission was delayed and thus the patients were severely affected. Eight patients died, five of the infants having already developed kernicterus on admission. All the deaths occurred in patients with ABO incompatibility. All of these patients were treated by the standard methods. In addition, on some patients, Chinese herbal medicine was tried. An herbal tea (composed of 15 mg of yin chen, 3 g of zhi dai huang, 9 g of huang lin, and 1.5 g of gan cao) was brewed and given to the infants in liquid form on a daily basis. The treatment was started as early as possible. Usually after 2–3 days of treatment clinical jaundice showed improvement. This prescription has been used for more than a 1000 years in the treatment of neonatal jaundice. Its effects are still subject to further evaluation.

1. Thalassemia in Chinese

Although they are found throughout the world, the α-thalassemias are more prevalent in Southeast Asia and in China. The reported incidence varies greatly. In studies from Thailand, the α-thalassemia gene was present in about 20% of the neonates tested (Kan *et al.*, 1976). Incidence in Chinese has been reported as 1.42% (Lin *et al.*, 1977) to 3% to 4% (Todd *et al.*, 1969), and 5.4% in Filipino newborns (Koenig and Vedvick, 1975).

In China this disease is most frequently seen in Guangdong and in Guangxi. It has recently been reported in Fujian, Jiangsu, Sichuan, and Tibet. The wider distribution may be attributed to the greater mobility of the population during the past 25 years, whereby α-thalassemia, which used to be endemic to certain ethnic groups, is now no longer so. In 1969, Todd *et al.* reported on their study of a random series of 500 samples of umbilical cord blood from Southern Chinese in Guangdong. Of the 500 samples, 16 showed HbBart's, but none showed HbH. One of the 16 was from a stillborn hydropic infant whose cord blood showed 75% HbBart's. In the remaining 15, all from live-birth infants, HbBart's varied from 3.1 to 9.8%. This frequency is similar to the frequency of 3.3% in Chinese and Indonesian Chinese, as reported by Lie-Injo (1959) but lower than that of 6.2% in Thailand, as reported by Weatherall (1963).

Lin *et al.* (1977) reporting a study of the cord blood of 3013 randomly selected newborns found 43 (1.4%) to have small amounts of HbBart's. The incidence in males was 19/1660 and in females 24/1388. The prevalence of heterozygous α-thalassemia in Southern Chinese (primarily from Guangdong and Fujian Provinces) has been reported to be about 3%. In Taiwan, however, Lin and co-workers' report included the children of parents coming from many parts of mainland China. Thus, those authors believe that the overall incidence among all Chinese as randomly represented in Taiwan imigrants may be closer to 1.42%. Unfortunately Lin and associates did not separate their study groups into those parents originating from Southern China and those whose parents originated from other parts of China, or those whose parents were native to Taiwan.

Recently, researchers in China have shown renewed interest in many aspects of thalassemia. Cheng and associates (1978) in a study of the Zhuang minority group in Guangxi Province reported 27 cases of HbCS disease. Xie and associates (1980) from the No. 2 Hospital of Hunan Medical College reported 48 cases of thalassemia for the years 1966 to 1979. Of this series, 44 were β-thalassemia, and 4 were α-thalassemia. More than 2 members had the disorder in 24 families and in one family, 10 persons suffered from the disorder.

Pan and associates (1980) reported 90 cases of thalassemia, 63 with α-thalassemia and 27 with HbH, at Sichuan Medical College between 1973 and

1978. The 90 patients came from 32 different districts in Sichuan Province. Among the 63 who had β-thalassemia, 46 were of Sichuan native origin, 15 were of families that had migrated from Guangdong, all but one were of Han descent. Among the 27 patients with HbH disease, 17 were of Sichuan native origin, 9 of Guangdong migrant families, 1 from a family of Fujian origin. One of the more interesting aspects of the recent research on these disorders by Chinese medical people is an interest in tracing the ethnographic factors in such conditions as thalassemia. In a 1978 report, Zhang and colleagues studied cases of α-thalassemia in the Ningxia region (the Northwest China). Reviewing old literature, they discovered evidence suggesting that cultural and commercial contact between China and Greece, Rome, and other Mediterranean countries had been established by 400–500 BC. They posit that the thalassemias entered China through the contacts made along one of the three routes linking ancient China with the Mediterranean world: the "silk-route"—a land route through the northwestern provinces; another land route through the southwestern provinces, i.e., Sichuan, Yunnan, Guizhou; or through a water route through the coastal provinces.

2. G6PD Deficiency in Chinese

Interest in abnormalities of human red blood cell glucose-6-phosphate dehydrogenase (G6PD), both as causes of various hemolytic disorders and as a useful genetic marker, has increased in recent years. One of the most common genetic enzymatic defects, the deficiency is manifested clinically by hemolysis, neonatal jaundice, and favism (Chan et al., 1964; Yue and Strickland, 1965). Deficiency due to abnormal alleles of the gene responsible for the synthesis of the G6PD molecule is inherited as an X-linked trait.

Original reports from China have been relatively scarce. Those that have appeared recently in Chinese medical literature focused mostly on the clinical aspects of this deficiency, primarily on neonatal hyperbilirubinemia and hemolytic anemia, but with a few on favism.

Favism, a result of G6PD deficiency in which the subjects show severe hemolysis soon after ingesting the fava bean, has long been recognized by rural peasants. In the early 1920's, the peasants of Sichuan Province called it "Hu dao Huan"—"Hu" bean jaundice (Z. X. Yang, personal communication). Since the early 1950's, cases of favism have been reported from Chengdu, Guiyang, Guilin, Shanghai, Guangdong, and Beijing (Du, 1964). The treatment initially was to avoid further ingestion of fava beans and to use herbal medicine to "hasten" the disappearance of jaundice. Because of the poor distribution of modern Western medicine during that period, the rural peasants of the interior provinces depended solely on folklore or village traditional doctors for care of their illnesses.

During the past several years, mass epidemiologic surveys, health education, and preventive measures were carried out in Guangdong Province and the incidence of favism has been dramatically reduced. A mass survey was conducted on the residents of Ningzhong and Nipo communes in the eastern part of Guangdong Province from 1962 to 1965 (Chungshan Medical College, 1977). These communes were chosen because they had the highest incidences of favism in their county. In Ningzhong commune, all 22,714 residents were examined. In Nipo commune, 15,728 were examined, a total that comprised only children less than 15 years of age and the families of school children who were known to be susceptible to fava beans. Incidence of G6PD deficiency in Ningzhong commune was 6.5% in Nipo commune, the incidence in the selected population was 8.2%. Of the 126 residents found to have a history of favism, 104 had G6PD deficiency.

None of the 32 new cases seen in the two communes in the year of the survey had abstained from fava beans, although they had known that they were susceptible. Nine ate a few fava beans with parental consent, five without parental permission, and two ate fava beans as staple food.

Worldwide in distribution, involving many millions of persons, the incidence and severity vary from ethnic group to ethnic group (Gilman, 1974; Jaffe, 1970; Yoshida and Beutler, 1978; Yoshida et al., 1971). Although more common in other ethnic groups, the disorder is not uncommon among Chinese (McCurdy et al., 1966). The deficiency occurs in 2–9% of all Chinese males, the incidence varying by geographic location, provincial residence, and ethnic composition (Chan et al., 1964; Du, 1964). A recent survey from Sichuan (Chinese Academy of Medical Sciences, 1980) of 923 school children (462 boys and 461 girls) reported 41 children with G6PD deficiency, an incidence of 4.4%. Tracing their family origins, part of them were Guangdong Hakka who had migrated to Sichuan. A report from Sichuan Medical College (Liao, 1978) of 91 children with G6PD deficiency (according to WHO standards) admitted to the hospital during the 5-year period from January 1973 to December 1977 found a male to female ratio of 4.7:1. Because the calculated ratio between hemizygous male and homozygous female in a large survey done in Guangdong Province was 24:1 (Du, 1964) the higher incidence of affected females in this group suggests that the heterozygous female from this area may also have hemolysis. Of the 91 children, 60 were from Sichuan Province, 30 from Hunan Province, and 1 from Jiangxi Province. Eighty-four suffered moderate-to-severe anemia. Duration between ingestion of drug, fava bean, or onset of infection and clinical appearance of hemolysis varied from 12 hours to 15 days. The average hemoglobin varied from 4.5 g/dl to 7.6 g/dl. The shorter the duration between precipitating cause and hemolysis, the more severe the hemolysis. Hemolysis followed drug ingestion in 37 cases. In 25 cases hemolysis was precipitated by infection. Fava bean ingestion, which was the cause of the most severe hemolysis and with the shortest time interval, was the precipitating factor in 25 cases.

Some reports state that Chinese newborns suffer more severe neonatal jaundice and kernicterus as a result of G6PD deficiency (Lu et al., 1966; Yeung and Field, 1969; Yue and Strickland, 1965). Yeung and Field reported that 18.5% of the cases of neonatal hyperbilirubinemia among Chinese newborns were caused by G6PD deficiency. The Chungshan Medical College Favism Study and Control Group (1972) reported the figure as 17.3%.

In Guangdong Province two hospitals reported studies on G6PD deficiency. One, for the period April 1974 to March 1975 (Huang and Wu, 1977), covered 123 admissions for neonatal hyperbilirubinemia (16.5% of total neonatal admissions). Of the 117 tested for G6PD deficiency, 54 (32 male and 22 female) were positive, accounting for 46.2% of the total neonatal hyperbilirubinemia. All of the patients came from the surrounding area of Guangzhou. Fourteen of these patients developed kernicterus.

The second Guangdong Province report covered the period of May 1976 to December 1977. Of the 87 patients admitted for neonatal hyperbilirubinemia, 39 had G6PD deficiency. The parents of all were native Guangdong residents. Fourteen of the 39 developed kernicterus. The usual age for developing kernicterus was 4 or 5 days. In addition to standard treatments, herbal medicine was tried on 12 cases. There were nine deaths (23.3%), seven among patients who had severe kernicterus on admission to the hospital who died between 5 and 17 hours after admission. One patient suffered sequelae from kernicterus.

In summary of these three reports, the first from Sichuan Province showed neonatal hyperbilirubinemia was not the main complaint, the provincial origin was two thirds native Sichuan, and no patients died. The second two reports, from Guangdong Province, showed that all were neonatal hyperbilirubinemia cases and all patients were native Guangdong residents who were readmitted after birth. In the two Guangdong Province hospitals, incidence of kernicterus was high (25.9 and 35.9%). In one Guangdong hospital, mortality was 23.3%, all from kernicterus, seven patients having been in a terminal state on admission. These reports confirm the earlier observation that neonatal hyperbilirubinemia of G6PD-deficient infants is extremely serious among Chinese, especially among those of Guangdong Province origin.

H. Lactose Malabsorption

In China, breast-feeding for infants is the rule today as it has been traditionally. If a nursing mother lacks an adequate milk supply for her baby, a friend who is nursing her own baby supplements the supply. Using cow's milk as a substitute for mother's milk is not a common practice, largely because dairy farms are scarce. Most milk substitutes are made from vegetable sources, mainly from soybeans. Once weaned, Chinese rarely drink milk, some people even considering milk-drinking "barbaric," and it has not been accepted widely as a part of the average adult's daily diet. The modern understanding of the nutritional value of milk has brought about some acceptance. Because so few mainland Chinese drink milk there has been little documentation in Chinese scientific or medical literature dealing with the problem of lactose malabsorption. Lactose malabsorption which manifests itself from the early postweaning period into adulthood, has been variously called "lactase deficiency," and "lactose maldigestion." Lactose, the only carbohydrate in milk, is hydrolyzed by the enzyme lactase within the brush border of the cells of the villus of the jejunum (Cajori, 1935). Lactase splits the disaccharide lactose into glucose and galactose. The released glucose is partially utilized directly by the cells of the villus; the remainder, together with galactose, is absorbed into the bloodstream and metabolized by the liver.

In fetal life, lactase begins to appear in the third trimester. Lactase activity reaches a peak level immediately after birth, falling thereafter to a lower level throughout the lactation period. By age 1½–3 years, it usually is almost completely absent (Kretchmer, 1972). In the postweaning population, lactose intolerance is considered the normal state of adults with lactose tolerance being considered statistically abnormal.

Nearly all the data on lactose malabsorption among Chinese, collected since 1963 has been from outside mainland China. The Chinese studies were in Singapore (Bolin et al., 1970), Taiwan (Sung and Shih, 1972), Australia (Bryant et al., 1970; Bolin and Davis, 1970), and the United States (Chung and McGill, 1968). Altogether the total number of subjects studied have been fewer than 200. The largest group consisted of 71 adults from Taiwan Province; the rest of the studies reported 20–30 subjects above the age of 5 years. From these reports, the prevalence of primary adult lactose intolerance among Chinese appear to be between 80 and 100%.

Simoons (1978) analyzed the prevalence rate around the world by geographic areas. In Southeast and East Asia, his composite prevalence rate, including Thai, Chinese, Malays, Japanese, Korean, Filipinos, and Indonesians, was 90%. His latest extensive geographic analysis serves as the evidence to support and supplement his earlier hypothesis, a variant genetic hypothesis he had called the "cultural-historical hypothesis" (Simoons, 1970; Johnson et al., 1974). Recently Simoons (1978) renamed his hypothesis the "geographic hypothesis." By grouping his subjects into ethnic or racial groups, he demonstrated that lactose malabsorption followed a pattern of biologic and cultural interrelationship. The relatively unmixed ethnic groups of the world seem to fall into two major population categories, the lactose malabsorbers (60–100% prevalences) and lactose absorbers (0–30%). A small group of intermediate prevalence is composed of a mixed absorber–malabsorber ancestry. By far the largest number of persons in the world belong to the malabsorber group.

Although lactose intolerance is a common phenomenon among Chinese, the scarcity of milk supply has protected most Chinese living within China from the discomfort of the symptoms. People have long learned from their own experience of milk intolerance either to abstain totally or to drink only small amounts of milk, or to change to sour milk or yogurt, the latter being more accepted as an adult food. Consequently this enzymatic disturbance has not been perceived there as a significant medical problem and has therefore occasioned academic interest primarily.

V. CONCLUSION

In this chapter I have barely touched the surface of biocultural factors of disease and of medical care in China. Some notable omissions include the application of acupuncture to induce analgesic effects and the integration of traditional Chinese methods with modern Western methods in the treatment of burns and of fractures. Nor have I discussed Chinese herbal medicine and "Tai Ji Quan" ("T'ai Chi Ch'uan"), the latter an ancient Chinese exercise regimen to achieve health and tranquility.

This discussion is intended only as an introductory reference for those interested in China and in medical trends there. After the disruption of the Cultural Revolution from 1965 to 1975, China is once again developing scientific inquiry into its diseases. To quote an old Chinese saying: *Pao Zhuan Yui Yu* ("It is hoped that by throwing a brick, one may get a gem in return").

REFERENCES

Bolin, T. D., and Davis, A. E. (1970). Lactose intolerance in Australian-born Chinese. *Aust. Ann. Med.* **19**, 40–41.

Bolin, T. D., Davis, A. E., Seah, C. S., Chua, K. L., Yong, V., Kho, M., Siak, C. L., and Jacob, E. (1970). Lactose intolerance in Singapore. *Gastroenterology* **59**, 76–84.

Bryant, G. D., Chu, Y. K., and Lovit, R. (1970). Incidence and etiology of lactose intolerance. *Med. J. Aust.* **1**, 1285–1288.

Buell, P. (1974). The effect of migration on the risk of NPC among Chinese. *Cancer Res.* **34**, 1189–1191.

Butterfield, F. (1979). After two decades of full control by Peking Tibetans find life better if a bit colonial. *New York Times* June 20, p. 5.

Cajori, F. A. (1935). The lactase activity of the intestinal mucosa of the dog and some characteristics of intestinal lactase. *J. Biol. Chem.* **109**, 159–168.

Chai, M. J. (1977). Recent progress in schistosomiasis control, Shanghai Institute of Parasitic Diseases. *Chin. Med. J. Peking* **3**, 95–99.

Chan, T. K., Rodd, D., and Wong, C. C. (1964). Erythrocyte G-6PD deficiency in Chinese. *Br. Med. J.* **ii**, 102.

Chen, J. (1937). "Xi Zang Wen Ti" (The Tibetan Problem). Commercial Press, Shanghai.

Chen, S. (1976). "Chang Lu Bao Ku—Guangxi" (Guangxi—The Evergreen Treasury), pp. 22-23. Zhong Hua Book Co., Hong Kong.

Cheng, G. F. *et al.* (1978). HbCS disease in Zhuang minority, Guangxi Province. *Chung-hua I Hsueh Tsa Chih (Peking)* **58**, 398-402.

Chinese Academy of Medical Sciences, Institute of Pediatric Research (1977). Survey of Chinese children's growth characteristics. *Chung-hua I Hsueh Tsa Chih (Peking)* **57**, 720-725.

Chinese Academy of Medical Sciences, Sichuan Branch Hospital (1980). Epidemiologic survey of G-6PD in Sichuan Jian Yang District. *Zhongguo Xueyebing Zazhi* **27**, 95-97.

Chu, C. J., and Tsui, T. Y. (1978). Pathologic study of metacarpal-interphalangeal joints in Kaschin-Beck disease. *Chin. Med. J. (Peking)* **4**, 309-313.

Chung, H. F. (1977). How schistosomiasis control work is run in New China. *Chin. Med. J. (Peking)* **3**, 86-94.

Chung, M. H., and McGill, D. B. (1968). Lactase deficiency in Orientals. *Gastroenterology* **54**, 225-226.

Chungshan Medical College, Department of Pathology (1977). Prevention of favism in the rural areas. *Chin. Med. J. (Peking)* **3**, 339-342.

Chungshan Medical College, Favism Study and Control Group (1972). Pathogenesis of favism III: Study of heterozygotes on G-6PD deficiency. *Sinxin Yixue (Guangzhou)* **6**, 26.

Chungshan Medical College, Health Statistics Section, Department of Public Health (1978). Epidemiological investigation of NPC among immigrants (with analysis of mortality). *Chung-hua I Hsueh Tsa Chih (Peking)* **58**, 167-1761.

DeSchryver, A., Friberg, S., Jr., Klein, G., Henle, W., Henle, G., de-Thé, G., Clifford, P., and Ho H. C. (1969). Epstein-Barr virus associated antibody patterns in carcinoma of the post nasal space. *Clin. Exp. Immunol.* **5**, 443-449.

Doll, R., Muir, C., and Waterhouse, J., eds. (1970). "Cancer Incidence in Five Continents." Springer-Verlag, Berlin and New York.

Du, C. S. (1964). Mass survey on hereditary G6PD deficiency in Kwangtung region. *Tianjin Xueyebing Zazhi Suppl.* **2**, 92.

Faust, E. C., and Meleney, H. E. (1924). Studies on *Schistosomiasis japonica. Am. J. Hyg., Monogr. Ser.* **3**, 1-399.

Gilman, P. A. (1974). Hemolysis in the newborn resulting from deficiency of red blood cell enzymes: diagnosis and management. *J. Pediatr.* **84**, 625.

Heilongjiang Endemic Disease Research Institute (1959). "Clinical Survey of Keshan Disease: Observation of 905 Cases." Heilongjiang Endem. Dis. Res. Inst., Heilongjiang, China.

Henle, W., Henle, G., Ho, H. C., Burtin, P., Cachin, Y., Clifford, P., de Schryver, A., de-Thé, G., Diehl, V., and Klein, G. (1970). Antibodies to Epstein-Barr virus in nasopharyngeal carcinomas, other head and neck neoplasms and control groups. *J. Natl. Cancer Inst.* **44**, 225-231.

Ho, J. H. C. (1972). Nasopharyngeal carcinoma. *Adv. Cancer Res.* **15**, 57-82.

Hsia, H. M., Hu, H. M., Chao, Y. L., Hu, C. J., and Niu, J. L. (1977). A survey of herdsmen's serum lipids in Inner Mongolia. *Chin. Med. J. (Peking)* **3**, 343-346.

Huang, S. L., and Wu, S. L. (1977). Acute hemolytic anemia and its relation to G6PD deficiency: report of eight cases. *Sinxin Yixue (Guangzhou)* **8**, 201.

Jaffe, E. R. (1970). Hereditary hemolytic disorders and enzymatic deficiencies of human erythrocytes. *Blood* **35**, 116-134.

Johnson, J. D., Kretchmer, N., and Simoons, F. J. (1974). Lactose metabolism: its biology and history. *Adv. Pediatr.* **21**, 197-237.

Kan, H. C., and Yao, Y. T. (1932). Some notes on the anti-*schistosomiasis japonicum* campaign in Chih-Huai-Pan Xian, Zhechiang. *Chung-hua I Hsueh Tsa Chih (Peking)* **48**, 323-336.

Kan, Y. W., Golbus, M. S., and Dozy, A. M. (1976). Prenatal diagnosis of α-thalassemia: clinical application of molecular hybridization. *N. Engl. J. Med.* **295,** 1165-1167.

Klein, G., Geering, G., Old, L. J., Henle, G., Henle, W., and Clifford, P. (1970). Comparison of the anti-EBV titre and the EBV-associated membrane reactive and precipitating antibody levels in the sera of Burkitt lymphoma and nasopharyngeal carcinomas patients and control. *Int. J. Cancer* **5,** 185-194.

Koenig, H. M., and Vedvick, T. A. (1975). α-Thalassemia in American-born Filipino infants. *J. Pediatr.* **87,** 756-758.

Kretchmer, N. (1972). Lactose and lactase. *Sci. Am.* **227** (4), pp. 71-78.

Ku, Y., and Liu, W. Y. (1959). Statistical analysis of 14,300 cases of tumor registered in Shanghai, 1958. *Chung-hua Ping Li Hsueh Tsa Chih* **4,** 177.

Lai, Y. F. (1960). Preliminary report of epidemiologic survey on concave finger nails in Jiang Zi District, Tibet. *Chung-hua Nei K'o Tsa Chih (Peking)* **8,** 119.

Lamm, S. H., and Sidel, V. W. (1974). Public health in Shanghai: an analysis of preliminary data. *In* "Chinese Medicine As We Saw It" (J. R. Quinn, ed.), pp. 109-144. U.S. Dep. Health, Educ. Welfare, Washington, DC.

Lederman, M. (1961). Its natural history and treatment. *In* "The Clinical Material in Cancer of the Nasopharynx" (M. Friedman, ed.), Chap. 1. Thomas, Springfield, Illinois.

Li, Q. L. (1979). Sudden death—a three-year retrospective survey. *Chung-hua Hsin Hsueh Kuan Ping Tsa Chih* **7,** 14-17.

Liao, C. K. (1978). Predisposing factors on hemolytic anemia due to G6PD deficiency. *Chung-hua Erh K'o Tsa Chih* **1,** 32-34.

Lie-Injo, W. E. (1959). Hemoglobin in newborn infants in Indonesia. *Nature (London)* **183,** 1125.

Lin, K. S., Liu, C. H., Lee, T. C., Blackwell, R. Q., and Huang, J. T. H. (1977). α-Chain thalassemia in Taiwan. *Clin. Pediatr.* **16,** 71-75.

Liu, S. G. (1978). Incidence of congenital anomalies in newborn infants. *Chung-hua I Hsueh Tsa Chih (Peking)* **58,** 24-28.

Liu, S. G. (1978). Incidence of congenital anomalies in newborn infants. *Chin. Med. J.* **58,** 24-28.

Lu, T. C., Wei, H., and Blackwell, R. Q. (1966). Increased incidence of severe hyperbilirubinemia among newborn Chinese infants with G-6-PD deficiency. *Pediatrics* **337,** 994-999.

Lu, Z.-n. (1978). Keshan disease in children, report of 25 cases of acute, severe type. *Sinxin Yixue (Guangzhou)* **9,** 384-385.

McCurdy, P. R., Kirkman, H. N., Naiman, J. L., Jim, R. T. S., and Pickard, B. M. (1966). A Chinese variant of G-6PD. *J. Lab. Clin. Med.* **67,** 374-385.

Mansfield, M. (1977). "China: A Quarter Century After the Founding of the People's Republic," U.S. Senate Report. U.S. Gov. Print. Off., Washington, D.C.

Muir, C. S., and Shanmugaratnam, K. (1967). The incidence of nasopharyngeal carcinoma in Singapore. *In* "Cancer of the Nasopharynx" (C. S. Muir and K. Shanmugaratnam, eds.), UICC Monogr. Ser., Vol. 1, pp. 47-53. Munksgaard, Copenhagen.

Pan, E. T., *et al.* (1980). Report of 90 cases of Mediterranean anemia from Sichuan Province. *Chung-hua Erh K'o Tsa Chih* **18,** 12-14.

Peking Children's Hospital, Editorial Committee (1975). Favism; Growth curves; Kaschin-Beck disease; Keshan disease. *In* "Practical Pediatrics," pp. 155-161; 174; 616-620; 689; 807. Zhong Wai Publ. Co., Beijing.

Simoons, F. J. (1970). Primary adult lactose intolerance and the milking habit; a problem in biologic and cultural interrelation, II, a cultural-historical hypothesis. *Am. J. Dig. Dis.* **15,** 695-710.

Simoons, F. J. (1978). The geographic hypothesis and lactose malabsorption: a weighing of the evidence. *Am. J. Dig. Dis.* **23,** 963-980.

Sullivan, W. (1979). China takes ambitious steps to end a deadly fever. *New York Times* Sept. 17, p. 10.

Sung, J. L., and Shih, P. L. (1972). The jejunal dissaccharidase activity and lactose intolerance of Chinese adults. *Asian J. Med.* **8,** 149–151.

Tan, X. Z. (1976). "Zhong Guo Shao Shu Min Zu Xin Mao" (The New Outlook of Minorities in China). Shanghai Book Co., Hong Kong.

Todd, D., Lai, M. C. S., Braga, C. A., and Soo, H. N. (1969). α-Thalassemia in Chinese cord-blood studies. *Br. J. Haematol.* **16,** 551–556.

U.S. Department of Health, Education and Welfare (DHEW) (1978). "Supply and Distribution of Physicians and Physician Extenders," DHEW Publ. No. HRA 78-11 U.S. Gov. Print. Off., Washington D.C.

Weatherall, D. J. (1963). Abnormal haemoglobins in the neonatal period and their relationship to thalassemia. *Br. J. Haematol.* **9,** 265.

Wen, C. P. (1974). Nasopharyngeal cancer. *In* "Chinese Medicine As We Saw It" (J. R. Quinn, ed.), pp. 287–344. U.S. Dep. Health, Educ. Welfare, Washington, D.C.

Wu, T. Y., Wen, G. Z., and Shen, S. D. (1978). An investigation of concave finger nails in Qinghai Province. *Chung-hua I Hsueh Tsa Chih (Peking)* **58,** 244.

Xie, Z. W., *et al.* (1980). Analysis of 48 cases of thalassemia in Hunan province. *Chung-hua Erh K'o Tsa Chih* **18,** 15–17.

Yeung, C. Y., and Field, C. E. (1969). Phenobarbitone therapy in neonatal hyperbilirubinemia. *Lancet* **ii,** 135.

Yoshida, A., and Beutler, E. (1978). Human G6PD variants: a supplementary tabulation. *Ann. Hum. Genet.* **41,** 347–355.

Yoshida, A., Beutler, E., and Motulsky, A. G. (1971). Table of human G6PD variants. *Bull. W. H. O.* **45,** 243–253.

Yue, P. C. K., and Strickland, M. (1965). G6PD deficiency and neonatal jaundice in Chinese male infants in Hong Kong. *Lancet* **i,** 350.

Zhang, G. H., *et al.* (1978). Survey on thalassemia in Ningxia region. *Zhongguo Xueyebing Zazhi* **2,** 8–11.

Zhao, Q. S., and Wang, X. Y. (1978). Shanghai Institute of Hypertension, a comparative study of epidemiology in the urban and rural areas of Shanghai. *Chung-hua Hsin Hsueh Kuan Ping Sa Chih* **7,** 14–17.

Zhu, D. E., *et al.* (1980). Study of abnormal Hb in Gongxi Province. *Zhongguo Xueyebing Zazhi* **1,** 66–71.

12

Diseases of Finland and Scandinavia

REIJO NORIO

I. INTRODUCTION

Finland, one of the northernmost countries of the world, is situated in northern Europe, between Scandinavia and the Soviet Union, and between latitudes 60 and 70 (Fig. 1). Its greatest length is more than 1100 km, its area about 337,000 km², and its population nearly 5 million, which gives a density of about 15 inhabitants to 1 km² of land area. Scandinavia includes Sweden and Norway, generally also Denmark, with 8, 4, and 5 million inhabitants, respectively. These four countries and Iceland are also called the Nordic countries.

The main task of this chapter is to describe the disease pattern of Finland, whereas the diseases of Scandinavia are dealt with superficially, as background

359

BIOCULTURAL ASPECTS OF DISEASE

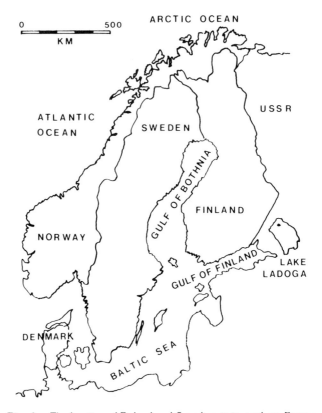

Fig. 1. The location of Finland and Scandinavia in northern Europe.

reference for the Finnish data. There are two reasons for this. First, the Finnish disease pattern is in many ways exceptional and therefore interesting, whereas no such singularity is known to exist in the Scandinavian countries. Second, the writer's nationality and research interests naturally conduct this report along such lines. Here, attention is focused mainly on genetic features.

The main topics to be discussed are as follows:

1. The specific pattern of rare hereditary diseases in Finland, or "the Finnish disease heritage."

2. The excessive mortality among the Finns, especially that from coronary heart disease and its uneven distribution within the country.

After the medical data on each topic are presented, aspects of the population history and structure are discussed to provide a background for understanding the exceptional circumstances.

TABLE I

Rare Recessive Diseases Accumulated in Finland[a]

| Disease | Number of patients known | | Estimated incidence in Finland |
	In Finland	Elsewhere	
Aspartylglucosaminuria	130	20	1:26,000
Autoimmune polyendocrinopathy— candidiasis—ectodermal dystrophy	40	100	1:30,000
Cartilage—hair hypoplasia	40	80	
Choroideremia (X linked)	90	200	
Congenital chloride diarrhea	30	30	1:30,000
Congenital nephrotic syndrome of Finnish type	200	200	1:8,000
Cornea plana congenita	50	20	
Diastrophic dysplasia	70	200	
Dystrophia retinae pigmentosa—dysacusis	200	?	1:30,000 (prevalence)
Hereditary fructose intolerance	20	100	
Hydrolethalus syndrome	30	—	1:20,000 (at least)
Hyperornithinemia with gyrate atrophy of the choroid and retina	40	30	
Inherited systemic amyloidosis with corneal lattice dystrophy (dominant)	210	?	
Lysinuric protein intolerance	30	10	1:60,000
Meckel's syndrome	40	100	1:10,000
Mulibrey nanism	30	5	
Muscle, eye and brain disease	15	1	
Neuronal ceroid lipofuscinosis			
Infantile type	70	30	1:13,000
Childhood (Jansky-Bielschowsky) type	20	?	
Juvenile (Spielmeyer-Sjögren) type	100	?	
Nonketotic hyperglycinemia	25	100	1:55,000
Polycystic lipomembranous osteodysplasia with sclerosing leukoencephalopathy	14	15	
Progressive myoclonus epilepsy	110	100	1:20,000
Retinoschisis (X linked)	220	100	
Salla disease	25	—	
Selective malabsorption of vitamin B_{12}	30	30	

[a] Based on data from several authors, cited in the text.

II. THE FINNISH DISEASE HERITAGE

The concept "the Finnish disease heritage" is about 10 years old. During that decade, more than 20 rare, mostly autosomal recessive diseases have been found to be unusually common in Finland; in many of the diseases, as shown in Table I, more cases are known in Finland than in the other parts of the world altogether. Some of them were first described in Finland. On the other hand, many inherited diseases that are quite common elsewhere are very rare if not absent in Finland.

Before discussing the causes of this peculiar situation, I will briefly describe the individual diseases in alphabetical order.

A. Rare Inherited Diseases Accumulated in Finland

Unless separately mentioned, the diseases described are transmitted by an autosomal recessive gene. Whereas Table I shows the numbers of known patients in Finland and elsewhere as well as the estimated incidences in Finland, Fig. 2 shows the geographical distribution within Finland.

Generally the descriptions are based on the data given by different authors for a poster exhibition at the Seventh Sigrid Juselius Symposium, "Population Genetic Studies on Isolates," in Mariehamn, Åland Islands (Norio and Nevanlinna, 1978). Those data as well as the papers of that symposium have also been published in "Population Structure and Genetic Disorders," edited by Eriksson *et al.* (1980). Pictures pertaining to the diseases will be found there and in two other references on hereditary diseases in Finland (Perheentupa, 1972c; Norio *et al.*, 1973).

1. Aspartylglucosaminuria (AGU)

A lysosomal storage disease with slowly progressive coarseness of the habitus and mental retardation, aspartylglucosaminuria, was discovered in Finland in connection with a search for phenylketonuria through the institutions for the mentally retarded. An unknown spot in urinary chromatographic analysis led to the tracks of this new disease (Palo, 1967). In the same year, Jenner and Pollitt (1967) described two affected siblings in Great Britain. In addition to the studies of Palo and co-workers (Palo and Matsson, 1970; Palo and Savolainen, 1973), the disease has been further investigated by the working group of Autio and Aula (Autio, 1972, 1980; Autio *et al.*, 1973a,b; Haltia *et al.*, 1975; Aula *et al.*, 1976).

Usually the patient develops normally in the first year of life, except for proneness to infections and hernias. The symptoms begin insidiously during

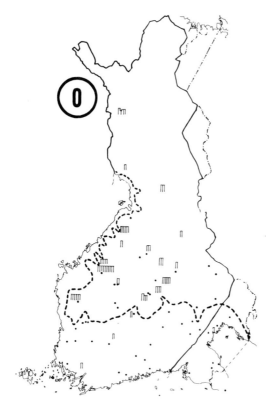

Fig. 2. The geographical distribution of the 24 diseases included in the Finnish disease heritage. The dots on the maps indicate the birthplaces of parents, grandparents, or great-grandparents of the patients. On some maps squares and parts of squares are used: a whole square indicates that all four grandparents of the obligatory heterozygotes (parents of the patients) were born in the same locality (= certain source of a gene); a part of a square shows how many such grandparents were born there (uncertain source of a gene). The eastern areas indicated in some maps by a broken line belonged to Finland before World War II. [Data from several authors cited in the text, published in the book "Population Structure and Genetic Disorders" (A. W. Eriksson *et al.*, eds.). Academic Press, London and New York, 1980.] (2/0) Background for the geographical distribution of the diseases. The broken line gives the northern and eastern boundary of the permanent settlement at the beginning of the 1500s. Schematic pedigrees show consanguinities between several parents of patients suffering from the congenital nephrotic syndrome (CNF); almost all of them are in the area of late settlement. The dots indicate the birth places of CNF parents who have not been found to be related to the other CNF parents. In most of the following maps the ancestry of the patients is situated mainly in the area of late settlement.

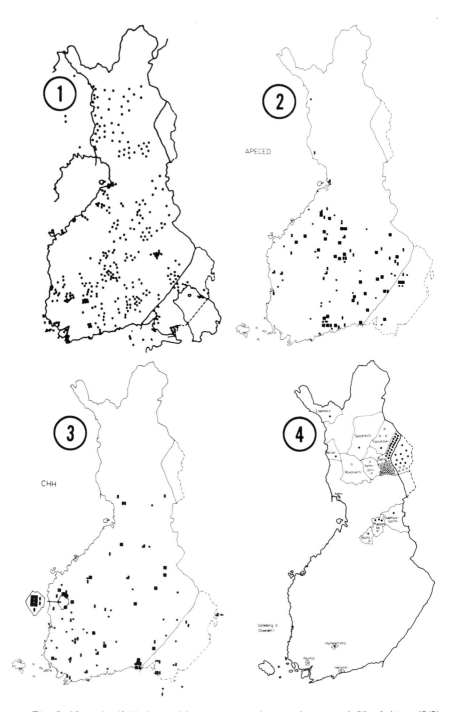

Fig. 2 (Cont.) (2/1) Aspartylglucosaminuria: the grandparents of 85 sibships. (2/2) Autoimmune polyendocrinopathy−candidosis−ectodermal dystrophy: the great-grandparents of 28 families. (2/3) Cartilage hair hypoplasia: the great-grandparents of 28 families. (2/4) Choroideremia (X-chromosomal); 40 mothers with affected sons (black dot) and 49 ophthalmoscopically detected carriers of the gene with no affected sons (circle).

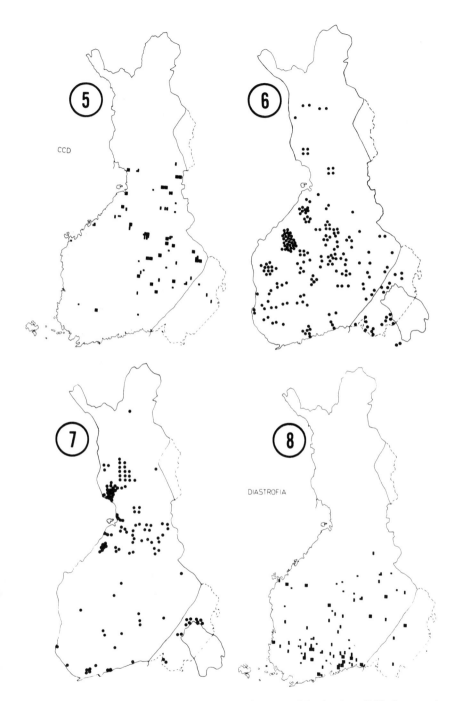

(2/5) Congenital chloride diarrhea: the great-grandparents of 21 families. (2/6) Congenital nephrotic syndrome of Finnish type: the grandparents of 57 families. (2/7) Corneal plana congenita: the grandparents of 32 families. (2/8) Diastrophic dysplasia: the great-grandparents of 25 families.

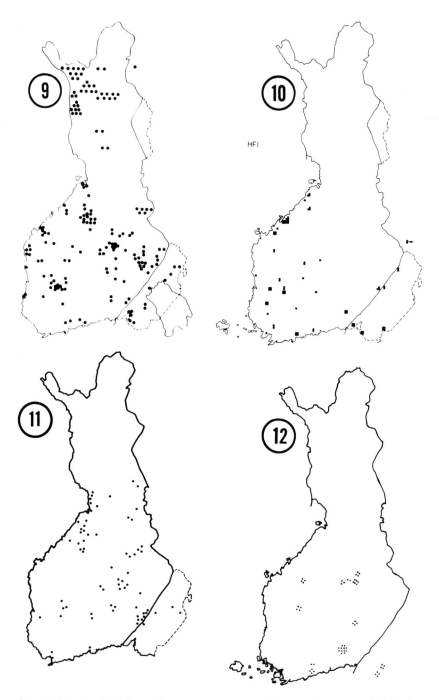

Fig. 2 (Cont.) (2/9) Dystrophia retinae pigmentosa–dysacusis: the parents of 89 families. (2/10) Hereditary fructose intolerance: the great-grandparents of 12 families. (2/11) Hydrolethalus syndrome: the grandparents of 18 families. (2/12) Hyperornithinemia with gyrate atrophy of the choroid and retina: the grandparents of 14 families.

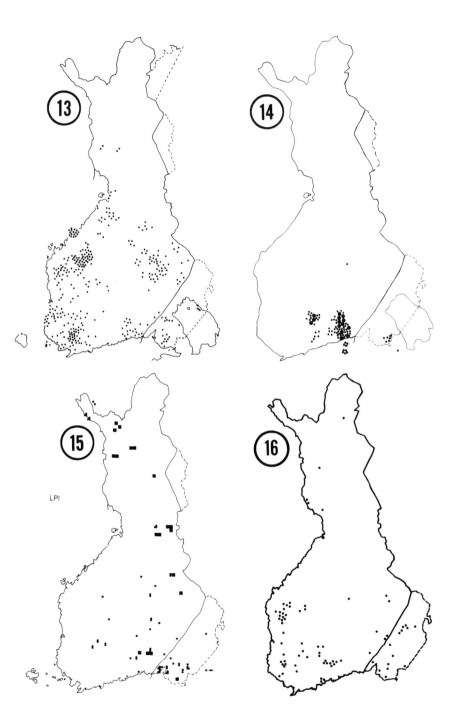

(2/13) Infantile type of neuronal ceroid-lipofuscinosis: the great-grandparents of 44 families.
(2/14) Inherited systemic amyloidosis with corneal lattice dystrophy (dominant): the affected
parents of 207 patients. A big dot indicates 10 parents. (2/15) Lysinuric protein intolerance:
the great-grandparents of 20 families. (2/16) Meckel's syndrome: the grandparents of 20 families.

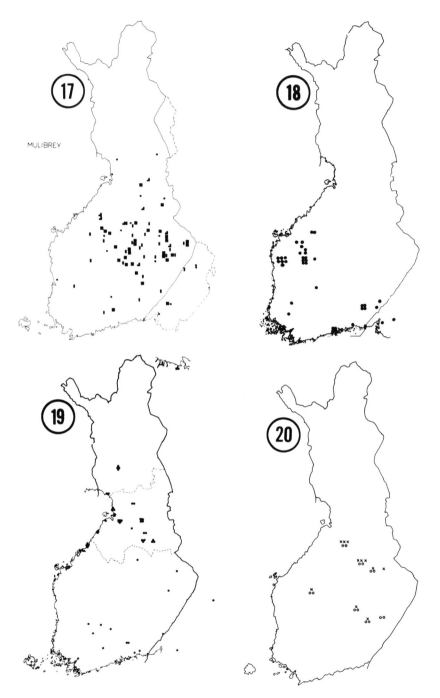

Fig. 2 (Cont.) (2/17) Mulibrey nanism: the great-grandparents of 28 families. (2/18) Muscle, eye, and brain disease: the grandparents of 10 families. (2/19) Nonketotic hyperglycinemia: the grandparents of 13 families. (2/20) Polycystic lipomembranous osteodysplasia with sclerosing leukoencephalopathy: the parents of 7 families (circle) and their children (cross).

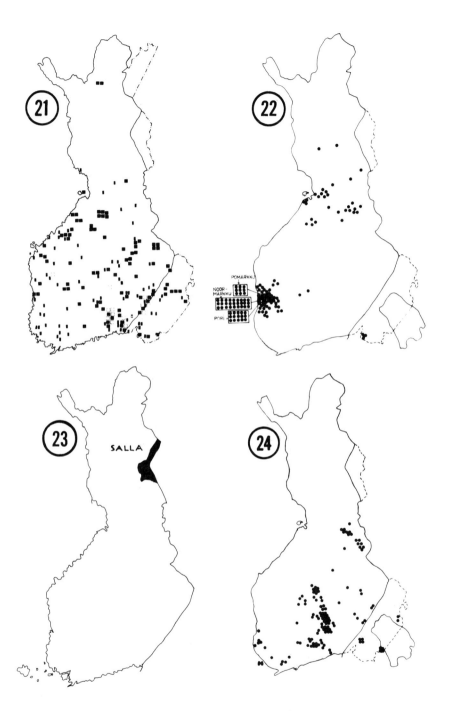

(2/21) Progressive myoclonus epilepsy: the grandparents of 74 families. (The white squares indicate the families found during the investigation.) (2/22) Retinoschisis X-chromosomalis: 127 mothers with affected sons. (2/23) Salla disease: most of the patients up to now originate from Salla. (2/24) Selective malabsorption of vitamin B_{12}: the great-grandparents of 16 families.

preschool age. Delayed speech, learning difficulties, stubborn and restless behavior, clumsiness, and hypotonia appear. In adults, the disease is characterized by severe retardation, poor speech, often short stature, and sometimes by erethistic or manic periods. Additional features are thick calvarium, osteoporosis, spontaneous fractures, and vertebral osteochondrosis. The afflicted person may die when less than 40 years of age. No specific treatment is available.

The diagnosis can be confirmed by the demonstration of aspartylglucosamine (2-acetamido-1(β-L-aspartamido)-1,2-dideoxy-glucose, AADG) in the urine by several chromatographic methods (Autio, 1972). Vacuolated lymphocytes and monocytes appear in the peripheral blood and the bone marrow specimen. The histological alterations of the brain are neuronal cell loss and gliosis, especially in the cortex. Storage lysosomes can be demonstrated in several tissues.

The pathogenetic basis is the defective activity of N-aspartyl-β-D-glucosaminidase (AADGase), demonstrable in peripheral blood lymphocytes and cultured skin fibroblasts, among others. This abnormality leads to the defective breakdown of the aspartylglucosamine and the intralysosomal storage of abnormal catabolites. In heterozygotes the activity of AADGase is intermediately low in blood lymphocytes and cultured skin fibroblasts. Prenatal diagnosis is possible by demonstrating the low activity of AADGase in the culture of amniotic cells. Until now, such tests have not been done, because the number of children in the family is usually "final" by the time this insidious disease is diagnosed in the proband.

2. Autoimmune Polyendocrinopathy–Candidosis–Ectodermal Dystrophy (APECED)

The long name characterizes well this disease, also called chronic mucocutaneous candidiasis with endocrinopathy (Amman and Fudenberg, 1976) or the syndrome of hypoparathyroidism, moniliasis, and adrenocortical insufficiency. Thorpe and Handley of the United States (1929) described it. In Finland, Visakorpi and Gerber (1963) gave the first report, Perheentupa and co-workers several more (Perheentupa, 1972b, 1980, 1981; Myllärniemi and Perheentupa, 1978; Perheentupa et al., 1981).

The clinical picture varies considerably. It consists of manifestations from three groups: dystrophic features of ectodermal tissues, signs of cellular immunity defects, and endocrine gland hypofunction due to autoimmune destruction. The dystrophic ectodermal findings include alopecia and vitiligo, punctate nail alterations, keratoconjunctivitis, and enamel hypoplasia of the permanent teeth.

As a sign of defective cellular immunity, a mucocutaneous candidiasis appears in most cases in varying extent and severity, often from infancy and before the endocrinological manifestations appear. Cheilosis (rhagades at the corner of the mouth) is a typical finding. Cutaneous anergy to tuberculin can often be demonstrated. Among the great variety of endocrine defects, hypoparathyroidism is the most common and often the first one. Hypoadrenocorticism, ovarian or testicular atrophy, diabetes mellitus, and hypothyroidism may appear in varying order and age. Steatorrhea and pernicious anemia are further signs of autoimmunity disorders.

The pathogenetic details and interconnections between the ectodermal and immunological phenomena are unknown.

Treatment that would stop the disease process is not available. Substitution therapy for endocrine deficiencies is essential; constant alertness is needed to detect and treat new endocrine defects. Topical antifungal treatment is useful. The prognosis *quoad vitam* is usually good but depends on the endocrinological components.

Heterozygotes are not demonstrable nor is prenatal diagnosis available.

3. Cartilage-Hair Hypoplasia (CHH)

Cartilage-hair hypoplasia is the original and easily remembered name for a considerable benign skeletal dysplasia, later named orthodoxically but not very imaginatively as metaphyseal chondrodysplasia, type McKusick. Maroteaux *et al.* (1963) and McKusick (1964) described it from the Amish isolate (see also McKusick *et al.*, 1965). Perheentupa (1972a) reported it as belonging to the Finnish disease heritage. Since then, a few detailed Finnish studies have come out (Rönning *et al.*, 1978; Virolainen *et al.*, 1978; Kaitila and Perheentupa, 1980), whereas a larger Finnish investigation of J. Kaitila and co-workers is in progress.

This disproportionate dwarfism is of rhizomelic type, i.e., the femora and humeri are particularly short. The hands and feet are short, the fingers pudgy and lax. The limitation of extension of the cubital articuli and bowlegs are common. On X ray metaphyseal splaying and irregular growth plates are seen; the alterations diminish by adulthood. The joints are almost unaffected.

Most patients have sparse and thin hair—eyebrows, beard, and axillary hair included. In infancy, intestinal malabsorption or colonic aganglionosis (Hirschsprung's disease) is often associated with CHH.

Exceptional reaction to·viral infections, such as severe and even fatal varicella or intractable infectious diarrhea, has been reported. These findings are not common in the Finnish patients. Alterations in cellular immune response are demonstrable (Lux *et al.*, 1970).

Although the adult height remains below 140 cm (4 ft 7 in.), the disease is in general "benign," without essential articular symptoms and compatible with "normal" life. Heterozygotes are not diagnosable and prenatal diagnosis has not been done; the shortness of the extremities, though recognizable in newborns, is hardly visible on X ray during the second trimester of pregnancy.

4. Choroideremia

This X-chromosomal eye disease was reported by Mauthner (1872), and the first time in Finland by Takki (1974b). Forsius and his group are working on an extensive study of large kindreds in northern Finland, the part of the country where most of the known patients come from (see also McCulloch and McCulloch 1948; Kurstjens, 1965; Forsius *et al.*, 1980a).

The affected men show symptoms resembling those of "retinitis pigmentosa": hemeralopia (with the first symptoms at school age), narrowing of the visual fields, and more or less pronounced blindness, even though usually at a rather late age (around 50 years). Ophthalmoscopically, increasing whitish atrophy of the retinal pigment layer and choriocapillaris is seen.

The carrier females are recognizable through progressive fundus changes that resemble those of retinitis pigmentosa but cause no or insignificant symptoms. The pathogenesis is unknown, as is specific treatment. Many patients are capable of doing their normal work until late middle age. The possibility of ophthalmoscopical detection of the carriers helps in genetic counseling. The carrier females should be told that they will not lose their vision, although every ophthalmologist, without knowing the correct diagnosis of the affected relative, would probably pronounce the fateful diagnosis of retinitis pigmentosa to her.

Prenatal diagnosis is not possible, but selective abortion of male fetuses may be considered after prenatal sex determination, if the family feel the burden of the disease to be heavy enough to justify abortion.

5. Congenital Chloride Diarrhea (CCD)

An inborn watery diarrhea, congenital chloride diarrhea, is characterized by excessive concentration of chloride ion in the colonic contents. Unless the condition is diagnosed correctly, the patients invariably die as newborns, whereas the correct diagnosis makes easy treatment and almost normal life possible. The disease was first described by Gamble *et al.* (1945) and Darrow (1945). The first

Finnish report was by Perheentupa *et al.* (1965). For further Finnish studies see Launiala *et al.* (1967), Norio *et al.* (1971a), Holmberg *et al.* (1977), and Holmberg and Perheentupa (1980); other references include Evanson and Stanburry (1965) and Bieberdorf *et al.* (1972).

The clinical picture in a newborn is typical and specific. Hydramnion is the first unfailing sign of the disease. Lack of meconium, excessive weight loss, dehydration, and neonatal icterus during the first few days of life are explained when the abundant watery diarrhea, often first mistaken for urine, is noticed. If the condition remains untreated, severe electrolyte disturbance develops—first hyponatremia, hypochloridemia, and acidosis and, later, hypokalemia and alkalosis (and hyperaldosteronism with renal histological alterations). High fecal chloride concentration (> 90 mmol/liter) confirms the diagnosis.

The basic defect is impaired active Cl^-/CHO_3^- exchange in the ileum and colon. Thus, an excess of chloride ion remains in the colon and causes osmotic diarrhea. This excess and defective secretion of bicarbonate ion secondarily lead to other disturbances of the fluid and electrolyte balance.

Without the correct diagnosis and treatment, the patients die during the first months of life. Adequate treatment—after correction of the fluid balance in the acute phase—consists of life-long oral replacement of NaCl, KCl, and water. This treatment probably maintains normal development and life despite moderate diarrhea.

Prenatal diagnosis is not available and its indications would apparently be controversial. The electrolyte concentrations in the amniotic fluid are normal.

6. Congenital Nephrotic Syndrome of Finnish Type (CNF)

This "prototype" of the Finnish disease heritage (see Section II,D,2) is a lethal nephrotic syndrome manifesting at an uncommon age for nephrosis. Before the first Finnish description of CNF by Hallman *et al.* (1956) several solitary case reports of possible CNF patients can be found (e.g., Ashby, 1901; Gautier and Miville, 1942). The disease has been actively studied by a large group of investigators close to Hallman (see Norio, 1966, 1980; Hallman *et al.*, 1970, 1973; Huttunen, 1976).

The first signs of the congenital character of the disease are the invariably large placenta (more than 25% of the birth weight) and often the premature birth of small-for-date baby. The signs of a nephrotic syndrome, namely, edema, heavy proteinuria, and nephrotic dysproteinemia, are found during the first days or at least during the first weeks of life. Further features are failure to thrive (patients never learn to walk), severe susceptibility to infections, bulging abdomen due to meteorism and ascites, resistance to medication, and death usually before age 2 years and always before 4 years. The immediate cause of death often remains unknown; often it is an infection, never uremia. The treatment is only symptomatic. Attempts at renal transplantation have failed.

The histological alterations of the kidneys cover a broad spectrum both qualitatively and quantitatively, showing glomerular, tubular, and interstitial changes. The most typical though not pathognomonic lesions are tubular dilatations (Hallman et al., 1973).

The pathogenesis is obscure. Some structural disturbances of the glomerular basement membrane have been proposed. The number of nephrons present is twice that of normal (Tryggvason and Kouvalainen, 1975).

Prenatal diagnosis is possible and has been done in Finland more than 20 times without a single mistaken diagnosis (Seppälä et al., 1976; Aula et al., 1978). The α-fetoprotein (AFP) concentration is elevated in the amniotic fluid, apparently due to fetal proteinuria. Thus, screening all pregnancies for AFP concentration in the maternal serum, to prevent the birth of newborns with neural tube defects, would eradicate CNF from the population in Finland. The diagnosis of CNF in an aborted mid-trimester fetus can be reached by electron microscopy (Aula et al., 1978) and, according to recent investigation, also by light microscopic examination (Rapola, 1981).

Several cases of CNF have been found in Minnesota, United States, where active immigration from Finland has taken place. There are also other types of familial infantile nephrosis (Vernier et al., 1957; Habib and Bois, 1973; Norio, 1981). Their exact place in disease classification is unclear. The "microcystic renal disease" presented by Oliver (1960) and misinterpreted by many, is probably not an etiological entity and thus should not be used as a synonym for CNF.

7. Cornea Plana Congenita

This congenital eye disease was described by Rübel of Germany (1912) and in Finland by Forsius (1957) (see also Forsius, 1961; Eriksson et al., 1973; Forsius et al., 1980b). The cornea is not flat but less convex than is usual, the radius of its convexity being similar to that of the sclera. The cornea is thin, the sclerocorneal boundary broad and hazy, resulting in microcornea, at least functionally. In the middle of the cornea an opaque area about 5 mm in diameter may be seen. A strong "arcus senilis" develops at an early age, probably caused by the alleviated transport of lipid particles into the extremely thin cornea. The visual acuity is more or less decreased permanently; hyperopia is a frequent sign. In severe cases, iris anomalies may occur. Also, a milder, dominant type of cornea plana is known.

8. Diastrophic Dysplasia

This severe disturbance of skeletal growth and development, described by Lamy and Maroteaux (1960) and mentioned the first time in Finland by Perheentupa (1972a), is at present subjected to a multidimensional nationwide study by Kaitila and co-workers in Finland (see also Langer, 1965; Walter, 1970; Walker *et al.*, 1972; Kaitila, 1980).

The disease is easily recognized from the bizarre complex of symptoms. The extremities are short from birth. Clubfootlike deformity, hitchhiker's thumb, stiffness of some phalangeal articuli in fingers, and the cystic swelling and later nodular deformations of the earlobes form a unique combination of signs. Cleft palate and a birdlike profile with roundish tip of nose and small chin often complete the picture. The large articuli are deformed, their mobility being at first too great but later on more and more limited, especially in the hips and knees. Severe kyphoscoliosis may develop.

X rays show the tubular bones to be short and thick, the epiphyses flattened and deformed. The first metacarpal is oval or triangular. Later, the mushroomlike deformity of hips with arthrotic changes is typical.

The pathogenesis is unknown, as is specific treatment. The prognosis depends on the function of the big articuli and on the possible kyphoscoliosis; the handicap may be severe. Active physiotherapy and follow-up is essential, whereas success with surgical treatment may be slight, except with the correction of foot deformity. The adult height is between 80 and 135 cm (32–53 inches). To my knowledge, the attempts at prenatal diagnosis have not been successful.

9. Dystrophia Retinae Pigmentosa – Dysacusis (DRD)

This combination of sensorineural hearing impairment and pigmentary retinal dystrophy was described by von Graefe of Germany (1858) and in Finland by Nuutila (1968, 1970; see also Forsius *et al.*, 1971; Nuutila, 1980).

The deafness is congenital, severe, and nonprogressive. The visual symptoms, typical for so-called retinitis pigmentosa, appear before or during school age and are progressive. They can be diagnosed by extinguished electroretinogram before the visual symptoms appear. Other possible signs of CNS involvement are secondary or incidental. The speed and grade of visual loss vary, but the loss is often severe at young adult age.

In Nuutila's opinion, the Finnish DRD is identical to syndromes described by Usher (1913–1914) of England, Hallgren (1959) of Sweden, and Lindenov (1945) of Denmark. In addition to the typical DRD, cases of milder and slower impairment of hearing and vision appear in Finland; their nosological position is not clear.

10. Hereditary Fructose Intolerance (HFI)

Froesch *et al.* (1957) described this disease from Switzerland, Perheentupa *et al.* (1962) from Finland. It is also called fructose-1-phosphate aldolase deficiency and, incorrectly, fructosemia. As with other intolerance diseases, the patient remains healthy unless he eats that for which he has an intolerance—in this condition, fructose (sucrose). Ingestion of fructose causes symptoms and signs ranging from poor thriving to sudden death. They derive from the small intestine (vomiting, anorexia, and poor thriving), from the liver (hepatomegaly, jaundice, hypoproteinemia, bleeding, tendency, and hypoglycemia that may be fatal), and from renal tubuli (proteinuria, glucosuria, aminoaciduria, and acidosis). The patients develop a strong aversion to sweet taste (Perheentupa, 1975, 1980; Froesch, 1978).

The primary fault is the defect of fructose-1-phosphate aldolase, normally present in the liver, kidneys, and the mucosa of the small intestine. From ingested fructose, fructose-1-phosphate accumulates in those organs, with depletion of adenine nucleotides, inhibition of glycogenolysis and glyconeogenesis, and other metabolic failures.

The patient's condition dramatically improves after fructose has been excluded from his diet. The diagnosis can be confirmed by an intravenous fructose test, which causes a fall in the serum phosphate and blood glucose concentration. The patients remain healthy if they can avoid fructose, whereas an infusion of fructose-containing fluid in parenteral fluid therapy may be fatal.

11. Hydrolethalus Syndrome

This lethal malformation syndrome was recently described by Salonen *et al.* (1981) in 28 newborn infants from 18 Finnish families. No patients have been reported from elsewhere. The name points to the three most obvious features: hydramnion, hydrocephalus, and lethality. The striking complex of malformations comprises an unusual structural alteration of the brain with lateral ventricles opening into the subarachnoidal space, a keyhole-shaped defect of the occipital bone, a very small mandible, polydactyly (usually postaxial in hands, preaxial or postaxial in feet), a heart malformation including ventricular septal defect, and anomalies of the larynx, trachea, and/or lungs. Contrary to their state in the Meckel syndrome (see page 379) the kidneys and liver are normal and not cystic.

Prenatal diagnosis has been done twice before the twentieth week of pregnancy by detecting the hydrocephaly ultrasonographically. The value of AFP-determination in amniotic fluid is not yet known.

The hydrolethalus syndrome represents a congenital hydrocephalic condition with an unusually high (25%) risk of recurrence in sibs. That is why it should be recognized by the pediatrician, obstetrician, and pathologist, who all share the responsibility of a stillborn or dying malformed infant.

12. Hyperornithinemia With Gyrate Atrophy of the Choroid and Retina (HOGA)

Gyrate atrophy of the choroid and retina has been known since the nineteenth century (Cutler, 1895), but the constant association of hyperornithinemia in that condition was detected by Simell and Takki (1973) of Finland (see also Takki, 1974a,b; Takki and Simell, 1974; Sipilä et al., 1980). This association has since then been confirmed by several investigators outside of Finland (McCulloch and Marliss, 1975; Berson et al., 1976; Valle et al., 1977; O'Donnell et al., 1978).

The ocular symptoms resemble those of "retinitis pigmentosa" having begun by the age of 5–9 years and leading to practical blindness by the early forties. The ophthalmoscopic picture is typical, with sharply demarcated whitish patches of chorioretinal atrophy that begin in the midperiphery of the eyeground, and enlarge, coalesce, and spread toward the posterior pole of the eye.

The patients also show a slightly decreased capacity in fast muscular performances but no ordinary muscular weakness or hypotonia. Electromyography reveals a myopathic pattern from a part of the fibers of the proximal muscles. Histologically, the type II fibers are decreased in number and show atrophic areas that on electron microscopy are filled with subsarcolemmal tubular aggregates. Abnormal systolic time intervals in the electrocardiogram of some patients are apparently signs of myocardial affection.

The hyperornithinemia is caused by the decreased activity of ornithine transaminase, which can be measured in cultured fibroblasts and lymphocytes. The high ornithine level inhibits the rate-limiting enzyme of creatine synthesis and probably leads to deficiency of creatine, creatine phosphate, and readily available energy.

Active attempts are in progress to find a preventive treatment for the visual loss. With a diet free from protein, ornithine, and arginine, the plasma ornithine concentration decreased to normal values and some visual functions of the patients improved (Valle et al., 1980; Kaiser-Kupfer et al., 1980). After supplementation of creatine, the amount of atrophic muscle fibers diminished and the visual deterioration seemed to be arrested (Sipilä et al., 1981). On the other hand, massive doses of vitamin B_6, the coenzyme of ornithine transaminase, did not give measurable response in Finnish patients.

In heterozygotes the activity of ornithine transaminase is half the normal mean in fibroblasts and lymphocytes. Prenatal diagnosis for homozygotes apparently is possible but has not been done so far. If preventive treatment becomes available, the neonatal screening of homozygotes would be sensible in Finland to prevent the visual loss in such patients.

13. Infantile Type of Neuronal Ceroid-Lipofuscinosis (INCL)

From the group of neuronal ceroid-lipofuscinoses, the childhood (Jansky–Bielschowsky) type and the juvenile (Spielmeyer–Sjögren) type are not infrequent in Finland and they are also well known in other countries. The adult type or Kufs' disease is extremely rare in Finland. On the other hand, the infantile (Santavuori-Haltia) type is surprisingly common in Finland and almost unknown in other countries. In fact, infants whose disease used to be diagnosed by Tay-Sachs disease in Finland have more likely suffered from this fatal degenerative brain disease. The first description came from Sweden (Hagberg *et al.*, 1968); many other reports have been published from Finland (Santavuori *et al.*, 1973, 1974; Haltia *et al.*, 1973; Santavuori, 1980).

After normal development in the first year of life, a rapid decline in psychomotor skills and development begins at the age of 12 to 18 months. Ataxia, myoclonic jerks, "knitting" movements of the hands, muscular hypotonia, and attacks of opisthotonic posture are typical. Extreme psychomotor deterioration is associated with the losses of hearing and vision, typical alteration of the eyegrounds with extinguished electroretinogram (Raitta and Santavuori, 1973), typical EEG changes with isoelectric pattern by age 3 years (Santavuori, 1973), and severe microcephaly. Spastic contractures with vita minima develop after the age of 5 years, and death usually occurs by age 10 years.

The striking histological feature is brain atrophy of an extraordinary degree, due to the loss of neurons. The remaining cells contain lipofuscin-like material (Haltia and Rapola, 1973). The pathogenesis is not known; an inborn error of arachidonic acid metabolism has been assumed (Svennerholm *et al.*, 1975). Prenatal diagnosis is not available.

14. Inherited Systemic Amyloidosis With Corneal Lattice Dystrophy

Corneal lattice dystrophy was described by Biber (1890) and later by many authors. Meretoja (1969) of Finland described a systemic amyloidosis in patients with corneal lattice dystrophy and characterized this disease in further extensive studies of 207 patients (for references, see Meretoja and Teppo, 1971; Meretoja, 1973; Collan and Meretoja, 1978). McKusick (1978) in his catalogue named it amyloidosis V (Finland or Meretoja type). Studies on both this disease and another type of corneal lattice dystrophy were also done in Finland by Kaunisto (1968, 1971, 1973).

The first manifestation of this autosomal dominant disease is corneal lattice dystrophy in the third decade of life. Other symptoms develop slowly, during decades. They are upper facial paresis and later on, other symptoms of cranial nerves, as well as cutaneous signs like cutis laxa with typical "hanging" face. The general symptoms of amyloidosis are slight, progress slowly, and apparently seldom shorten life. At autopsy, accumulation of amyloid is found in various organs. Visual acuity remains fairly good until about the age of 65 years. Simple glaucoma occurs in a fourth of the cases.

The affected ancestors of the patients come from a limited area (Fig. 2/14), apparently due to one mutation some hundreds of years ago.

15. Lysinuric Protein Intolerance (LPI)

After the first report by Perheentupa and Visakorpi (1965) from Finland, several investigations have appeared in Finland by Kekomäki and co-workers (for references, see Norio et al., 1971b) and by Simell and associates (for references, see Simell et al., 1975; see also Simell et al., 1980). For studies from other countries see Awrich et al. (1975), Kato et al. (1976), and Carson and Redmond (1977).

The affected infants tolerate mother's milk well, but after weaning they get symptoms of protein intolerance: failure to thrive, anorexia, vomiting, diarrhea. Without the right diagnosis and therapy, short stature, weak muscles, hepatosplenomegaly, osteoporosis, and susceptibility to infections and fractures develop. A few patients are moderately mentally retarded. Forced ingestion of protein may result in a coma.

The patients develop an aversion to protein-rich food, which protects them from grave symptoms. Urinary excretion of ornithine, arginine, and especially lysine is increased, and their plasma concentrations are decreased. Anemia, leukocytopenia, thrombocytopenia, as well as increased serum levels of lactate dehydrogenase and ferritin are additional laboratory findings.

The basic pathogenetic lesion is impaired intestinal absorption and tubular reabsorption and defective uptake into liver cells of the diamino acids lysine, ornithine, and arginine. This impairment causes deficiency of ornithine in the urea cycle, which in turn retards the function of the urea cycle and leads to hyperammonemia after protein load. The shortage of lysine may contribute to the growth failure and to the histological liver changes. Recent studies (Rajantie et al., 1980) suggest that the defect in epithelial cells is localized at the basolateral cell membrane.

The treatment consists of citrulline supplementation that corrects the ornithine deficiency and allows a moderate ingestion of protein and nearly symptomless life. One of the oldest Finnish patients recently graduated from high school with good results and was accepted into the medical faculty of the University of Oulu.

Heterozygous manifestations and prenatal diagnosis are not known.

16. Meckel's Syndrome

Recently, Meckel's syndrome, also called Gruber's syndrome and dysencephalia splanchnocystica, has been found to be surprisingly common in Finland. This perinatally lethal malformation syndrome was described by Meckel as early as 1822 (Meckel, 1822; see also Opitz and Howe, 1969; Mecke and Passarge,

1971) and in Finland by Aula *et al.* (1977). A nationwide study of R. Salonen and co-workers is in progress (see also Norio *et al.*, 1980).

The main triad of malformations in Meckel's syndrome is gross neural tube defect (anencephalus, encephalocele, or hydrocephalus), postaxial polydactyly, and dysplastic kidneys, which are usually large and cystic. This main triad is often accompanied by other malformations, such as cleft lip–palate, ocular abnormalities, congenital heart defects, hypoplastic adrenal glands, ambiguous genitalia, and clubfeet. Often, the placenta is large. All patients die perinatally; hence, obstetricians and pathologists should recognize this recessive disorder, the recurrence risk of which is high as compared with similar syndromes involving multiple anomalies. Trisomy of chromosome 13 should be kept in mind as a differential diagnostic alternative.

Prenatal diagnosis by aid of increased α-fetoprotein concentrations of the amniotic fluid has been reported several times in cases with open neural tube defect (Aula *et al.*, 1977; Shapiro *et al.*, 1977; Seller, 1978; Friedrich *et al.*, 1979). Large cystic kidneys can be traced by ultrasound scanning in the second trimester of pregnancy. The possible alterations of amniotic fluid due to renal abnormalities are not known; raised AFP values without open neural tube defects have also been reported (Chemke *et al.*, 1977).

17. Mulibrey Nanism

This multisymptomatic proportional growth disturbance had been first described in Finland by Perheentupa and co-workers (Perheentupa *et al.*, 1973, 1975; Raitta and Perheentupa, 1974; Tuuteri *et al.*, 1974; Perheentupa, 1980c). Only a few patients have been described from elsewhere (Thorén, 1973; Cumming *et al.*, 1976; Voorhess *et al.*, 1976).

The term mulibrey nanism is an acronym for *mu*scle, *li*ver, *br*ain, and *ey*e. The proportionate growth failure has a prenatal onset. The muscles are hypotonic and gracile. The liver is enlarged due to congestion. The skull is large and dolichocephalic, the sella long and J-shaped. Intelligence is often of low normal or slightly subnormal range. The eyegrounds show yellowish dots and pigment dispersion. Triangular face, high forehead, and cutaneous nevi flammei, cystic fibrous dysplasia of tibiae, and squeaky voice are prominent features. The strangest and most important finding is constrictive pericardial fibrosis that may not only lead to raised venous pressure and hepatomegaly but also to severe cardiac failure and death. Spontaneous abortions are frequent in the families.

Nothing is known about the common denominator of this bizarre complex of findings. The prognosis varies; some patients die of heart failure at the age of a few months, others reach adulthood with hardly any handicap. Surgical treatment of the constrictive pericardium may be life-saving.

18. Muscle, Eye, and Brain Disease (MEB)

This disease was described by Santavuori *et al.* (1977) from Finland; one case is reported from elsewhere. It consists of a combination of severe mental retardation, severe congenital muscular hypotonia, and some congenital abnormalities of the eye. In addition to the severe mental retardation, the brain findings present as feeding difficulties, slight spasticity despite muscular hypotonia, myoclonic jerks and/or convulsions, and abnormal EEG. The muscular features are severe early hypotonia, retarded motor development, diminished or absent tendon jerks, elevated serum creatine kinase levels, myopathic EMG, and histology compatible with muscular dystrophy. The eye findings are varying combinations of severe congenital myopia, congenital glaucoma, and hypoplasia of optic discs and/or retina (Raitta *et al.*, 1978; see also Santavuori and Leisti, 1980).

The pathogenesis is unknown, as is therapy and prenatal diagnosis. The data on prognosis and survival time are scanty because of the short follow-up time so far.

19. Nonketotic Hyperglycinemia (NKH)

This severe and rapidly progressive metabolic brain disease was described in the same year in the United States by Gerritsen *et al.* (1965) and in Finland by Visakorpi *et al.* (1965). The two siblings reported by Mabry and Karam (1963) probably also had NKH. The disease, typical for northern Finland, has been investigated in Oulu by Similä, von Wendt, and co-workers (Similä and Visakorpi, 1970; von Wendt *et al.*, 1978, 1979; von Wendt and Similä, 1980).

Pregnancy, delivery, and usually the first day of life of the affected infants are normal. On the second or third day of life, signs of severe neurological damage appear: hypotonia and lethargy, irritability and myoclonic jerks, diminishing reaction to pain, and severe progressive respiratory failure. If the patient survives the neonatal period, a rapid and severe mental and motor deterioration into a decerebrated state is inevitable. The EEG may be almost isoelectric already at the age of a few days, showing the burst suppression pattern (Seppäläinen and Similä, 1971).

The concentration of glycine is elevated in the urine, plasma, and especially in the cerebrospinal fluid, in the absence of ketosis or metabolic acidosis. The proportion of glycine concentrations in plasma as compared with that in the cerebrospinal fluid is pathognomonically low (11 ± 6, normally 55 ± 26).

The enzyme defect causing defective degradation of lysine is not known (de Groot *et al.*, 1970; Perry *et al.*, 1977). Prenatal diagnosis is not available. Glycine concentration of the amniotic fluid remains unchanged during NKH pregnancy. The heterozygotes have shown elevated concentrations of glycine in the urine and serum, and they have shown slightly pathological findings in neurological and neurophysiological examinations (EEG, ENG, ERG).

20. Polycystic Lipomembranous Osteodysplasia With Sclerosing Leukoencephalopathy (PLO-SL)

This neuro-osteological disease was described in Finland by Järvi, Hakola, and co-workers (Järvi *et al.*, 1964, 1968, 1980; Hakola, 1972; Hakola and Karjalainen, 1975); Terayama (1961) had reported two patients from Japan.

After a symptomless childhood and adolescence, the patient's first symptoms are the pain and swelling of ankles and wrists due to minor fractures after stress and injury at about age 20 years. The increasing bone lesions consist of systemic cysts filled with necrotic fat tissue in which fatty acid crystals and autofluorescent membranes with phospholipids can be found.

The neurological symptoms appear after age 30 years. These are progressive dementia with a prefrontal syndrome, signs of upper motor neuron involvement, agnostic–apractic–aphasic symptoms, myoclonic twitching, and epileptic seizures. The EEG pattern is typical. The main findings in the brain are atrophy and sclerosis of the white matter, generalized demyelination, gliosis, and enlarged ventricles. Mean lifetime is about 40 years.

According to the pathogenetic hypothesis of the Finnish group, the structural changes of the nervous system and bones are due to vascular changes; narrowed, altered vessels with perivascular edema can be seen in both brain and bone cysts. According to Nasu *et al.* (1973) and Ohtani *et al.* (1979) from Japan, the disease is a disorder of lipid metabolism. However, thorough lipid analyses of bone cysts and brain tissue of the Finnish patients has not revealed any abnormalities (L. Svennerholm, 1978, unpublished data).

21. Progressive Myoclonus Epilepsy (PME)

First described by Unverricht (1891) of Estonia and from Finland by Harenko and Toivakka (1961), this neurological disease has been extensively investigated during the last few years by Koskiniemi and co-workers (Koskiniemi *et al.*, 1974a, 1980).

The Finnish PME is identical with the Unverricht–Lundborg type and clearly distinguishable from the Lafora type (Norio and Koskiniemi, 1979). The grand mal seizures and myoclonic jerks begin about age 10 years and occur particularly in the mornings. Unsteadiness in walking, dysarthric speech, and other neurological symptoms appear. The EEG is typical (Koskiniemi *et al.*, 1974b). The stimulus-sensitive myoclonus becomes more and more generalized and finally prevents all activities of the patients. Intelligence is only slightly affected, if at all (Koskiniemi, 1974). Survival varies: many patients live for decades. Lafora bodies have never been found.

In contrast, in the Lafora type onset is at around the age of 15 years; dementia and psychotic symptoms are common. The course is rapid, leading to death within 10 years, and Lafora bodies are found in brain specimen.

Because the course of the Finnish PME may be slow and benign, rehabilitative treatment is important "to keep the patients living." The myoclonic attacks are controlled better with sodium valproate and clonazepam than with conventional anticonvulsive medication.

22. Retinoschisis X-Chromosomalis

This X-chromosomal eye disease is the most common cause of bilateral amblyopia in boys in northern Finland. The first description of the disease was by Haas (1898). In Finland it has been investigated by Forsius and his group (Forsius et al., 1962, 1973; Eriksson et al., 1967; Vainio-Mattila et al., 1969; Forsius and Eriksson, 1980).

Retinoschisis does not mean a colobomatous cleft of the retina but a microcystic degeneration of the retinal nerve fiber layer; this degeneration leads to the splitting of the retina into layers. The disease exists from infancy, but the severity varies greatly. The visual acuity is 0.6–0.1 at young age and decreases slowly with age. However, the visual handicap is usually mild until 40–50 years of age. The ophthalmoscopic picture in mild cases shows macular degeneration resembling a wheel with spokes. Moderate cases show also semitranslucent vitreous veils, mainly in the lower temporal quadrant of the retina; they consist of detached pieces of the superficial layers of the retina. In severe cases detachment or roll-shaped peeling of the retina leads to its total destruction and blindness.

The carrier females show no manifestations of the gene. The offspring of carrier females oddly enough show a male preponderance (167:100; Eriksson et al., 1967).

Prenatal diagnosis is not possible. Selective abortion of boys after prenatal sex determination is possible, but its indication is debatable because of the relative mildness of the visual impairment.

23. Salla Disease

Salla disease is one of the latest newcomers among the Finnish disease heritage. Most of the patients come from the same northern region, Salla. The disease was described from Finland by Aula et al. (1979); see also Aula and Autio, 1980; no reports are known from elsewhere.

Salla disease was discovered as a by-product of studies on aspartylglucosaminuria—in the same way as aspartylglucosaminuria was found when searching for phenylketonuric patients. It is a lysosomal storage disease. Its main features are progressive and finally severe mental retardation, impaired speech, motor clumsiness, and ataxia, whereas facial features are mostly normal. The onset of symptoms occurs between ages 6 and 18 months, slow psychomotor development, muscular hypotonia, and ataxia being the main symptoms. The deterioration happens sooner or later, during the second decade at the latest. Vacuolated lymphocytes are found in the peripheral blood, storage lysosomes in skin biopsy specimens, and cultured fibroblasts. The urinary excretion of free sialic acid is increased about tenfold. This increase can be demonstrated also by thin-layer chromatographic method (Renlund *et al.*, 1979).

The pathogenesis is unknown, as is specific treatment. The survival time is not known yet; the oldest known patient is more than 60 years old.

24. Selective Malabsorption of Vitamin B_{12} (SMB$_{12}$)

Described in the same year by Gräsbeck *et al.* (1960) in Finland and by Imerslund (1960) in Norway, this disease is characterized by megaloblastic anemia due to the lack of vitamin B_{12} and proteinuria. The symptoms begin insidiously during the first few years of life. An absorption defect of vitamin B_{12} can be demonstrated by the Schilling test, but the activity of the intrinsic factor in the gastric juice is normal, as are other intestinal absorptive functions. The mechanism of proteinuria is poorly understood. Parenteral administration of vitamin B_{12} corrects the anemia but not the proteinuria. Without parenteral treatment, the patient with this disease would die (Visakorpi and Furuhjelm, 1968; Furuhjelm and Nevanlinna, 1973; Nevanlinna, 1980).

B. Rare Inherited Diseases That Are Exceptionally Rare in Finland

Despite the abundance of some recessive diseases, Finland can hardly be considered to be a country especially prone to sickness. As a compensation for the accumulation of the "Finnish" diseases, many other disorders, common in other countries, are extremely rare, if not absent, here. The most striking example is the nearly total absence of phenylketonuria (PKU). A careful search through the institutions for the mentally retarded yielded only three PKU patients, and the screening of 71,000 newborn babies did not uncover a single case of PKU (Visakorpi *et al.*, 1971). Thus, neonatal screening programs based on the search for PKU at first hand and for other diseases as its by-product are not sensible in Finland. It is also difficult to render an incidence figure for PKU in Finland; perhaps something like < 1:100,000 could be given.

Galactosemia, maple syrup urine disease, cystinosis, histidinemia, and Pendred's syndrome (deafness with goiter) have apparently never been found. Tay-Sachs disease, Gaucher's disease, Hartnup disease, Fabry's disease, and some glycogenoses have been diagnosed, each in one or two instances. One sibship is known to be suffering from homocystinuria (Norio and Westerén, 1972). Cystic fibrosis is also among the diseases seldom found. About ten living patients were known of in 1977, and in a screening of 6400 newborns, none were found to be affected (though showed 40 false-positive tests) (Isolauri *et al.*, 1979). Although an accurate incidence figure cannot be estimated, most probably it does not exceed 1:20,000 or is at least ten times smaller than the average estimate in Europe (Stephan *et al.*, 1975).

C. Data on Some "Classical" Inherited and Allied Diseases in Finland

1. Autosomal Dominant Disorders

By 1976, there were 107 patients with acute intermittent porphyria (AIP) and 45 patients with variegated porphyria known in Finland. Their prevalence was calculated as 2.4 and 1.0/100,000 inhabitants (Mustajoki and Koskelo, 1976), whereas in Sweden the prevalence of AIP is 7:100,000. Hereditary angioneurotic edema is known to exist in 33 symptomatic and 25 asymptomatic members of 7 kindreds, most of them in southern and southeastern Finland (Ohela, 1977). Dominant and X-linked ichthyoses are not so rare. They have been investigated in northern Finland by Kuokkanen (1969). Dominant "adult" type of polycystic disease of kidney and liver is not rare, either. Peltokallio (1970) has described 117 patients, most of whom were from central Finland. They were actually presented as patients having liver cysts, whereas renal and other parenchymal cysts were reported only in some of them. Probably this is not a disease in and of itself. Some patients with Alport's syndrome (Kouvalainen and Pasternack, 1962) and nail-patella syndrome (Hakosalo *et al.*, 1968) are known. Myotonic dystrophy is known in 250 patients from 43 kindreds (Wikström *et al.*, 1978). Tuberous sclerosis and neurofibromatosis (Recklinghausen's disease) are not rare.

2. Autosomal Recessive Disorders

Congenital hypothyroidism, notably the iodine organification defect (Mäenpää, 1972) and congenital adrenal hypoplasia, most patients presenting with 21-hydroxylase deficiency (Perheentupa, 1972b), are often seen in pediatric hospitals, as is mucopolysaccharidosis type I. Four patients with mucolipidosis II (I-cell disease) and seven with mannosidosis (Autio, 1975; Autio *et al.*, 1973a; Nordén *et al.*, 1974) are known. The perinatal form of the recessive, childhood type of cystic disease of kidneys and liver is fairly common, at least in eastern and northern Finland (Uhari and Herva, 1979); it could be considered to be included in the Finnish disease heritage. The neonatal, infantile, and juvenile subtypes, on the other hand, are very rare. About ten cases of nephronophthisis are known. The Shwachman syndrome, or exocrine insufficiency of pancreas with bone marrow dysfunction, has been seen more than ten times; necrotic and fibrotic cardiac alterations resembling myocarditis are often seen in this disease (J. Rapola, personal communication). Leber's congenital amaurosis is seen frequently and total achromatopsia, sometimes. The so-called retinitis pigmentosa is not rare. Most patients with that condition may have an autosomal recessive disease. [X-linked retinitis pigmentosa has probably never been found. The data of Voipio *et al.* (1964) are frequently cited in ophthalmological literature, giving figures of 37% of autosomal recessive, 19.5% for autosomal dominant, 4.5% for X-linked recessive, and 39% for "sporadic" retinitis pigmentosa in Finland. In fact, this information is grossly wrong: the figures do not at all concern Finnish patients but are based on an erroneous citation of a congress report (H. Voipio, personal communication).] Congenital lamellar ichthyosis may be seen more often than epidermolysis bullosa dystrophica. Krabbe's disease and the metachromatic leukodystrophies are rare. The prevalence of lactose malabsorption is 17% in Finland, 4% in Denmark, less than that in Sweden, and over 30% in the Finnish Lapps (Sahi, 1974, 1978). Little is known about α-antitrypsin deficiency in Finland.

3. X-Chromosomal Recessive Disorders

As can be supposed, hemophilia is relatively common (Ikkala, 1960). (The autosomal dominant Willebrand disease, which was first described in the Åland Islands, occurs also on the mainland.) Progressive muscular dystrophy, both Duchenne and, less frequently, Becker types, is not rare. Some cases of Norrie's disease, Menkes' syndrome, Lowe's syndrome, and Wiskott-Aldrich syndrome are known. Recently Renpenning's syndrome (X-chromosomal mental retardation) has occasionally been diagnosed.

4. Other Rare Disorders

Anencephaly incidence is one of the lowest figures in the world; according to Granroth *et al.* (1977) it is 0.32/1000 births. Oral clefts show an average incidence of 1.72:1000, but their division is unusual: the incidence of cleft lip with or without cleft palate is low, 0.83:1000, whereas the incidence of cleft palate is one of the highest reported, 0.86:1000 for the whole of Finland and 1.47:1000 for the easternmost province of North Karelia (Saxén and Lahti, 1974). The prevalence of multiple sclerosis in Finland is high: 40/100,000 inhabitants. A cluster with a prevalence up to 60:100,000 occurs in the western province of Vaasa; in the cluster area, 13% of the cases are familial (Wikström and Palo, 1975; Wikström, 1975). The prevalence figure for myasthenia gravis is 5.6:100,000, or 1:18,000 (which is an average frequency), whereas 7% of cases were familial, which is a high figure (Pirskanen, 1977).

The blood groups and other polymorphisms remain outside the scope of this presentation. Reference is given to Streng (1935, 1937), Mustakallio (1938), Mourant (1954), Seppälä (1965), Nevanlinna (1972, 1973a,b), Nevanlinna *et al.*

(1980), Nevanlinna and Pirkola (1973), Eriksson (1973), and Steinberg *et al.* (1974).

D. The Population Basis of the Finnish Disease Heritage

The concept of the Finnish disease heritage has two sides: an accumulation of some peculiar, mostly autosomal recessive disorders that are very uncommon elsewhere, and the lack of many "classical" recessive diseases. The explanation for this heritage must include a cause for these two circumstances: the existence of the peculiar genes (and the lack of some other genes) and some mechanism that easily leads two carriers of the same rare recessive genes into a common marriage—or favors the chance meeting of two similar rare genes into a homozygous state. These causes are the national and the regional isolation of a small population.

1. National Isolation

Although accurate data on the early history and origin of the Finns are scanty (cf. Section IV, C), one thing is certain: the number of the "original" Finns, say 2000 years ago, must have been small—hundreds or thousands rather than hundreds of thousands, to say nothing of millions. The ancient Finns cannot have brought all possible recessive genes to Finland but only an assortment of them. This same rule must apply to many other small nations and tribes. The exceptional fact is that the existence of this assortment has survived throughout history in the national isolation. Finland is situated on the margin of the inhabited world, between two contrasted cultures, i.e., between Sweden and Russia. The Finno-Ugrian language of the Finns differs fundamentally from both Swedish and Russian. Most of the population has belonged first to the Roman Catholic and then to the Protestant Lutheran Church, like the Swedes but unlike the Russians. Although Finland belonged to the Swedish Kingdom until 1809 and to the Czarist Russia from 1809 to 1917, immigration from either side has been minimal through history. Neither have migrations of peoples taken place in northern Europe. Thus the "original" assortment of rare genes has been well preserved—or become accentuated by the regional isolation.

2. Regional Isolation

The excessive occurrence of peculiar autosomal recessive diseases cannot be due solely to the existence of peculiar genes but demands an excessive number of homozygotes, or excessive possibilities for heterozygotes having one and the same gene to marry each other. In Finland this circumstance is due to an uneven geographical distribution of rare genes, a geographical clustering of heterozygotes.

The first time this fact arose was when the heredity of the congenital nephrotic syndrome was investigated (Norio, 1966). The ancestors of the 57 affected sibships were not evenly distributed throughout the country but were concentrated in more or less dense clusters in a big area that was not permanently populated before the sixteenth century AD (Fig. 2/0). A remarkable "biocultural aspect," namely the admirable population register kept by the Lutheran Church, made it possible to trace back the ancestors six to ten generations. Many of the parents of the affected infants were shown to be consanguineous not only with their own spouses (29% of the marriages) but with two to ten other parents of the affected infants. The consanguinities were mostly remote, whereas first-cousin marriages were totally lacking.

In fact, incredible as it may seem, a large part of Finland, northward and eastward from the broken line in Fig. 2/0, was permanently settled as late as the sixteenth century, and the northernmost parts later still. The settlement of individual regions was begun by a few families that migrated into the wilds from South Savo, the mid-southeastern part of today's Finland. In such circumstances, due to chance or genetic drift or founder effect, some genes of the newcomers became firmly established in the next few generations and some others were lost. The gene clusters with such an origin were then maintained by the population structure. Thus, the population remained sparse for the large area of the country, being 400,000 in the seventeenth century, 1.6 million in 1850, and 2.6 million in 1900. Long distances, vast forests, and innumerable lakes, all typical of Finland, separated the villages from each other, forming isolation by distance, or better still, isolation by population density. Most of the population—94% in 1850, 79% in 1930, and 49% in 1970—had lived in rural communes (parishes) until the active industrialization of the last decades.

Little need existed for internal migration, not least because of the little industry. After World War II, an active migration to cities and especially to the south of Finland occurred. The native inhabitants of individual rural communes in the areas of late settlement are even now descendants of those few immigrants from the sixteenth century, i.e., from 15 to 20 generations back. Therefore they are remotely related to each other (Fig. 3), which also means that the frequencies of some rare genes of the original immigrants are even now surprisingly high in some small areas and nonexistent in most other regions. Thus, the intermarriage of two heterozygotes with the same "rare" gene is not so rare an event in such a population.

The same isolated basic structure of the rural population also exists, to a great extent, in the older settlement on the southern side of the boundary in Fig. 2/0, excepting the southern and southwestern parts of the country. The population density is highest in the south and decreases gradually northwards, being sparse in Lapland. The maps showing the distribution of the ancestry in 24 Finnish diseases (Fig. 2) are in principle inverse to the density of population; most

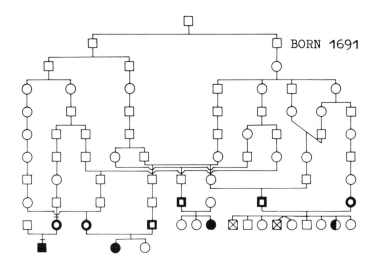

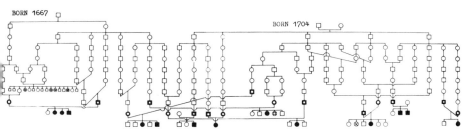

Fig. 3. Typical Finnish pedigrees showing mostly remote consanguinities between several parents (thick squares and circles) of patients (black squares and circles) suffering from congenital nephrotic syndrome. (According to Norio, 1966.)

ancestors originate from the areas of late settlement. The few maps of dominant and X-linked diseases (Fig. 2/4, 2/14, and 2/22) clearly show the small amount of population movement, although these genes, contrary to autosomal recessive ones, need no isolation to become manifest.

The number of remotely consanguineous marriages between parents of affected children has been shown to be great in many diseases, namely, 5/10 = 50% in lysinuric protein intolerance (Norio et al., 1971a), 6/14 = 43% in congenital chloride diarrhea (Norio et al., 1971b), 4/17 = 24% in selective malabsorption of vitamin B_{12} (Furuhjelm and Nevanlinna, 1973), 15/68 = 22% in progressive myoclonus epilepsy (Norio and Koskiniemi, 1979), and 8/44 = 18% in infantile neuronal ceroid lipofuscinosis (Norio and Santavuori, 1981).

The remote consanguineous marriages can be demonstrated by tracing the ancestors through the church records: the more generations are traced back, the more marriages can be shown to be consanguineous. The "original" settlers of the 1500s cannot be reached, however, because the oldest church records date from the end of the seventeenth century, and thus a gap of four to ten generations remains untraceable. Another type of pedigrees obtained from church records studies shows remote consanguinities between groups of parents of affected children from different sibships. These pedigrees depict a possible route of a gene from one common ancestor to some of today's heterozygotes, but the oldest common ancestor that can be traced need not be the only source of that gene in that area (Fig. 3).

Marriages between first cousins are not common in Finland; they were prohibited by law until 1872. For the same reason the few inbreeding coefficients calculated so far are small: 0.0006 for 57 sibships with congenital nephrosis, 0.0017 for their parents (Norio, 1966), and 0.0087 for 60 members of a rural isolate, who were born about 1900 (Nevanlinna, 1972).

Systematical studies on the structure of the Finnish population have been done by Nevanlinna (1972, 1973a,b; see also Norio *et al.,* 1973). He has shown enormous differences of blood group frequencies between the villages of the same commune, due to the founder effect. Thus, for example, the extreme frequencies of blood group B were 15.5 and 49.9%, and of transferrin D_{chi} 0.5 and 13.3%. Nevanlinna also studied the size and character of breeding units, consanguinity, and loss of ancestors. He created the theory of superisolates that have dynamically been divided into smaller population units. He stressed the significance of the smallness (and common origin) of the basic population and the great role of the first immigrants to the genetic pool and to the accumulation and compensatory losses of rare genes. His estimate was that one-third of the children born in the last decade have parents who both were born in the same rural area.

III. OUTLINE OF RARE HEREDITARY DISEASES IN SCANDINAVIA

Contrary to the situation in Finland, I have never heard anyone speak of the Swedish or Norwegian disease heritage. It does not mean that rare hereditary diseases, as well as more or less "own" diseases, do not exist in those countries. They too are sparsely populated and partly isolated, whereas Denmark, with its small area, dense population, and closeness to central Europe may not be a suitable soil for recessive diseases. Contrary to conditions in Finland, perhaps the diseases in Sweden and Norway occur more locally (see Sjögren and Larsson, 1957), and perhaps they and the population structure in those countries have escaped "institutionalization." If that were so, it is not my place or task to attempt to account for it here.

Most disorders of the Finnish disease heritage are extremely rare in Scandinavia, or they can be found in Sweden, among the many Finns who have moved to Sweden after World War II. In northern Norway, in a region called Finnmark, some cases of aspartylglucosaminuria have been found. Three diseases make an exception, however. Dystrophia retinae pigmentosa—dysacusis (see Section II, A, 9), investigated in Sweden by Hallgren (1959) and in Denmark in Lindenov (1945), is almost as common there as in Finland, with an estimated prevalence of 3/100,000 in Denmark, 2.4/100,000 in Sweden, and 3.5/100,000 in Finland. The other interesting exception is progressive myoclonus epilepsy (PME), or Unverricht–Lundborg disease. Lundborg (1901, 1903) described 18 patients having this autosomal recessive disorder, all being descendants of an extremely inbred kindred in southern Sweden. Since then, as far as is known, only solitary patients have been described from Sweden. In Finland more than 100 patients are known (see Section II, A, 21). The first described patients with PME, the eight patients from two sibships of Unverricht (1891, 1895) lived in Estonia. As far as can be judged, all these patients had the same so-called non-Lafora type of PME (Norio and Koskiniemi, 1979). A tempting thought is that the gene in those three countries would have a common source, especially as Sweden, Estonia, and Finland have had many interconnections both in history and prehistoric times. The third exception is selective malabsorption of vitamin B $_{12}$ (see Section II, A, 24); data on at least 12 patients with this disease have been published from Norway (Imerslund, 1960).

Leber's congenital amaurosis, described in Sweden by Alström (1957) as "Heredo-retinopathia congenitalis monohybrida recessiva autosomalis," and juvenile neuronal ceroid-lipofuscinosis or the Spielmeyer–Sjögren disease (Sjögren, 1931) occur frequently in both Sweden and Finland.

Other rare hereditary diseases described from Sweden are the Sjögren–Larsson syndrome (mental retardation, spasticity + ichthyosis-like skin changes; Sjögren and Larsson, 1957; Jagell et al., 1981), cystinuria (Boström and Hambraeus, 1964), and torsion dystonia (Larsson and Sjögren, 1966).

The following diseases reported from Norway deserve to be mentioned: the X-linked Aarskog syndrome, or faciogenital dysplasia (seven patients in one kindred; Aarskog, 1970, 1971); acrodermatitis enteropathica (Brandt, 1936; Danboldt and Closs, 1942); several types of epidermolysis bullosa (more than 100 patients; Gedde-Dahl, 1970, 1978), lecithin–cholesterol acyltransferase (LCAT) deficiency (seven affected in three families; Gjone et al., 1978); Refsum's syndrome, or heredopathia atactica polyneuritiformis (Refsum, 1946, 1977); and Seip's syndrome, or generalized lipodystrophy (six patients in five families; Seip, 1971, 1975).

Studies on population genetics in Sweden have been done by Beckman (1959) and Alström (1963), among others, and in Norway by Gedde-Dahl (1973, 1974).

IV. EXCESS MORTALITY AMONG THE FINNS FROM
CORONARY HEART DISEASE AND OTHER CAUSES

A. Excess in General Mortality

It has been said that Finland has the healthiest children and sickest men in Europe. In fact, the infant mortality figures in Finland and the Scandinavian countries are the lowest in the world, i.e., $8.3\%_{00}$ in Sweden, $9.6\%_{00}$ in Finland, $10.4\%_{00}$ in Denmark, and $11.1\%_{00}$ in Norway in 1975 (World Health Statistics Annual, 1978; Statistical Year Book of Finland, 1977). In Finland the main reason for this, apart from the high standard of pediatrics in general, may be the Infant and Maternity Health Care Center arrangement begun more than 50 years ago by private organizations and united to the Public Health Care system after World War II. This service, available in every village and used by nearly all families, has effectively spread health education to the families and provided services of preventive medicine.

All the more strange is the fact that these healthy infants become sick adults. Compared with those of the Scandinavian countries, whose climates, socioeconomic bases, and standards of medical care are similar, most mortality curves of the Finns are the highest. This concerns the overall mortality figures in different age-groups as well as most figures showing groups selected for causes of death. The excess mortality applies especially to middle-aged Finnish men. In Table II, some numbers are given; illuminating graphs, in addition to detailed numerical data, are presented by Bolander (1971) (see also Fig. 4).

B. Excess Mortality from Coronary Heart Disease

1. National Situation

The most striking and significant component in the Finnish excess mortality is coronary heart disease (CHD). Finnish men are on top in the world lists for coronary mortality, whereas women rank eighth, after Scotland, North Ireland, Israel, Australia, the United States, New Zealand, and Ireland (Pyörälä and Valkonen, 1981). CHD kills Finnish men when young; in the period 1966 to 1968, CHD accounted for 41% of the deaths among men aged 50–54 years. The average age at death for men was 65.3 years and for women 73.6 years, and mortality from CHD for men aged 45 and 50 years was as great as it was for women aged 60 and 64 years, respectively (Bolander, 1971). The standardized death rates from CHD for men aged 45–74 in 1966–1968 were 1077 for Finland and 585, 636, and 677 for Sweden, Norway, and Denmark, respectively (Bolander, 1971). As in many countries (Epstein and Pisa, 1979), the mortality from CHD has also shown a declining trend during the 1970s in Finland (Pyörälä and Valkonen, 1981).

TABLE II

Figures on Natality and Mortality in Finland, Sweden, Norway, and Denmark

	Finland	Sweden	Norway	Denmark
Natality per 1000, live born[a]	14.1	12.7	14.1	14.2
General mortality per 1000[a]	9.4	10.8	10.0	10.1
Infant mortality per 1000[b]	9.6	8.3	11.1	10.4
Expected age at death, at the age of 0 years[c]				
—Males	65.4	71.6	71.0	70.3
—Females	72.6	75.7	76.0	74.5
Standardized death rates for the age group 45–74 years[d]				
All natural causes				
Males	2630	1506	1636	1765
Females	1332	947	939	1091
Neoplasms				
Males	627	385	381	504
Females	314	323	310	400
Cerebrovascular diseases				
Males	288	136	180	145
Females	247	116	150	113
Motor vehicle accidents				
Males	54	30	21	46
Females	16	12	8	16

[a] 1975 (World Health Statistics Annual, 1977, 1978).
[b] 1975 (as above; Statistical Yearbook of Finland, 1977).
[c] Bolander (1971); based on period mortality for 1961–1965.
[d] Bolander (1971); the standard population applied is the total population of both sexes in the four countries by 5-year age-groups in 1966–1968.

2. Regional Differences Within Finland

Also remarkable are the regional differences of CHD frequency within Finland. It has been customary to speak about an eastern–western difference. In fact, in the southwestern part of Finland the death rates are not high but resemble other European figures, in contrast to rates in the remaining parts of the country, whereas two provinces in the mideastern part of Finland have the highest CHD figures. The east–west difference is seen also in the female CHD mortality (Fig. 5).

3. Role of General Risk Factors

Do the differences of individual CHD risk factors give an explanation for the Finnish situation either inter- or intranationally? Giving an accurate answer to this question is difficult, not least because data from various sources are difficult to compare. A rough answer is that, although the deviations from the mean in

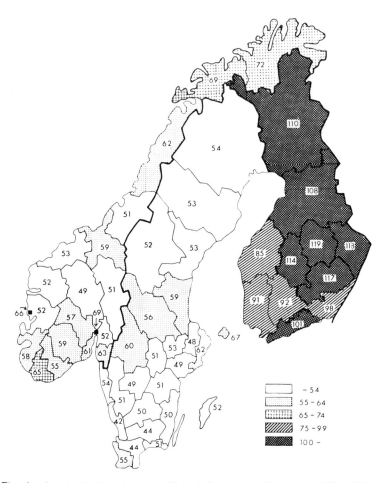

Fig. 4. Standardized death rates in Finland, Sweden, and Norway in 1970–1971 among males aged 5–64 years by provinces (in relation to the national rate in Finland = 100). (From Valkonen and Notkola, 1977; courtesy of the authors of the Population Research Institute, Helsinki.)

many risk factors have a logical tendency, none of them have thus far given quantitatively satisfactory explanation for the specific situation in Finland.

Thus, the serum cholesterol and triglyceride concentrations are considerably high (260–280 mg/100 ml in middle-aged men) in Finland, slightly (5–7 mg/100 ml) higher in eastern than in western Finland, but by no means do they give an explanation to the CHD difference between Finland and Scandinavia (Aromaa *et al.*, 1975; Björkstén *et al.*, 1975; Karvonen *et al.*, 1967; Pyörälä and Valkonen, 1981). Representative data on HDL-cholesterol are not yet available.

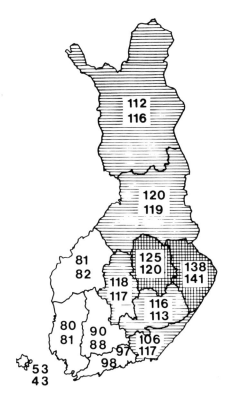

Fig. 5. Age-adjusted mortality from coronary heart disease by provinces for men aged 35–64 years (upper numbers) and for women aged 35–74 years (lower numbers). The figures are indexes related to index 100 for the whole country. (According to Valkonen and Niemi, 1978.)

Hypertension does not explain the international CHD discrepancy but is in some correlation with the east-west difference in Finland (Aromaa *et al.*, 1977). The use of tobacco was common in the 1910–1920s, and smoking habits were unhealthy; this might have some correlation with at least the international CHD excess (Rimpelä, 1978). Obesity does not at all correlate with CHD mortality; it is more usual in the West and might even be interpreted as being a protective factor (A. Aromaa, unpublished data).

Differing opinions exist about the significance of diet, especially of the considerably high consumption of animal fats and table salt (Keys *et al.*, 1970; Pyörälä and Valkonen, 1981). A comprehensive investigation on the mineral element composition of Finnish foods has recently been completed (Koivistoinen, 1980). According to it, the interesting deviations in the daily intake from the overall values and the recommendations by the U.S. Food and Nutrition

Board, 1980, are excess of calcium (1500 pro 800 mg/day) and phosphorus (2000 pro 800 mg/day), and lack of selenium (30 pro 50–200 μg/day) and chromium (20 pro 50–200 μg/day). Comparisons between western and eastern Finland have not been done. Drinking water was not included in the figures presented.

The role of trace elements in the soil and ground water is the object of diverse opinions (Punsar et al., 1975; Karppanen et al., 1978), but no certain conclusions can be drawn. During the glacial period, which ended 10,000 years ago, the conditions were different in the eastern and western parts of the country as concerns ice and water (i.e., from melted ice). A nationwide study of the geochemical composition of the soil and ground water is being done by the Geological Survey of Finland (P. Lahermo, personal communication).

The recent hypothesis about the protective effect of abundant consumption of wine (St. Leger et al., 1979) might well be suitable for Finland as a whole but hardly fits in with the east–west difference; in Finland, in the absence of vine, the consumption of wine has really been small. (Apropos, the peculiar drinking habits of the Finns—the consuming of strong liquors to become inebriated instead of using milder drinks moderately—are greatly due to this climatic-biocultural reality.)

The influence of socioeconomic factors on the geographical variation of mortality (and thus mainly of mortality from CHD) has been studied by Valkonen and Notkola (1977) (see also Fig. 4). According to them, the general standard of living is an important determinant of mortality, especially if that level is not rather high, as was the case some decades ago, at least in some parts of Finland and Scandinavia. If the standard of living is a determinant, the fact that modern cultural and socioeconomic development, industrialization, and urbanization took place in Finland some decades after a similar development in Scandinavia could be a not unimportant factor in the respective national and regional differences of CHD.

During 1972–1977, a comprehensive community program (the North Karelia project) was carried out in the eastern province of North Karelia, the "blackest" CHD area in Finland. The aims were to reduce three risk factors of CHD, i.e., smoking, serum cholesterol concentration, and raised blood pressure among the population, and thus reduce the morbidity and mortality from CHD. For the results assessed so far, which may be regarded as positive with certain reservations, see Puska et al. (1979) and Salonen et al. (1979). At present, a multicenter study of atherosclerosis precursors in Finnish children is in progress, conducted by H. K. Åkerblom, J. Viikari, and M. Uhari.

4. Role of Possible Genetic Factors

CHD is certainly a multifactorial disease. The role and character of genetic factors is widely unknown, as is the question of possible "major genes" among other genetic components.

In Finland, attempts at explaining the east–west difference by genetic factors have been few, if not altogether neglected. However, Pesonen *et al.* (1975) showed that intimal thickenings of the left coronary arteries of those who died at less than 1 year of age were greater and more frequent in infants whose grandparents originated from eastern Finland. Valkonen and Notkola (1977), in their conclusion about regional mortality differences, assume that some systematic regional variation is likely to remain unexplained by the known environmental factors studied; as such a factor, the genetic composition of the population could be relevant.

If some genetic factor, perhaps a single gene or the lack of one, were to explain the regional difference of CHD mortality in Finland, this factor ought to be common in the population. Regional isolation, inbreeding, or uneven distribution of rare genes, which readily explain the accumulation of rare recessive diseases, cannot be responsible for such a common phenomenon as CHD. Instead a genetic explanation would presuppose a ''racial'' difference between inhabitants of those regions and thus the different origins and composition of the respective populations. The ''absolute'' origin of the Finns and their relation to other Finnic nationalities may have little relevance in this context. But is there any evidence for a genetic difference between the eastern and western population of Finland?

C. The Origin and Composition of the Finnish Population

1. The Finnish Population Today

The population of Finland today is, at least superficially, very homogeneous. Most persons are Finnish-speaking Finns. Some (7%) of the population speak Swedish; a part of them belong to the rural population in the western and southern coastal region. Their ancestors probably moved from Sweden at the beginning of the second millennium, although opinions are divided about the details and significance of this immigration. A specific minority is the population of the Åland Islands of the Baltic Sea, southwest of the Finnish mainland. That population is totally Swedish speaking and most probably originates mainly from Sweden. The population differs in many respects from the rest of the Finns and has been the object of extensive population genetic studies, especially by Eriksson and co-workers (see Eriksson *et al.*, 1973a,b; Mielke *et al.*, 1976). In the northernmost part of Finland, Lapland, live fewer than 3000 Lapps. The majority of the Lapps live in northern Norway, Sweden, and the Soviet Union. Their ethnic origin is uncertain; their own language is related to Finnish. Extensive studies on the genetic constitution of the Lapps have been done by the working group of Forsius and Eriksson, among others (see Eriksson, 1973; Steinberg *et al.*, 1974; Eriksson *et al.*, 1975; Aromaa *et al.*, 1975; Björkstén *et al.*, 1975). None of these minorities as such is likely to have essential significance in the origin of the Finnish populations as concerns CHD.

2. The Unitary and Dualistic Theories on the Inhabitation of Finland

According to the classical theory on the inhabitation of Finland, the first Finns came from the south, from Estonia across the Gulf of Finland during the first centuries AD, settled in the southwestern part of the country, and spread out during the first millennium AD eastward along a zone of about 200 km wide to Lake Ladoga, and northward along a narrow strip on the coast of the Gulf of Bothnia. As they proceeded, they forced the few nomadic ''Lapps'' out of the way northward. By the 1500s the boundary shown in Fig. 2/0 was reached. The remaining part of the country was settled as described in Section II, D,2.

If this unitary theory is correct, genetic difference between the eastern and western populations would be incredible. Recently, however, another theory, a dualistic one, has gained general support among archaeologists, historians, and linguists. According to that theory, the immigrants came from two sources, one group via the Lake Ladoga region. Both populations may have been more or less ''Finnic,'' but from different sources and different wanderings. Moreover, before these immigrations there may have been a considerable basic population that then, at least in part, became ''acculturated,'' merged into the newcomers. This basic population, with a probable continuity since the Stone Age, may have had a considerable influence on the Finnish genetic pool (Meinander, 1973), which in turn means that its origin is interesting in this context. The main part of the population may have come from eastern Europe according to the distribution of the comb ceramic culture (about 3500–1500 BC). The later boat-axe culture (about 2000 BC) found in western Europe and southern Scandinavia reached only to the southwestern parts of Finland. According to this and later archaeological and linguistic findings, southern and western Finland may have more Germanic and Scandinavian influence than the eastern parts. According to some historians and linguists (Kerkkonen, 1971; Itkonen, 1972), it is not even out of the question that the immigration from Estonia to southwestern Finland was limited to a small area only, whereas the settlement of the neighboring midsouthern area, Häme, consisted mainly of the basic Finnic population. What relationship this basic population has with the Lapps of today is an unsettled but interesting question. Whatever the situation, archaeological, historical, and linguistic studies clearly leave plenty of possibilities for the dualistic or pluralistic population basis and also for explaining the east–west difference of CHD on genetic background. Further evidence in favor of the dualism may be offered by the similarity of the

---

Fig. 6. (*opposite*) Boundaries showing differences between "eastern" and "western" Finland. (A) Anthropological types (according to Kajanoja, 1971). (B) Dialect groups (according to Rapola, 1961). (C) Five folkloristic differences in agricultural tools, vehicles or foods (according to Talve, 1972). (D) The boundary of permanently settled and unsettled parts of the country around 1500 AD; the area marked "late settlement" was populated after 1500, mainly by the people from south Savo (according to Jutikkala, 1933).

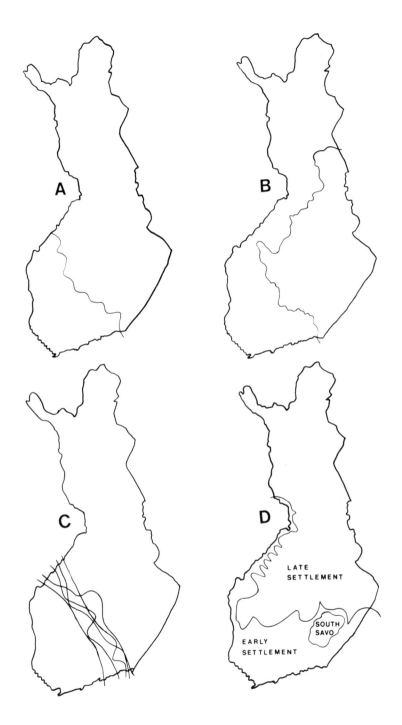

boundaries between eastern and western CHD regions, dialects (Rapola, 1961), some folkloristic divisions (Talve, 1972) and anthropological types (Kajanoja, 1971; see also Chit, 1972; Mark, 1972; Subow, 1972) (cf. Figs. 5 and 6).

But the dualism can be derived even from so young and really historical an event as the settlement of large parts of Finland during the 1500s; if the main group of the migrating people, the population of south Savo (Fig. 6), were of eastern origin (or had come from the Lake Ladoga region), then the young settlement area added with the southeastern parts of Finland is in good congruence with the "black" CHD area.

Have we any genetic evidence for or against the unitary or dualistic population theories? Extensive blood group studies have been done in the 1930s by Streng (1935, 1937) and Mustakallio (1938), among others, and recently by Nevanlinna (1972, 1973a,b). The first-mentioned writers interpreted their own results to show a difference, even if not a big one, between eastern and western Finland. Seppälä (1965) in his study on transferrin groups in Finland found a lower frequency of the "Asiatic" Tf D_{chi} gene in southwestern Finland as compared with frequencies from other parts of the country. Nevanlinna found extremely great blood group differences between villages, great differences between rural communes (parishes), but only slight differences between provinces (e.g., in the southwestern province of Turku and Pori and for the mideastern province of Kuopio, the blood group frequencies were 43.55 and 46.08% for A, 15.75 and 16.15% for B, and 31.36 and 28.3% for O, respectively; the numbers of tested persons were 845 and 805, respectively). Nevanlinna interpreted this last finding as strong evidence for the unitary population theory. It would be interesting to compare and reanalyze the data of these investigations in closer detail in the light of different population theories.

Another piece of evidence forwarded by Nevanlinna in favor of the unitary theory is the geographical distribution of some extremely rare dominant and recessive blood groups (Nevanlinna, 1972, 1973a). They have been found mainly in southwestern Finland and its near surroundings, whereas no such blood group genes have been found in eastern Finland (Fig. 7). Because the rarest genes are likely to be found only in the near vicinity of the original immigrants, this would show that all the Finns today originate from the immigrants to southwestern Finland.

On the other hand, the geographical distribution of the ancestors of the Finnish recessive diseases show several kinds of patterns (Fig. 2). The overall feature is that the ancestors disperse unevenly and mostly to the area of the more recent population from the 1500s. The population in Finland is dense in the south and becomes sparser northward, whereas the diseases often show overrepresentation in the sparsely populated areas (Fig. 2, maps 3, 7, 9, 11, 15, 17, and 19 i.a.). Many of them can well be explained by the settlement movement of the 1500s: some ancestors are found in the original region of the active movers in the midsouthwestern part of the country (south Savo), and a random clustering of

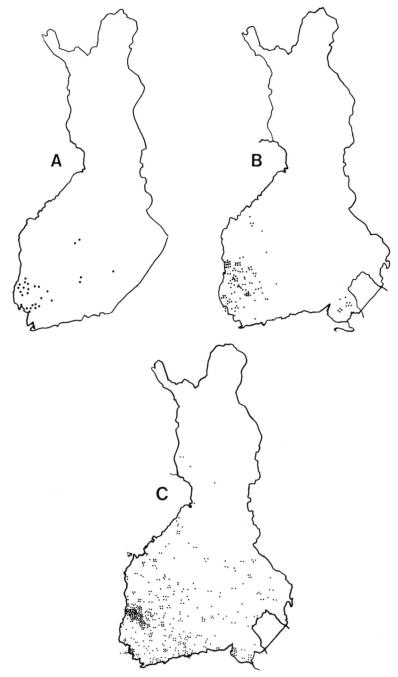

Fig. 7. Geographical distribution of some rare blood groups. (A) P^k (autosomal recessive); birthplaces of parents of 15 proposita. (B) A^{Fin} (autosomal dominant); birthplaces of parents of 60 proposita. (C) Rh gene r″ (cdE); birthplaces of parents of 568 proposita. (According to Nevanlinna *et al.*, 1981.)

ancestors occurs in the central, eastern, and northern parts of the country (Fig. 2, maps 5, 11, 15, 20, and 24 i.a.). If the disease is not very rare, the points are more scattered, though sparse in the southern and southwestern areas (old settlement) and with clusters here and there in the late settlement area (Fig. 2, maps 6, 9, and 21 i.a.). There are three remarkable exceptions. The map of infantile ceroid-lipofuscinosis (Fig. 2, Map 13) shows a wide cluster in southwestern Finland and two others in the young area of settlement, one in the west, one in the east. Whereas in the last two regions extensive pedigrees can be drawn showing remote consanguinities between several INCL parents, in southwestern Finland such consanguinities are not found. Such evidence shows that in this old, densely settled population the abundant occurrence of INCL is not based on isolated structure of population (which does not exist there) but on a really great general frequency of the INCL gene (R. Norio and P. Santavuori, unpublished data). The map of aspartylglucosaminuria (Fig. 2/1) shows a long zone of ancestry from southern Häme to Lapland. Interesting is the map of diastrophic dysplasia (Fig. 2/8), which outlines the contours of the assumed ancient area of the Häme Finns.

Thus, although few actual facts are known about the population history of the Finns of the prehistoric times (before 1000 AD), the opinion of most representatives of different branches of science concerned tends to favor the dualistic or pluralistic origin of the settlement in Finland. However, a divergent opinion based on population genetic studies is represented by Nevanlinna. Unbiased attempts at comparing and associating the observations and theories in different branches of science would be important. Nevertheless, the door is open for genetic investigations to help in the solving of the etiological problem of CHD.

V. CONCLUSION

During the last few years, Finland has appeared as the Promised Land of rare recessive disorders. There are three simultaneous reasons for this: a primitive population structure, an advanced level of medicine, and excellent church records for drawing pedigrees. The national and late regional isolation of a small population in a large area has created accumulations of unique recessive disorders and losses of many well-known diseases; "rare flora grows in rare soil."

Minimal infant mortality is characteristic of all Nordic countries, whereas Finland differs from the others by the excess mortality of middle-aged men. The main reason for this, though not the only one, is coronary heart disease, which in turn shows great differences between the eastern and western areas of the country. This difference is not satisfactorily explained in relation to known risk factors. To know whether genetic dualism could be the basis for this difference demands further, multiscientific studies and insights.

A partial cause of the excess mortality may be directly or indirectly found in the biological and cultural youngness of the Finnish population of today, in the late but rapid social, economical, cultural, and psychical development of the last decades and centuries. While Michelangelo was painting the Sistine Chapel in the Vatican, the greatest part of Finland was still an uninhabited wilderness. The adaptation of adult life takes its own time.

ACKNOWLEDGMENTS

I am grateful to Professor Jan Lindsten of Stockholm, Professor Kåre Berg and Dr. Tobias Gedde-Dahl of Oslo, and to Dr. Margareta Mikkelsen of Copenhagen for fruitful discussions. The experts on many nonmedical branches of science gave valuable knowledge and new ideas. The collaboration of numerous colleagues, experts on various Finnish diseases, including coronary heart disease, was of inestimable value. My sincerest thanks belong to Miss Liisa Savolainen for taking such trouble in preparing the manuscript.

REFERENCES

Aarskog, D. (1970). A familial syndrome of short stature associated with facial dysplasia and genital anomalies. *J. Pediatr.* **77**, 856.

Aarskog, D. (1971). A familial syndrome of short stature associated with facial dysplasia and genital anomalies. *Birth Defects, Orig. Artic. Ser.* **7**(6), 235.

Alström, C. H. (1957). Heredo-retinopathia congenitalis monohybrida recessiva autosomalis; a genetical–statistical study. *Hereditas* **43**, 1.

Alström, C. H. (1963). Population movements in Sweden from a genetic point of view. *Acta Psychiatr. Scand.* **39**, 41.

Amman, A. J., and Fudenberg, H. H. (1976). Chronic mucocutaneous candidiasis (with and without endocrinopathy). *In* "Basic and Clinical Immunology" (H. H. Fudenberg, D. P. Stites, J. L. Caldwell, and J. V. Wells, eds.), p. 344. Lange Med. Publ., Los Altos, California.

Aromaa, A., Björkstén, F., Eriksson, A. W., Maatela, J., Kirjarinta, M., Fellman, J., and Tamminen, M. (1975). Serum cholesterol and triglyceride concentrations of Finns and Finnish Lapps. I. Basic data. *Acta Med. Scand.* **198**, 13.

Aromaa, A., Maatela, J., and Pyörälä, K. (1977). Prevalence and incidence of hypertension in Finland; The Social Insurance Institution's study on Finnish population groups. *Nord. Counc. Arct. Med. Res. Rep.* No. 19, p. 88.

Ashby, H. (1901). A case of nephritis in a newly born infant. *Rep. Soc. Study Dis. Child.* **1**, 129.

Aula, P., and Autio, S. (1980). Salla disease. *In* "Population Structure and Genetic Disorders" (A. W. Eriksson *et al.*, eds.) p. 677. Academic Press, London and New York.

Aula, P., Raivio, K., and Autio, S. (1976). Enzymatic diagnosis and carrier detection of aspartylglucosaminuria using blood samples. *Pediatr. Res.* **10**, 625.

Aula, P., Karjalainen, O., Rapola, J., Lindgren, J., and Seppälä, M. (1977). Prenatal diagnosis of the Meckel syndrome. *Am. J. Obstet. Gynecol.* **129**, 700.

Aula, P., Rapola, J., Karjalainen, O., Lindgren, J., Hartikainen, A.-L., and Seppälä, M. (1978). Prenatal diagnosis of congenital nephrosis in 23 high-risk families. *Am. J. Dis. Child.* **132**, 984.

Aula, P., Autio, S., Raivio, K., Rapola, J., Thodén, C. J., Koskela, S. L., and Yamashina, I. (1979). "Salla disease." A new lysosomal storage disorder. *Arch. Neurol.* **36**, 88.

Autio, S. (1972). Aspartylglucosaminuria. Analysis of thirty-four patients. *J. Ment. Defic. Res., Monogr. Ser.* No. 1.

Autio, S. (1975). Clinical features of mannosidosis. *J. Pediatr.* **86,** 814.

Autio, S. (1980). Aspartylglucosaminuria. In "Population Structure and Genetic Disorders" (A. W. Eriksson *et al.,* eds.) p. 577. Academic Press, London and New York.

Autio, S., Nordén, N. E., Öckerman, P. A., Riekkinen, P., Rapola, J., and Louhimo, T. (1973a). Mannosidosis: Clinical, fine-structural and biochemical findings in three cases. *Acta Paediatr. Scand.* **62,** 555.

Autio, S., Visakorpi, J. K., and Järvinen, H. (1973b). Aspartylglucosaminuria. Further aspects on its clinical picture, mode of inheritance and epidemiology based on a series of 57 patients. *Ann. Clin. Res.* **5,** 149.

Awrich, A. E., Stackhouse, J., Cantrell, J. E., Patterson, J. H., and Rudman, D. (1975). Hyperdibasicaminoaciduria, hyperammonemia and growth retardation: Treatment with arginine, lysine and citrulline. *J. Pediatr.* **87,** 731.

Beckman, L. (1959). A contribution to the physical anthropology and population genetics of Sweden; variations of the ABO, Rh, MN and P blood groups. *Hereditas* **45,** 1.

Berson, E. L., Schmidt, S. Y., and Rabin, A. R. (1976). Plasma amino-acids in hereditary retinal disease. Ornithine, lysine, and taurine. *Br. J. Ophthalmol.* **60,** 142.

Biber, H. (1890). Über einige seltene Hornhauterkrankungen: Die oberflächliche gittrige Keratitis. Dissertation, A. Diggelmann, Zürich.

Bieberdorf, F. A., Gorden, P., and Fordtran, J. S. (1972). Pathogenesis of congenital alkalosis with diarrhea. *J. Clin. Invest.* **51,** 1958.

Björkstén, F., Aromaa, A., Eriksson, A. W., Maatela, J., Kirjarinta, M., Fellman, J., and Tamminen, M. (1975). Serum cholesterol and triglyceride concentrations of Finns and Finnish Lapps. II. Interpopulation comparisons and occurrence of hyperlipidemia. *Acta Med. Scand.* **198,** 23.

Bolander, A. M. (1971). A Comparative Study of Mortality by Cause in Four Nordic Countries, 1966-1968, with Special Reference to Male Excess Mortality. *Statistical Reports, Ser. Be.* No. 9. Natl. Centr. Bur. Stat., Stockholm.

Boström, H., and Hambraeus, L. (1964). Cystinuria in Sweden VII. Clinical, histopathological and medico-social aspects of the disease. *Acta Med. Scand., Suppl.* No. 411.

Brandt, T. (1936). Dermatitis in children with disturbances of the general condition and the absorption of food elements. *Acta Derm.-Venereol.* **17,** 513.

Carson, N. A. J., and Redmond, O. A. B. (1977). Lysinuric protein intolerance. *Ann. Clin. Biochem.* **14,** 135.

Chemke, J., Miskin, A., Rav-Acha, Z., Porath, A., Sagiv, M., and Katz, Z. (1977). Prenatal diagnosis of Meckel syndrome: alpha-fetoprotein and beta-trace protein in amniotic fluid. *Clin. Genet.* **11,** 285.

Chit, H. L. (1972). Über das Hautleistensystem der Bevölkerung Finnlands. *Ann. Acad. Sci. Fenn., Ser. A5* No. 151.

Collan, Y., and Meretoja, J. (1978). Inherited systemic amyloidosis (Finnish type): Ultrastructure of the skin. *Ann. Clin. Res.* **10,** 43.

Cumming, G. R., Kerr, D., and Ferguson, C. C. (1976). Constrictive pericarditis with dwarfism in two siblings (Mulibrey nanism). *J. Pediatr.* **88,** 569.

Cutler, C. W. (1895). Drei ungewöhnliche Fälle von Retino-Chorioideal Degeneration. *Arch. Augenheilkd.* **30,** 117.

Danboldt, N., and Closs, K. (1942). Acrodermatitis enteropathica. *Acta Derm.-Venereol.* **23,** 127.

Darrow, D. C. (1945). Congenital alkalosis with diarrhea. *J. Pediatr.* **26,** 519.

de Groot, C. S., Troelstra, J. A., and Hommes, F. A. (1970). Nonketotic hyperglycinemia: an *in vitro* study of the glycine-serine conversion in liver of three patients and effect of dietary methionine. *Pediatr. Res.* **4,** 238.

Epstein, F. H., and Pisa, Z. (1979). International comparisons of ischaemic heart disease mortality.

In "Proceedings of the Conference on the Decline in Coronary Heart Disease Mortality" (R. J. Havlik and M. Feinleib, eds.), National Heart, Lung and Blood Institute, Bethesda, Maryland, 24–25 October 1978, NIH Publication No. 79–161, U.S. Department of Health, Education and Welfare.

Eriksson, A. W. (1973). Genetic polymorphisms in Finno-Ugrian populations. Finns, Lapps and Maris. *Isr. J. Med. Sci.* **9**, 1156.

Eriksson, A. W., Vainio-Mattila, B. A., Krause, U., Fellman, J., and Forsius, H. (1967). Secondary sex ratio in families with X-chromosomal disorders. *Hereditas* **57**, 373.

Eriksson, A. W., Eskola, M.-R., Workman, P. L., and Morton, N. E. (1973a). Population studies on the Åland Islands. II. Historical population structure: Inference from bioassay of kinship and migration. *Hum. Hered.* **23**, 511.

Eriksson, A. W., Lehmann, W., and Forsius, H. (1973b). Congenital cornea plana in Finland. *Clin. Genet.* **4**, 301.

Eriksson, A. W., Fellman, J. O., Workman, P. L., and Lalouel, J. M. (1973c). Population studies on the Åland Islands. I. Prediction of kinship from migration and isolation by distance. *Hum. Hered.* **23**, 422.

Eriksson, A. W., Forsius, H., and Fellman, J. (1975). Populationsgenetiska undersökningar i Lappland. *Fin. Läkaresällsk. Handl.* **119**, 15.

Eriksson, A. W., Forsius, H. R., Nevanlinna, H. R., Workman, P. L., and Norio, R. K. (eds.) (1980). "Population Structure and Genetic Disorders." Academic Press, London and New York.

Evanson, J. M., and Stanburry, S. M. (1965). Congenital chloridorrhoea or so called congenital alkalosis with diarrhoea. *Gut* **6**, 29.

Forsius, H. (1957). Cornea plana and embryotoxon corneae posterius. *Acta Ophthalmol.* **35**, 63.

Forsius, H. (1961). Studien über Cornea plana congenita bei 19 Kranken in 9 Familien. *Acta Ophthalmol.* **39**, 272.

Forsius, H. R., and Eriksson, A. W. (1980). Retinoschisis X-chromosomalis. *In* "Population Structure and Genetic Disorders" (A. W. Eriksson *et al.*, eds.) p. 673. Academic Press, London and New York.

Forsius, H., Vainio-Mattila, B., and Eriksson, A. W. (1962). X-linked hereditary retinoschisis. *Br. J. Ophthalmol.* **46**, 678.

Forsius, H., Eriksson, A., Nuutila, A., Vainio-Mattila, B., and Krause, U. (1971). A genetic study of three rare retinal disorders: Dystrophia retinae dysacusis syndrome, X-chromosomal retinoschisis and grouped pigments of the retina. *Birth Defects, Orig. Artic. Ser.* **7**(3), 83.

Forsius, H. R., Krause, U., Helve, J., Vuopala, V., Mustonen, E., Vainio-Mattila, B., Fellman, J., and Eriksson, A. W. (1973). Visual acuity in 183 cases of X-chromosomal retinoschisis. *Can. J. Ophthalmol.* **8**, 385.

Forsius, H. R., Eriksson, A. W., and Kärnä, J. (1980a). Choroideremia. *In* "Population Structure and Genetic Disorders" (A. W. Eriksson *et al.*, eds.) p. 592. Academic Press, London and New York.

Forsius, H. R., Eriksson, A. W., and Lehmann, W. (1980b). Cornea plana congenita. *In* "Population Structure and Genetic Disorders" (A. W. Eriksson *et al.*, eds.) p. 605. Academic Press, London and New York.

Friedrich, U., Hansen, K. B., Hauge, M., Hägerstrand, I., Kristoffersen, K., Ludvigsen, E., Merrild, U., Nørgaard-Pedersen, B., Petersen, G. B., and Therkelsen, A. J. (1979). Prenatal diagnosis of polycystic kidneys and encephalocele (Meckel syndrome). *Clin. Genet.* **15**, 278.

Froesch, E. R. (1978). Essential fructosuria and hereditary fructose intolerance. *In* "The Metabolic Basis of Inherited Disease" (J. B. Stanbury, J. B. Wyngaarden, and D. S. Fredrickson, eds.), p. 121. McGraw-Hill, New York.

Froesch, E. R., Prader, A., Labhart, A., Stuber, H. W., and Wolf, H. P. (1957). Die hereditäre Fruktoseintoleranz, eine bisher nicht bekannte kongenitale Stoffwechselstörung. *Schweiz. Med. Wochenschr.* **87**, 1168.

Furuhjelm, U., and Nevanlinna, H. R. (1973). Inheritance of selective malabsorption of vitamin B_{12}. *Scand. J. Haematol.* **11**, 27.

Gamble, J. L., Fahey, K. R., Appleton, J., and MacLachlan, E. (1945). Congenital alkalosis with diarrhea. *J. Pediatr.* **26**, 509.

Gautier, P., and Miville, D. (1942). Syndrome de néphrose lipóidique congénitale. *Rev. Med. Suisse Romande* **62**, 740.

Gedde-Dahl, T., Jr. (1970). "Epidermolysis Bullosa; A Clinical, Genetic and Epidemiological Study." Universitetsforlaget, Oslo.

Gedde-Dahl, T., Jr. (1974). Population structure of Norway in view of rare recessives. *Bull. Eur. Soc. Hum. Genet.* Oct., p. 15.

Gedde-Dahl, T., Jr. (1978). Classification of epidermolysis bullosa. *In* "Pädiatrische Dermatologie" (J. J. Herzberg and G. W. Korting, eds.), p. 65. Schattauer, Stuttgart.

Gerritsen, T., Nyhan, W. L., Rehberg, M. L., and Ando, T. (1965). Metabolism of glyoxalate in nonketotic hyperglycinemia. *Pediatr. Res.* **3**, 269.

Gjone, E., Norum, K. R., and Glomset, J. A. (1978). Familial lecithin-cholesterol acyltransferase deficiency. *In* "The Metabolic Basis of Inherited Disease" (J. B. Stanbury, J. B. Wyngaarden, D. S. Fredrickson, eds.), p. 589. McGraw-Hill, New York.

Gräsbeck, R., Gordin, R., Kantero, I., and Kuhlbäck, B. (1960). Selective vitamin B_{12} malabsorption and proteinuria in young people. *Acta Med. Scand.* **167**, 289.

Granroth, G., Hakama, M., and Saxén, L. (1977). Defects of the central nervous system in Finland, I. Variations in time and space, sex distribution, and parental age. *Br. J. Prev. Soc. Med.* **31**, 164.

Haas, J. (1898). Über das Zusammenvorkommen von Veränderungen der Retina und Chorioidea. *Arch. Augenheilkd.* **37**, 343.

Habib, R., and Bois, E. (1973). Hétérogéneité des syndromes néphrotiques à début précoce du nourisson. (Syndrome nephrotique "infantile.") Etude anatomoclinique et génétique de 37 observations. *Helv. Paediatr. Acta* **28**, 91.

Hagberg, B., Sourander, P., and Svennerholm, L. (1968). Late infantile progressive encephalopathy with disturbed polyunsaturated fat metabolism. *Acta Paediatr. Scand.* **57**, 495.

Hakola, H. P. A. (1972). Neuropsychiatric and genetic aspects of a new hereditary disease characterized by progressive dementia and lipomembranous polycystic osteodysplasia. *Acta Psychiatr. Scand., Suppl.* No. 232.

Hakola, P., and Karjalainen, P. (1975). Bone mineral content in PLO. *Acta Radiol.* **16**, 385.

Hakosalo, J., Similä, S., Vesa, L., and Järvi, J. (1968). Renal abnormalities in hereditary onychoosteodysplasia. *Ann. Paediatr. Fenn.* **14**, 55.

Hallgren, B. (1959). Retinitis pigmentosa with congenital deafness; vestibulo-cerebellar ataxia and mental abnormality in a proportion of cases. A clinical and genetico-statistical study. *Acta Psychiatr. Scand.* **138**, 34.

Hallman, N., Hjelt, L., and Ahvenainen, E. K. (1956). Nephrotic syndrome in newborn and young infants. *Ann. Paediatr. Fenn.* **2**, 227.

Hallman, N., Norio, R., Kouvalainen, K., Vilska, J., and Kojo, N. (1970). Das kongenitale nephrotische Syndrom. *Ergeb. Inn. Med. Kinderheilkd.* **30**, 3.

Hallman, N., Norio, R., and Rapola, J. (1973). Congenital nephrotic syndrome. *Nephron* **11**, 101.

Haltia, M., and Rapola, J. (1973). Infantile type of so-called neuronal ceroid-lipofuscinosis. Histological and electron-microscopic studies. *Acta Neuropathol.* **26**, 257.

Haltia, M., Rapola, J., Santavuori, P., and Keränen, P. (1973). Infantile type of so-called neuronal ceroid-lipofuscinosis. Part 2. Morphological and biochemical studies. *J. Neurol. Sci.* **18**, 269.

Haltia, M., Palo, J., and Autio, S. (1975). Aspartylglucosaminuria: A generalized storage disease. Morphological and histochemical studies. *Acta Neuropathol.* **31**, 243.

Harenko, A., and Toivakka, E. (1961). Myoclonus epilepsy (Unverricht-Lundborg) in Finland. *Acta Neurol. Scand.* **37**, 282.

Holmberg, C., and Perheentupa, J. (1980). Congenital chloride diarrhea. *In* ''Population Structure and Genetic Disorders'' (A. W. Eriksson *et al.*, eds.) p. 596. Academic Press, London and New York.

Holmberg, C., Perheentupa, J., Launiala, K., and Hallman, N. (1977). Congenital chloride diarrhea. A clinical analysis of 21 Finnish patients. *Arch. Dis. Child.* **52**, 255.

Huttunen, N. P. (1976). Congenital nephrotic syndrome of Finnish type. A study of 75 cases. *Arch. Dis. Child.* **51**, 344.

Ikkala, E. (1960). Haemophilia: A study of its laboratory, clinical, genetic and social aspects based on known haemophiliacs in Finland. *Scand. J. Clin. Lab. Invest., Suppl.* No. 45.

Imerslund, O. (1960). Idiopathic chronic megaloblastic anaemia in children. *Acta Paediatr. (Stockholm), Suppl.* No. 119.

Isolauri, J., Uitti, J., and Visakorpi, J. K. (1979). Kystisen fibroosin seulonta vastasyntyneistä. (Neonatal screening for cystic fibrosis: A pilot study with meconium test.) *Duodecim* **95**, 16. (Engl. sum.)

Itkonen, T. (1972). Historiantakaiset Häme ja Suomi kielentutkijan näkokulmasta. (Prehistoric ''Häme'' and ''Finland'' from a linguistic viewpoint.) *Historiallinen Aikakauskirja* **70**, 85.

Jagell, S., Gustavson, K. H., and Holmgren, G. (1981). Sjögren-Larsson syndrome in Sweden; a clinical, genetic and epidemiological study. *Clin. Genet.* **19**, 233.

Järvi, O. H., Lauttamus, L. L., and Solonen, K. A. (1964). Membranous reticulin dysplasia of bones, probably a new disease entity (only title). *Proc. Scand. Congr. Pathol. Microbiol., 14th* p. 51. Universitetsforlaget, Oslo.

Järvi, O. H., Hakola, H. P. A., Lauttamus, L. L., Solonen, K. A., and Vilppula, A. H. (1968). Cystic capillary-necrotic osteodysplasia. A systemic bone disease probably caused by arteriolar and capillary necrosis. Relation to brain affection. *Int. Congr. Int. Acad. Pathol., 7th, State Univ. Milan* Abstr., p. 291.

Järvi, O., Hakola, P., Sourander, P., Kormano, M., Nevalainen, T., and Kalimo, H. (1980). Polycystic lipomembranous osteodysplasia with sclerosing leukoencephalopathy. *In* ''Population Structure and Genetic Disorders'' (A. W. Eriksson *et al.*, eds.) p. 656. Academic Press, London and New York.

Jenner, F. A., and Pollitt, R. J. (1967). Large quantities of 2-acetamido-1-(β-L-aspartamido)-1,2-dideoxyglucose in the urine of mentally retarded siblings. *Biochem. J.* **103**, 48.

Jutikkala, E. (1933). Asutuksen leviäminen Suomessa 1600-luvun alkuun mennessä. *In* ''Suomen Kulttuurihistoria I'' (G. Suolahti *et al.*, eds.), p. 51. Gummerus, Jyväskylä-Helsinki.

Kaiser-Kupfer, M., Monasterio, F. M. de, Valle, D., Walser, M., and Brusilow, S. (1980). Gyrate atrophy of the choroid and retina: improved visual function following reduction of plasma ornithine by diet. *Science* **210**, 1128.

Kaitila, I. (1980). Diastrophic dysplasia. *In* ''Population Structure and Genetic Disorders'' (A. W. Eriksson *et al.*, eds.) p. 610. Academic Press, London and New York.

Kaitila, I., and Perheentupa, J. (1980). Cartilage–hair hypoplasia. *In* ''Population Structure and Genetic Disorders'' (A. W. Eriksson *et al.*, eds.) p. 588. Academic Press, London and New York.

Kajanoja, P. (1971). A study in the morphology of the Finns and its relation to the settlement of Finland. *Ann. Acad. Sci. Fenn., Ser. A5* No. 146.

Karppanen, H., Pennanen, R., and Passinen, L. (1978). Minerals, coronary heart disease and sudden death. *Adv. Cardiol.* **25**, 9.

Karvonen, M. J., Blomqvist, G., Kallio, V., Orma, E., Punsar, S., Rautaharju, P., Takkunen, J., and Keys, A. (1967). Epidemiological studies related to coronary heart disease; characteristics of men aged 40–59 in seven countries. C 4. Men in rural East and West Finland. *Acta Med. Scand., Suppl.* No. 460, p. 169.

Kato, T., Tanaka, E., and Horisawa, S. (1976). Hyperdibasicaminoaciduria and hyperammonemia in familial protein intolerance. *Am. J. Dis. Child.* **130**, 1340.

Kaunisto, N. (1968). Dystrophia reticulata corneae. *Duodecim* **84**, 853. (In Finn.)

Kaunisto, N. (1971). Sarveiskalvon verkkomainen dystrofia. (Lattice dystrophy of the cornea.) *Duodecim* **87**, 1257. (Engl. sum.)

Kaunisto, N. (1973). Lattice dystrophy of the cornea. Its connection with preceding episodes of crystals and with subsequent amyloidosis. *Acta Ophthalmol.* **51**, 335.

Kerkkonen, M. (1971). Esihistorialliset Häme ja Suomi. (Prehistoric Häme and Finland.) *Historiallinen Aikakauskirja* **69**, 213.

Keys, A., ed. (1970). Coronary heart disease in seven countries. *Circulation* **41**, Suppl. No. 1.

Koivistoinen, P. (ed.) (1980). Mineral element composition of Finnish foods: N, K, Ca, Mg, P, S, Fe, Cu, Mn, Zn, Mo, Co, Ni, Cr, F, Se, Si, Rb, Al, B, Br, Hg, As, Cd, Pb, and ash. *Acta Agricult. Scand. Suppl.* **22**.

Koskiniemi, M. (1974). Psychological findings in progressive myoclonus epilepsy without Lafora bodies, *Epilepsia* **15**, 531.

Koskiniemi, M., Donner, M., Majuri, H., Haltia, M., and Norio, R. (1974a). Progressive myoclonus epilepsy. A clinical and histopathological study. *Acta Neurol. Scand.* **50**, 307.

Koskiniemi, M., Toivakka, E., and Donner, M. (1974b). Progressive myoclonus epilepsy. Electroencephalographical findings. *Acta Neurol. Scand.* **50**, 333.

Koskiniemi, M., Donner, M., Toivakka, E., and Norio, R. (1980). Progressive myoclonus epilepsy. *In* "Population Structure and Genetic Disorders" (A. W. Eriksson *et al.*, eds.) p. 669. Academic Press, London and New York.

Kouvalainen, K., and Pasternack, A. (1962). Alportin oireyhtymä (Alport's syndrome). *Duodecim* **78**, 1022. (Engl. sum.)

Kuokkanen, K. (1969). Ichthyosis vulgaris; A clinical and histopathological study of patients and their close relatives in the autosomal dominant and sex-linked forms of the disease. *Acta Derm.-Venereol., Suppl.* No. 62.

Kurstjens, J. H. (1965). Choroideremia and gyrate atrophy of the choroid and retina. *Doc. Ophthalmol.* **19**, 1.

Lamy, M., and Maroteaux, P. (1960). Le nanisme diastrophique. *Press Med.* **68**, 1977.

Langer, L. O. (1965). Diastrophic dwarfism in early infancy. *Am. J. Roentgenol.* **93**, 399.

Larsson, T., and Sjögren, T. (1966). Dystonia musculorum deformans; A genetic and clinical population study of 121 cases. *Acta Neurol. Scand., Suppl.* No. 17.

Launiala, K., Perheentupa, J., Pasternack, A., and Hallman, N. (1967). Familial chloride diarrhea—chloride malabsorption. *Mod. Probl. Pediatr.* **11**, 137.

Lindenov, H. (1945). The aetiology of deaf-mutism with special reference to heredity. Thesis, Copenhagen, Opera ex Domo Univ. Hafniensis, No. 8.

Lundborg, H. (1901). "Über Degeneration und degenerierte Geschlechter in Schweden. I. Klinische Studien und Erfahrungen hinsichtlich der familiaren Myoklonie und damit verwandter Krankheiten." Isaac Marcus' Boktr.-Aktiebolag, Stockholm.

Lundborg, H. (1903). "Die progressive Myoclonus-Epilepsie (Unverrichts Myoclonie)." Almqvist & Wiksell, Uppsala.

Lux, S. E., Johnston, R. B., August, C. S., Say, B., Penschaszadeh, V. B., Rosen, F. S., and McKusick, V. A. (1970). Chronic neutropenia and abnormal cellular immunity in cartilage-hair hypoplasia. *N. Engl. J. Med.* **282**, 231.

Mabry, C., and Karam, E. (1963). Idiopathic hyperglycinemia and hyperglycinuria. *South. Med. J.* **56**, 1944.

McCulloch, C., and McCulloch, R. J. P. (1948). A hereditary and clinical study of choroideremia. *Trans. Am. Acad. Ophthalmol. Otolaryngol.* **52**, 160.

McCulloch, C., and Marliss, E. B. (1975). Gyrate atrophy of the choroid and retina with hyperornithinemia. *Am. J. Ophthalmol.* **80**, 1047.

McKusick, V. A. (1964). Metaphyseal dysostosis and thin hair: A "new" recessively inherited syndrome? *Lancet* **1**, 832.

McKusick, V. A. (1978). "Mendelian Inheritance in Man." Johns Hopkins Press, Baltimore, Maryland.

McKusick, V. A., Eldridge, R., Hostetler, J. A., Ruangwit, U., and Egeland, J. A. (1965). Dwarfism in the Amish. II. Cartilage-hair hypoplasia. *Bull. Johns Hopkins Hosp.* **116**, 285.

Mäenpää, J. (1972). Congenital hypothyroidism. Aetological and clinical aspects. *Arch. Dis. Child.* **47**, 914.

Mark, K. (1972). A contribution to the physical anthropology of the Finns. *Ann. Acad. Sci. Fenn., Ser. A5* No. 152.

Maroteaux, P., Savart, P., Lefebvre, J., and Royer, P. (1963). Les formes partielles de la dysostose métaphysaire. *Presse Med.* **71**, 1523.

Mauthner, H. (1872). Ein Fall von Chorioideremia. *Ber. Naturmed. Ver. Innsbruck* **2**, 191.

Mecke, S., and Passarge, E. (1971). Encephalocele, polycystic kidneys and polydactyly as an autosomal recessive trait simulating certain other disorders: the Meckel syndrome. *Ann. Genet.* **14**, 97.

Meckel, J. F. (1822). Beschreibung zweier durch sehr ähnliche Bildungsabweichung entstellter Geschwister. *Dtsch. Arch. Physiol.* **7**, 99.

Meinander, C. F. (1973). The problem of the Finno-Ugrian peoples' origin on the base of archaeological data. *In* "Studies in the Anthropology of the Finno-Ugrian Peoples," Stencil No. 7. Archaeol. Inst., Univ. of Helsinki, Helsinki.

Meretoja, J. (1969). Familial systemic paramyloidosis with lattice dystrophy of the cornea, progressive cranial neuropathy, skin changes and various internal symptoms. A previously unrecognized heritable syndrome. *Ann. Clin. Res.* **1**, 314.

Meretoja, J. (1973). Genetic aspects of familial amyloidosis with corneal lattice dystrophy and cranial neuropathy. *Clin. Genet.* **4**, 173.

Meretoja, J., and Teppo, L. (1971). Histopathological findings of familial amyloidosis with cranial neuropathy as principal manifestation. *Acta Pathol. Microbiol. Scand., Sect. A* **79**, 432.

Mielke, J. H., Workman, P. L., Fellman, J., and Eriksson, A. W. (1976). Population structure of the Åland Islands, Finland, *Adv. Hum. Genet.* **6**, 241.

Mourant, A. E. (1954). "The Distribution of the Human Blood Groups." Blackwell, Oxford.

Mustajoki, P., and Koskelo, P. (1976). Hereditary hepatic porphyrias in Finland. *Acta Med. Scand.* **200**, 171.

Mustakallio, E. (1938). Untersuchungen über die M-N-, A_1-A_2- und O-A-B- Blutgruppen in Finnland. *Acta Soc. Med. Fenn. Duodecim, Ser. A* **20**, 1937.

Mylläriniemi, S., and Perheentupa, J. (1978). Oral findings in the autoimmune polyendocrinopathy-candidosis syndrome and other forms of hypoparathyroidism. *Oral Surg.* **45**, 721.

Nasu, T., Tsukahara, G., and Terayama, K. (1973). A lipid metabolic disease "membranous lipodystrophy"—an autopsy case demonstrating numerous peculiar membrane structures composed of compound lipid in bone and bone marrow and various adipose tissues. *Acta Pathol. Jpn.* **23**, 539.

Nevanlinna, H. R. (1972). The Finnish population structure; A genetic and genealogical study. *Hereditas* **71**, 195.

Nevanlinna, H. R. (1973a). Further evidence of the inhabitation in a marginal population. *Hereditas* **74**, 127.

Nevanlinna, H. R. (1973b). Suomen väestorakenne. Geneettinen ja genealoginen tutkimus. *Kansanalekelaitoksen Julk., Sär. A* No. 9.

Nevanlinna, H. R. (1980). Selective malabsorption of vitamin B_{12}. *In* "Population Structure and Genetic Disorders" (A. W. Eriksson *et al.*, eds.) p. 680. Academic Press, London and New York.

Nevanlinna, H. R., and Pirkola, A. (1973). An inherited blood group A variant in the Finnish population. II. Population studies. *Vox Sang.* **24**, 404.

Nevanlinna, H. R., Hekali, R., Sistonen, P., Pirkola, A., and Virtaranta, K. (1980). Polymorphic and rare markers in Finland. *In* "Population Structure and Genetic Disorders" (A. W. Eriksson *et al.*, eds.) p. 665. Academic Press, London and New York.

Nordén, N.-E., Lundblad, A., Svensson, S., and Autio, S. (1974). Characterization of two mannose-containing oligosaccharides isolated from the urine of patients with mannosidosis. *Biochemistry* **13**, 871.

Norio, R. (1966). Heredity in the congenital nephrotic syndrome; A genetic study of 57 Finnish families with a review of reported cases. *Ann. Paediatr. Fenn., Suppl.* No. 27.

Norio, R. (1980). Congenital nephrotic syndrome of Finnish type. *In* "Population Structure and Genetic Disorders" (A. W. Eriksson *et al.*, eds.) p. 600. Academic Press, London and New York.

Norio, R. (1981). Nephrotic syndrome. *In* "The Principles and Practice of Medical Genetics". (A. E. H. Emery and D. L. Rimoin, eds.). Churchill Livingstone, Edinburgh (in press).

Norio, R., and Koskiniemi, M. (1979). Progressive myoclonus epilepsy; Genetic and nosological aspects with a special reference to 107 Finnish patients. *Clin. Genet.* **15**, 382.

Norio, R., and Nevanlinna, H. R., eds. (1978). Rare Hereditary Diseases and Markers in Finland. Poster Exhibition, the 7th Sigrid Juselius Symposium "Population Genetic Studies on Isolates," Aug. 13-16, 1978. Mariehamn, Finland.

Norio, R., and Santavuori, P. (1981). To be published.

Norio, R., and Westeren, L. (1972). Homocystinuria; the first recognized case in Finland. *Scand. J. Clin. Lab. Invest., Suppl.* No. 122, p. 54.

Norio, R., Perheentupa, J., Launiala, K., and Hallman, N. (1971a). Congenital chloride diarrhea, an autosomal recessive disease. Genetic study of 14 Finnish and 12 other families. *Clin. Genet.* **2**, 182.

Norio, R., Perheentupa, J., Kekomäki, M., and Visakorpi, J. K. (1971b). Lysinuric protein intolerance, an autosomal recessive disease; A genetic study of 10 Finnish families. *Clin. Genet.* **2**, 214.

Norio, R., Nevanlinna, H. R., and Perheentupa, J. (1973). Hereditary diseases in Finland; Rare flora in rare soil. *Ann. Clin. Res.* **5**, 109.

Norio, R., Aula, P., and Rapola, J. (1980). The Meckel syndrome. *In* "Population Structure and Genetic Disorders" (A. W. Eriksson *et al.*, eds.) p. 637. Academic Press, London and New York.

Nuutila, A. (1968). Neuropsychiatric and genetic aspects of the dystrophia retinae pigmentosa-dysacusis syndrome. Thesis, Univ. of Helsinki, Helsinki.

Nuutila, A. (1970). Neuropsychiatric and genetic aspects of the dystrophia retinae pigmentosa-dysacusis syndrome. *J. Genet. Hum.* **18**, 57.

Nuutila, A. (1980). Dystrophia retinae pigmentosa-dysacusis syndrome. (1980). *In* "Population Structure and Genetic Disorders" (A. W. Eriksson *et al.*, eds.) p. 614. Academic Press, London and New York.

O'Donnell, J. J., Sandman, R. P., and Martin, S. R. (1978). Gyrate atrophy of the retina: Inborn error of L-ornithine: 2-oxoacid aminotransferase. *Science* **200**, 200.

Ohela, K. (1977). Hereditary angioneurotic oedema in Finland; Clinical, immunological and genealogical studies. *Acta Med. Scand.* **201**, 415.

Ohtani, Y., Miura, S., Tamai, Y., Kojima, H., and Kashima, H. (1979). Neutral lipid and sphingolipid composition of the brain of a patient with membranous lipodystrophy. *J. Neurol.* **220**, 77.

Oliver, J. (1960). Microcystic renal disease and its relation to "infantile nephrosis." *Am. J. Dis. Child.* **100**, 312.

Opitz, J. M., and Howe, J. J. (1969). The Meckel syndrome (dysencephalia splanchnocystica, the Gruber syndrome). *Birth Defects, Orig. Artic. Ser.* **5**(2), 167.

Palo, J. (1967). Prevalence of phenylketonuria and some other metabolic disorders among mentally retarded patients in Finland. *Acta Neurol. Scand.* **43**, 573.

Palo, J., and Matsson, K. (1970). Eleven new cases of aspartylglucosaminuria. *J. Ment. Defic. Res.* **14**, 168.

Palo, J., and Savolainen, H. (1973). Biochemical diagnosis of aspartylglucosaminuria. *Ann. Clin. Res.* **5**, 156.

Peltokallio, V. (1970). Non-parasitic cysts of the liver: A clinical study of 177 cases. *Ann. Chir. Gynaecol. Fenn., Suppl.* No. 174.

Perheentupa, J. (1972a). Kolme periytyvää kasvuhäiriötä. (Cartilage–hair hypoplasia, diastrophic nanism and mulibrey nanism.) *Duodecim* **88**, 60. (Engl. sum.)

Perheentupa, J. (1972b). Kaksi ryhmää lisämunuaiskuoren periytyviä vajaatoimintatiloja. (Congenital adrenal hyperplasia, and the syndrome of hypoparathyroidism, Addison's disease and candidiasis.) *Duodecim* **88**, 119. (Engl. sum.)

Perheentupa, J., ed. (1972c). Suomalainen tautiperintö. (Symposium on inherited disease in Finland.) *Duodecim* **88**, 1. (Engl. sum.)

Perheentupa, J. (1975). Hereditary fructose intolerance. *In* "Endocrine and Genetic Diseases in Childhood and Adolescence" (L. I. Gardner, ed.), p. 986. Saunders, Philadelphia, Pennsylvania.

Perheentupa, J. (1980a). Autoimmune polyendocrinopathy-candidosis-ectodermal dystrophy. *In* "Population Structure and Genetic Disorders" (A. W. Eriksson *et al.*, eds.) p. 583. Academic Press, London and New York.

Perheentupa, J. (1980b). Hereditary fructose intolerance. *In* "Population Structure and Genetic Disorders" (A. W. Eriksson *et al.*, eds.) p. 617. Academic Press, London and New York.

Perheentupa, J. (1980c). Mulibrey nanism. *In* "Population Structure and Genetic Disorders" (A. W. Eriksson *et al.*, eds.) p. 641. Academic Press, London and New York.

Perheentupa, J. (1981). In preparation.

Perheentupa, J., and Visakorpi, J. K. (1965). Protein intolerance with deficient transport of basic amino acids: another inborn error of metabolism. *Lancet* **11**, 813.

Perheentupa, J., Pitkänen, E., Nikkilä, E. A., Somersalo, O., and Hakosalo, J. (1962). Hereditary fructose intolerance. A clinical study of four cases. *Ann. Paediatr. Fenn.* **8**, 221.

Perheentupa, J., Eklund, J., and Kojo, N. (1965). Familial chloride diarrhoea ("congenital alkalosis with diarrhoea"). *Acta Paediatr. Scand., Suppl.* No. 159, p. 119.

Perheentupa, J., Autio, S., Leisti, S., Raitta, C., and Tuuteri, L. (1973). Mulibrey nanism, an autosomal recessive syndrome with pericardial constriction. *Lancet* **11**, 351.

Perheentupa, J., Autio, S., Leisti, S., Raitta, C., and Tuuteri, L. (1975). Mulibrey nanism: Review of 23 cases of a new autosomal recessive syndrome. *Birth Defects, Orig. Artic. Ser.* **11**(2), 3.

Perheentupa, J., Tiilikainen, A., and Lokki, M. (1981). In preparation.

Perry, T. H., Urquhart, N., and Hansen, S. (1977). Studies of the glycine cleavage enzyme system in brain from infants with glycine encephalopathy. *Pediatr. Res.* **12**, 192.

Pesonen, E., Norio, R., and Sarna, S. (1975). Thickenings in the coronary arteries in infancy as an indication of genetic factors in coronary heart disease. *Circulation* **51**, 218.

Pirskanen, R. (1977). Genetic aspects in myasthenia gravis; A family study of 264 Finnish patients. *Acta Neurol. Scand.* **56**, 365.

Punsar, S., Erämetsä, O., Karvonen, M. J., Ryhänen, A., Hilska, P., and Vornamo, H. (1975). Coronary heart disease and drinking water. A search in two Finnish male cohorts for epidemiologic evidence of a water factor. *J. Chronic Dis.* **28**, 259.

Puska, P., Tuomilehto, J., Salonen, J. Neittaanmäki, L., Mäki, J., Virtamo, J., Nissinen, A., Koskela, K., and Takalo, T. (1979). Changes in coronary risk factors during comprehensive five-year community programme to control cardiovascular diseases (North Karelia project). *Br. Med. J.* **2**, 1173.

Pyörälä, K., and Valkonen, T. (1981). The high ischaemic heart disease mortality in Finland; international comparisons, regional differences, trends and possible causes. *In* "Medical Aspects of Mortality Statistics.'' Skandia International Symposia, Almqvist and Wiksell, Stockholm (in press).

Raitta, C., and Perheentupa, J. (1974). Mulibrey nanism; An inherited dysmorphic syndrome with characteristic ocular findings. *Acta Ophthalmol., Suppl.* No. 123, p. 162.

Raitta, C., and Santavuori, P. (1973). Ophthalmological findings in so-called infantile neuronal ceroid-lipofuscinosis. *Acta Ophthalmol.* **51**, 755.

Raitta, C., Santavuori, P., Lamminen, M., and Leisti, J. (1978). Ophthalmological findings in a new syndrome with muscle, eye and brain involvement. *Acta Ophthalmol.* **56**, 465.

Rajantie, J., Simell, O., and Perheentupa, J. (1980). Basolateral-membrane transport defect for lysine in lysinuric protein intolerance. *Lancet* **1**, 1219.

Rapola, M. (1961). ''Johdatus Suomen murteisiin'' (An Introduction to the Finnish Dialects), Tietolipas 4. Suom. Kirjallisuuden Seura, Helsinki.

Rapola, J. (1981). Renal pathology of fetal congenital nephrosis. A light microscopic study of 15 cases. *Acta Pathol. Microbiol. Scand. (A)* **89**, 63.

Refsum, S. (1946). Heredopathia atactica polyneuritiformis: A familial syndrome not hitherto described. A contribution to the clinical study of the hereditary diseases of the nervous system. *Acta Psychiatr. Scand., Suppl.* No. 38.

Refsum, S. (1977). Heredopathia atactica polyneuritiformis, phytanic acid storage disease (Refsum's disease) with particular reference to ophthalmological disturbances. *Metab. Ophthalmol.* **1**, 73.

Renlund, M., Chester, A., Lundblad, A., Aula, P., Raivio, K. O., Autio, S., and Koskela, S. L. (1979). Increased urinary excretion of free N-acetylneuraminic acid in thirteen patients with Salla disease. *Eur. J. Biochem.* **101**, 245.

Rimpelä, M. (1978). Aikuisväestön tupakointitavat Suomessa 1950-1970-luvuilla (Adult Use of Tobacco in Finland in the 1950-1970's). *Kansanterveystieteen Julk.* (Dept. of Health, Univ. of Tampere) *Ser. M, No. 40.*

Rönning, O., Myllärniemi, S., and Perheentupa, J. (1978). Craniofacial and dental characteristics of cartilage-hair hypoplasia. *Cleft Palate J.* **15**, 49.

Rübel, E. (1912). Kongenitale familiäre Flachheit der Kornea (Cornea plana). *Klin. Monatsbl. Augenheilkd.* **50**, 427.

Sahi, T. (1974). Lactose malabsorption in Finnish-speaking and Swedish-speaking populations in Finland. *Scand. J. Gastroenterol.* **9**, 303.

Sahi, T. (1978). Intestinal lactase polymorphisms and dairy foods. *Hum. Genet., Suppl.* No. 1, p. 115.

St. Leger, A. S., Cochrane, A. L., and Moore, F. (1979). Factors associated with cardiac mortality in developed countries with particular reference to the consumption of wine. *Lancet* **1**, 1017.

Salonen, J. T., Puska, P., and Mustaniemi, H. (1979). Changes in morbidity and mortality during comprehensive community programme to control cardiovascular diseases during 1972-7 in North Karelia. *Br. Med. J.* **2**, 1178.

Salonen, R., Herva, R., and Norio, R. (1981). The hydrolethalus syndrome: delineation of a ''new,'' lethal malformation syndrome based on 28 patients. *Clin. Genet.* **19** (in press).

Santavuori, P. (1973). EEG findings in the infantile type of so-called neuronal ceroid-lipofuscinosis. *Neuropaediatrie* **4**, 375.

Santavuori, P. (1980). Infantile type of neuronal ceroid-lipofuscinosis. *In* ''Population Structure and Genetic Disorders'' (A. W. Eriksson *et al.*, eds.) p. 626. Academic Press, London and New York.

Santavuori, P., and Leisti, J. (1980). Muscle, eye and brain disease. *In* ''Population Structure and Genetic Disorders'' (A. W. Eriksson *et al.*, eds.) p. 647. Academic Press, London and New York.

Santavuori, P., Haltia, M., Rapola, J., and Raitta, C. (1973). Infantile type of so-called neuronal ceroid-lipofuscinosis. Part 1. A clinical study of 15 patients. *J. Neurol. Sci.* **18**, 257.

Santavuori, P., Haltia, M., and Rapola, J. (1974). Infantile type of so-called neuronal ceroid-lipofuscinosis. *Dev. Med. Child Neurol.* **16**, 644.

Santavuori, P., Leisti, J., and Kruus, S. (1977). Muscle, eye and brain disease: A new syndrome. *Neuropaediatrie* **8**, Suppl., p. 553.

Saxen, I., and Lahti, A. (1974). Cleft lip and palate in Finland: Incidence, secular, seasonal, and geographical variations. *Teratology* **9**, 217.

Seip, M. (1971). Generalized lipodystrophy. *Ergeb. Inn. Med. Kinderheilkd.* **31**, 59.

Seip, M. (1975). The syndrome of generalized lipodystrophy. *Birth Defects, Orig. Artic. Ser.* **11**(2), 325.

Seller, M. J. (1978). Meckel syndrome and the prenatal diagnosis of neural tube defects. *J. Med. Genet.* **15**, 462.

Seppälä, M. (1965). Distribution of serum transferrin groups in Finland and their inheritance. *Ann. Med. Exp. Biol. Fenn.* **43**, Suppl. No. 4.

Seppälä, M., Aula, P., Rapola, J., Karjalainen, O., Huttunen, N. P., and Ruoslahti, E. (1976). Congenital nephrotic syndrome: prenatal diagnosis and genetic counselling by estimation of amniotic-fluid and maternal serum alphafetoprotein. *Lancet* **11**, 123.

Seppäläinen, A. M., and Similä, S. (1971). Electroencephalographic findings in three patients with nonketotic hyperglycinemia. *Epilepsia* **12**, 101.

Shapiro, L. J., Kaback, M. M., Toomey, K. E., Sarti, D., Luther, P., and Cousins, L. (1977). Prenatal diagnosis of the Meckel syndrome: use of serial ultrasound and alphafetoprotein measurements. *Birth Defects, Orig. Artic. Ser.* **13**(3D), 267.

Simell, O., and Takki, K. (1973). Raised plasma-ornithine and gyrate atrophy of the choroid and retina. *Lancet* **1**, 1031.

Simell, O., Perheentupa, J., Rapola, J., Visakorpi, J. K., and Eskelin, L. E. (1975). Lysinuric protein intolerance. *Am. J. Med.* **59**, 229.

Simell, O., Rajantie, J., and Perheentupa, J. (1980). Lysinuric protein intolerance. *In* "Population Structure and Genetic Disorders" (A. W. Eriksson *et al.*, eds.) p. 633. Academic Press, London and New York.

Similä, S., and Visakorpi, J. (1970). Clinical findings in three patients with nonketotic hyperglycinemia. *Ann. Clin. Res.* **2**, 151.

Sipilä, I., Simell, O., and Takki, K. (1980). Hyperornithinaemia with gyrate atrophy of the choroid and retina. *In* "Population Structure and Genetic Disorders" (A. W. Eriksson *et al.*, eds.) p. 620. Academic Press, London and New York.

Sipilä, I., Rapola, J., Simell, O., and Vannas, A. (1981). Supplementary creatine as treatment in gyrate atrophy of the choroid and retina. *N. Engl. J. Med.* (in press).

Sjögren, T. (1931). Die juvenile amaurotische Idiotie; klinische und erblichkeitsmedizinische Untersuchungen. *Hereditas* **14**, 197.

Sjögren, T., and Larsson, T. (1957). Oligophrenia in combination with congenital ichthyosis and spastic disorders. *Acta Psychiatr. Neurol. Scand., Suppl.* No. 113.

Statistical Year Book of Finland (1977). Cent. Stat. Off., Helsinki.

Steinberg, A. G., Tiilikainen, A., Eskola, M.-R., and Eriksson, A. W. (1974). Gammaglobulin allotypes in Finnish Lapps, Finns, Åland Islanders, Maris (Cheremis), and Greenland Eskimos. *Am. J. Hum. Genet.* **26**, 223.

Stephan, U., Busch, E. W., and Kollberg, H. (1975). Cystic fibrosis detection by means of a test-strip. *Pediatrics* **55**, 35.

Streng, O. (1935). Die Blutgruppenforschung in der Anthropologie. *Acta Soc. Med. Fenn. Duodecim, Ser. A No. 17.*

Streng, O. (1937). Blutgruppenforschung und Anthropologie. *Z. Rassenphysiol.* **9**, 97.

Subow, A. A. (1972). Einige Angaben der dentalen Anthropologie über die Bevölkerung Finnlands. *Ann. Acad. Sci. Fenn. Ser. A5* No. 150.

Svennerholm, L., Hagberg, B., Haltia, M., Sourander, P., and Vanier, M.-T. (1975). Polyunsaturated fatty acid lipidosis (PFAL); Lipid biochemical studies. *Acta Paediatr. Scand.* **64**, 489.

Takki, K. (1974a). Gyrate atrophy of the choroid and retina associated with hyperornithinemia. *Br. J. Ophthalmol.* **58**, 3.

Takki, K. (1974b). Differential diagnosis between the primary total choroidal vascular atrophies. *Br. J. Ophthalmol.* **58**, 24.

Takki, K., and Simell, O. (1974). Genetic aspects in gyrate atrophy of the choroid and retina with hyperornithinaemia. *Br. J. Ophthalmol.* **58**, 907.

Talve, I. (1972). "Suomen kulttuurirajoista ja alueista" (Aspects of cultural boundaries and regions in Finland). Esitelmät pöytäk., Suom Tiedeakat., Helsinki.

Terayama, K. (1961). Two cases of cystic bone disease showing peculiar features. *Nippon Seikeigeka Gakkai Zasshi* **35**, 626.

Thorén, C. (1973). So-called mulibrey nanism with pericardial constriction. *Lancet* **11**, 731.

Thorpe, E. S., Jr., and Handley, H. E. (1929). Chronic tetany and chronic mycelial stomatitis in a child aged four and one half years. *Am. J. Dis. Child.* **38**, 328.

Tryggvason, K., and Kouvalainen, K. (1975). Number of nephrons in normal human kidneys and kidneys of patients with the congenital nephrotic syndrome; A study using a sieving method for counting of glomeruli. *Nephron* **15**, 62.

Tuuteri, L., Perheentupa, J., and Rapola, J. (1974). The cardiopathy of mulibrey nanism, a new inherited syndrome. *Chest* **65**, 628.

Uhari, M., and Herva, R. (1979). Polycystic kidney disease of perinatal type. *Acta Paediat. Scand.* **68**, 443.

Unverricht, H. (1891). "Die Myoclonie." Deuticke, Vienna.

Unverricht, H. (1895). Über familiäre Myoclonie. *Dtsch. Z. Nervenheilkd.* **7**, 32.

Usher, C. H. (1913–1914). On the inheritance of retinitis pigmentosa with notes of cases. *R. London Ophthalmol. Hosp. Rep.* **19**, 130.

Vainio-Mattila, B., Eriksson, A. W., and Forsius, H. (1969). X-chromosomal recessive retinoschisis in the region of Pori. An ophthalmo-genetical analysis of 103 cases. *Acta Ophthalmol.* **47**, 1135.

Valkonen, T., and Niemi, M.-L. (1978). Sepelvaltimotautikuolleisuuden alueelliset erot Suomessa. (The regional differences of mortality from coronary heart disease in Finland.) *Suom. Lääkärilehti* **33**, 1978.

Valkonen, T., and Notkola, V. (1977). Influence of socioeconomic and other factors on the geographic variation of mortality in Finland, Sweden and Norway. *Yearb. Popul. Res. Finl.* **15**, 9.

Valle, D., Kaiser-Kupfer, M. I., and del Valle, L. A. (1977). Gyrate atrophy of the choroid and retina: deficiency of ornithine aminotransferase in transformed lymphocytes. *Proc. Natl. Acad. Sci. U.S.A.* **74**, 5159.

Valle, D., Walser, M., Brusilow, S. W., and Kaiser-Kupfer, M. (1980). Gyrate atrophy of the choroid and retina. Amino acid metabolism and correction of hyperornithinemia with an arginine-deficient diet. *J. Clin. Invest.* **65**, 371.

Vernier, R. L., Brunson, J., and Good, R. A. (1957). Studies on familial nephrosis. *Am. J. Dis. Child.* **93**, 469.

Virolainen, M., Savilahti, E., Kaitila, I., and Perheentupa, J. (1978). Cellular and humoral immunity in cartilage-hair hypoplasia. *Pediatr. Res.* **12**, 961.

Visakorpi, J., and Furuhjelm, U. (1968). Selective malabsorption of vitamin B_{12}. *Mod. Probl. Pediatr.* **11**, 150.

Visakorpi, J. K., and Gerber, M. (1963). Hypoparathyroidism with steatorrhoea and some features of pernicious anaemia in a 5-year-old girl. *Ann. Paediatr. Fenn.* **9**, 129.

Visakorpi, J. K., Donner, M., and Norio, R. (1965). Hyperglycinuria with severe neurological manifestations. *Ann. Paediatr. Fenn.* **11**, 114.

Visakorpi, J. K., Palo, J., and Renkonen, O.-V. (1971). The incidence of PKU in Finland. *Acta Paediatr. Scand.* **60**, 666.

Voipio, H., Gripenberg, U., Raitta, C., and Horsmanheimo, A. (1964). Retinitis pigmentosa; A preliminary report. *Hereditas* **52**, 247.

von Graefe, A. (1858). Exceptionelles Verhalten des Gesichtsfeldes bei Pigmententartung der Netzhaut. *Albrecht von Graefes Arch. Ophthalmol.* **4**, 250.

von Wendt, L., and Similä, S. (1980). Nonketotic hyperglycinemia. *In* "Population Structure and Genetic Disorders" (A. W. Eriksson *et al.*, eds.) p. 652. Academic Press, London and New York.

von Wendt, L., Similä, S., Hirvasniemi, A., and Suvanto, E. (1978). Nonketotic hyperglycinemia. A clinical analysis of 19 Finnish patients. *Monogr. Human Genet.* **9**, 58.

von Wendt, L., Hirvasniemi, A., and Similä, S. (1979). Heterozygotes of nonketotic hyperglycinemia. A genetical analysis of 13 Finnish families. *Clin. Genet.* **15**, 411.

Voorhess, M. L., Husson, G. S., and Blackman, M. S. (1976). Growth failure with pericardial constriction. The syndrome of mulibrey nanism. *Am. J. Dis. Child.* **130**, 1146.

Walker, B. A., Scott, C. I., Hall, J. G., Murdoch, J. L., and McKusick, V. A. (1972). Diastrophic dwarfism. *Medicine (Baltimore)* **51**, 41.

Walter, H. (1970). Der diastrophische Zwergwuchs. *Adv. Hum. Genet.* **2**, 31.

Wikström, J. (1975). Studies on the clustering of multiple sclerosis in Finland. II: Microepidemiology in one high-risk county with special reference to familial cases. *Acta Neurol. Scand.* **51**, 173.

Wikström, J., and Palo, J. (1975). Studies on the clustering of multiple sclerosis in Finland. I: Comparison between the domiciles and places of birth in selected subpopulations. *Acta Neurol. Scand.* **51**, 85.

Wikström J., Aho, K., Jokelainen, M., Karli, P., and Matell, R. (1978). Epidemiology of multiple sclerosis and optic neuritis, stroke, amyotrophic lateral sclerosis, dystrophia myotonica and myasthenia gravis in Finland. *Acta Neurol. Scand., Suppl.* No. 67, p. 290.

World Health Statistics Annual Vol. 1. (1977, 1978). WHO, Geneva.

13
Culture and Disease in Britain and Western Europe

D. F. ROBERTS

BIOCULTURAL ASPECTS OF DISEASE
Copyright © 1981 by Academic Press, Inc.
ISBN 0-12-598720-X

I. INTRODUCTION

Disease in man can be seen as a continuous spectrum. At one extreme are conditions due entirely to extraneous causes, such as skin destruction after burns and skeletal fractures as a result of accident, that occur in patients irrespective of their genetic constitution. At the other extreme are diseases due to the genetic constitution of the individual irrespective of his environment, e.g., Duchenne muscular dystrophy, Huntington's chorea. Most diseases occur somewhere between these two extremes.

In infections, microorganisms successfully invade human tissues and produce disease. Yet millions of microorganisms are to be found in some parts of the human body without adverse effect, and indeed often confer benefit. If, however, they become established in other tissues they can cause serious pathology. Soon after birth the pneumococcus colonizes the back of the nose and throat, without ill effect. But later in life the organism sometimes descends into the lungs, where it may cause pneumonia, or ascends into the brain, where it may cause meningitis; some patients survive, some die. Obviously individuals differ in the ability to cope with such colonizations, even within themselves at different times. In genetic disease relatively few cases are manifest at birth or in early childhood. A woman in Newcastle may appear to be healthy but genetically a porphyriac; if she takes a holiday on the Mediterranean, or if she chooses a regimen of the contraceptive pill, the frank manifestation of the disorder may be triggered. The pattern of disease in any community is complex. It may vary with change in the genetic constitution of the population, or change in the environment, or both. A major factor in environmental change is culture, and the whole complex of attitudes, beliefs, behavior, living practices, and possessions that culture implies.

Northwest Europe is a cultural area distinctly different from anywhere else. It shares certain features with other regions, but nowhere is the combination exactly duplicated. It is a region of dense population (in some localities extremely so), with great urban concentrations. Opportunity for close personal contact is far greater than anywhere else at any time in human history. The standard of living is high. Most homes are warm, clean, and weather-proof. Sanitary conditions are generally adequate, and sewage disposal and clean water supply efficient. There is gross local pollution of the atmosphere by dense motor traffic and industrial gases, and of the natural waters by effluents. Ignorance about personal hygiene and the spread of infection is widespread. Nevertheless, the pattern of mortality has grossly changed during the last century, with the eradication of deaths from diphtheria, smallpox, whooping cough, typhoid, and other diseases that were previously such terrible scourges. The populations have access to highly efficient methods of infection control, whose widespread misuse is in turn producing problems. Indeed, the armament of procedures for combating, diagnosing, and prediagnosing conditions is the strongest ever in human history. The people are highly susceptible to indoctrination via the communications media and personal contact from schooldays, through working life and into old age. This combination of conditions has produced a characteristic disease pattern, from which excellent illustrations can be found of biocultural interaction.

II. MAJOR CAUSES OF DEATH IN WESTERN EUROPE

Death statistics are not the most reliable data. Errors may occur in diagnosis, and personal, local, or national recording practices and interpretations may differ. However, they do provide some indication of the disease pattern.

Table I lists the ten leading causes of death in 1971 for 14 countries in western Europe, together with the percentage of deaths for which each accounts (World Health Organization, 1974). Admittedly, each category includes a number of different diseases, and international comparisons of mortality by cause are difficult because interpretations of the International Classification of Diseases differ from one country to another. But the general pattern is clearly similar in each country. In all, heart disease is the leading cause of death, followed by malignant neoplasms, and then cerebrovascular disease. In seven countries, the first two categories account for more than 50% of the deaths and in five countries the first three account for more than 65%. After these, accidents, accounting for about 5% of deaths, are the fourth most frequent cause in nine countries, whereas the remaining categories vary in rank from country to country. Of the respiratory disorders, the acute (influenza and pneumonia) account for 4% of deaths and the chronic (bronchitis, emphysema, and asthma) for about 3%, and these vary at about fifth or sixth rank. The remaining categories contribute 1 or 2% each and are more variable in rank; cirrhosis of the liver varies from fourth to below tenth and suicide from sixth to below tenth. But the general similarity is striking, both in the limited number of categories that appear among the top ten and the proportions for which they account.

A. Age

The causes of death differ, of course, among age-groups. In the age-group 1–4 years in all countries, accidents are the leading cause, accounting for about one-third of all deaths, followed closely by malignant neoplasms or congenital anomalies or influenza and pneumonia (Table II). In nine countries these first four categories account for more than 60% of the deaths. In the 5–14 year age-groups, accidents are consistently the leading cause of death, and malignant neoplasms the second in all the 14 countries. Congenital anomalies are third in 12 of the 14 and influenza and pneumonia fourth in 11. The first two categories

TABLE I

The Ten Leading Causes of Death in Selected Countries for All Ages[a]

Cause of death	Austria	Belgium	Denmark	France	German Federal Republic	Greece	Ireland	Italy	Netherlands	Norway	Spain	Switzerland	England and Wales	Scotland
Heart disease B25–29	27.9	27.0	34.5	20.2	27.6	19.8	32.2	28.9	30.3	33.5	22.3	28.2	33.2	34.5
Malignant neoplasms B19	19.8	19.7	23.5	19.7	19.9	16.1	17.8	19.0	23.3	18.8	15.7	22.0	20.6	20.7
Cerebrovascular disease B30	15.1	13.5	10.5	13.9	14.8	14.8	14.3	13.9	11.0	15.3	14.1	11.5	14.1	16.2
Accidents BE47–48	6.3	5.4	4.8	7.2	5.3	4.6	4.0	4.9	5.7	5.2	4.1	6.8	3.0	3.7
Influenza and pneumonia B31–2	3.3	3.4	2.4	2.5	2.4	4.2	5.7	3.5	2.7	6.4	5.9	3.7	7.1	3.8
Cirrhosis of the liver B37	2.4	1.0	0.9	3.2	2.1	1.9		3.1			2.6	1.7		
Bronchitis, emphysemia, and asthma B33	2.2	2.5	2.6	1.1	3.1	2.9	5.4	3.5	3.0	1.3	4.3	2.2	5.0	4.2

Suicide BE49	1.7	1.3	2.5	1.4	1.8	2.7	1.0	2.4	1.0	0.8		2.0	0.7	0.6
Diabetes mellitus B21	1.4	3.0	1.4	1.4					2.2	0.8	1.9	2.8	0.9	1.1
Congenital anomalies B42		0.7	0.9				1.3	0.8	1.1	0.8		0.9	0.8	1.0
Benign tumors B20					0.9	1.2			0.9	0.6				
Nephritis and nephroses B28						1.7	0.6				1.4			
Birth injuries B43							0.9	1.1						0.8
Tuberculosis B5–6	1.0										1.2			
Peptic ulcer B34													0.7	
Intestinal obstruction and hernia B36				0.8										

[a] As percentage of all deaths.

TABLE II

The Ten Leading Causes of Death in Selected Countries: 1–4 Years

Cause of death	Austria	Belgium	Denmark	France	German Federal Republic	Greece	Ireland	Italy	Netherlands	Norway	Spain	Switzerland	England and Wales	Scotland
Accidents	35.4	30.7	36.1	32.6	33.0	20.7	27.7	23.0	38.8	47.4	17.9	36.5	27.5	35.1
Malignant neoplasms	10.3	9.5	18.3	7.5	10.1	10.9	12.9	11.1	9.5	8.0	8.8	8.7	10.7	9.9
Congenital anomalies	8.5	11.1	17.3	10.0	13.6	8.6	12.9	10.2	15.3	15.0	6.5	16.3	17.9	11.5
Influenza and pneumonia	6.3	5.9	3.5	4.4	5.6	16.8	14.4	13.1	3.3	4.2	11.5	3.7	10.3	8.8
Meningococcal infection, B11	2.3	5.5	1.5	1.1	2.4	2.3	1.5	3.8	1.9	0.5	5.7	3.4	1.5	3.1
Measles, B14	1.9	1.4		0.9	1.3		3.5	1.8	0.5	1.4		1.4		0.8
Meningitis, B24	1.4		2.0	2.4	1.8		2.0	1.8	1.9	1.9	3.7	1.4	1.6	1.5
Appendicitis, B35	1.4		0.5							0.5				
All other external causes, BE50	1.4	1.2		1.7	1.3	1.3		1.4	1.9			0.8	1.9	1.9
Benign neoplasms	1.2	1.2	0.5	1.8	1.8						2.1	0.6		
Cerebrovascular disease		2.2				2.7					5.8		1.6	
Heart disease		1.2	0.5	2.6		2.3	5.4	5.7	2.7	4.7	2.0		3.3	5.3
Enteritis and other diarrhea, B4			2.0		1.5	5.7								
Anemias, B23								3.2						
Tuberculosis						1.1	1.0				1.7			
Bronchitis, emphysema, and asthma							2.0		0.5	1.4		0.8	2.0	1.1

[a] As percentage of all deaths.

together account for more than 60% of deaths in this age-group in eight of the countries.

In the younger adult age-group (15–44 years, Table III), accidents remain the leading cause of death in all of the countries except England and Wales, where they are supplanted by malignant neoplasms, which consistently occupy second place in the remainder of the countries. Heart disease accounts for more than 10% in ten countries, occupying third place, and in the remainder, third rank is taken by suicide. Cerebrovascular disorders attain more than 2% in most countries, though cirrhosis of the liver exceeds this figure in several. In the later adult age-group (45–64 years) malignant neoplasms rise to first rank in ten countries, heart disease in four, and together they account for more than 55% of the deaths in 11 countries. Cerebrovascular diseases occupy third place in 11, a little less than 10%, and accidents are the fourth or fifth rank, at about 5%. In the over-65 year group, heart disease occupies first rank consistently, accounting for about a third of all deaths, followed by malignant neoplasms or cerebrovascular diseases, accounting for about a fifth. In this age-group also occur, among the ten leading causes of death, conditions not represented in the earlier adult groups, namely, nutritional deficiency, hyperplasia of the prostate, and intestinal obstruction.

Age, then, influences the major pattern of disease mortality. Although accidents in the youngest age-group are preponderant, many infants die of congenital anomalies, of inability to cope with infection, and of unsuccessful control of neoplastic growth. This pattern is maintained in the 5- to 14-year-old group, though at a lower level, and here appear for the first time suicide and organic disorders at a low percentage in some countries. In the younger adult age-group, where accidents and cancers predominate, suicide emerges as a distressing major cause, the infections are relegated to minor rankings, but organic pathologies become more important. In the later adult age-group (45–64 years), malignant neoplasms predominate, again relatively few infections occur, but deterioration of organ function emerges as of greatly increased importance. Finally, in old age, the aging of organs brings heart and cerebrovascular disease to the fore, accompanying malignant neoplasms, but also infections appear to be re-establishing their command, presumably through deterioration of the body's capacity to withstand them, and other disorders occur because the elderly are unable to look after themselves. For example, they may be nutritionally deficient or have intestinal obstruction. Differences in age structure among populations, then, can be expected to have pronounced effects on the patterns of disease mortality, and so any cultural modification that alters age composition will alter the disease pattern.

B. Population Variations in Mortality

Comparisons between populations are not simple, because the data are relative. The fact that Norway has the highest infant accident mortality, or that

TABLE III

The Ten Leading Causes of Death in Selected Countries: 15–44 Years[a]

Cause of death	Austria	Belgium	Denmark	France	German Federal Republic	Greece	Ireland	Italy	Netherlands	Norway	Spain	Switzerland	England and Wales	Scotland
Accidents	36.7	33.5	25.3	35.8	30.6	26.3	26.3	28.0	31.6	33.4	25.3	33.3	27.7	24.5
Malignant neoplasms	15.6	18.8	25.3	14.7	15.8	22.1	23.0	22.0	22.1	21.1	16.9	18.2	23.8	20.8
Suicide	11.5	7.3	16.5	7.2	12.2	2.8	3.5	3.9	6.2	8.3	2.1	15.0	6.1	5.2
Heart disease	8.7	11.3	8.0	5.9	10.0	12.0	13.1	12.5	11.5	10.9	15.6	9.0	17.0	17.4
Cirrhosis of liver	3.4	1.2	1.2	5.6	3.2	1.9		4.9		1.0	3.5	1.8		
Cerebrovascular disease	2.6	3.2	2.1	3.1	2.3	3.7	5.6	3.2	3.1	3.6	4.2	1.6	4.8	5.9
Tuberculosis	1.5			1.0	1.0	2.4		1.7			3.4			
Influenza and pneumonia	1.5	1.8	0.9	0.8	1.3	1.7	3.8	1.7	1.0	0.8	3.3	2.1	2.8	2.2
All other external causes	1.1	1.6	3.2	2.0	1.9		4.4		1.1	1.1		1.6	2.7	4.3
Nephritis and nephroses	1.0					3.3	1.9	1.6			2.3		1.2	1.0
Bronchitis, etc.		1.4					2.7		1.0		1.1		2.1	2.4
Congenital anomalies	1.4	0.9	1.9	1.4			1.4		1.8	1.5		1.4	1.7	1.3
Benign neoplasms						2.2			1.5					
Diabetes	0.9	2.3	2.3	1.4	1.5					1.8		0.9		
Complications of pregnancy, B41								1.5						

[a] As percentage of all deaths.

England has the highest mortality from congenital malformations, does not mean that mothers are less careful in Norway than in other countries, or that the English are particularly prone to congenital malformation; instead, those health services are more successful in restricting mortality from other causes. It is difficult to disentangle the cultural from other elements. For example, the fact that deaths from cirrhosis of the liver in young adults are most frequent in France (5.6%), Italy (4.9%), Spain (3.5%), and Austria (3.4%) can only reflect the cultural pattern with the enhanced alcohol consumption in those countries; yet the emergence of cirrhosis of the liver as the tenth cause of death in Spanish 5- to 14-year-olds suggests either precocity in adult habits or a nonenvironmental element—perhaps a largely genetic form of cirrhosis such as occurs in India. Conversely, the mortality from anemias in infancy in Greece (5.7%) and Italy (3.2%) certainly includes the genetic contribution of deaths from thalassemia, the hemoglobinopathies, and possibly glucose-6-phosphate dehydrogenase (G6PD) deficiency, but the possibility of enhancement from nutritional inadequacy cannot be eliminated. Similarly, the high frequency of deaths from the respiratory disorders in Ireland (11.1%), England (12.1%), and Spain (10.2%) suggests some effect of location on the western European seaboard, but the inflated levels in infants in Greece suggest that an element of the quality of health care may be contributing to these figures.

Comparing distributions on a more local scale, which removes some of the artifacts of data compilation and gross cultural variation, is more rewarding, but even restricting study to a single country does not remove such complications totally. In Britain, for example, the distribution of mortality from several causes suggests that the adequacy of the Health Services is a variable in mortality and morbidity. The highest mortalities from cancer of the uterus occur in Scotland and the more remote rural areas of England, and seem to reflect the accessibility of the gynecological services and early detection programs. Here too there may be an additional cultural factor; women in these areas may be more reluctant to avail themselves of these services. Similar reluctance may contribute to the pattern of infant mortality in Britain. Infant mortality is often taken as an index of living standards, for Woolfe and Waterhouse (1945) among others showed that infant mortality was related to unemployment, low pay, and overcrowding. It is much higher than any of the disease-specific causes and has shown a satisfying gross decline. During 1954–1958, the average yearly number of deaths in Britain in children under 1 year of age was 22,689, giving an average national infant mortality of 27.5/1000 live births. Corresponding figures for 1959–1963 were 21,055, or 22.5/1000 live births. But rates vary by region and locale, tending to be higher in Northern Ireland than in Scotland and higher in both than in England and Wales. Areas of highest infant mortality were south and west Wales, the industrial conurbations of northeast England, west Yorkshire, the Midlands, Lancashire, and the western part of central Scotland.

Such variations are, however, useful pointers to cultural effects. Social class differences in mortality remain conspicuous, and, although mortality generally has fallen, the decrease is less in social class 5 than in class 1. The rates of age-groups 1–4 and 5–9 years for social class 5 are more than double those in class 1. Socioeconomic factors, such as the proportion of houses with more than one person per room, the percentage of houses occupied by their owners, and the percentage with inadequate plumbing facilities, were compared with mortality rates in the county boroughs in England (Lambert, 1976). Both in the young adult (15–44 years) and older (45–54 years) age-groups, mortality was correlated significantly with socioeconomic indicators. There were significant positive cor-relations in both these age-groups with the proportion of unemployed respon-dents, the proportion in social classes 4 and 5, increased numbers of people per room, absence of inside toilet, and absence of bath, whereas significant negative correlations occurred with proportion in social class 1, the domestic rating per household (local taxes), and the proportion with their own toilet facilities. Partial correlations eliminating the effect of social class removed many of the significant associations in the younger age-group, but not in the older. Apparently socioeconomic variables in urban areas in England affect adult mortality (Bren-nan, 1978a).

III. CULTURAL ELEMENTS AND RESPIRATORY DISORDERS IN BRITAIN

The distribution of mortality from specific causes (Howe, 1970) in Britain shows patterns that help in understanding interaction between disease and cul-tural factors. Each year from 1954 to 1958, on average, 17,346 males and 2973 females died of cancer of the trachea, lung, and bronchus in the United King-dom, giving death rates of 599 per million for males, and 102 per million for females. In 1959–1963, rates rose to 947 and 373 per million, respectively. When standardized for differences in age structure, mortality is highest in Lon-don and southeast England, the Midlands, southern Lancashire, west Yorkshire, northeast England, and central Scotland. All the areas of highest mortality from this cause are associated with foci of industry or dense population. The deaths in females, though fewer, show a similar pattern to that in males. For both sexes a regular declining gradation of mortality is seen from the overcrowded industrial areas through the provincial conurbations, large, middle-sized, and small towns, to the rural districts, which are the least affected.

Whether this gradation of mortality from cancer of the respiratory tract is due to some fundamental distribution of cancer deaths as a whole can be examined by comparing its distribution with that from cancer of the stomach. In 1954–1958 the number of annual deaths from stomach cancer averaged 9036 males and 7175 females, with a United Kingdom death rate of 361/million for males and 263/ million for females, which remained almost unchanged during 1959–1963 at 346 and 254 million, respectively. Howe's (1970) maps show first a clear gradient; the heaviest mortality occurs in Wales, particularly in the north, and the mountain areas of northern England, and southwest Scotland, whereas the south and east of the United Kingdom show generally lower rates. A second generalization is that ratios in the urban districts of practically every county are higher than those for the surrounding rural districts. The areas with the highest ratios relate to large areas of almost empty country where mortality experience is small and the calculated ratios are based on a small number of deaths, so they may be of varying reliability. But if sampling error were responsible, much more variation from locality to locality and a more random distribution would be expected than is in fact observed, so the pattern of distribution is taken as a reasonable representation of what actually occurs. It differs considerably from that for the respiratory tract.

One can, therefore, conclude that the mortality distribution from respiratory cancers is not part of a general cancer pattern, but is a characteristic of the site of lesion. The association with industrial location, urbanization, and density of population indicates the importance of cultural variables in the development of this disorder and mortality from it. The precise variables in the etiology remain to be identified, but ample evidence supports the importance of inspiration of polluted air.

A. Smoking

Smoking is a habit that spread rapidly after its introduction into Europe in the sixteenth century, and particularly since the introduction of the cigarette at the end of the nineteenth century, though it has only recently become as established among women as among men in Britain. The initial investigation of Doll and Bradford Hill (1956) remains classic. They sent questionnaires to more than 40,000 male and female physicians in Britain to ascertain their smoking habits, and subsequently analyzed their causes of death. They found "a marked and steady increase in the death rate from lung cancer as the amount smoked increases" from a death rate of 0.07/1000 in nonsmokers, 0.47/1000 in light smokers (1–14 g/day), and 0.86 in medium (15–24 g/day) to 1.66 in heavy smokers (over 25 g/day); death rates in the heavy smokers were approximately 20 times those in nonsmokers. This increase was observed in all age-groups older than age 35 years. For all deaths attributed to cancer of the lung, the diagnosis was confirmed by the certifying practitioner. In addition, the cases were divided into those in which histological evidence was or was not sought, and the increased incidence was found in both groups. Smoking habits did not differ among subjects resident in large cities or elsewhere, so the results were not due to differential exposure to atmospheric pollutants other than those of smoking. Similar trends emerged for cancers of the upper respiratory and upper digestive tracts, and for bronchitis, but not for other disorders. Subsequent work has not only established this relationship, but it has been taken as the basis of a public health campaign against smoking. Though the campaign has had some effect in the more educated groups, its impact on the mass of the population in Britain has so far been relatively slight.

Here is one cultural variable, then, the habit of cigarette smoking, that is shown to be directly responsible for specific morbidity and mortality. It is unlikely, however, to account for the differences between European countries in their bronchitis rates, because no evidence exists that cigarette smoking is any greater in the United Kingdom than in France or Germany. Nor is any real evidence yet available that the pattern of geographic variation in respiratory cancer mortality in Britain is due to differences in habits of cigarette smoking. Although smoking is indeed a likely contribution, and probably elevates the rates in all areas, other factors must also be responsible, e.g., general pollution of the atmosphere in the overcrowded industrial areas remains a distinct possibility.

B. Atmospheric Pollution

The great London smog of 5–9 December 1952 provided confirmatory evidence of the importance of atmospheric pollution on respiratory mortality and morbidity. Again it is a classic example. An intensive anticyclone covered the greater part of western Europe, no pressure gradients existed and, therefore, no winds occurred, so over the lower Thames basin the establishment of a temperature inversion led to a rapid concentration of dense smoke-polluted fog, which persisted for 4 days. In central London for 48 hours, smoke-pollution averaged more than 4500 and sulfur dioxide more than 3800 mg/m³. The greater part of this pollution came from house chimneys (the open coal-burning fireplace was the focus of so much of domestic life in Britain), and relatively little was from industry. Deaths began to increase on the first day of the fog and continued to increase until the last day, but fell again immediately after the atmosphere cleared. Over these four days the death rate in London more than doubled, with an excess of some 4000 deaths above the usual number for the time of year, and sickness rates similarly increased. The deaths occurred in people already suffering from serious respiratory or cardiac disease, mostly the elderly and a few in the young. Similar incidents had occurred earlier, e.g., in the Meuse Valley in Belgium in 1930. As a result of the London incident, deaths and meteorological conditions were monitored, and in the years 1958–1960 respiratory morbidity and mortality were clearly correlated with smoke and sulfur dioxide pollution during the winter months (Martin, 1964), and a clear association was shown between the daily condition of chronic bronchitis patients and the degree of pollution (Lawther *et al.*, 1970). Similar epidemiological investigations have been continued in order to measure the effects of the Clean Air Act (Waller *et al.*, 1969), and, from the sharp reduction in smoke and the improved indices of health, some toxic element apparently has been removed from the atmosphere, or at least its toxicity has been diminished.

C. Occupation

Such acute incidents are dramatic and point to the type of factor that is involved in the etiology of respiratory conditions. But their precise effects are much more difficult to establish—for example, to distinguish the effects of atmospheric pollution from those of tobacco smoking, occupation, and socioeconomic status (Royal College of Physicians, 1970). Useful evidence comes from occupational health data. Gas, asbestos, and chromate workers have increased risks of lung cancer (Doll, 1952), and apparently the hazards of their occupation, the exposure of their respiratory tracts to noxious substances, produces the site-specific cancer. It is not that the respiratory tissue is particularly susceptible, for similar findings come from other industries; for example, among chemical workers exposed to β-naphthylamine, mortality from bladder cancer is elevated (Case, 1954). Gas workers at the top of old-fashioned horizontal retorts were found to inhale concentrations of the carcinogenic polycyclic aromatic hydrocarbons a hundred times that usual in urban atmospheres, and the incidence of cancer in this group of workers was elevated, though not as high as might have been expected (Doll *et al.*, 1965) perhaps because of the delay in manifestation. Comparisons of respiratory disease in a given occupational group working in areas of high and low pollution but of otherwise similar socioeconomic backgrounds are particularly informative. They demonstrate that pollution and bronchitis are clearly related (Reid and Fairbairn, 1958), and that nonsmokers are much less affected by pollution than are smokers. These comparisons all suggest that it is chronic exposure that is important. Therefore, atmospheric pollution may well affect respiratory conditions as the result of development of lung tissue damage in childhood, which becomes noticeable in the later years of life through the aggravation of disease. It is not known whether the urban effect is due to continued daily exposure to slightly increased levels of pollution or to repeated exposure to episodes of high pollution, each producing a massive deterioration.

As a measure to mollify such effects, smoke abatement in Britain has been successfully introduced, primarily through the control of domestic coal consumption but also of industrial chimney emissions. There is much greater control of occupational health hazards, leading up to the recent Health and Safety at Work Act in Britain. Little has yet been done to restrict toxicity from motor-exhaust fumes, perhaps because even in localities of particularly high concentrations or in people particularly exposed to traffic, a major effect has been difficult to identify. In the latter group, for instance, the carboxyhemoglobin saturation of the blood in nonsmokers is only a fraction as high as in smokers (Lawther and Commins, 1970). Certainly the respiratory disorders in Britain indicate the importance of cultural variables in morbidity and mortality, particularly those associated with urban industrial society.

IV. CULTURAL ELEMENTS AND CARDIOVASCULAR DISEASE

About half of all cardiovascular deaths are due to ischemic heart disease, in Britain as in much of western Europe, and hypertension is the other main cause, though it is not so pronounced as it is, for example, in Japan. Rheumatic heart disease only accounts for 2% of such deaths, and congenital heart disease 1%. Again the type varies with age with most deaths from heart disease in persons less than 15 years of age being congenital; between 20 and 35 years, rheumatic; and more than 35 years, coronary or hypertensive. Pulmonary heart disease is essentially restricted to males aged 45 years and over.

Annual deaths from arteriosclerotic heart disease, including coronary disease, during the period 1954–1958 in Britain averaged 53,806 males and 32,213 females, and during 1959–1963, 66,525 males and 42,074 females, so that death rates for both sexes rose by almost 13%, from 2025 and 1198 to 2610 and 1545/million in half a decade. Howe's (1970) maps show that in males the most obvious feature of the geographic distribution is the concentration of high mortality ratios in the north of the country and low in the south. Particularly unfavorable mortality areas for arteriosclerotic heart disease are southwest and central Scotland, Tyneside, Teesside, the south Lancashire conurbation, the West Riding of Yorkshire, and south Wales. A similar pattern emerges for females. The southeast of England tends to be economically favored, so the distribution is unusual in that it appears to reverse the international trend in which coronary mortality is positively correlated with prosperity. Diagnostic practice undoubtedly varies, but coronary disease is so common a cause of death that the geographic pattern cannot be attributed to that factor. Again the mortality experience is better in the rural areas than in the corresponding urban ones.

Regional differences in mortality from vascular lesions affecting the central nervous system in Britain show a pattern somewhat similar to that for arteriosclerotic heart disease. Standardized mortality ratios greater than the national average occur in Britain north of the line from the Severn to the Humber estuaries, with greatest mortalities in urban localities in south Lancashire, central Scotland, northeast England, and west Yorkshire. London has a favorable mortality experience similar to the remainder of the southeast. Again in Britain during the period 1959–1963 the death rate from stroke was high, averaging

36,384 males and 52,884 females annually, a rise of 8% for males and 6% for females in half a decade.

A. Smoking

Nicotine is the principal, or possibly the sole, physiologically active ingredient in tobacco smoke. It is rapidly absorbed in the lungs of cigarette smokers who inhale, but less rapidly through the epithelium of the mouth of pipe and cigar smokers who tend not to inhale because of the stronger tobacco. The effect of nicotine is to cause a small and consistent increase in heart rate, blood pressure, cardiac output, and stroke volume, with shorter isometric periods of left ventricular contraction, reduced skin temperature, and reduced blood flow. After smoking, the coronary blood flow, blood pressure, and left ventricular output all increase, and if coronary disease is already present this increased cardiac work is not met by any increased coronary arterial flow.

Although there is little convincing experimental evidence that smoking damages tissue of the cardiovascular system, the epidemiological evidence is striking. A large excess of cardiovascular deaths occurs in heavy cigarette smokers, which became obvious first in men and then in women. Consumption of 20 cigarettes or more per day increases the risk of myocardial infarction to three times that in nonsmokers. In populations highly susceptible to coronary heart disease, cigarette smoking contributes powerfully to the risk. Conversely, cessation of smoking leads to reduced mortality, as was shown by the follow-up study of physicians in the United Kingdom (Royal College of Physicians, 1971).

Much of the evidence is physiological. In young smokers endurance is clearly impaired, and evidence is consistent that oxygen debt increases even after moderate exercise, although the level becomes normal again after abstaining from smoking. Nonsmokers who inhale carbon monoxide are similarly impaired and have the same carboxyhemoglobin levels that are found in smokers. In heavy smokers with their increased concentrations of carboxyhemoglobin, the oxygen dissociation curve of hemoglobin is displaced. This means that their oxygen requirements need to be met by increased blood flow, and in obstructive disease of the coronary arteries the flow is likely to be impeded.

B. Occupation

Occupational exposure to toxic substances is relatively unimportant in cardiovascular disease, although some interesting associations occur. Persons with coronary atherosclerotic heart disease, working in explosives factories, and exposed to nitroglycol, a highly volatile substance that is absorbed rapidly by the lungs and skin, were affected on weekends with angina pectoris, which disappeared on returning to work. Thus, they were liable to sudden death during the weekends when deprived of the vasodilator effects of the nitroglycol present during the working week (Lob, 1965).

Much more important, however, is the association of coronary atherosclerotic heart disease and differences in occupational activity. Farmers tend to have a lower incidence of coronary heart disease. Coronary heart disease occurs more commonly among postal clerks, telephonists, and post office executives than among the more active postmen. In a prospective study of middle-aged London busmen, the physically active conductors had less symptomatic ischemic heart disease than the comparable sedentary drivers, and the levels of blood pressure and serum cholesterol were the predominant predictive factors. Comparative studies of samples with similar dietary intake show a greater incidence of is-chemic heart disease and myocardial infarction in the sedentary than in the physically active workers, whereas a prospective study of male executive civil servants after an examination of their exercise pattern showed fewer deaths from coronary heart disease during the next eight years in those who had reported vigorous daily exercise (Chave *et al.*, 1978).

Men in sedentary occupations tend to have fatal myocardial infarctions at an average age several years younger than those whose occupations include consid-erable physical activity, irrespective of their economic status. However, exam-ination of postmortem material from accident cases shows that rates of pathologi-cal signs of coronary atherosclerosis are comparable in those engaged in seden-tary and in physically active occupations; so apparently, it is not the presence of the disease but how rapidly it kills that is related to occupational activity. Post-mortem analyses in middle-aged men dying of noncoronary causes showed no relation between increased physical activity of occupation and coronary artery wall atheroma. Some had a slight negative relation with occlusion of the coro-nary artery lumen, and others had a strongly negative relation with ischemic myocardial fibrosis; it seems that physical activity is protective against the pro-gression of coronary atherosclerotic heart disease.

C. Emotional Stress

Evidence indicates the importance of emotional stress associated with occupa-tional responsibility. In the London busmen referred to above, not only were the drivers more sedentary, but they were also more subject to stress in the driving through difficult London traffic. But proving the association remains difficult. Traditionally thought to occur among persons with heavy responsibilities and worry, clinical coronary atherosclerotic heart disease nonetheless shows no ele-vated incidence among executive and top management personnel when compared with the incidence in other sedentary workers.

Emotional stimuli may profoundly influence the cardiovascular system through their effects on the autonomic nervous control. Emotional situations such as stressful interview, criticism, or pain cause increased vascular resistance in the kidneys, splanchnic area, and skin and decreased vascular resistance in muscle, so that there is a nonspecific hemodynamic response as in muscular exercise but without the obligatory increase in cardiac output. Alternatively, such situations may give rise to circulatory collapse, with decreased heart rate, arterial pressure, and peripheral resistance. But such interactions are transient; the effects of acute emotional stress and the effects of prolonged stress are not established. Many studies of populations living under differing circumstances produced no good evidence that life in western Europe is more stressful than among primitives, and there is not clear concordance that stressful occupations produce a high incidence of coronary disease. Certainly attacks of angina pectoris may be precipitated by emotional stress, for example, of blazing anger or intense but concealed emotion. But evidence is insubstantial that coronary thrombosis and occlusion are due to emotional stress, although it seems probable that emotional and physical stress may lead to myocardial infarction or sudden death in persons with pre-existing coronary disease.

V. SUBCLINICAL AND CHRONIC DISEASE

The suggestion, therefore, is that frank disease in many cases is merely the visible part of the iceberg and many more individuals in a population carry physiological signs of a disorder without appreciating it, or signs of a previous manifestation from which they have recovered, or in whom the trigger to convert a mere predisposition to frank disorder has not yet been set off. Similarly, mortality is not the best indicator of disease distribution; it merely indicates those who do not recover, and for most disorders how many survive. Such survival is well shown by the distribution of ischemic heart disease in a community (Tunbridge *et al.*, 1977).

A. Ischemic Heart Disease

In a recent epidemiological study in Whickham, a suburb of Newcastle, England, a one-in-six sample of adults was obtained from the electoral register of 1972. Cooperation was excellent—82.4% of the sample agreeing to participate. The age and sex distribution is similar to that of Britain as a whole, except for a slight deficiency in the numbers of both sexes less than 25 years of age, and a slight excess of males aged 45–54 years and females aged 25–34 years. Each subject was questioned and investigated.

A history of angina or myocardial infarction occurred in 7.5% of males and 4.8% of females. The frequency increased with age, from 0.4% in males aged 25–34 years, to 28.5% in males aged 65–74 years. Seven percent of both sexes had chest pain on effort, the frequency increasing with age in both sexes. Possible infarction had occurred in 5.4% of males and 3.8% of females, again increasing with age in both sexes. Major ECG changes were seen in 4.7% of both sexes, again the frequency increasing with age from less than 1% of those less than 45 years of age to 20–25% of those more than 75 years of age. Combination of criteria from history and examination showed probable heart disease in 11% of each sex, and the rate rose from less than 3% of those aged 45 years or less to some 30% of those aged more than 65 years. Possible heart disease occurred in a further 6.5% of males and 10.4% of females (Table IV). Firm diagnosis of ischemic heart disease by the methods employed is of course impossible, for even when confirmed at the time of the attack by serial ECG and enzyme changes, these do not persist in many patients. But whether cardiovascular disease is identified by the most restrictive criterion (major ECG changes) or history, or some combination thereof, a situation in which at least 1 in 20, and more likely 1 in 10, of the adult population has experienced the disorder represents indeed an appreciable concealed morbidity load. For, though many patients may feel totally recovered or some may not know that they have had an acute episode, from the preceding discussion (Sections IV, C and V, A) this load appears to confer a greater risk of early mortality.

B. Rheumatic Diseases

Such episodes may or may not have left permanent effects on performance. By contrast, the rheumatic diseases are a source of chronic distress and are among the most important causes of loss of work and limitation of activity. In 1955, the rheumatic diseases caused the loss of 27 million working days in England and Wales. In sample surveys of adults in northwest England carried out in 1954–1959, 35% of those interviewed said that they had rheumatic symptoms at the time, and 64% said they had experienced them at some time. More than 25% had lost at least a week's work from rheumatic complaints, and 9% had been incapacitated for more than three months, the most frequent complaint-site being the back, especially the lumbar region. In those losing one or more weeks of work, the cause in men was most frequently intervertebral disc degeneration, usually associated with low back pain, while in females it was usually rheumatoid arthritis associated especially with pain in the fingers and in the cervicobrachial distribution. Of the total days lost (107,268) by the 653 males and 689 females in the sample, 49,469 were due to inflammatory polyarthritis.

Rheumatoid arthritis can be defined by the American Rheumatism Association criteria, and these have been applied in surveys of different populations. One such study of a combined urban/rural population in northwest England covered 1060 males and 1174 females aged 15–64 years. In the males, 0.5% were definitely

TABLE IV

Age and Sex Distribution (%) of Ischemic Heart Disease in Whickham (Newcastle-upon-Tyne) by Varying Criteria

Age	Number	Past history (A)	Chest pain on effort (B)	Possible infarction (C)	Major ECG changes (D)	Minor ECG changes (E)	Probable IHD (B ± D)	Possible excluding probable IHD (C ± E)
Males								
18–24	110	0	1.8	0.9	0.9	0	2.7	0
25–34	233	0.4	1.3	1.7	0.4	1.7	1.7	3.4
35–44	255	1.6	2.0	3.5	0.4	1.6	2.4	3.5
45–54	290	4.5	6.6	3.4	3.1	3.8	8.3	4.5
55–64	210	16.2	13.3	11.4	7.6	14.3	19.5	13.3
65–74	130	28.5	24.6	14.6	14.6	17.7	35.4	12.3
75+	57	14.0	10.5	5.3	24.6	19.3	33.3	15.8
Total	1285	7.5	7.4	5.4	4.7	6.5	11.1	6.5
Females								
18–24	128	0	0.8	0.8	0	3.9	0.8	4.7
25–34	323	0	0.9	1.9	0.9	4.0	1.9	5.3
35–44	275	1.5	2.5	2.5	1.5	7.3	3.6	8.4
45–54	240	2.9	8.4	2.9	3.7	10.8	11.7	10.4
55–64	266	6.8	13.2	4.9	6.4	15.8	16.9	12.8
65–74	182	13.7	20.9	9.3	11.5	23.1	26.9	19.2
75+	80	22.5	16.2	7.5	20.0	20.0	28.8	18.8
Total	1494	4.8	7.8	3.8	4.7	11.0	10.8	10.4

affected, and in females, 1.6%. If to these figures are added the number of subjects falling in the "probable" category, the prevalence rises to 2.5% in males and 6% in females. An increase occurs in the older (over 45 and 55 years, respectively) age-groups to more than twice these figures. Surveys in different parts of western Europe show little difference in general prevalence among populations.

In lumbar disc degeneration, the occupation appears to be a particularly important factor in males. Degeneration of grades 3–4 was present by age 40 in 50% of miners, 30% of dock workers, but only 5% of more sedentary clerks, whereas rural laborers showed a similar figure to the miners. In females the condition was more frequent and more severe in rural than urban localities. Apparently the amount of degeneration varies with the amount of lifting that is involved in the work (Lawrence, 1955).

Osteoarthrosis was examined by routine X rays in the northwest of England sample. At least one affected joint was shown in 50% of males and 52% of females and again an age increase occurred, from 11% at age 15–24 years to 96% in those aged more than 75 years in both sexes. Again an occupational association is apparent. Osteoarthrosis of the knee is five times as frequent in underground miners as in office workers; osteoarthrosis of the arm is especially prevalent in laborers using pneumatic drills, and of the fingers in cotton operatives and diamond cutters. In Europe a geographic gradient is apparent, the prevalence being least in the most northerly samples.

Gout affected 0.3% of males and no females in a sample in northwest England (Kellgren *et al.*, 1953). A more detailed survey by X rays and examination of serum uric acid levels showed the figure of 0.2% in males. The hyperuricemia was more frequent, occurring in a Yorkshire sample at 5% in males and 1% in females; this condition was particularly associated with upper social class, for in Manchester patients with the complaint, 31% occurred in each of social classes 1 and 2, whereas in the general population of patients these classes were only represented by 14 and 15%.

The rheumatic diseases cause varying degrees of disability, and the degree of handicap experienced by a patient varies from time to time as well as from person to person. The example shows the strong effect of aging, as well as the relatively high general level in the population, and emphasizes once again the importance of occupation in the etiology. Rarely does the sufferer feel himself free of disease, so that this group of diseases illustrates another facet of the interrelationship of culture and disease. The discussion so far has centered on the effect of cultural variables on the disease pattern. This group of diseases serves as a reminder that an effect in the opposite direction also exists; the way of life of the sufferer may be profoundly changed, and his contribution to society greatly altered.

VI. DAY-TO-DAY ILLNESSES

Mortality and chronic morbidity give only one view of the disease load in a community. Another extremely important component is the group of diseases that account for so much of the sickness experience of most persons and contribute so heavily to the day-to-day work of a family doctor. Dr. W. Pickles, who was in a rural practice in Yorkshire for many years, kept a record of the cases of epidemic disease seen over a period of 15 years before World War II. Influenza was at the top of the list, followed by gastrointestinal infections (Table V). The list of infections seen by the family doctor would be much the same today (Table VI), except that there would be fewer cases of measles, fewer whooping cough, and no diphtheria, as a result of the immunization measures that are so much a part of preventive medicine in Britain (Office of Population Censuses, 1974). Few of these infections would have proved lethal, so that their frequency is not evident from the study of mortality reports. Nevertheless, it is such illnesses that account for so much of the time lost from work or school and so restrict the economic output of the person.

Some of the clearest indications of how patterns of living affect morbidity

TABLE V

Cases of Epidemic Disease in 15 Years of a Wensleydale Practice

Disease	No. of cases
Influenza	1112
Diarrhea and vomiting	1018
Measles	510
Febrile catarrh	407
Chickenpox	318
Whooping cough	295
Tonsillitis	289
Mumps	233
German measles	175
Herpes zoster	140
Hepatitis	122
Scarlet fever	117
Lobar pneumonia	41
Glandular fever	41
Bornholm disease	25
Diphtheria	12
Total	4855

TABLE VI

**Patient Consulting Rates in General Practice
in England and Wales 1970-1971,
per 1000 Population**

Illness	Rate
Influenza	5.8
Intestinal infection	18.0
Measles	4.8
Catarrh	15.0
Chickenpox	4.2
Whooping cough	2.1
Mumps	1.6
German measles	5.0
Herpes zoster	4.0
Hepatitis	0.8
Scarlet fever and streptococcal sore throat	1.5
Lobar pneumonia	3.3
Bornholm disease	0.2
Diphtheria	0

come from the studies of the development and progress of infectious epidemics. For this purpose "rural districts, where the population is thin and the lines of intercourse are few and easily traced, offer opportunities ... which are not met with in the crowded haunts of large towns" (William Budd). The following study, told by Pickles (1948), of the effect of a village fete illustrates this (Fig. 1). The occurrence of an epidemic of hepatitis in his practice was brought to his attention by symptoms in five patients within a single week. He discovered that they had one experience in common—they had all been present at a village fete on August 28. Somebody transmitting the disease had probably been present. After prolonged search, he found that a young girl (B in Fig. 1) in whom the disease manifested on August 23 and whom he had seen in her bed on the morning of the fete, never dreaming that she would or could have left it, had actually attended the festivities. She spent the afternoon with patient E, and was in the house of Mrs. C, so it seems highly likely that she infected these two and the other three persons. Patient E, who was a maidservant in another village, had spent the afternoon with B, returned home, and subsequently infected her admirer (M), her employer's small son (H), his friend (J), and her own great-aunt (P). M and J subsequently infected other relatives and friends (K, L, N, O). The history clearly indicates an incubation period of about a month, and suggests a short period of infectivity, while the method of spread was by personal contact, probably by droplet infection. But it is as an indicator of the way of life in this rural community that the account is particularly relevant. One young girl, deter-

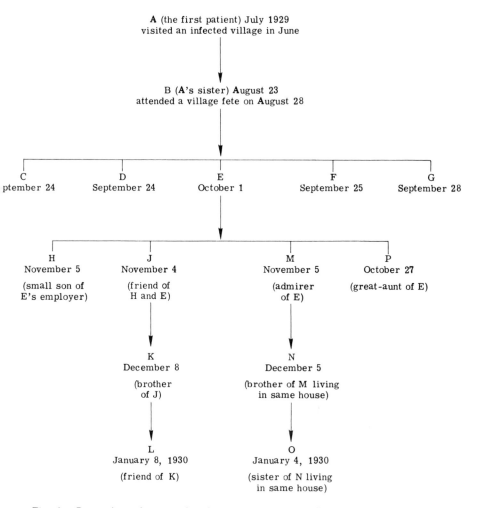

Fig. 1. Dates of manifestation of epidemic hepatitis among villagers who attended a fete, and their contacts.

mined to have what she considered her legitimate amusement, was responsible for 13 other sufferers. A fete in a village was regarded as so important that a girl who was ill felt that she just had to go, and not only was it attended by the villagers themselves, but also by visitors from elsewhere. The pattern of family living meant the distribution of the infection throughout the family, and contact was sufficiently close between family and maidservant that she infected her employer's small son.

Dr. Pickles relates similar anecdotes for other infectious diseases, one showing the role of the village inn as a place to while away a few spare minutes casually talking with friends and acquaintances, and incidentally transmitting infection. In a village well removed from the prevailing epidemic of measles, a man (A) showed symptoms. Twelve days previously, B, a friend of his, had called at a doctor's surgery (office) and instead of waiting had visited the nearby inn, and there had a drink with A. On B's return to the surgery he was found to have the measles. During his short visit to the inn, he had clearly infected his companion (A); the incubation period was 12 days.

The limited communication between villages meant that Dr. Pickles in many cases was able to identify the person responsible for introducing the virus to the village from outside. For example, a school mistress returning from spending Christmas in 1936 with her parents in Scarborough must have brought the virus with her, for she attended school on the first day after the vacation before succumbing herself, and was responsible for 78 cases of influenza among her pupils and their families. This example illustrates the attitude, still prevalent today, that Christmas is a time for family reunion.

VII. RURAL MORBIDITY

The fact that so much of the disease pattern in western Europe is associated with industry and urbanization must not be taken to indicate that no morbidity is associated with rural life. There remain large agricultural populations, 800,000 workers in Britain who each have wives and families. But the illnesses prevalent in rural areas in Britain as late as the 1920s differed in many ways from those met today (Barber, 1974). Far more were due to poverty and deficiency. Often old people and children in large families tended to be short of food, badly clothed, and poorly housed. The most prevalent diseases were bronchitis and rheumatism. The "rheumatics" was accepted by the farm laborer—it was the outcome of endless insults to his joints through carrying heavy loads over rough ground in any sort of weather, and often not being completely dry for weeks on end. No immunization programs were organized, so that the infectious diseases were killers; diphtheria was, therefore, a dreaded disease, as were scarlet fever with its consequent mastoids, nephritis, and valvular heart disease. Tuberculosis was common, the pulmonary type nearly always ending in a lingering death, whereas the bovine type caused septic neck glands and joint diseases. Osteomyelitis was frequent in children, and after surgery and the long period of drainage and dressings, the child was often left with a permanent disability. Rheumatic fever with heart disease turned healthy children into permanent semi-invalids. Some rickets occurred and was particularly serious in women who had experienced it in childhood and whose pelvises had been narrowed by the pressure of their hip joints to produce the characteristic "clover-leaf" effect.

Today, infections from contact with animals are common, although the more severe forms are fortunately rare. Anthrax is comparatively rare but may occur in men handling carcasses, skins, hides, or hair of animals that have been infected. Glanders occasionally comes from contact with sick horses. Of ringworms, *Ectothrix trichophyta* are derived from animals and birds and are found in cowmen and animal breeders, where their lesions in the form of agminate folliculitis may be seen. Brucellosis occurs in men handling cattle or pigs or their carcasses; in west Somerset, of 38 patients with undulant fever, 23 had had habitual contact with cows, 17 worked on farms, and 5 were veterinary surgeons (Boycott, 1964). Tularemia in Europe, a general infection of small rodents, is confined to Scandanavia; in outbreaks in 1966 in Sweden, farmers were infected from voles invading their barns in search of food. Q fever occasionally occurs among farmers, abattoir workers, and veterinary surgeons. Of 96 workers in the Edinburgh abattoir (Schonell *et al.,* 1966), 27 had antibodies to *Coxiella burneti,* all of whom appeared to be symptomless. Louping-ill, a natural disease of sheep well known in Scotland and the north of England, occasionally occurs in shepherds and farmers, veterinary officers, and carcass workers, and is transmitted by a tick. Ornithosis is transmitted not only by cage birds but in the poultry and wild bird populations; in Hungary between 1950 and 1962 occurred 550 cases among workers engaged in processing ducks.

In those rural areas in Great Britain where rainfall is high occurs the condition called farmer's lung, a respiratory disease arising from the handling of moldy hay and straw, due to the inhalation of the dust. The acute illness is short, but the subacute phase may be more incapacitating, lasting several months after removal from contact with the dust. Should it progress through the chronic phase to pulmonary fibrosis with emphysema, it becomes irreversible.

Because of the wide variety of tasks done by a farmer or farmworker, the risk of accident is wide and varied. Accidents come from the use of field and barn machinery, handling of animals, gunshot wounds, falls, cuts from hand tools, and electrocution. Animal accidents include the sudden savage and unexpected attacks by bulls, so serious in their effects—in 1964 in Britain four such accidents were fatal and 102 nonfatal. More frequent are the smaller injuries, for example, when the foot is trodden on in leading horses or cows, or from pig attacks. But the increased use of mechanization has produced most morbidity. In Britain a decade ago more than 25,000 accidents occurred per year from the use of tractors.

The pattern of agricultural morbidity has clearly changed during the last few decades. The more widespread use of artificial insemination has reduced the number of bull accidents. Educational campaigns directed to farmworkers on the proper use of tractors have had some effect. The greater knowledge of veterinary medicine and the improved standards of health of animals generally, supported by rigorous animal health legislation, have reduced the load of infections. The variation in these measures accounts for much of the variation in the health of agricultural workers in western Europe.

VIII. THE DISEASE PATTERN AND RECENT CULTURAL CHANGE

A. Venereal Disease

The pattern of venereal disease (VD) in western Europe since World War II is depressing. As a result of improved health, hygiene, and social conditions, the number of cases of syphilis that are acquired without sexual contact has fallen, and the same factors have virtually eliminated chancroid. But the sexually transmitted diseases are now more prevalent than at any other time since the war. At first syphilis declined in almost every country, sharply until 1952 and continued to fall more slowly thereafter (World Health Organization, 1970, 1975). But then the trend reversed. In 1955, France began an increase from about 42% of the 1950 level, rising sharply in 1964. In the United Kingdom the upturn began later, at about 1958 (15% of the 1950 figure), and the peak was in 1965, at about 40%. Norway reached the same percentages but again slightly later, with the trough in 1961 and a peak in 1967. From the latest figures available (1973), Austria and Germany had the highest prevalence.

Gonorrhea is still more of a problem and has reached epidemic proportions (World Health Organization, 1975). Almost all countries in western Europe show an increase by comparison with the 1950 figures, except for France and Italy, which have shown slight declines. In the United Kingdom, the 1968 figure was double that for 1950, and so it was in Norway, both showing a fairly steady increase. Sweden has shown a massive increase, from an incidence of 150/100,000 in 1950 to 381/100,000 in 1968, although a slight fall was shown in the latest figures available (1974), while Norway and Denmark have continued to increase, the latter now (1973) having the highest incidence in western Europe at 330. One country cannot be compared exactly with another since facilities and reporting procedures are different, but levels today in all give great cause for concern.

Besides gonorrhea and syphilis many other diseases are transmitted sexually. Those caused by viruses, bacteria, protozoa, fungi, spirochetes, and parasites are rarely recorded. Yet in England and Wales, where information on nongonococcal urethritis in males is available, its prevalence now exceeds that of gonorrhea. Syphilis and gonorrhea together account for only one-fourth of new cases among persons attending VD clinics.

Cultural Factors on the Increase

In a population with an increasing number of young people, a greater number of young people must be at risk. But the increase in cases of gonorrhea is far greater than that expected from the population increase. Another factor is increased movement of individuals from home to take up employment elsewhere and also from one center to another in the course of their employment, both within their own countries as well as by migration. Another element of movement is that associated with holiday and business travel. Once outside the immediate home environment the opportunity for sexual contact may be enhanced or at least inhibitions against it reduced. The most conspicuous factor accounting for the increase in sexually transmitted disease is cultural, the change in attitude and change in behavior with the arrival of the "permissive" society. Sex is emphasized in newspapers, television, advertising, films. Concomitantly the inhibitions of the restraining influences of family, public opinion, religion, fear of VD, and fear of conception have been eroded. These themselves reflect other cultural changes—the decreased interest in religion and attendance at churches; the weakening of family links; the movement away from home leading, on the one hand, to loneliness and, on the other, to the absence of friends, family, and neighbors to express opinions; and the increased availability of simple treatments for VD.

Whereas all age-groups have been affected by the rise in VD, the increase in the youngest (those in their teens and in their early twenties) is most conspicuous. At the same time, the increased acceptability of abnormal sexual practices is shown in the increased numbers of homosexual patients and the anatomical distribution of the lesions.

B. Unemployment

An unfortunate feature of western European culture in the 1970s is the widespread rise in unemployment rates. Involuntary unemployment affects the health of those concerned, as is well shown by prospective enquiries, following workers from the trauma of being told that they are to be dismissed (e.g., when a factory is to be closed) to their subsequent re-employment or final despair at its impossibility. In addition to psychological effects, notably depression, blood pressure and other indicators of stress tend to rise and remain high until the workers have settled into a new post (Kasl and Cobb, 1972). Despite improved benefits, unemployment is still typically productive of poverty with its characteristic higher morbidity and mortality levels (Draper *et al.*, 1979). That consequence is also reflected in higher childhood mortality, especially in the age-group 0-4 years, where the correlation remains after allowance for social class (Brennan and Lancashire, 1978); and in childhood morbidity, with a doubling of hospital admission rates (Brennan, 1978b).

C. Oral Contraception

A major change in cultural habits in the last decade has been the increasing use of the contraceptive pill. Progestogen-only pills appear to be without serious risks to health, but the more widely used estrogen/progestogen combined pill affects subsequent mortality; although from the large numbers of women who have been followed in controlled prospective studies the actual number of deaths is small, the trends are clear. The number of deaths in young women that caused concern in the late 1960s, from pulmonary embolism secondary to venous thrombosis, has declined since the recommendation to reduce the daily intake of estrogen in combined pills. A more serious effect emerged in respect to acute myocardial infarction (Mann and Inman, 1975), pill users having a greater risk of this after allowing for the effects of other factors (Table VII).

Deaths that occurred among pill users (Royal College of General Practitioners, 1977; Vessey *et al.*, 1977) indicated the importance of cerebrovascular disease including subarachnoid hemorrhage and a possible deleterious effect on cardiac function in cases of heart disease. Overall age-specific mortality rates are indeed low (Table VIII), but the trends with independent cultural factors, particularly age, duration of use, and smoking, are clear (Royal College of General Practitioners, 1977).

Much more important is morbidity (Table IX), for the range of side effects in which estrogen is implicated is enormous. Those effects are important on account of the frequency of occurrence and the severity of their consequences. The cardiovascular problems if not fatal can lead to serious disablement. Multiple pulmonary emboli may cause young women to become respiratory cripples, and

TABLE VII

Relative Risks of Myocardial Infarction
in Pill Users
after Allowing for Different Variables

After allowing for	Relative risk
Obesity	4.4[a]
Hypertension	4.1[a]
Pre-eclamptic toxemia	3.9[b]
Cigarette smoking	3.2[b]

[a] Significant at 0.001.
[b] Significant at 0.01.

TABLE VIII

Increase in Mortality Risks in Pill Users

Variable	Category	Excess annual mortality rate in pill users (per 100,000 users)
Age	15–34	5
	35–44	33
	45–49	140
Duration of use	<5 years	13
	≥5 years	50
Smoking	Nonsmokers	10
	Smokers	33

the occurrence of cerebral hemorrhages or vascular occlusions may lead to defects of special senses, speech, limb function, or mental function. Increasing demands on the heart may precipitate cardiac failure in women with existing heart lesions. Retrospective studies (Mann and Inman, 1975) on myocardial infarction show the marked interaction of the pill with underlying risk factors—age, smoking, obesity, presence of diabetes, hypertension, or familial hyperlipidemia. The risk of cerebrovascular accidents is enhanced in the presence of hypertension, and often there are warning signs, e.g., symptoms similar to migraine, temporary blindness, transient limb paralyses. Pill users may slowly develop raised blood pressure, and this can lead to malignant hypertension and vascular lesions. Cervical erosions are frequent (Vessey *et al.*, 1976). Pill users have increased plasma lipids, such as cholesterol and triglycerides, and the occurrence of gallstones is doubled. In some women psychological effects are apparent, particularly depression and attempts at suicide.

TABLE IX

Increase in Morbidity Risk in Pill Users

Side effect	Excess risk in pill users (per 1000 woman/years of use)
Cervical erosion	5.19
Gall bladder disease	0.74
Migraine	0.70
Poisoning	0.54
Venous thrombosis and embolism	0.51
Cerebrovascular disease	0.40

Although the continuing use of the pill carries a slightly increased risk of mortality and serious morbidity, so varying the general population pattern, the risk can be greatly reduced by careful monitoring of the patients and excluding anyone who appears to be developing undesirable symptoms. But again the influence is two-way, for not only does the cultural change alter the disease pattern but also the possible effects mean a change in patterns of consultation with family doctors.

D. Congenital Malformations

Undoubtedly the high proportion of early mortality accounted for by congenital malformations in most countries in western Europe is to be attributed to cultural advances leading to the control of other causes of death. However, a small proportion is due to environmental teratogens, exposure to which results from the technical advances of western European culture. Progress in teratoepidemiology is disappointingly slow (Klingberg and Papier, 1979) and detection of teratogenic relationships has not kept pace with the ever-increasing sources of potential hazards.

1. Drugs

Few drugs have been shown to be definitely teratogenic in man. Apart from thalidomide, these include the androgenic steroid hormones, which cause virilization in the female embryo, and folate antagonists, which cause a variety of abnormalities and fetal death. Establishing such relationships is difficult, because of the restricted time in development at which the fetus is susceptible, possible involvement of genetic predisposition in susceptibility, varying teratogenicity according to drug dosage, the added complication of possible synergistic effect among drugs, or simply determination of whether the malformation is due to the drug or to the disease that the drug treats. Epileptic mothers will be treated with anticonvulsants, and of these phenytoin is a more potent teratogen than phenobarbitone, but in combination the effect is synergistic. The defects produced are skeletal, cardiac, facial, digital, and central nervous system and mental abnormalities. Comparison of offspring of two groups of epileptic women, pre- and postanticonvulsant usage, showed the postanticonvulsant group to have a rate of malformation five times that of the preanticonvulsant group (Visser et al., 1976). Elevation of risk is also seen in the infants of treated diabetic mothers, although the experimental evidence is less good, because no nondiabetic controls received insulin. However, treated diabetic mothers seem to have a fetal malformation rate five times that of normal mothers. Of the anticoagulant drugs, Warfarin appears to produce nasal hypoplasia, optic atrophy, skeletal abnormalities, and mental retardation.

Alcohol consumption, when chronic and heavy, is associated with a specific group of defects in the fetus, dysfunctions of the central nervous system, growth deficiencies, characteristic facial abnormality, and other varying defects, to which the name "fetal alcohol syndrome" has been given (Streissguth, 1978).

2. Sex Hormones

Exposure to sex hormones, used in pregnancy tests or to induce withdrawal bleeding in nonpregnant women, is frequent in early pregnancy. Their effects on the fetus are reported to be congenital heart disease, central nervous system malformations, and limb-reduction deformities, at a risk double that of the general population; that risk is sufficiently high to warrant the discontinuation of hormonal pregnancy tests. For oral contraceptives the evidence is less clear. The increase is slight, but not consistent, in chromosome anomalies among the offspring of women conceiving immediately after using oral contraceptives. Similarly in prospective studies, some report cardiovascular defects or minor malformations, whereas others do not. Apparently oral contraceptives present no major teratogenic hazard except in those mothers who continue to take the pill during early embryogenesis.

The latent carcinogenic effect of the nonsteroidal estrogen diethylstilbestrol (DES) in daughters of women who took the drug to prevent miscarriage is well established. Folic acid antagonists, particularly aminopterin, have been associated with a variety of functional and structural defects in fetuses exposed to the drug in the first trimester.

3. Industrial Physicochemical Factors

Adverse pregnancy outcomes have been reported when parents have been exposed to lead, vinylchloride, organic solvents, and anesthetic gases. Europe has little to compare with the catastrophic exposures that have occurred in Japan to methyl mercury, cadmium, and polychlorinated biphenyls, but the 1976 chemical plant explosion at Seveso (Italy), giving large-scale contamination by TCDD (2,3,7,8-tetrachlorodibenzo-p-dioxin), caused extensive damage to both animals and humans, and particularly cases of chloracne, although more serious effects have not been documented.

Microcephaly is the most common malformation resulting from intrauterine radiation exposure, along with mental retardation. A dose of 10 rads to the fetus at any time during gestation seems to be the threshold for the induction of congenital defects.

4. Infections

Various infections produce congenital defects if the mother is exposed at a critical time in pregnancy. The changed pattern of exposure, as a result of public health measures, means that fewer children are naturally immunized and may, therefore, be at risk as adults. The rubella virus is teratogenic, with the highest risk to the developing fetus at 8-10 weeks, producing cardiovascular, eye, skin, and skeletal defects, brain damage, speech and hearing defects, and growth retardation; furthermore, the neonatal mortality rate is high. Cytomegalovirus is the most common fetal viral infection, and fetuses exposed during the first or second trimesters tend to show the most severe symptoms (Monif *et al.*, 1972), including deafness, hepatosplenomegaly, encephalitis, microcephaly, cerebral calcification, mental retardation, and cerebral palsy. Venezuelan equine encephalitis may cause hydrocephalus and cataract. *Herpes simplex* may produce microcephaly, microphthalmia, cerebral calcification, psychomotor retardation, retinal dysplasia, cutaneous lesions, and congenital heart defects. Infection with *varicella* or *Herpes zoster* may result in limb reduction deformities, encephalomyelitis, or lesions of the eye and the central nervous system. But the whole impact of infection accounts for only 2-3% of all malformations (Wilson, 1973).

IX. GENETIC DISEASE

As with congenital malformations, genetic morbidity and mortality have also come to assume increased importance in the disease pattern in western Europe through advances in controlling other diseases. The problems these genetic consequences have brought, however, are of concern for a different reason, for they affect not only immediate morbidity but also that of future generations. Moreover, in modern human society deleterious genes assume an importance beyond that which they confer on the life of the individual himself. They present a far wider range of problems than mere survival and reproduction imply, problems not only of treatment—often expensive and long-continued—but also of day-to-day care and maintenance. Society itself is adversely affected by the presence of deleterious genes.

In Britain as in many other western European countries, the burden of morbidity and mortality that genetically determined disease imposes on our health resources is already high. Stevenson (1959) endeavored to measure the genetic disease burden in terms of demands on personnel. He found that in Northern Ireland approximately 6% of all consultations with family doctors and 8% of consultations with specialists were by patients with hereditary and congenital disease, 26% of all institutional beds were occupied by such patients, and 2/1000 of the population were occupied fully in caring for these patients.

A study of child mortality in Newcastle hospitals provided yet more disturbing figures (Roberts *et al.*, 1970). The data were collected from the reports of deaths of children during 1960-1966 among five hospitals in Newcastle-upon-Tyne. In that city, all ill children admitted to hospital would come to one of those hospitals.

Of the total number of children's deaths in the series (1067), 26 were discarded because the information was insufficient for any classification to be possible. For each case of the total usable series (1041) the causes of mortality and details of associated conditions were reviewed. The genetic disease was not necessarily the immediate cause of death; for instance, in children with fibrocystic disease of the pancreas, the immediate cause of death may have been pneumonia, but there is little doubt that the fibrocystic disease was fundamental. The cases were classified into five categories.

1. Single-gene effects. Diseases due to a replacement of one allele by another at a particular locus show the classical patterns of dominant or recessive or co-dominant inheritance. Some 1300 conditions are well established as being due to such single-gene substitutions, and for a similar number the evidence is strongly suggestive. The frequencies of some of these, including the most common, in western Europe from Carter's (1977) compilation are shown in Table X. Although individually rare, in combination they add up to an appreciable load affecting all body systems. Their impact is shown by the fact that, of the present series of children's deaths, 88 cases (8.5%) involving such simple genetic diseases could be identified (Table XI). Of those, 74 were recessive, 2 dominant, and 3 sex-linked.

2. Chromosome disorders. Disorders in which chromosomal irregularities appear as secondary phenomena, e.g., chronic myeloid leukemia, were not included in this category. Twenty-five of the deaths in the series (2.5%) occurred in children having associated numerical chromosomal aberrations. The most frequent was Down's syndrome, with or without associated defects, which accounted for 22 of the cases. This total is regarded as an underestimate, because at that time chromosomal examination was not done routinely.

3. Disorders of complex genetic etiology. Here were included (a) those disorders in which a genetic component is detectable by reason of its tendency to familial occurrence, but in which the pattern of hereditary transmission is not that observed in the case of single-gene effects; and (b) those in which a strong but complex genetic component seems likely (because of the specificity of the development disorder in the absence of common extrinsic factors) and those due to persistence of some earlier embryonic stage of development, again unassociated with any detectable maternal pregnancy disorder. Both the latter disorders may be interpreted as deriving from genetic mechanisms controlling development. Diseases in this category can be regarded as due to a number of genes interacting with each other and with other factors of the milieu of development; hence, the name multifactorial applies to this type of inheritance. Altogether these cases number 326 (31%), the most frequent being disorders of the central nervous system, closely followed by various congenital heart conditions.

TABLE X

Estimates of Birth Frequencies of Some Genetic Disorders
in Western European Populations per 100,000 Live Births

Dominant
  Nervous system
    Huntington's chorea 50
    Neurofibromatosis 40
    Myotonic dystrophy 20
    Basilar impression 3
    Tuberous sclerosis 1
  Intestines
    Multiple polyposis coli 10
  Kidney
    Polycystic disease of the kidneys 80
  Skeletal system
    Diaphysial aclasia 50
    Osteogenesis imperfecta 4
    Marfan's syndrome 4
    Achondroplasia 2
    Ehlers-Danlos syndrome 1
    Osteopetrosis tarda 1
  Sight
    Dominant forms of blindness 10
    Retinoblastoma 5
  Hearing
    Dominant forms of early childhood onset deafness .. 10
    Dominant otosclerosis (adult onset) 100
  Circulation
    Monogenic hypercholesterolemia 200
  Teeth
    Dentinogenesis imperfecta 10
    Amelogenesis imperfecta 2
  Blood
    Congenital spherocytosis 20
  Metabolism
    Acute intermittent porphyria 1
    Porphyria variegata 1
Recessive
  Metabolism
    Cystic fibrosis 50
    Phenylketonuria classical 10
  Nervous system
    Neurogenic muscle atrophies 10
  Endocrine glands
    Adrenal hyperplasias 10
  Hearing
    Severe congenital deafness 20
  Sight

(*continued*)

TABLE X (Cont.)

Recessive forms of blindness	10
Mental retardation, severe	
Nonspecific recessive forms	50
X-linked	
Locomotor system	
Duchenne muscular dystrophy	30
Blood clotting	
Hemophilia A	12
Skin	
Ichthyosis	10
Mental retardation	
Nonspecific X-linked	10

TABLE XI

Simple Genetic Disease

Disease	Mode of inheritance	Number of cases
Fibrocystic disease of the pancreas	Recessive	37
Hemolytic disease of the newborn	—	9
Werdnig-Hoffman disease	Recessive	7
Endocardial fibroelastosis	Recessive	7
Polycystic kidney (infantile)	Recessive	3
Galactosemia	Recessive	3
Adrenogenital syndrome	Recessive	2
Cystinosis	Recessive	2
Pierre Robin syndrome	Recessive	2
Diffuse cerebral sclerosis	X-linked	2
Gargoylism	Recessive	1
Christmas disease	X-linked	1
Zollinger-Ellison syndrome	Dominant	1
Albinism	Recessive	1
Glycogen storage disease	Recessive	1
Inborn error of metabolism (probably maple syrup urine disease)	Recessive	1
Epidermolysis bullosa lethalis	Recessive	1
Wolman's disease	Recessive	1
Terminal myopathy (juvenile distal)	Dominant	1
Neonatal thrombocytopenia	Recessive	1
Krabbe's disease	Recessive	1
Phenylketonuria	Recessive	1
Hyperoxaluria	Recessive	1
Spontaneous hypoglycemia	Recessive	1
Total		88

4. The fourth category concerns those diseases of doubtful etiology, virtually composed of two broad categories, first, the various neoplasms including leukemia and, second, low birth weight, and these accounted for 17%.

5. In the final category of deaths genetic factors did not seem to be primarily implicated, and these accounted for about 41%.

This series suggests that 42% of children's deaths have an appreciable genetic component. Such a series of deaths in specialist hospitals cannot be used to quantitate the genetic component in child mortality in general. In the classifications used a degree of subjectivity exists, the five categories are not clearly distinct, and of course the series is not a random sample, because complex and unusual cases would have been referred from the whole hospital region. However, the study does indicate a heavy genetic contribution to present-day child mortality in Newcastle.

By comparison with the earlier survey of Carter (1956), the genetic burden appears to be increasing. In a 1914 necropsy series of children at Great Ormond Street Hospital, London, two-thirds of all deaths were from diseases such as pneumonia, tuberculosis, and various infections, and only 16% were attributable to genetic or part-genetic causes. By 1954, more than one-third were identified as wholly or partly due to genetic causes. The present series, although not directly comparable in view of the differing nature of the two hospital populations, suggests further elevation.

The Newcastle survey says nothing of the genetic contribution to morbidity, but one can reasonably assume that genetic morbidity is pursuing a parallel course. Little direct evidence exists, but, for example, in 1922 the Board of Education surveyed schoolchildren on the causes of blindness and found that 37% of cases were due to congenital and hereditary anomalies. A similar survey in 1950 showed that, whereas the total rate of blindness had been halved, the figure for blindness due to congenital and hereditary anomalies had risen from 37 to 68%. Retinoblastoma incidence appears to have doubled in several countries during the last generation. Adults who as infants were diagnosed presymptomatically as suffering from phenylketonuria, and were successfully treated, have now begun to reach reproductive age and are passing on their genes to the next generation, so an absolute increase in incidence is occurring. A similar increase is occurring in those genetic diseases formerly restricted to low frequencies by nonsurvival but for which improved methods of treatment now allow survival and reproduction of those affected.

These results illuminate a number of urgent problems at the interface of culture and disease—the need for genetic advisory services, the need for knowledge on which these services are based, and the need for early diagnosis for rendering appropriate treatment.

Social Implications

Genetic disorders vary in severity; the effects may be minimal in the less severe, but in others they may be profound. Among the many babies with serious genetic defects who in former days would have died young, now, thanks to modern knowledge and treatment, a large proportion survive the early years of life, and similar improved survival is seen in adults with late-onset genetic disorders. Their defects impose varying degrees of disability on them. Not only do their medical problems increase the demand on health services, but the disablement to which they give rise produces many personal problems, emotional, social, and economic.

The educational and economic difficulties experienced by hemophiliacs in Britain until recently were extensive (Boon and Roberts, 1970). They affected the life of the whole family. They led to family limitation by the parents. The interaction between siblings often led to a strong bond of affection between the affected and unaffected children but in some cases caused great friction between them. Many a family was unable to go on holiday, either because they could not afford it or because they were too worried about the health of the hemophiliac boy to risk traveling any distance. Many mothers were unable to take part in activities or seek employment outside the home, and this reduced the social and economic potential of the family. For the hemophiliac, good education was essential because the nature of the disease prevented him from undertaking many forms of manual labor. But in the past, professional opportunities were denied to hemophiliacs, because of the succession of interruptions of school life resulting from their bleeding episodes. Against this background of incomplete and interrupted education, the employment problems were not surprising. Only one-fourth of the affected men had had steady occupations throughout their working lives. Some employers were reluctant to employ a man with hemophilia, for repeated absences from work were obviously a nuisance. To the hemophiliac workers, security was an important factor, and they were satisfied with work below their potential, for although they realized that the scope was limited, that work gave the all-important security.

It is usual for all serious cases of genetic disease to be referred to hospital sooner or later for diagnosis, assessment, and treatment. Such referral may involve numerous visits for continuing supervision, resulting in a strain on family life, both financial and otherwise (Boon, 1978). In those families where the family history is clear, the carriers frequently have a guilt complex. The shock to the parents, when the diagnosis is made in childhood, and to the patient when made later in life, is profound, requires to be recognized and managed. The patient's nursing or treatment at home may be intensely worrying. Intense too may be the concern about the patient's education, ultimate employment, and his ability to lead a normal life. With time comes the realization of the constrictions placed on family life. With these superimposed on the worry regarding the inherited aspects of the disease, it is no wonder that many families disintegrate.

Individuals suffering from serious genetic disease are not contributing fully to society and may prevent their families from doing so, partly because of the nature of the disease and partly because society itself is not organized to allow them to do so, to recognize their special needs, and to make allowances for them. Here much more can be done by social measures to diminish the gap between the patient's potential and his actual contribution. Similarly worrying are the implications for posterity of the increasing frequency of deleterious genes. That increase will continue until new equilibrium frequencies are attained, and the levels will depend on the changed fitness of the individuals concerned under modern conditions of treatment and management. In that changed fitness lies the hope for the resolution of the biological part of this problem. For if those to whom modern medicine has given their own lives, or those of their children, can be educated to reproduce responsibly, that is to say, to restrict their reproduction to a level below that of the population as a whole, then the maintenance of their genetic fitness at a lower level will prevent the new equilibrium gene frequency from rising to too high a point, and the total burden that society must face will be correspondingly reduced. Clinical genetics is a rapidly growing branch of modern medicine, and the number of genetic advisory centers at which information can be imparted to those at risk is increasing. Because of the intricate interdigitation and interaction of biological and social factors in western European culture, such centers, together with those for diagnosis and treatment, must consider the day-to-day problems of living for the individual and family unit with as much care as the genetic problems.

X. CONCLUSIONS

Examples are presented of different facets of the interaction between culture and disease in Britain and western Europe.

The major causes of death show considerable similarity in all western European countries, both in the categories of disease that are the preponderant causes, and the proportions for which they account. The mortality pattern varies consistently between age-groups, so differences in age structure between populations and any cultural changes that bring these about alter the disease pattern.

Comparison of mortality patterns, although not straightforward, provides useful pointers to the effects of culture on disease. Respiratory cancers show a characteristic distribution in Britain: heaviest in the overcrowded industrial areas, diminishing through the provincial conurbations, large, middle-sized, and small towns, to the least-affected rural districts. In this distribution the cultural variables of smoking habits, atmospheric pollution, and occupation are major contributing factors. Cardiovascular disease, approached in the same way, also shows the importance of smoking habits, occupation, and, less clearly, emotional stress.

Frank morbidity and mortality represent only part of the disease burden of the community. The examples of ischemic heart disease and rheumatic disease show the existence of a heavy chronic age-associated morbidity. In ischemic heart disease that morbidity is concealed, but confers a greater risk of early mortality if, often, little immediate handicap. In rheumatic disease the associations with occupation and social class are strong, but the degree of disability, although variable, is high in many cases. Both illustrate the opposite facet of culture-disease interaction, that the disease affects the culture by changing profoundly the way of life of the sufferer and restricting his contribution to society generally.

Day-to-day illness contributes greatly to the morbidity burden, and the infectious diseases, particularly in rural areas, provide a clear example of how patterns of living affect health. Of special importance is the limited intervillage travel and the role of the inn and village gatherings on disease transmission. Rural morbidity shows how the pattern of disease has changed with the cultural advances of the last three generations, not only those primarily directed to human health and hygiene, but also the educational campaigns on the proper use of agricultural machinery, the greater knowledge of veterinary medicine, and the introduction of animal health legislation.

For the distressing rise in venereal disease, recent cultural changes are essentially responsible—changes in attitude and changes in behavior with the arrival of the permissive society, the emphasis on sex, and the decrease in inhibitory influences on unselfdisciplined or abnormal behavior. The increase in congenital malformations, and the proportion of early deaths for which they account, is mainly due to cultural advance leading to the control of other causes of death, but is also partly attributable to teratogens that have been produced intentionally and unintentionally during recent technical advances (e.g., drugs, industrial physicochemical products). The teratogenicity attributable to infecting organisms has been influenced by the changed pattern of exposure as the result of public health measures, so that fewer children are infected and, therefore, come to be at risk as adults. Other minor effects of recent cultural changes on the health pattern are illustrated with reference to unemployment and the use of oral contraceptives.

Although most genetic diseases are individually rare, in total their effect is extensive, and today they contribute heavily to the morbidity and mortality patterns of western Europe. They are particularly important for their implications for the health of generations yet to come. The amount of genetic morbidity is already high and an appreciable proportion of services of hospitals caring for children are already preempted by society's deleterious genes. But such morbidity is increasing and, therefore, will require yet more services. The burden falls not only on the health services, but particularly on the families concerned, for genetic disease affects the quality of life of the family as well as the patient himself. The development of genetic advisory centers to allow them to fulfill their roles in preventive and family medicine is a step toward containing this increase.

The examples show the extensive and fundamental influence of culture on the health pattern in Britain and western Europe, and conversely the effects of disease on society. These interactions are manifest at all levels from survival and well-being in prenatal life to old age, and indeed to that of future generations. Some of the disease burden is outside the control of the individual, but many instances occur where he has a conscious choice to indulge or not indulge in a particular behavior and so affect his later health. Perhaps more of the vast resources of western Europe should be devoted to educating people of all ages to make such choices wisely.

REFERENCES

Barber, G. (1974). "Country Doctor." Boydell, Ipswich.

Boon, A. R. (1978). Genetic disorders: Their impact on the family. *In* "Perimeters of Social Repair" (W. H. G. Armytage and J. Peel, eds.), pp. 59–72. Academic Press, New York.

Boon, A. R., and Roberts, D. F. (1970). The social impact of haemophilia. *J. Biosoc. Sci.* **2,** 237–264.

Boycott, J. A. (1964). Undulant fever as an occupational disease. *Lancet* **i,** 972.

Brennan, M. E. (1978a). Patterns of mortality and the alienation of life. *In* "Perimeters of Social Repair" (W. H. G. Armytage and J. Peel, eds.), pp. 73–79. Academic Press, New York.

Brennan, M. E. (1978b). Children, poverty and illness. *New Sci.* **36,** 681.

Brennan, M. E., and Lancashire, R. (1978). Association of childhood mortality with housing status and unemployment. *J. Epidemiol. Community Health* **32,** 28–33.

Carter, C. O. (1956). Changing patterns in the causes of death at the Hospital for Sick Children. *Great Ormond Street J.* No. 11, p. 65.

Carter, C. O. (1977). Monogenic disorders. *J. Med. Genet.* **14,** 316–320.

Case, R. A. M. (1954). Cancer risk. *Br. Med. J.* **ii,** 987.

Chave, S. P. W., Morris, J. N., Moss, G., and Semmance, A. M. (1978). Vigorous exercise in leisure time and the death rate. *J. Epidemiol. Community Health* **32,** 239–243.

Doll, R. (1952). The causes of death among gas workers. *Br. J. Indust. Med.* **9,** 180–185.

Doll, R., and Bradford Hill, A. (1956). Lung cancer and other causes of death in relation to smoking. *Br. Med. J.* **ii,** 1071–1081.

Doll, R., Risher, R. E., and Gammon, E. J. (1965). Mortality of gas workers with special reference to cancers of the lung and bladder, chronic bronchitis, and pneumoconiosis. *Br. J. Indust. Med.* **22,** 1–12.

Draper, P., Dennis, J., Griffiths, J., Partridge, J., and Papay, J. (1979). Microprocessors, macroeconomic policy and public health. *Lancet* **i,** 373–375.

Howe, G. M. (1970). "National Atlas of Disease Mortality in the United Kingdom," 2nd ed. Nelson, London.

Kasl, S., and Cobb, G. (1972). Changes in reported illness and illness behavior related to termination of employment: A preliminary report. *Int. J. Epidemiol.* **1**, 111.

Kellgren, J. H., Lawrence, J. S., and Aitken Swan, J. (1953). Rheumatic complaints in an urban population. *Ann. Rheum. Dis.* **12**, 5–15.

Klingberg, M. H., and Papier, C. M. (1979). Teratoepidemiology. *J. Biosoc. Sci.* **11**, 233–258.

Lambert, P. (1976). Perinatal mortality: social and environmental factors. *Popul. Trends* **4**, 4–8.

Lawrence, J. S. (1955). Rheumatism in coal miners. *Br. J. Indust. Med.* **12**, 249–261.

Lawther, P. J., and Commins, B. T. (1970). Cigarette smoking and exposure to carbon monoxide. *Ann. N.Y. Acad. Sci.* **174**, 135–147.

Lawther, P. J., Waller, R. E., and Henderson, M. (1970). Climate, air pollution and chronic bronchitis. *Thorax* **25**, 525–539.

Lob, M. (1965). Angine de poitrine et carence en nitroglycol dans les fabriques d'explosifs. *Rev.Med.Suisse Romande* **85**, 489.

Mann, J. I., and Inman, W. H. W. (1975). Oral contraceptives and death from myocardial infarction. *Br. Med. J.* **ii**, 245–248.

Martin, A. E. (1964). Mortality and morbidity statistics and air pollution. *Proc. R. Soc. Med.* **57**, 969–975.

Monif, G. R. G., Egan, E. A., Held, B., and Eitzman, D. V. (1972). Correlation of maternal cytomegalovirus infection during gestation and with neonatal involvement. *J. Pediatr.* **80**, 17–20.

Office of Population Censuses and Surveys (1974). "Morbidity Statistics from General Practice; Second National Study, 1970–71." HM Stationery Off., London.

Pickles, W. (1948). Epidemiology in country practice. *N. Engl. J. Med.* **239**, 419–427.

Reid, D. D., and Fairbairn, A. S. (1958). The natural history of bronchitis. *Lancet* **i**, 1147.

Roberts, D. F., Chavez, J., and Court, S. D. M. (1970). The genetic component in mortality. *Arch. Dis. Child.* **45**, 33–38.

Royal College of General Practitioners (1977). Oral contraception study. *Lancet* **i**, 970.

Royal College of Physicians (1970). "Air Pollution and Health." London.

Royal College of Physicians (1971). "Smoking and Health Now." London.

Schonell, M. E., Brotherston, J. G., Burnett, R. C. S., Campbell, J., Coghlan, J. D., Moffat, M. A., Norval, J., and Sutherland, J. A. W. (1966). Occupational infections in the Edinburgh abattoir. *Br. Med. J.* **ii**, 148–150.

Stevenson, A. C. (1959). The load of hereditary defects in human populations. *Radiat. Res., Suppl.* No. 1, p. 306–325.

Streissguth, A. P. (1978). Fetal alcohol syndrome. *Am. J. Epidemiol.* **107**, 467–487.

Tunbridge, W. G. M., Evered, D. C., Hall, R., Appleton, D., Brewis, M., Clark, F., Grimley Evans, J., Young, E., Bird, T., and Smith, P. A. (1977). Lipid profiles and cardiovascular diseases in the Whickham area with particular reference to thyroid failure. *Clin. Endocrinol.* **7**, 495–508.

Vessey, M. P., Doll, R., Peto, R., Johnson, B., and Wiggins, P. (1976). A long-term follow-up study of women using different methods of contraception—an interim report. *J. Biosoc. Sci.* **8**, 373–427.

Vessey, M. P., McPherson, K., and Johnson, B. (1977). Mortality among women participating in the Oxford/Family Planning Association contraceptive study. *Lancet* **ii**, 731.

Visser, G. H. A., Huisjes, H. J., and Elshove, J. (1976). Anticonvulsants and fetal malformations. *Lancet* **1**, 970.

Waller, R. E., Lawther, P. J., and Martin, A. E. (1969). Clean air and health in London. *Proc. Clean Air Conf., Eastbourne, London Natl. Soc. Clear Air* **1**, 71.

Wilson, J. G. (1973). "Environment and Birth Defects." Academic Press, New York.

Woolf, B., and Waterhouse, J. (1945). Studies of infant mortality. *J. Hyg.* **44**, 67–98.

World Health Organization (1970). Treponematoses research. *W. H. O. Tech. Rep. Ser.* No. 455.
World Health Organization (1974). The ten leading causes of death for selected countries in North America, Europe and Oceania, 1969, 1970 and 1971. *World Health Stat. Rep.* **27**, 563–652.
World Health Organization (1975). Current data: infectious diseases. *World Health Stat. Rep.* **28**, 423–426.

14

Diseases of Eastern Europeans

V. SIMKO AND B. KROMPHOLZ

Despite our present-day technological competence, obtaining information pertinent to eastern and central European countries is difficult, largely because of the limitations of availability of data and their inaccessibility through customary resources. Furthermore, some countries—specifically the vast Union of Soviet Socialist Republics, which itself contains more than 100 ethnic groups—have populations that are so heterogeneous that each region could be the subject of a separate chapter. Our attempt here, then, is merely to survey the information available for the nine countries, Albania, Bulgaria, Czechoslovakia, the German

459

BIOCULTURAL ASPECTS OF DISEASE
Copyright © 1981 by Academic Press, Inc.
All rights of reproduction in any form reserved.
ISBN 0-12-598720-X

Democratic Republic, Hungary, Poland, Rumania, Yugoslavia, and the Soviet Union, of which East Europe is comprised.

In toto, we will refer to these as East European countries not only because of their political alliance but because they are so listed in the 1980 U.S. National Library of Medicine Medical Subject Headings Tree Structures.

We will attempt to systematize the data preliminary to later attempts by others at greater comprehensiveness and refinement. The need for such a survey is obvious; the latest (fifth) edition of McKusick's (1978) comprehensive book, "Mendelian Inheritance in Man," has no listing for the ethnic distribution of diseases for the countries covered in this chapter.

I. HISTORIC, ETHNIC, AND SOCIOECONOMIC BACKGROUND

For more than 2000 years, farmers and warriors have moved across eastern Europe, producing a rich genetic pool of Slavic, Germanic, Hungarian, Central Asian, and other peoples. Here we briefly summarize the extraordinary ethnic heritage of the East European states.

A. Ethnic Clustering, Migration, and Settlement

Throughout history many sovereignties and other political systems have affected the stability of peoples of the area. The Hapsburg Empire, for example, until its fall in 1918 represented a multinational central European state, with its German, Hungarian, Slavic, and Italian ethnic groups locked essentially in the same regional areas they had reached by extensive migration toward the end of the tenth century BC. However, the ethnic groups originally present in East Europe did not all later become part of the ethnic pool of the Hapsburg state.

The Finns, Estonians, Livonians, Latvians, and Lithuanians resided in the area of the Baltic littoral from earliest times. The Germans and Slavs, more inclined to wander, were thus less indigenous to certain areas (Fischer-Galati, 1970). After the downfall of the Roman Empire, Slavs and other newcomers from the Urals and the Caspians displaced some German tribes from extensive areas of eastern Europe. In the fifth century AD bands of Huns and Avars moved along the Danube Valley into the heart of Europe, only to be absorbed by other ethnic groups. Slavic migration reached the classical frontiers of the Roman Empire and Greece. White Russians and Great Russians settled in what is now the western Soviet Union. The Little Russians went farther west to areas of the modern western Ukraine and Galicia. Czech, Slovak, and Polish tribes settled permanently in the heart of Europe. Slavic tribes of Wends and Serbs migrated as far west as the River Elbe and to the area of Berlin but later were almost entirely absorbed by Germans. The Slavic tribes of Slovenes, Croatians, Serbs, and Montenegrins moved toward the western littoral of the Balkan Peninsula. In the ninth century they were separated from the Slavic tribes in central Europe by a forceful invasion of Magyars who settled in the Great Danubian Plain.

Besides Magyars and Germans, other important non-Slavic ethnic groups settled in what is now East Europe. Along the Danube inflow settled the Rumanians with their basic Latin culture. In the seventh century, Bulgars moved into the Balkan Peninsula, later to be completely absorbed by the Slavs. The Turkish Khazars established in the eighth century a highly civilized empire north of the Black Sea. Their Khan converted to Judaism, and the Khazars, although later Moslems and Christians, are believed by some to be the ancestors of many of the Russian Jews (see Chapter 10).

By the tenth century, colonization of central and eastern Europe was essentially completed, but repeated forceful invasions from the east during the next millenium prevented cultural and economic integration of the area with the more-advanced countries of western Europe.

Mongols from China and central Asia who raided Europe in the eleventh century reached Bohemia and central Europe by the thirteenth century. The Ottoman Turks, from the fourteenth century on, gradually moved across the Balkan Peninsula, occupying Bulgaria, Serbia, Albania, Rumania, and Hungary in turn, and then, in 1683, besieged Vienna. Almost 150 years of Turkish rule over Hungary, and several hundred years of domination by the Ottoman Empire over Serbia, Albania, Rumania, and Bulgaria led to important economic, social, and cultural consequences. That domination undoubtedly left genetic footprints on the population of the conquered areas.

After the Turks were driven back beyond the Danube, the Hapsburg rulers tried to colonize the devastated land with Germans and also with some Slavic tribes. German craftsmen and miners formed small ethnic groups in several areas in East Europe. The Swabians settled along the lower Danube.

B. The Nine Nations

Numerous ethnic groups are included in the nine nations of East Europe. Ottoman domination and its major religion, Islam, influenced Albania more than any foreign power. Among Albania's major ethnic groups are the Serbs and Montenegrins.

By the ninth century, the Bulgars, a Turkish tribe that took control of an area south of the River Danube, had fully merged with the Slavs. After a succession of rises and declines as a power and empire, Bulgaria became the first European nation to be taken into the Ottoman Empire. In the nineteenth century, with help from Rumania and Serbia, Bulgaria again became an independent state.

Czechoslovakia includes Slovakia and the traditional Czech lands of Bohemia,

Moravia, and the Czech Silesia. Today that nation's population is about 65% Czech, 28% Slovak, and lesser amounts of Hungarian and German. The Czechs and Slovaks differ in their history, religion, and culture.

By composition, the German people, including persons living in the Democratic Republic (East Germany) and the Federal Republic of Germany (West Germany), is the great ethnic complex of Europe. Both Germanies derived from many barbaric tribes that spread over Europe in the first 1000 years AD. East Germany includes the former states of Brandenburg, Mecklenburg, Thuringia, Saxony, and the Saxony-Anhalt.

The populations of the other eastern European countries also had various origins. The population of Hungary is about 60% rural and relatively homogeneous. The Magyars, originally a Finno-Ugric people from beyond the Urals, constitute about 96% of the population. Poland is also composed of a relatively homogeneous population, derived from the Polians who had hegemony over other Slavic tribes that occupied the country in the ninth to the tenth century.

Rumania is derived from seven historic and geographic regions: Walachia, Moldavia, S. Bukovina, Dobruja, Transylvania, Crisana-Maramures, and Banat. Most of the population is Rumanian, but the country has many ethnic minorities.

Today, Yugoslavia is a federation of six peoples' republics: Serbia, Croatia, Macedonia, Slovenia, Montenegro, and Bosnia-Hercegovina. Each of the republics except the latter has maintained some measure of ethnic individuality by historical and cultural factors.

The Soviet Union which spans 11 time zones, comprises 15 republics, the most important and largest of which is the Russian Soviet Federated Socialist Republic. Others are Estonia, Latvia, Lithuania, Belorussia, Ukraine and the Moldavian, Georgian, Armenian, Azerbaijan, Kazakh, Tadzhik, Uzbek, Turkmen, and Kirghiz SSRs. The later five republics are in the Asian part of the Soviet Union. The Soviet Union is a multiethnic state with more than 100 ethnic groups and languages. The Slavic group, consisting of Russians, Ukrainians, and Belorussians, is the largest and accounts for about three-fourths of the total population.

An anticlimax to the cultural and intellectual development of East Europe during the past 700 years has been the geopolitical fragmentation and political developments of the twentieth century. The outbreak of World War I accelerated the breakdown of the Austro-Hungarian monarchy and led to the creation of the small, strongly nationalistic countries unable to withstand the pressure of strong expansionist neighbor countries.

The events of World Wars I and II were more destructive to the countries of East Europe than to any other parts of the world. Civilian losses during World War I in the Austro-Hungarian monarchy and Serbia were one million persons, with another 800,000 lives lost by Rumania (Taylor, 1973–1974a). In World War II, Poland alone lost 4,320,000 lives, and Yugoslavia 1,700,000. The racial policy of the Third Reich alone resulted in a mass extermination of 4 million East European Jews (Taylor, 1973-1974b). Furthermore, political turbulence after World War II led to the forced displacement of millions of ethnic Germans from the countries of eastern Europe, Poland, the Danube delta, and Czechoslovakia. The human consequences of mass extermination, starvation, epidemics of contagious diseases, emotional stress, and displacement of entire ethnic groups and nations must inevitably reflect in the biomedical statistics for generations to follow.

After 1945, Europe was divided politically into East and West (eliminating the important transitional zone of Central Europe). Thus Prague, East Berlin, and parts of Germany farther west than Munich are considered to be within East Europe, whereas Vienna, former heart of the Austro-Hungarian empire, is considered part of the West.

Today, cultural differences between countries like Albania and Czechoslovakia in East Europe are far greater than those between, for example, Portugal and West Germany. Western Europe has no country such as Albania. Travel to Albania from other East European countries is limited, replicating the pattern of lack of exchange among the Soviet-block countries until the early 1960s. Travel between Yugoslavia and most other East European countries had been restricted because of differences in official political platforms. Such travel limitations are an important factor in considering both the exchange of biomedical information and the spread of communicable diseases. Massive seasonal movements of migrant workers, for example, typical for some areas of western Europe, are virtually unknown in East Europe. An exception is the job flux of Yugoslavs to western Europe, mostly to Germany and Sweden.

II. DISEASE PREVALENCE IN EAST EUROPE

During 1980, the first phase of an ambitious effort to develop a uniform system for collecting health information in East Europe will have been completed. Being undertaken by the Health Committee of the Warsaw Pact, it will permit systematic collection and analysis of data on morbidity, mortality, and natality and allow for comparison of age-specific prevalence and incidence of disease and mortality among participant countries (Makovicky, 1978). Some basic demographic data for previous years for the nine East European countries are given in Table I.

The present lack of standardized criteria for classification, reporting, and coding necessitates caution when interpreting data on diseases prevalent in these countries. However, World Health Organization statistics for selected countries allow us to assume that heart disease, malignant neoplasms, and cerebrovascular disease are the leading causes of death in East European countries. High frequen-

TABLE I

Basic Demographic Data on Nine East European Countries

Category	Albania	Bulgaria	Czechoslovakia	German Democratic Republic	Hungary	Poland	Rumania	Yugoslavia	Soviet Union
Population in millions (Census 1970–1974)[a]	1.6	8.2	14.3	17.1	10.3	32.6	19.1	20.5	241.7
Population density per km^2 (1974)[b]	84.0	78.0	115.0	157.0	114.0	108.0	89.0	83.0	—
Life expectancy at birth (Male)	64.9	68.2	67.2	68.9	66.7	67.0	67.2	67.7	64.0
(Female)	67.0	73.5	73.6	74.5	73.1	74.9	71.6	72.6	74.0
	(1966)	(1971)	(1975)	(1976)	(1977)	(1976)	(1977)	(1976)	(1971)
Live births per 1000 population (1974)	33.4	17.2	19.8	10.6	17.8	18.4	20.3	18.1	3.4
Infant mortality (under 1 year of age per 1000 live births) (1974)	—	25.5	20.4	15.9	34.3	23.5	35.0	40.9	27.7
Deaths (except infants per 1000 population) (1974)[a]	8.1	9.8	11.7	13.5	12.0	8.2	9.1	8.4	9.5

[a] From Demographic Yearbook (1977).
[b] From Statistical Yearbook (1976).

cies of respiratory diseases—bronchitis, emphysema, asthma, influenza, and pneumonia—are reported as next most frequent causes of death. The frequency of suicide among Hungarian and Czechoslovak adults is striking, the more so when coupled with high rates of death by accident, in which category one may assume many self-inflicted deaths are reported.

Many East European countries are now undergoing massive industrialization, centrally planned and organized by the state bureaucracies. Although environmental protection is considered to have been ensured by applying state regulations, air and water pollution and their consequences are still considerable. Morbidity and mortality data may reflect the environmental and social stresses of urbanization. Diseases such as obesity and emotional disorders are now becoming important contributors to the health pattern of East European countries. A shift away from infectious diseases has occurred with improved standards of public health in the more populous regions. Nevertheless, tuberculosis, viral hepatitis, bacillary dysentery, and streptococcal infections remain prominent problems. In Poland and Yugoslavia in particular, high mortality from ''all other causes'' is observed, perhaps reflecting problems of data collecting. Accidents are on the increase, and, although significant advances have occurred in perinatal care, infant death rates remain relatively high.

In general, the populations of Czechoslovakia and the German Democratic Republic have the highest levels of health care among the East European countries, reflecting not only an overall higher living standard but a longer tradition of medical care and public health practices. A survey of East German recruits by Jaschke (1968), revealed prominent disability related to juvenile hypertension, conditions related to inflammatory heart disorder, and viral hepatitis, tuberculosis, and disorders of the musculoskeletal system. In Poland, where medical facilities are less adequate to meet the needs of a still largely rural population, infectious diseases continue to influence morbidity and mortality data disproportionate to statistics for the more-urbanized countries. Nonetheless, the impact of urban stress may be observed here too: in a recent survey of 1000 journalists by Kopcynski and Mrozowa (1978), more coronary heart disease and myocardial infarction were observed than in the average population. A higher rate also was found for tuberculosis. Lower-than-average incidences of rheumatic disorders and obesity were reported. Similarly, Hungarian data reveal the preponderance of degenerative over infectious diseases, with infant mortality remaining relatively high.

Because emigration and migration do not contribute significantly to the population structure of East European countries, two events, births and deaths, determine the demographic composition of East Europe (Table I). The population structure, however, is undergoing an aging process similar to that occurring in western countries. Between 1950 and 1970, the proportion of Czechoslovaks aged 60 years or more increased by 50%, as did the proportion of those 80 years or more (Zaremba and Zavazalova, 1979). In 1975, 12.9% of the population was more than 65 years, and a rapid increase of this geriatric segment is projected to the end of the century. In the 70+ age-group, 90% have at least one chronic condition, with an average of 2.7 conditions per person.

III. SPECIFIC DISEASES

A. Nutrition-Related Diseases

Major efforts have been taken to compare nutrition and health indices in technologically developing communities with those of the more traditional rural areas. Several studies in Czechoslovakia (Kajaba et al., 1966; Kajaba, 1969) reported on persisting differences in the nutritional status of children in different areas (in disfavor of the less-developed parts of the country). On the other hand, negative consequences of industrialization were found to be increased caloric consumption in the form of simple carbohydrates and fats, increased obesity, and rising plasma cholesterol levels. As in other technologically developed countries, classical cases of nutritional deficiency were rarely encountered. Curiously, plasma cholesterol levels in children were reported to be somewhat higher than the values published for similar age-groups in the United States. Kajaba (1973), studying a rural population aged 40–75 years in the Slovak part of Czecho-slovakia, found that their diet was slightly above recommended standards in caloric content and fat (34% of total calories) but was considered deficient in vitamin A, riboflavin, and ascorbic acid. Mean plasma cholesterol levels for the fifth, sixth, and seventh decades were 208, 203, and 200 mg/dl for men and 189, 199, and 202 mg/dl for women.

A report from the Polish Academy of Sciences (Wolanski, 1975) examined the development and physical fitness of Poles of different age-groups. Men and women in 19–20 years age-group had increased their average height by 4.2 cm and average body weight by 4 kg in the last 80 years. Comparing data from 1938, World War II, and the postwar period resulted in impressive declines in the indices of height and weight among growing Poles. Wide regional differences were noted in recently obtained somatometric indices. Persons in the areas with better health care (Warsaw and Szczecin) were noted to have better indices than those living in parts of Poland exposed to environmental pollution with sulfur compounds and dust (Upper Silesia); whereas, somatometric differences in War-saw children seemed to relate to social class.

In 1962–1963, three republics of Yugoslavia (Serbia, Slavonia, and Dalmatia) participated in a multinational epidemiological study related to coronary heart disease, coordinated by Dr. Ancel Keys and funded by the U.S. Public Health Service and the American Heart Association. (Four other European countries, the

United States, and Japan also participated in this project.) More than 2000 subjects in Serbia (Djordjevic *et al.*, 1965) and another 1476 men aged 40–59 years in Slavonia and Dalmatia (Buzina *et al.*, 1966) were studied. Dietary studies were done on randomly selected subgroups. Although caloric proportions of the main nutrients ingested were similar in Slavonia and Dalmatia (54% carbohydrates, 14% protein, 32% fat), subjects in Dalmatia ingested about twice the amount of polyunsaturated fatty acids and had correspondingly lower plasma cholesterol levels, although subjects in Slavonia had relatively low cholesterol levels compared with West European standards. Hypertension was somewhat less common in Dalmatia. About 40% of men in both areas were nonsmokers. In the Serbian study, one subgroup comprised 654 university professors in Belgrade. These were matched with groups of peasants and factory workers. The professors had a daily intake of 200 calories in excess of recommended standards, whereas the peasants had 700 calories and the workers 200 calories below the recommended intake. Accordingly, the relative body weight of peasants was 10% below, and that of the professors 5% above, ideal body weight. Daily fat intake was 25% of total calories in peasants and 35% in professors. Mean plasma cholesterol levels were 159 mg/dl for the peasants, 171 mg/dl for the workers, and 166 mg/dl for the professors, all considerably below the cholesterol levels observed in technologically advanced countries. The group of peasants consistently had a lower frequency of arterial hypertension than the other groups.

B. Heart Disease

Several recent epidemiological surveys show the increase of coronary heart disease in East European countries. Laznicka *et al.* (1974) studied 658 patients hospitalized in a rural northwestern Czechoslovakian area and drawn from a referred pool of 75,000 persons. In men and women, the highest frequency of transmural infarctions (33% of all infarcted patients) occurred in the seventh decade of life. Women were affected by the disease at a later age than were men, but after age 80 years the incidences for the sexes did not differ. Forty-four percent of patients were hospitalized within the first 24 hours after the onset of symptoms. In the first year after an intensive care unit was established (1972), mortality from myocardial infarction in this district hospital dropped from 30 to 22%. Using retrospective data and the same referral sample, the authors reported the incidence of myocardial infarctions for the years 1969–1973 to be fourfold that of 10 years earlier, and 16-fold that of data from 31 years earlier. Although variances in data-collection procedures may contribute to vastly increased reporting of myocardial infarctions, modern hospitalization practices and changes in health status obviously play primary roles.

Useful descriptive data were obtained in an area of rural Rumania that is undergoing rapid development (Cucuianu, 1973). Focusing on atherosclerosis and coronary heart disease, investigators found rural farmers still had serum cholesterol levels as low as 160 mg/dl, whereas the incidence of myocardial infarction increased eightfold in the past five decades.

According to Simonson and Berman (1972), myocardial infarction in persons under 40 years of age is not rare and has been increasing faster than in the older population since 1950 in the Soviet Union. The incidence of myocardial infarction in patients under 40 years of the total infarction population has been estimated to be from 2.7 to 20%. The male to female ratio is significantly greater in the younger than in the older patients.

C. Neoplasms

As noted in Table II, major differences exist in cancer mortality in East Europe, when compared with those of the technologically advanced countries of western Europe and the United States (World Health Organization, 1972–1973). Czechoslovakia had the sixth highest mortality due to cancers of all sites. Among the 44 countries listed, Rumania had the fifth and Hungary the seventh highest uterine cancer mortality. Hungary had the fourth highest death rate for stomach cancer among males, preceded only by Japan, Chile, and Costa Rica. Poland was fifth, Czechoslovakia seventh, Bulgaria eleventh, Rumania twelfth, and Yugoslavia eighteenth in mortality from gastric cancer in males. No sex-related differences in gastric cancer were noted. Bulgaria, Hungary, Poland, Yugoslavia, and Czechoslovakia are among the leading countries of the world in mortality for primary cancer of the liver (World Health Organization, 1978).

TABLE II

Age-Adjusted Death Rates for Cancer (All Sites)

Country	Mortality[a]		
	Total	Male	Female
1. Hungary (1977)	249.3	278.8	221.5
2. Czechoslovakia (1975)	230.2	272.3	190.1
3. East Germany (1974)	225.0	242.8	209.5
4. Poland (1976)	160.2	181.1	140.4
5. Bulgaria (1977)	145.4	173.4	117.4
6. Rumania (1977)	135.7	147.7	116.2
7. Yugoslavia (1976)	119.9	135.8	104.4
8. West Germany (1977)	260.8	273.7	249.1
9. England and Wales (1977)	257.4	283.1	233.0
10. France (1975)	230.2	271.2	190.7
11. United States (1976)	178.0	198.8	158.2

[a] Rates per 100,000.

D. Gastrointestinal Disease

In some of the East European countries the incidence of peptic ulcer and ulcerative colitis have been reported to be extremely high. A retrospective study of 8050 persons more than 60 years of age in rural Poland by Modzelewski and Zaczek-Modelewska (1978) found 2% had peptic ulcer. Of that number, 73% had gastric ulcer and 27% duodenal ulcer. Although these authors did not comment on the differential diagnosis with regard to gastric cancer, they suggested that among Polish men in early or mid-adulthood duodenal ulcer occurs more frequently than does gastric ulcer. Polish women, on the other hand, have gastric ulcer more frequently at all ages. Gastric ulcer is more commonly found after age 60 years in both sexes.

Mazur (1978), studying the ulcer diseases in adolescents and younger children in rural Poland found 33% had gastric ulcer, and 67% duodenal ulcer, with the diagnosis determined by an upper GI series. Of the patients, 57% had histories of peptic ulcer in the families. In more than half of the patients, the parasite *Giardia lamblia* was detected in the duodenal fluid (reflecting, probably, high prevalence of giardiasis in the general population).

Although some unpublished reports cite the disease's increasing frequency in East Europe, Crohn's disease (regional enterocolitis) is found relatively infrequently in East European countries. This low frequency may relate partly to the dramatic decrease of Jewish population in East Europe in the last five decades. In a study of 34 adult Czechoslovak patients with resections of the bowel, Crohn's disease was the underlying disorder in only four cases (Dvorsky *et al.*, 1970).

E. Cirrhosis of the Liver

Compared with data for several other European countries, mortality for cirrhosis of the liver is relatively low in East Europe. Nevertheless, it remains a substantial public health problem, reflecting the incidence of alcohol abuse in the population. High incidence of virus B and non A–non B hepatitis in East Europe may be another contributing factor to liver cirrhosis. Czechoslovakia (38.7 per 100,000 for men and 9.2 for women) and Hungary (28.5 for men and 10.1 for women) have the highest mortality from cirrhosis in East Europe, the number of fatalities among men being greater than those among women, as expected. Nonetheless, overall death rates are significantly lower than those reported for western Europe (e.g., 79.9 for French men and 34.8 for French women) and the United States (46.3 for men and 22.8 for women).

F. Infectious Diseases

Some of the more common infectious diseases in East Europe are discussed below.

1. Tuberculosis

Although communicable diseases in East Europe have been largely contained, they continue to pose serious social and public health problems. Tuberculosis is typical. Although deaths per 100,000 are decidedly low in Czechoslovakia (6.9) and the German Democratic Republic (4.0), other East European countries experience notable morbidities and mortalities. Among 27 European countries, the highest incidence was recorded for Poland (18.4), followed by Yugoslavia (17.3), Hungary (15.8), Rumania (14.0), and Bulgaria (8.9).

2. Hepatitis

Viral hepatitis is common in East Europe. As such, it is a serious public health problem, with health service professionals at higher risk than the rest of the population. In a region of western Czechoslovakia, the incidence of viral hepatitis in persons more than age 15 years varied between 0.106 and 0.325% (Truksova, 1976). In Rumania the annual incidence of viral hepatitis in the general population was reported as 0.21%, but in the personnel of regional blood banks, 2% (Apateanu et al., 1971).

In Poland, the Department of Infectious Diseases of the Medical School in Cracow treated 3301 patients for acute viral hepatitis in the years 1965 to 1974 (Sowa and Mossor-Ostrowska, 1976). Health service workers represented 13% of all patients with acute viral hepatitis. Comparing the incidence of viral hepatitis in the same area in the years 1955 to 1964, those authors claimed an 80% increase in the number of patients hospitalized for acute viral hepatitis.

Important outbreaks of water-borne infectious hepatitis in rural Yugoslavia in recent years have been of extreme concern to public health officials (Gaon, 1973). Achieving a peak morbidity of 307 cases per 100,000 population, the epidemics occurred in villages that drew their water supplies from contaminated wells, and affected all age-groups and social classes. Relatively short durations of 28–83 days characterized the water-borne outbreaks, as contrasted with the longer duration of contact-type hepatitis. The significance of these outbreaks in a country where 60% of the rural population draws its water supply from drilled or dug wells and where the water is of poor quality cannot be overestimated. These rural localities have much more water-borne infectious hepatitis than was originally supposed.

3. Giardia lamblia

This flagellate protozoan parasite is commonly associated with diarrhea, abdominal discomfort, and sometimes malabsorption. Although giardiasis occurs most frequently in Africa and India, it has been frequently observed in travellers coming from the Soviet Union, especially Leningrad (Brodsky et al., 1974; Wright et al., 1977; Levinson and Nastro, 1978). One study reported the attack rate of giardiasis in two groups of U.S. travellers to the Soviet Union to be 29 and 51%, respectively (Walzer *et al.*, 1971). Returning travellers from the Soviet Union had eggs of *Ascaris lumbricoides* in their stools. Drinking water in Leningrad hotels was considered the most likely vehicle of the parasite. This finding was related to the report that *Ascaris* is the most common helminth in the inhabitants of the Leningrad area (Babaeva *et al.*, 1969). Parasitic infection with *Giardia* may show no symptoms in the population residing in the area. It is possible that prolonged infection leads to acquired immunity and to an asymptomatic carrier state.

An especially high incidence of *Giardia lamblia* in the stool was reported in a study from northcentral Czechoslovakia (Pazdziora, 1972). The parasite was found in 7.6% of 883 children of three nursery schools, the frequency of positive findings being related to the length of attendance at the nursery school. Family contacts of parasite-positive children were parasite positive in 9.8%, whereas families of parasite-negative children had parasites in the stool of 3.2%. Nursery staff were 4.5% parasite positive. In more than half of the cases, no clinical symptoms related to the presence of *Giardia*.

G. Emotional Disorders

A rapid introduction of technology to previously rural areas has increased the emotional stresses on large portions of the population, as have the higher incidences of disrupted families, divorce, and abortion that have accompanied the industrialization and urbanization of the East Europe countries. With more than half of the labor force composed of women, who, in addition to their occupational or agricultural tasks, continue to bear major responsibility for homemaking and childrearing in traditional patrilineal societies, the incidence of stress-induced emotional disorders among females is of importance. A report from the German Democratic Republic describes a 12.4% incidence of psychoneurotic disorders in 3000 outpatient visits among an agricultural population of 3780 men and women (Scheerer, 1973). Women were affected three times more often than were men. However, we must emphasize that women appear to be more willing to present themselves for psychiatric treatment than are men, who enter treatment more commonly for severer manifestations of psychopathology. In this study, precipitating factors in women were observed to be excessive work loads. Neurotic disorders occurred with less frequency in rural areas of East Germany than among industrial plant employees of urban populations, where the incidence of neurosis was reported to be in excess of 30% of all patient visits. Neurotic disorders were frequent among intellectuals and managers, old retired persons, and women employed in agriculture.

A recent report on the incidence of neurotic problems in a population of almost 1500 subjects of a multiethnic Hungarian village concluded that neurotic disor-

TABLE III

Mortality from Suicide and Self-Inflicted Injuries, 15-44 Years[a]

Country	Mortality[b]	Percentage of all causes
Bulgaria	7.9	5.5
Czechoslovakia	24.0	15.2
France	11.5	7.2
Hungary	29.5	17.8
Ireland	3.9	3.5
Norway	9.0	8.3
Poland	14.1	8.4
Spain	2.7	2.1

[a] From World Health Organization (1974).
[b] Rates per 100,000.

ders occurred with the same frequency in rural and urban populations, more in women than in men, and more among poorly educated persons (Tenyi and Ozsvath, 1978).

The above frequencies for psychoneurotic disorders are consistent with cross-national epidemiological reports and patient data from practitioners, and vary only slightly from those of western countries. However, in one important area the experience of East European countries is noteworthy: suicide rates are extremely high in Hungary and Czechoslovakia (Table III). In those countries, they are, respectively, the second and third leading causes of death among adults aged 15-44 years. Hungary had the highest suicide rate for men among 14 European countries. Speculating on the reason for the high rate is difficult. Increased rates of suicide have been positively correlated with situations involving stress, instability, and real or threatened deprivation. Whether sociopolitical and economic stresses are influential in producing suicides must await the results of careful epidemiological studies, as must conclusions on the relative importance of genetically transmitted affective disorders.

IV. UNIQUE DISEASES IN EAST EUROPE

Possibly owing to the movement of peoples across central and eastern Europe for many centuries as well as past and present integration with the rest of the continent, and possibly due to the limitations of available data, few diseases have been reported to be specific to East Europe.

A. Balkan Endemic Nephropathy

Some authors (Bruckner *et al.*, 1967) believe Balkan nephropathy (endemic nephropathy, or chronic Balkan nephritis) to be distinct from other known types of chronic renal disease. It affects a relatively high percentage of the inhabitants of some areas in Rumania, Yugoslavia, and Bulgaria, the endemic areas bordering one another in the vicinity of the Danubian Iron Gates tributaries. This disorder has the characteristics of a chronic renal insufficiency not associated with arterial hypertension or edema. It has a high familial correlation and is typified by severe bilateral renal atrophy and, invariably, death, usually within 5 years of diagnosis. The earliest information about an increased endemic incidence of renal disease in Bulgaria was reported in 1941, but the first large-scale epidemiologic investigation was done in 1956 (Puchlev, 1967). The region of endemic nephropathy in northwestern Bulgaria is about 70 × 30 km, including a mountainous and hilly area, 3 towns, and 77 villages. The mortality caused by renal diseases in 14 of the endemic villages was 34%, compared with 1.2% in all other regions. The highest incidence of the disease was for persons between ages 30 and 69 years, especially between 40 and 59 years. It has not been definitively diagnosed in children and adolescents. Occurrence among families of different social standards and living conditions has been demonstrated.

During World War II physicians in rural parts of Serbia (Yugoslavia) observed a high frequency of death from uremia among certain families in several villages (Danilovic and Stojimirovic, 1967). During a 15-year period, in some villages located 40–70 km from Belgrade, 37 members in 12 families died of uremia, and of 44 survivors, 23 had chronic kidney disease. Yet in a nearby small town not a single case of chronic renal disease was reported. Similar rural distributions have been noted in Rumania (Moroeanu, 1967). Persons affected were mostly farmers living in seasonally flooded areas. In Bosnia (Yugoslavia), as many as 9% of the inhabitants of endemic villages were affected, mostly of the agricultural population of the valleys and plains but infrequently the inhabitants of hilly areas as well (Gaon, 1967). Similarly, the disease was reported to be more common in women than in men, to have increasing incidence with age, and to decrease in frequency in the mountainous areas. No cases were reported in villagers not directly engaged in agriculture (e.g., teachers, drivers, managers).

Balkan nephropathy usually starts insidiously with headaches, fatigue, and anorexia. The skin of affected persons may display xanthochromia, especially on the palms and soles. Although proteinuria is usually not prominent and hematuria not frequent, anemia does occur early. Prominent hematuria usually signals a tumor of the urinary tract, an unusually frequent complication of the disorder (e.g., in 32% patients treated for the disease in Sofia, Bulgaria) (Puchlev, 1967). Pyuria is relatively infrequent, although urine cultures were positive in one-third of the patients. Progression of the disorder is accompanied by decreased creatinine clearance, metabolic acidosis, and electrolyte imbalance. Electrophoretic and gel immunodiffusion analyses of urinary proteins show the proteinuria to be a "mixed" type (Bruckner *et al.*, 1967).

Advanced Balkan nephropathy is marked by a bilateral reduction of the mass of the kidneys to about 40 g each (normal weight of an adult kidney is approximately 150 g). In about 35% of patients the renal parenchymal disease was found at autopsy to be accompanied by papilloma and carcinoma of the pelvis, ureter, and urinary bladder.

Histopathological studies (autopsy and biopsy) in the early stages reveal dystrophic and necrotic changes in the renal tubular epithelium, mainly in the loops of Henle (Puchlev, 1967). Thickening of the basement membrane and proliferation of the perivascular connective tissue are frequent. However, tubular and interstitial changes precede glomerular damage; even in patients with grossly sclerotic kidneys the glomeruli may appear normal. Apostolov *et al.* (1975), summarizing the histopathology of renal biopsies in seven patients, described glomerular mesangial and segmental thickening besides degenerative tubular changes.

The cause of Balkan nephropathy continues to be an enigma. An environmental cause is suggested by the fact that the disease is absent in family members who move from the endemic area early in life. It takes more than 10 years of residence in the endemic region for the early manifestations of the disorder to become prominent. Many possible causes of the disease have been listed, including infection by streptococci, leptospiras, and viruses, contamination with fertilizers or pesticides, heavy-metal poisoning, and an allergic or toxic reaction to fungus present in food.

Numerous cytoplasmic vesicles having coronavirus characteristics were found in the kidneys of persons with Balkan nephropathy (Apostolov *et al.*, 1975). This has led some investigators to suggest, that, because the disease almost exclusively affected subjects having close contacts with pigs and because pigs are carriers of coronavirus, Balkan nephropathy is due to a slow coronavirus infection. However, doubt was cast on a viral cause by Georgescu *et al.* (1977). They noted that the viruses identified from ticks, wild mice, and ground squirrels living in the endemic area did not share the electron microscope features of the viruslike particles detected in the kidneys of affected patients. The resemblance of many features of Balkan nephropathy to analgesic nephropathy encouraged the belief that the causative agent may be an undetected nephrotoxin. Investigation of the use of handling of fertilizers and pesticides in persons affected with Balkan nephropathy has provided no clues. Hypotheses linking heavy metals (lead and uranium) or trace elements (zinc and cadmium) with the disease also have not been substantiated.

Austwick (1975) described contamination of food with fungi, e.g., *Penicillium verrucosum* var. *cyclopium,* in the endemic areas. Interesting contributions to the possible cause of this fascinating disease were made by Barnes *et al.* (1977), who produced strikingly similar renal tubular lesions in rats force-fed with *P. verrucosum* and Elling and Krogh (1977), who produced fungal nephropathy in rats and pigs with fungal ochratoxin-A. However, a major discrepancy exists between the wide distribution of the fungus and the endemic pattern of the disease (Editorial, 1977). As a possibly preventive measure, avoiding ingestion of food contaminated with the fungus in the endemic area has been suggested.

At present the fascinating and challenging epidemiological and clinical problem of Balkan nephropathy remains unresolved.

B. Endemic Respiratory Illness in Bosnia (Yugoslavia)

The existence of high rates of cor pulmonale and of chronic nonspecific respiratory illness in the Yugoslavian rural mountainous areas of Bosnia has attracted epidemiological attention in recent years. Zarkovic (1973) surveyed 12,000 adults and 10,000 schoolchildren of Bosnia and Herzegovina, selecting those with respiratory or heart symptoms for medical examination. Although smoking habits were strongly influential in chronic respiratory illness, they were regarded as an insufficient explanation for the high prevalence rates of cor pulmonale and nonspecific disease in the rural, atmospherically unpolluted mountains. Occupational dust exposure and "farmer's lung" were similarly rejected as primary causative factors.

V. CONGENITAL DEFORMITIES

The incidence of certain congenital abnormalities in some of the East European countries is high (Table IV).

In Hungary nearly all deliveries take place in hospitals and the reporting of congenital malformations has been compulsory since 1962. Czeizel (1978) and his many collaborators have published extensively on the prevalence of congenital deformities in Hungary. Czeizel *et al.* (1972a) estimated the incidence of congenital heart defects in Budapest in 1963–1965 to be 7.06/1000 births. The most frequent type of heart defect was ventricular septal defect, with an incidence of 1.85/1000 births. Atrial septal defects accounted for 0.91/1000.

The incidence of congenital dislocation of the hip of 27.5/1000 in Budapest infants recorded between 1962 and 1967 is conspicuously high (Czeizel *et al.*, 1972b). The authors noted the occurrence of the defect was significantly higher in first births in infants of mothers above 40 years of age, and in those children of mothers living in good socioeconomic conditions. The latter may be correlated

TABLE IV

Congenital Anomalies[a] in Seven East European Countries

	Albania	Bulgaria	Czechoslovakia	German Democratic Republic	Hungary	Rumania	Yugoslavia
Congenital anomalies	5.8	9.0	6.6	11.1	11.4	9.7	5.7
Congenital anomalies of heart	2.5	4.1	2.3	4.0	4.9	4.6	2.5
Spina bifida	0.4	0.2	0.2	0.9	0.4	0.5	0.2

[a] Rates per 100,000.

with its greater incidence in infants of high birth weight. In the same population Czeizel and Tusnadi (1972) found the incidence of cleft lip with or without cleft palate and without other defects to be 1.03/1000 births, and the incidence of posterior cleft palate without other defects to be 0.27/1000 births. They found first-degree relatives had 47 times, second-degree 7 times, and third-degree 3 times the incidence of the malformation compared with that for the general population. Also consanguineous marriages occurred more frequently in the affected population.

VI. GENETIC DISEASES

Genetic studies in East European countries have been seriously hampered for many decades, first by the official doctrines of the fascist ideology and then by the restrictive teachings of Lysenkoism in the Soviet Union. For many years, the Soviet school of genetics opposed the theories of heredity accepted by most geneticists throughout the rest of the world. In East Europe genetic problems have been considered a highly political, and thus an extremely sensitive, matter. The consequence is a great paucity of reliable data on genetic diseases in this part of Europe. The first Department of Human Genetics in Poland was not established until 1963. Even in Czechoslovakia, the birthplace of Mendel, only since 1970 has genetics been officially restored to its position as a legitimate field of medical inquiry. However, acceptance of genetic causation of disease has been slow, and scientists have generally considered caution advisable. For example, a recent extensive article on the origin of family disorders in children published in a leading Czechoslovak pediatric journal failed to list genetic disorders among the causes, although physical or emotional instability of one or both the parents was considered (Dunovsky, 1978).

Investigations have begun to establish prevalence rates and to explore causative factors of several genetic disorders. For example, in an epidemiological survey in Czechoslovakia, 1292 members who gave birth to children with Down's syndrome during a 12-year period (1960–1971) were studied as to their health before and during gravidity (Cernay *et al.*, 1977). Compared with a control group, the study group had increased morbidity and more than three times the rate of complications during pregnancy. Although average age of the study group was greater than the controls (32.2 years versus 25.9 years), subgroups of study mothers and controls matched for age showed increased morbidity of mothers of children with Down's syndrome before and during pregnancy. Morbidity during pregnancy was striking—62.9% for the study subgroup but only 12.5% for the controls. Unfortunately, data were not provided for the specific diseases or difficulties.

A review of human genetics in Poland by Horst (1973) failed to list any new or unusual genetic diseases.

A relatively high frequency of the autosomal recessively inherited, alkaptonuria, has been reported in Slovakia of eastern Czechoslovakia (Srsen and Varga, 1978). This inborn error of phenylalanine and tyrosine metabolism due to a constitutional lack of homogentisic acid oxidase has been the object of comprehensive study for more than a decade. Preliminary data estimate a frequency of about 1/25,000.

Zitnan and Sitaj (1963) described a rare disease, articular chondrocalcinosis, characterized by multiple calcifications both of the joints and of the intervertebral disks. Until their report, only 32 cases of the disease had been described in the world medical literature. Of 27 patients they described, 21 were members of five different families residing in one locality in eastern Czechoslovakia, where most of the population was more or less akin. In each family investigated, the disorder occurred in only one parent (Valsik *et al.*, 1963). The disease was more common in daughters than in sons. The authors concluded that articular chondrocalcinosis was a genetic disorder, probably due to an autosomal dominant gene. The genetic investigation was hindered by the fact that the disease manifests itself only in the later adult life. Earliest clinical manifestations were described as occuring in the third decade of life. In the disease the ground substance of the cartilage is altered with deposits of mineral salts in the altered cartilage. The mineral incrustations in the cartilage (mainly carbonate apatite) lead to recurrent attacks of arthritis and to early polyarticular osteoarthrosis and spondylosis.

Reports on high incidence of gastric and duodenal ulcer in Poland (Modzelewski and Zazcek-Modelewska, 1978; Mazur, 1978) has raised the possibility of a hereditary disorder. Peptic ulcer is known to occur more frequently among siblings, in monozygotic twins, and in persons with the blood group O. However, a closer look at the blood groups in populations of different areas of Europe does not explain the high incidence of peptic ulcer in parts of Europe. Blood group O seems to be less prevalent in East Europe. The incidence of group B steadily increases from western Europe to Asia and from northern Europe to Africa, mostly at the expense of group O (Candela, 1942). This ''gene flow'' is considered the result of population migration, especially related to the invasion of Europe by Mongols, who have a high frequency of group B.

Other important aspects of genetics in this part of Europe include efforts to eliminate chemical and radiation pollutants thought to be genetically dangerous. Such efforts are consistent with attempts to ''improve the species'' through improvement of the physical and socioeconomic environment under the socialist system, where official belief is that some characteristics acquired through environmental influences are inherited. For example, an analysis of delivery records as a means of determining a possible effect of external environment on the genetic load of the population was conducted on parents who worked with chemical compounds. The frequency of congenital abnormalities in the children of chemical workers achieved statistical significance over that for the children of a control group, with talipes the most common anomaly, followed by morbus Down.

VII. COMMENT AND CONCLUSION

Theoretical and applied economics and politics influence all cultures. Each group survives, commingles, or perishes, depending on its responses to those and other influences. As science advances, with ostensible objectivity, data should accumulate on the importance of specific factors to individual and group consequences from simplistic cause and effect at the molecular level to complex combinations of factors leading to bizarre results. Foods ingested in early life; cultural patterns in homelife, work, and recreation; prescribed social activities; changes in environment resulting from industrialization, and the superimposition of inexplicable human attitudes all contribute to individual and group potential, development, survival, morbidity, and mortality.

As we, objective scientists, look at the information that accumulates or isolates individual cultures and whole groups, the evidence should become more apparent in a comparison of differences, one group to the other. Today's deficiency in bioculture diseases data from the East European countries should reduce in the coming years to allow for greater comparability with other-group data, whereby conditions, factors, and behavioral patterns that have been poorly studied or ignored become important clues to prevention or treatment of diseases in the future.

REFERENCES

Apateanu, V., Popovici, C., Ricman, T., Calarasu, E., and Dacu, M. (1971). The incidence of viral hepatitis and Australia antigen among personnel of transfusion centers. *Rev. Roum. Inframicrobiol.* **8**, 3–7.

Apostolov, K., Spasic, P., and Bojanic, M. (1975). Evidence of a viral etiology in endemic (Balkan) nephropathy. *Lancet* **ii**, 1271–1273.

Austwick, P. K. C. (1975). Balkan nephropathy. *Proc. R. Soc. Med.* **68**, 219–221.

Babaeva, E. N., Kalinkovsky, I. S., and Antykova, I. P. (1969). On helmintic fauna and prevalence of helmintic diseases among the population of the Leningrad region (in Russian). *Med. Parazitol. Parazit. Bolezni* **38**, 138–141.

Barnes, J. M., Carter, R. L., Peristianis, G. C., Austwick, P. K. C., Flynn, F. V., and Aldridge, W. M. (1977). Balkan (endemic) nephropathy and a toxin-producing strain of *Penicillium verrucosum* var. *cyclopium:* an experimental model in rats. *Lancet* **i**, 671–675.

Brodsky, R. E., Spencer, H. C., and Schultz, M. G. (1974). Giardiasis in American travelers to the Soviet Union. *J. Infect. Dis.* **130**, 319–323.

Bruckner, I., Stoica, G., and Serban, M. (1967). Studies on urinary proteins in endemic nephropathy. In "The Balkan Nephropathy" (G. E. W. Wolststenholme and J. Knight, eds.), pp. 84–99. Little, Brown, Boston, Massachusetts.

Buzina, R., Keys, A., Brodarec, A., Anderson, J. T., and Fidanza, F. (1966). Dietary surveys in rural Yugoslavia: Chemical analyses of diets in Dalmatia and Slavonia. Voeding **27**, 31–36.

Candela, P. B. (1942). The introduction of blood group B into Europe. Hum. Biol. **14**, 413–443.

Cernay, J., Bircak, J., and Hudakova, G. (1977). Diseases and abortions in mothers of children with Down's syndrome (in Slovak). Bratisl. Lek. Listy **68**, 559–567.

Cucuianu, M. (1973). Some aspects of the organization of medical research in Rumania. In "Medical Research Systems in Europe," Ciba Found. Symp., No. 21, p. 187. Elsevier Excerpta Med., Amsterdam.

Czeizel, A. (1978). The Hungarian congenital malformation monitoring system. Acta Paediatr. Acad. Sci. Hung. **10**, 225–230.

Czeizel, A., and Tusnadi, G. (1972). An epidemiological study of cleft lip with or without cleft palate and posterior cleft palate in Hungary. Hum. Hered. **21**, 17–38.

Czeizel, A., Kamaras, J., Balough, O., and Szentpeteri, J. (1972a). Incidence of congenital heart defects in Budapest. Acta Paediatr. Acad. Sci. Hung. **13**, 191–202.

Czeizel, A., Vizkelety, R., and Szentpeteri, J. (1972b). Congenital dislocation of the hip in Budapest, Hungary. Br. J. Prev. Soc. Med. **26**, 15–22.

Danilovic, V., and Stojimirovic, B. (1967). Endemic nephropathy in Kolubara, Serbia. In "The Balkan Nephropathy" (G. E. W. Wolstenholme and J. Knight, eds.), p. 44–50. Little, Brown, Boston, Massachusetts.

Demographic Yearbook (1977). 28th ed. United Nations, New York.

Djordjevic, B., Simic, B., Simic, A., Straser, T., Josipovic, V., Macarol, V., Klinc, L., and Nedeljkovic, S. (1965). Dietary studies in connection with epidemiology of heart disease: results in Serbia. Voeding **26**, 117–127.

Dunovsky, J. (1978). Family disorders and their diagnosis by a pediatrician (in Czech). Cesk. Pediatr. **33**, 352–364.

Dvorsky, A., Chorvathova, V., and Ovecka, M. (1970). "Status after Resection of Intestine and Their Nutritional Treatment with Special Reference to Fat Intake," Selected Papers. Inst. Hum. Nutr., Bratislava, Czechoslovakia.

Editorial (1977). Balkan nephropathy. Lancet **i**, 683–684.

Elling, F., and Krogh, P. (1977). Fungal toxins and Balkan (endemic) nephropathy (Letter). Lancet **i**, 1213.

Fischer-Galati, S. (1970). "Man, State, and Society in East European History." Prager, New York.

Gaon, J. A. (1967). Endemic nephropathy in Bosnia. In "The Balkan Nephropathy" (G. E. W. Wolstenholme and J. Knight, eds.), pp. 51–71. Little, Brown, Boston, Massachusetts.

Gaon, J. A. (1973). The role of drinking water in epidemics of infectious hepatitis in rural Yugoslavia. In "Uses of Epidemiology in Planning Health Services 1" (A. M. Davies, ed.), pp. 276–286. Savrem. Administracija, Belgrade.

Georgescu, L., Litvac, B., Diosi, P., Plavosin, L., and Herzog, G. (1977). Viruses in Balkan nephritis. Am. Heart J. **94**, 805–806.

Horst, A. (1973). Human genetics in Poland. Hum. Biol. **45**, 1–21.

Jaschke, G. (1968). Various conclusions from the recruit examination of 1964 to 1967 (in German). Z. Aerztl. Fortbild. **62**, 284–286.

Kajaba, I. (1969). Clinical-biochemical indices of the nutritional status of the population patterns of children and adults (in Slovak). Bratisl. Lek. Listy **51**, 17–26.

Kajaba, I. (1973). Selected parameters of the lipid metabolism in rural population of Slovakia (in Slovak). Bratisl. Lek. Listy **59**, 7–20.

Kajaba, I., Osancova, K., and Hejda, S. (1966). Comparison of selected parameters of the nutritional status of children from Bohemia and Slovakia (in Slovak). *Cesk. Gastroenterol. Vyz.* **20,** 498–504.

Kopcynski, J., and Mrozowa, E. (1978). Health Status of Warsaw journalists (in Polish). *Przegl. Epidemiol.* **32,** 36–380.

Laznicka, M., Sercl, J., and Samohyl, M. (1974). Incidence of myocardial infarction in a rural district (in Czech). *Cas. Lek. Ces.* **113,** 1359–1362.

Levinson, J. D., and Nastro, L. J. (1978). Giardiasis with total villous atrophy. *Gastroenterology* **74,** 271–275.

McKusick, V. A. (1978). ''Mendelian Inheritance in Man,'' 5th ed. Johns Hopkins Press, Baltimore, Maryland.

Makovicky, E. (1978). Scientific and technical surveillance of the population defined by the Warsaw pact (in Slovak). *Cesk. Zdrav.* **26,** 289–294.

Mazur, A. (1978). Gastric and duodenal ulcer in children and adolescents from rural areas (in Polish). *Pediatr. Pol.* **53,** 1211–1214.

Modzelewski, A., and Zaczek-Modelewska, T. (1978). Peptic ulcer among elderly rural population (in Polish). *Wiad. Lek.* **31,** 1043–1045.

Moroeanu, S. B. (1967). Epidemiological observations on the endemic nephropathy in Rumania. *In* ''The Balkan Nephropathy'' (G. E. W. Wolstenholme, and J. Knight, eds.), pp. 4–16. Little, Brown, Boston, Massachusetts.

Pazdziora, E. (1972). Epidemiological aspects of lambliasis in nursery schools (in Czech). *Cesk. Epidemiol., Mikrobiol., Imunol.* **21,** 271–276.

Puchlev, A. (1967). Endemic nephropathy in Bulgaria. *In* ''The Balkan Nephropathy'' (G. E. W. Wolstenholme and J. Knight, eds.), pp. 28–43. Little, Brown, Boston, Massachusetts.

Scheerer, S. (1973). Incidence of functional and neurotic disorders in rural ambulatory care (in German). *Z. Aerztl. Fortbild.* **67,** 235–237.

Simonson, E., and Berman, R. (1972). Myocardial infarction in young people. Experience in U.S.S.R. *Am. Heart J.* **84,** 814–822.

Sowa, J., and Mossor-Ostrowska, J. (1976). Incidence of viral hepatitis among health workers in the last decade (in Polish). *Pol. Tyg. Lek.* **31,** 1517–1519.

Srsen, S., and Varga, F. (1978). Screening for alkaptonuria in the newborn in Slovakia. *Lancet* **ii,** 576.

Statistical Yearbook (1976). 27th ed. United Nations, New York.

Taylor, A. J. P., ed. (1973–1974a). ''History of World War I.'' Phoebus, London.

Taylor, A. J. P., ed. (1973–1974b). ''History of World War II.'' Phoebus, London.

Tenyi, J., and Ozsvath, A. (1978). Epidemiology of neuroses in a rural areas (studies in a Hungarian village) (in German). *Z. Gesamte Hyg.* **24,** 360–363.

Truksova, B. (1976). Viral hepatitis in health workers (in Czech). *Cesk. Epidemiol., Mikrobiol., Immunol.* **25,** 105–112.

Valsik, J., Zitnan, D., and Sitaj, S. (1963). Chondrocalcinosis articularis. Section II: Genetic study. *Ann. Rheum. Dis.* **22,** 153–157.

Walzer, P. D., Wolfe, M. S., and Schultz, M. G. (1971). Giardiasis in travellers. *J. Infect. Dis.* **124,** 235–237.

Wolanski, N. (1975). The biological state of the Polish population: Somatic development and physical fitness. *Sante Publique (Bucur)* **18,** 341–352.

World Health Organization (1972–1973). ''World Health Statistics Annual.'' WHO, Geneva.

World Health Organization (1974). ''World Health Statistics Report,'' Vol. 27, No. 3/4. WHO, Geneva.

World Health Organization (1978). ''World Health Statistics, Quarterly Report.'' WHO, Geneva.

Wright, S. G., Tomkins, A. M., and Ridley, D. S. (1977). Giardiasis: clinical and therapeutic aspects. *Gut* **18**, 343–350.

Zaremba, V., and Zavazalova, H. (1979). Long term care of the elderly (in Czech). *Cesk. Zdrav.* **27**, 67–72.

Zarkovic, G. (1973). Etiology of non-specific chronic respiratory illness and cor pulmonale in Bosnia and Hercegovina. *In* "Uses of Epidemiology In Planning Health Services 2" (A. M. Davies, ed.), pp. 623–651. Savrem. Administracija, Belgrade.

Zitnan, D., and Sitaj, S. (1963). Chondrocalcinosis articularis. Section I: Clinical and radiological study. *Ann. Rheum. Dis.* **22**, 142–152.

15
Illness in Black Africans

ROBERT R. FRANKLIN, CLAUDE F. JACOBS,
AND WILLIAM E. BERTRAND

BIOCULTURAL ASPECTS OF DISEASE
Copyright © 1981 by Academic Press, Inc.
ISBN 0-12-598720-X

I. INTRODUCTION

To those who deal on a regular basis with the health problems of black Americans, it is of interest to focus on that part of the world that provided the genetic and cultural basis for this population. Although the linkage is far from direct, an understanding of the cultural and biological diversity of the people who make up sub-Saharan Africa can only aid a health professional in dealing with the problems of persons in the United States who spring from this rich heritage.

During the three and a half centuries in which the Atlantic slave trade was operative, an untold number of Africans reached the New World in a movement of people that has been called the most dramatic in recent history. Estimates of the number of blacks taken captive range from 12 million to 20 million or more. The identification of their place of origin in Africa has been an intriguing question. Although earlier researchers described the trade as having been limited to areas along the west coast of the continent and the region of the Congo (present day Zaire), it now appears that in the continual search for new sources of slaves, penetration was deeper into these sections than previously believed and included areas of southeast Africa as well.

The African continent can generally be thought of as composed of two different worlds, one north of the Sahara and other to its south. Stretching along the Mediterranean, north of the earth's largest desert, are modern nation states of the world of Islam. In what is sometimes referred to as the Maghreb, people are generally thought of as being Arabs or whites. The rest of the continent, sub-Saharan Africa, is alternately known as Black Africa. It is an immense area with a wide variety of terrains, climates, and peoples. In addition, an overlay of recently created nations has contributed increased complexity to a web of traditional cultures.

The division of the continent by the Sahara, however, has not prevented contacts between peoples on either side. This occurred historically in both western and eastern regions. A network of caravan trade routes connected the Mediterranean coast with the Niger River and Lake Chad. The Nile Valley linked Egypt and the Horn of Africa. Although there was a movement of goods and individuals along these corridors, the contacts did not create a common way of life but left two rather distinct areas of culture and types of people.

To understand either sub-Saharan Africa itself or its patterns of disease, one must consider three interacting forces: the region's environment, which is particularly harsh; the biology of its people, who are genotypically and phenotypically unique; and the way of life, which has been culturally traditional. Although patterns of health and illness in the region must be understood as outcomes of the interaction of all three of these factors, for the purposes of this analysis, environment, culture, and population biology will be discussed separately, followed by examples of the relationship that each has to the diseases that occur in this

area. Although this approach has limitations, it at once demonstrates the complexity of the situation while simplifying it for discussion along a discrete
number of approaches.

II. THE SUB-SAHARAN AFRICAN ENVIRONMENT

Africa is the most tropical of the world's continents, extending from 37°N to
35°S of the equator. Eighty percent of its surface is found within the tropical zone.
It comprises one-fifth of all the earth's land, being exceeded in size only by Asia
(Carlson, 1973; Murdock, 1959; de Blij, 1964).

The sub-Saharan African environment has been a major influence in determining the current health status of black Africans through several mechanisms.
Perhaps most important, the natural barriers to its penetration have significantly
influenced the history of the area, including its technological development.

Although the continent has 16,000 miles of coastline, maritime approaches to
it are difficult because there are sand bars and swift currents close to shore and
few natural ports. Topographically, the subcontinent consists of a massive block
containing a series of plateaus surrounded by narrow coastal plains and bordered
by the Sahara Desert on the north. Between and among the higher plateaus, there
are wide depressions such as the Zaire basin near the center of the continent and
Lake Chad in the north.

Two outstanding features break what Murdock (1959) characterizes as the
continent's surface monotony. In East Africa, there are continuously snowcap-
ped extinct volcanoes such as Mounts Elgon, Kenya, and Kilimanjaro, which
tower as high as 19,400 feet above sea level. Also in this region there are the rift
valleys, north–south fractures thousands of feet deep in the earth's surface.

Because of the sharp descent in elevation from the plateau to the sea, none of
the major rivers, such as the Zaire, Niger, and Zambesi, is navigable very far
inland from the ocean. All plunge over steep rapids or cataracts, the highest
being the Zambesi River's Victoria Falls, which is twice the height of Niagara
Falls. Such barriers meant that in the past the outside explorers who wanted to
penetrate the continent had to travel overland routes rather than utilize the major
waterways. This alternative resulted in their contending with deserts, dense
forests, and swamps (Fordham, 1972).

Moreover, there were severe obstacles to settlement. African disease patterns
frequently discouraged many Europeans and early colonizers experienced exceedingly high death rates (Hartwig and Patterson, 1978). One English attempt to
colonize Portuguese Guinea left 91 willing settlers ashore in 1792. Of these, 66
died from fever, probably malarial, in less than 18 months (Gourou, 1966).

In light of such obstacles to settlement, it is not difficult to understand why
European colonists favored less severe, more rewarding environments in the

Americas and Asia. This meant that most of sub-Saharan Africa did not come into contact with white man's diseases or with technological developments, including those influencing health care and disease prevention, until much later than other parts of the world.

Africa has a range of climates varying from extreme heat to polar, containing massive deserts as well as impenetrable swamps (Carlson, 1973). Typically, the African environment is described as containing tropical rain forest, savanna, steppe, and desert. Savanna is the most common type of environment on the continent and it is in these savanna zones that most Africans live (de Blij, 1964).

The critical factor in Africa's climate and in distinguishing one ecological zone from the other is rainfall. The intertropical weather front, or zone along the equator where the air masses of the northern and southern hemispheres meet, controls the climate of much of the continent. Because there is no range of mountains to control the pattern of movement of fronts, both the quantity and timing of yearly rains fluctuate considerably. An area that receives abundant rain one year may experience little precipitation during the next. Therefore, rather than average rainfall, the frequency and severity of the drought years determine the population density, types of vegetation, and agricultural production.

While some regions have a high annual precipitation, such as in parts of West Africa where rainfall reaches 400 inches per year, these comprise a relatively small sparsely populated part of the continent. More common are the regions with at least some water shortage. For example on the eastern plateaus, rainfall near the equator drops to 34 inches per year (de Blij, 1964). If North Africa is included, nearly three-fifths of the continent is arid to semi-arid and has to confront a lack of water at some point each year (Carlson, 1973). Since the dry land appears to be increasing in area, the problems that this sort of environment poses will become more significant in future years.

Throughout most of the continent, the pattern of rainfall in these tropical and semi-tropical climates has led to a leaching of soluble elements from the soil. The result is soil that is poor in mineral matter, phosphorus, and humus, and that is not very productive agriculturally. It has been estimated that whereas in the United States humus is 10–12% or more of soil volume in farming areas, in tropical soil it is 1.8% or less (Wilson, 1977). Even with the addition of manure, the benefit is reduced to a period of months instead of years, as would be the case in temperate areas.

The traditional cultural adaptation to these conditions has been to practice shifting cultivation combined in places with migratory life styles. Therefore, population densities are usually correspondingly low because of the poor food yield (Gourou, 1966).

The sub-Saharan environment also appears to be well suited for an extremely wide variety of infectious disease organisms. High temperatures, humidity, extensive surface water in many places all provide the necessary conditions for the development of complexes in which man, animals, insects, and microbes or larger parasites can interact closely (Gourou, 1966). The area's water and soil are often filled with disease-causing agents. In addition, both domestic and wild animals serve as hosts for disease as well as reservoirs of infection.

In traditional culture areas, the major diseases that are closely associated with the environment tend to be spread mainly by insect vectors. Whereas in modern settings, the environmental factors that lead to disease tend to be more frequently associated with the increased density of people in urban areas (Fordham, 1972).

Physical environmental influences such as these partly explain the basis for the current socioeconomic conditions present in sub-Saharan Africa. Table I summarizes World Bank basic indicators for the continent. The most striking overall observation is that 25 of 39 African nations are currently on the World Bank's list of low-income countries. These countries, which are the world's poorest, have less than $360.00 per capita income. No other area of the world has so high a proportion of its countries listed among the World Bank's (1980) low income countries.

While the rate of inflation is generally high, the indicator that best reflects the relationship between economic development and overall health status is the Physical Quality of Life Index (PQLI). This index combines infant mortality, literacy, and life expectancy at age one in a single measure which reflects overall quality of life (Morris, 1979). Sub-Saharan Africa stands out as the area of the world where conditions are the most substandard. All African countries have PQLI indices no higher than 55, with more than one-half having indices below 30 (developed world = 90). The relationship of Africa to the rest of the world is illustrated in Fig. 1, a map of the world comparing PQLI scores in different areas. One glance at the map quickly shows the difficulties that Africa faces. Twenty-five of the thirty-nine African nations fall in the lowest third of all nations on the PQLI index. Data such as these seem to indicate that the environment has had a major influence on the health of black Africans, which in turn acted as an obstacle to technological development.

III. CULTURES OF BLACK AFRICA

The population of Africa, numbering greater than 300 million people, supports a wide variety of cultures. However, within this diversity, there exists a degree of commonality in patterns, themes, and ways of life. This cultural unity has been labeled by Maquet (1972) as "Africanity" and is based on widespread similarities of social institutions, belief systems, and world views.

Several features are particularly significant in producing this unity. First, the relative isolation of the peoples of Black Africa has been reinforced by an environment resistent to penetration by outsiders.

TABLE I

Basic Indicators for Africa[a]

Area[b]	Population (millions) mid-1978	GNP per caput		Average annual rate of inflation (%)		Adult literacy rate (%) 1975c	Life expectancy at birth (years) 1978
		Dollars 1978	Average annual growth (%) 1960–1978	1960–1970a	1970–1978b		
Algeria	17.6	1260	2.3	2.3	13.4	37	56
Angola*	6.7	300	1.2	3.3	22.0	—	41
Benin*	3.3	230	0.4	1.9	7.4	11	46
Burundi*	4.5	140	2.2	2.8	10.1	25	45
Cameroon	8.1	460	2.9	3.7	9.8	—	46
CAR*	1.9	250	0.7	4.1	9.0	—	46
Chad*	4.3	140	−1.0	4.6	7.4	15	43
Congo	1.5	540	1.0	5.4	10.6	50	46
Egypt	39.9	390	3.3	2.7	7.0	44	54
Ethiopia*	31.0	120	1.5	2.1	4.0	10	39
Ghana	11.0	390	−0.5	7.6	35.9	30	48
Guinea*	5.1	210	0.6	1.7	6.4	—	43
Ivory Coast	7.8	840	2.5	2.8	13.9	20	46
Kenya*	14.7	330	2.2	1.5	12.0	40	53
Lesotho*	1.3	280	5.9	2.5	11.2	55	50
Liberia	1.7	460	2.0	−1.9	9.7	30	48

Libya†	2.7	6910	6.2	5.2	20.7	50	55
Madagascar*	8.3	250	-0.3	3.2	9.6	50	46
Mali*	6.3	120	1.0	5.0	7.8	10	42
Malawi*	5.7	180	2.9	2.4	9.1	25	46
Mauritania*	1.5	270	3.6	1.6	10.4	17	42
Morocco	18.9	670	2.5	2.0	7.1	28	55
Mozambique*	9.9	140	0.4	2.8	10.9	—	46
Niger*	5.0	220	-1.4	2.1	10.7	8	42
Nigeria	80.6	560	3.6	2.6	18.2	—	48
Rwanda*	4.5	180	1.4	13.1	14.7	23	46
Senegal*	5.4	340	-0.4	1.7	8.0	10	42
Sierra Leone*	3.3	210	0.5	2.9	10.8	15	46
Somalia*	3.7	130	-0.5	4.5	10.7	60	43
South Africa	27.7	1480	2.5	3.0	11.7	—	60
Sudan*	17.4	320	0.1	3.7	7.4	20	46
Tanzania*	16.9	230	2.7	1.8	12.3	66	51
Togo*	2.4	320	5.0	1.7	7.4	18	46
Tunisia	6.0	950	4.8	3.7	7.1	55	57
Uganda*	12.4	280	0.7	3.0	27.3	—	53
Upper Volta*	5.6	160	1.3	1.3	9.6	5	42
Zaire*	26.8	210	1.1	29.9	26.2	15	46
Zambia	5.3	480	1.2	7.6	5.7	39	48
Zimbabwe	6.9	480	1.2	1.3	7.6	—	54

[a] From World Bank (1980) (World Bank, Oxford University Press, New York, 1980).
[b] (*) Low-income countries—per caput GNP 360 or less in 1978; (†) capital surplus oil exporter.

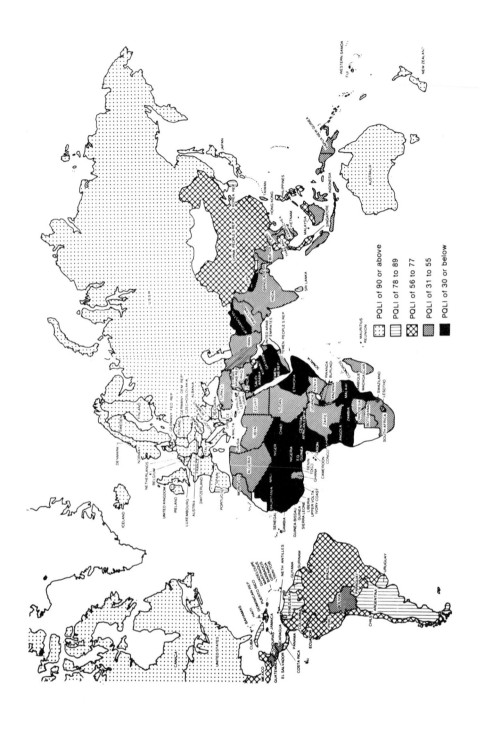

PQLI of 90 or above

PQLI of 78 to 89

PQLI of 56 to 77

PQLI of 31 to 55

PQLI of 30 or below

Second, the environment within which Africans have lived and worked has been relatively hostile. The habitats have proved basically unfavorable to agriculture, hunting, and animal domestication (Maquet, 1972). At the same time, the environment has posed severe health problems for humans in terms of endemic tropical illnesses that lower the capacity to work.

Third, Africans have experienced a significant amount of "moving about" or migration. As Maquet stated, almost every African population is from elsewhere. The Bantu expansion and southward migration of the Cushites perhaps present the best examples of this sort of pattern (Murdock, 1959).

Fourth, kinship is important everywhere on the continent. It not only gives the individual a setting in which he is socialized, but determines his behavior toward others in later life as well. It also provides solidarity and security. Maquet (1972) stated that ancestor cults merely reflect ritually what the individual knows: he is a member of a certain descent group and everything has come to him through this chain of ancestors.

Fifth, religion and ritual rites of passage orient the individual to the gods, to the invisible world, and to the life of the group. Surgical circumcision for boys and excision for girls have been steps to adulthood. Maquet (1972) noted that Africans do not want improvisation, but rather the production of personality types that will not bring tension to the group. Therefore, ceremonies and ritual events become key elements in the process of socialization.

However, there is also a wide variety of cultures. The extent of diversity among African cultures is perhaps best illustrated by examining the data of linguists who have worked in the area. Greenberg (1966) classified 730 native languages and acknowledges that the actual number may be more than 800. Another reported estimate of active indigenous languages places the figure at 1500 (Owusu, 1978). To assist in this discussion, the hundreds of languages may be classified into four major language groups: Niger-Congo, Khoisan, Nilo-Saharan, and Afro-Asiatic.

Niger-Congo is both the largest language group and the one containing the languages spoken over the greatest geographical area of the continent. These languages are spoken by peoples living along the Guinea coast, throughout Central Africa, and along both coasts from the mid-region to the south. It has six main branches, the best known being the Benue-Congo branch, which includes the Bantu languages. The Khoisan, or "click" languages are spoken in Southwest Africa among the San and Khoi-Khoi. The Nilo-Saharan languages are found from the Central Sudan to the Great Lakes region. This group includes among its branches the Nilotic languages and Songhai. The Afro-Asiatic languages are spoken along the northern boundary of black Africa and in the region of the horn. There are two main branches of this group: Chad, which includes Hausa, spoken in northern Nigeria, and the Cushitic languages of northeast Africa.

In the face of this multilingualism, *linguae francae* have developed. Throughout eastern and central Africa where present day Tanzania, Kenya, Uganda, Mozambique, and parts of Zaire are located, Swahili has come to fill this role. Other languages used in this fashion include Hausa in West Africa, northern Nigeria, Niger, and Ghana; Bemba in central Africa; and Lingala and Kongo in and around Zaire.

The similarities that are seen in African cultures are partly related to basic patterns of subsistence. Bohannan and Curtin (1971) suggested that more than any other factor, these patterns correlate with cultural activities such as work habits of men and women, diet, trade, and size and composition of social groups. Four major subsistence areas can be identified and classified by source of staple food product: the root area, banana area, grain area, and herding area.

Roots form the staple in an area along the Guinea coast that continues across central Africa in a broad belt in the region of the Congo basin. Bananas are the major dietary item of central Africa in a narrow band that crosses the continent, transecting the region where roots are a staple. The grain area is found primarily in East Africa along the coast south of the horn and extends toward central Africa below the root production area.

Herding is the primary mode of subsistence in the southeast and along the northern border of Black Africa. Although the principal domestic herd animals are cattle, goats are frequently found on the Serengeti plain, as are camels in the north. Both milk and blood are items used in the diet in these areas.

Descriptions written by the earliest travelers to the continent utilized the idea of "tribes" as mutually exclusive groups to form categories of people. The fluid nature of these units was not recognized. Bohannan and Curtin (1971) pointed out that the term tribe has come to be used in several different ways: to define social groups living in units comparable to city states; to discuss empires with large numbers of inhabitants living on significant amounts of territory; to distinguish language groups; and to facilitate administrative problems by forming indiscriminate classifications of people. Several analyses of tribal groups have developed. Murdock's (1959) "Africa: Its People and Their Culture History" contains tribal maps of the continent that are considered by many to be the best reference.

There was considerable confusion during the 1950s and 1960s over the use of the terms tribe and ethnic group among students of African culture. Some researchers used tribe to refer to social groups in a rural setting, but used ethnic group to refer to residents of urban settings. Among these writers, tribalism came to refer to traditional social organization, but persistence of loyalties and values was seen as ethnicity (Du Toit, 1978). The process of possible detribalization in urban areas and the emergence of urban groups based on social class, labor unions, or other voluntary associations is seen as an important focus in contemporary social settings (Little, 1957). As Du Toit stated, the fluidity of boundaries among groups of people was beginning to be recognized in terms of its social, biological, and interactional implications.

The classification of the cultures of Africa has been a particularly complex problem. Seligman (1966), in "Races of Africa" divides the continent's people into Bushmen, Hottentots and Nigritos, the true Negro, Hamites, half-Hamites, and Bantu. The classification became familiar to many students of Africa, but the system was criticized for constantly shifting from race to language to culture as the basis for making its distinctions.

Herskovits (1962) proposed a classification of traditional African cultures based on the concept of "culture area," without regard to the semi-independent factors of physical type and language. He argued that it is a way of accounting for all aspects of culture as well as ecology while not being restricted to relying on arbitrarily selected single features such as kinship patterns.

Herskovits proposed three areas composed of cultures whose economics are based on food gathering and herding, i.e., the Khoisan area, the East Africa cattle area, and the Eastern Sudan, and three areas composed of cultures based on agriculture, i.e., the Congo, the Guinea Coast, and the Western Sudan. These areas are outlined on the map of Africa in Fig. 2.

A. The Khoisan Area

The Khoisan area is inhabited primarily by the San (Bushmen) and descendents of the Khoi-Khoi (Hottentots). They differ from other Africans principally by their culture, and the extent of their absorption by neighbors (Wilson, 1977). Mixing of these indigenous people either with Africans of Bantu origin or with Europeans has been extensive. The Khoi-Khoi especially have come to constitute a major part of the detribalized population known as the Cape Colored in the Union of South Africa. The groups of Khoi-Khoi involved in this mixture include the Grigriqua, Attaqua, and Kora.

In their traditional cultural settings, these groups have presented classic examples of basic subsistence patterns: the San as hunters and gatherers, and the Khoi-Khoi as herders. The social structure is fairly simple. Marriage is monogamous, descent is bilateral, and there is a system of clans. There is no political superstructure; decisions are made within the individual groups by the elders (Herskovits, 1962).

Ethnographic descriptions of the Nama indicate that the Khoi-Khoi had a slightly more secure subsistence pattern with cattle raising as the typical occupation along with the collection of vegetable food from wild plants. This resulted in seasonal migrations to find adequate pasture and water. The relative security allowed the development of a more complex social structure than that of the San. The traditional Khoi-Khoi tribal organization was headed by chiefs. Descent was patrilineal and organized the group into essentially independent exogamous clans

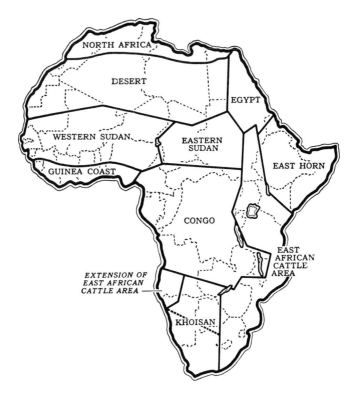

Fig. 2.   Culture Areas of Africa. (Drawn by William A. Norman, Herskovits, Alfred A. Knopf, Inc., 1962.)

that, during disputes, could separate themselves from the tribe with which they were originally affiliated (Herskovits, 1962).

B. The East African Cattle Area

The East African cattle area stretches along the east coast from the extreme south to the Great Lakes region and beyond. It also includes a small region of southwestern Angola. The most characteristic feature of the area is the cattle complex, which combines elements of social structure, economics, politics, and ritual. For example, the use of cattle as bride-wealth has been described extensively.

Social structure is based on patrilineal descent groups. Marriage is polygynous and residence is patrilocal. The outstanding feature is the system of age-grading to form age-groups. This form of organization cuts across kin groups to erect hierarchies based on residence and age. Because age is considered to be equal to wisdom, as these age-groups move through time they assume more power. There is little specialization of labor, except that which takes place along sex lines and that of iron workers. Without a system of money or markets, the distribution of goods is largely a process of exchange within the extended family. The political structures of the area have varied with those groups in the south, such as the Zulu and Ngwato, characterized as exhibiting a state form of organization and those in the north, such as the Logoli and Nuer, as stateless (Fortes and Evans-Pritchard, 1940).

C. The Eastern Sudan

The Eastern Sudan reaches from the Nile to Lake Chad in the area west of the northern part of the East African cattle area. Including both savanna and desert it covers parts of Sudan, Chad, the northern part of the Central African Republic, and northern Nigeria. The Eastern Sudan includes agriculturalists and herders similar to its neighbors, but these patterns are not as well developed.

Moving from east to west, the importance of cattle is replaced to some extent by camels among tribes in the northern Wadai. In certain areas in the west, among the Beni Helba and the Habbania, the horse is put to considerable use. Around Lake Chad, cattle assume exchange rather than prestige value (Murdock, 1959).

Descent is largely unilateral with persons having rights and obligations within the families of both parents, regardless of the side from which lineage is reckoned. The area is characterized by political, ethnic, and linguistic fragmentation. Markets are generally absent except in the western part of the area. Islam plays an important role, although numerous spirit cults such as those of the Nuer make up the religious life of the area (Herskovits, 1962).

D. The Congo

The Congo area embraces the heart of Africa and includes peoples of Angola, Zaire, south Cameroon, and the southern strip of the Sudanese Republic and the Central African Republic (Herskovits, 1962). Agriculture dominates the region and there is an absence of herding animals. Hunting and fishing, however, are significant activities. Based on the exchange of goods, a symbiotic relationship exists between Pygmies and other people in the area.

Descent is largely matrilineal and residence matrilocal in the south, whereas patterns are patrilineal and patrilocal in the north. Although the extended family is everywhere, clans are not generally present. Political groups in the area have included stable kingdoms in the past that covered large areas such as the Kongo and Lunda empires, tribal states as among the Bemba and Kuba, and groups where control is in the hands of kin groups and there is minimal formal organization as in the case of the Makonde and Mwera (Murdock, 1959).

E. The Guinea Coast

The Guinea Coast follows the line of the West African littoral from the Bight of Biafra to the southern portion of the Republic of Guinea. It is essentially a long and narrow forested belt (Herskovits, 1962). Within the area, population is dense and subsistence is agriculturally based. There is a significant degree of work specialization, institutional complexity, and trade in markets, especially in the geographical center of the region stretching from Ghana to western Nigeria.

Descent is usually partilineal and residence is patrilocal, although matrilineal groups are found occasionally in the western section. Polygyny is common and depends on a man's economic position. Some age-groups exist but not to the same extent as in East Africa. Numerous secret societies, religious cults, and cooperative groups are found in this area. Among the best known groups of people in this area are the Twi, Kru, Ibo, and Yoruba (Murdock, 1959).

F. The Western Sudan

The Western Sudan stretches roughly from the forested belt along the coast to the desert. It includes most of what was formerly French West Africa except the southern Ivory Coast, Togo, and Dahomey (Herskovits, 1962). The area varies considerably, but in many respects it resembles the Guinea Coast in terms of population and institutional complexity, although it has larger domesticated animals. Within the region, there are agriculturalists and herders such as the Gurunsi, agriculturalists and traders such as the Mande-Diula, and pastoralists such as the Fulbe (Murdock, 1959).

In terms of social organization, it is largely patrilineal with patrilocal residence. Polygyny is common. The nuclear family is central and clans are not prominent. The village units are clearly linked to kin groups without a significant sense of larger political entities. Voluntary associations, cooperative societies, and craft guilds are important. Religious patterns are a mixture of traditional beliefs and adopted Islamic ideas and rituals.

IV. THE BIOLOGICAL UNIQUENESS OF BLACK AFRICANS

Any discussion of the biological diversity of *Homo sapiens* in Africa must acknowledge the biological history of the species on the continent as well. It is here that the oldest skeletal remains of man's ancestors have been found in an evolutionary sequence of physical types and cultures that suggests that

Africa is the "cradle of mankind" (Murdock, 1959). Current archaeological evidence points to the savannas in the north and southeast as possible places for the species' origin, with subsequent movement into the immense forested areas of the continent.

The environment has been a major influence on the biological diversity of the sub-Saharan African. The geographical barriers discussed earlier have prevented any large-scale penetration of the subcontinent and have limited gene flow into the area to very modest amounts, mostly from the Arabs or North Africans. These barriers, however, have not prevented internal migrations and expansions, which have occurred since the earliest times. These population movements have resulted in modifications of gene frequencies through genetic drift, interbreeding between isolated groups, and a limited introduction of new traits. In addition, the wide variety of environments within the subcontinent has produced selective forces for certain physical characteristics. This combination of factors produced what Alland (1973) describes as a land characterized by a wide variety of people linguistically, ethnically, and genetically.

The diversity of physical characteristics among the sub-Saharan populations is extreme and can be illustrated with the following examples. In terms of population means, the tallest and shortest peoples in the world are found in Africa, as are those with the thickest and thinnest lips. Variations in mean nose width and head diameter include 92 and 80% of the world range, respectively. Serologically, the frequency of alleles that define hemoglobin S and C vary from zero to the highest in the world and the variation in alleles of the Rh blood group system covers 24–84% of the world range (Hiernaux, 1975).

Other genetic markers point to further distinctions among groups of Africans, and between Africans and peoples of other parts of the world; several will be discussed here. Frequencies of the ABO blood groups vary greatly; some phenotypes are nonexistent or exhibit low frequencies. Phenotype A is present in a lower frequency than in Europe, its highest frequency being in southwest Africa. The frequency of phenotype B is similar to the distribution of phenotype A in Europeans. Phenotype O is high throughout Africa (Mourant et al., 1976). In the MNS system, alleles M and N appear in about equal frequency but the S allele is relatively rare (Tobias, 1966; Mourant et al., 1976). Rh_0 is characteristic of all of Black Africa with frequencies reaching 100% among some groups of the San. High frequencies are also found among the Khoi-Khoi, Hadza, Nuer, Dinka, and Pygmies. The lowest frequencies occur in West Africa (Mourant et al., 1976).

The Henshaw antigen is present in all tested populations, with the Khoisan having the highest frequencies. The Kell-Cellano antigen occurs in low percentages in most groups, but again its highest rates appear among the Khoisan. The Diego antigen has not been reported in Africa whereas the Lutheran antigen has been reported only in low frequencies and appears to be absent among the

Khoisan. In the Duffy system, the phenotype Fy (a-b), which is very rare in Europeans, is prevalent in most parts of Africa (Ssebabi, 1975). However, Tobias (1966) reports that the presence of the Duffy antigen does rise to moderate rates among the Khoisan.

Haptoglobins among Africans offer a contrast to much of the world's populations. Most Africans have a higher rate of the gene Hp^1 than Hp^2. Hp^1 reaches its highest frequencies among the Yorubas of Nigeria in West Africa, and low frequencies of Hp^1 characterize the Pygmies and San, a characteristic shared by hunting and herding groups in other parts of the world such as the Alaskan Eskimos, Swedish Lapps, and Australian Aborigines. Equal frequencies of Hp^1 and Hp^2 are seen among the Zulu, Xhosa, Ibo, and Khoisan. Ahaptoglobinemia appears with high frequency in Africa (Tobias, 1966).

Glucose-6-phosphate dehydrogenase (G6PD) deficiency occurs in low frequencies among the southern Bantu, San, and Pygmies. Color blindness ranges from 1.7 to 2.7% among eastern Bantu, and 2.8 to 4.6% in the southern Bantu, and affects 2.7% of the San (Tobias, 1966).

In total, about 1000 biologically distinct populations have been identified in sub-Saharan Africa. Complete quantitative physical anthropological data, however, have been assembled for only a few (Hiernaux, 1975). Numerous classification schemes that combine local groups into larger units have been proposed but none has been found completely satisfactory.

Murdock (1959) emphasizes that racial factors are not considered relevant in explanations of cultural variations in Africa and acknowledges that the value of using anthropometric and somatological criteria for making such distinctions is highly questionable. In spite of these limitations he maintains that divisions produced in this fashion can be useful for historical reconstructions in archaeology and ethnology. Therefore, in a section of his work specifically devoted to the topic, he discusses the continent's population in terms of five races: Bushmanoid, Caucasoid, Mongoloid, Negroid, and Pygmoid. Descriptions in terms of stature, skin color, lips, and head, nose, and hair forms are used as bases for differentiations among these groups.

Alland's (1973) comparison of the classification schemes of Coon (1965) and Montagu (1960) demonstrates two distinct approaches to the subject. He points out that whereas Coon's research emphasizes the uniformity in the populations of Black Africa based on divisions that are purely biological, Montagu's work splits them into a number of subpopulations based on a mixture of biological and cultural traits. The outcome of these positions is that Coon considers his divisions as biologically real and believes that they should be labeled as ''races.'' On the other hand, the biological diversity that Montagu illustrates does not lead him to make absolute divisions among groups above the population level.

Much of Hiernaux's recent research has consisted of attempts to use matrix analysis of genetic diversity combined with environmental and historical data to derive clusters that would establish groups between the levels of population and species. He maintains, however, that his results throw considerable doubt on the concept of race as a classificatory device and indicate that such groupings work only minimally. According to Alland (1973), Hiernaux's research clearly illustrates that genetic variation appears to fall into a series of continuums on which the different traits are differentially distributed; therefore, no single ordering of the data is possible.

From the biological diversity in Africa, Hiernaux (1975) believes that a number of relatively independent homogeneous population sets have evolved over a long period. One line of evolution led to the Khoisan; another or several lines produced the present-day populations of western and central Africa as well as the Bantu expansionists; one or more lines gave rise to the various physically elongated, narrow-headed populations of East and West Africa. Using biological data modified by cultural and linguistic factors, he classifies sub-Saharan African populations into these basic groups for constructing biological histories: Khoisan people, Pygmies and Pygmoids, elongated Africans and Nilotes, people of the Western Sudan and the Guinea Rain Forest, and Bantus (Hiernaux, 1975).

A. Khoisan Peoples

The term Khoisan, originally a linguistic one, is used, however, to refer to two populations, the San and the Khoi-Khoi, which together are biologically distinct from other sub-Saharan populations.

Physically the Khoisan have small stature that is thought to be of selective advantage for the muscle leverage needed for archery. The women demonstrate steatopygia, a protruding accumulation of fat on thighs and buttocks, a condition that has a skeletal basis in lordosis, which is present in both sexes. The Khoisan are also found to have macronymphia (*tablier*, Hottentot apron), an elongation of the labia minora in the women, which is apparently of genetic origin, and the condition of permanently semi-erect penis in the males. Eye folds with palpebral fissures (slitlike lids) give an Asian appearance to the face. The skin color is yellow-brown and the hair is peppercorn or tufted, representing the extreme form of African hair. There is also a very high frequency of the R_0 allele and a low r in the Rh system of blood groups (Hiernaux, 1975).

B. Pygmies and Pygmoids

The Mbuti Pygmies live as seminomadic hunter–gatherers in the Ituri Forest in northeastern Zaire. Their most marked characteristic is diminished stature, probably of genetic origin, averaging 137 cm in women and 144 cm in men. The height is believed to be an adaptation to life in the equatorial forest. Other physical characteristics include a large head relative to body size, a broad nose and wide mouth, and marked subnasal prognathism. The Pygmies also have relatively light-colored skin and excessive pilosity (hairiness).

For a number of genetic blood traits, the Pygmies represent the far "ultra-African" spectrum, distinct from European and Arab values. These traits imply a long history of genetic isolation from other sub-Saharan African groups (Hiernaux, 1975).

The Pygmoids inhabit areas of the equatorial rain forest extending from Uganda and Burundi to Gabon and the Cameroons. They live as hunter–gatherers in association with Bantu agriculturalists. Physically, all Pygmoids have a mean stature between 150 and 160 cm, which is between that of the Pygmies and their agriculturalist neighbors. One of the best known Pygmoid groups is the Twa.

C. Elongated Africans and Nilotes

Most Elongated Africans and Nilotes live as pastoralists and nomads in a geographic area that transects the continent extending from Kenya and Ethiopia in the east to Mauritania in the northwest. They have an elongated body build with narrow heads, faces and noses, dark skin, and spiraled hair. The features apparently represent a genetic adaptation to the dry air of the semi-arid crescent at the northeastern limit of sub-Saharan Africa. Well-known groups include the Masai, Ful, Tutsi, and Hima. The Nilotes represent the extreme of this group, having narrow heads with wider, lower noses, and being taller and more slender than the other groups (Hiernaux, 1975).

D. Inhabitants of Western Sudan and the Guinea Rain Forest

Little is known about the pre-Neolithic inhabitants of this area. Climatic change and large-scale trade undoubtedly have modified this group biologically, but there are few pre-Neolithic fossil records in existence to demonstrate the extent of change. One probable modification was gracilization, or the "fining down" of the skeleton resulting from changes in living conditions associated with the evolution of hunter–gatherers to agriculturalists. The population groups in this area display a great deal of biological variation, much of which is associated with their physical environment. Examples of ethnic groups living in this area include the Dogon in Mali, the Ibo and Yoruba of Nigeria, and the Ashanti of Ghana (Hiernaux, 1975).

E. Bantu

"Bantu" is originally a linguistic designation indicating a secondary branch of Niger-Congo in the classification of African languages. The speakers of Bantu languages migrated east and south from an area in what is now Nigeria to cover the great majority of the continent south of a line from Cameroon to Somalia. The expansion began about 2000 years ago and was rapid. It was assisted by an iron technology and an agricultural system that were superior to the Late Stone Age technology and food-gathering techniques then present in the region.

Although linked by similarities in language, the current Bantu peoples are morphologically diverse. They have been strongly influenced both by genetic interbreeding with other groups and by selective forces in the wide variety of environments encountered in the areas in which they settled. The groups most morphologically similar are the Basa, Ewando, and northern Fong of Cameroon, the Birra and Luba of northeastern and southeastern Zaire, respectively, and the Nyomwezi of western Tanzania. These groups are probably slightly modified descendents of the original nuclear Bantu.

Within and between these groups, anthropologists have begun a search for clines as evidence of gene flow or differential selection in cases where environmental gradients can be demonstrated. According to Hiernaux (1977), a number of anthropometric characteristics presents a cline of values associated with a climatic scale from the arid zone to the equatorial forest of the continent. Higher stature with relatively longer legs, narrower head, face, and nose, narrower shoulders and wider hips are associated with higher levels of heat and dryness. A shorter stature and a relatively broader nose, face, and head are associated with a moister climate with lower levels of heat and dryness. Similar clines within groups have been described in a manner suggested by Cavalli-Sforza (1977) to explain morphological and genetic differences between western and eastern Pygmies.

The significance of these differences in terms of population adaptation remains open to discussion. Although the function and spread of the adaptive polymorphism HbS have been demonstrated by Livingstone (1958), similar explanations for polygenetic traits that are thought to have some adaptive value, such as skin color, stature, and hair texture, are less certain and remain open to question (Alland, 1973).

V. DISEASES ASSOCIATED WITH THE ENVIRONMENT

The sub-Saharan African environment supports an extremely wide variety of diseases that are noted for their high prevalence and incidence, and are frequently dependent on the environment for one or more steps in their transmission cycles. Infectious diseases, followed by nutritional disorders, are the most important of these in terms of impact on human population through mortality (World Health Organization, 1977, 1979). Most of the major infectious diseases can be grouped according to the public health measures necessary to control them: arthropod control, sewerage and water treatment, immunization programs, and others. Although it is not possible to discuss all of the diseases, examples from each group will be examined in detail to demonstrate their impact on the health of black Africans and the problems that arise in attempting to control them. Nutritional disorders, because of their close association with cultural practices, will be discussed later.

A. Arthropod Control

Arthropod-borne diseases probably have had the greatest influence of any group of diseases in sub-Saharan Africa and much of this impact has been due to malaria. Malaria is present in all areas of sub-Saharan Africa, except for parts of the southernmost states, and is probably the major health problem in many states (Young, 1976). The highest mortality rates due to the disease tend to occur in the youngest age-groups, usually ages 7 months to 5 years (Morley, 1973). Morbidity due to malaria, however, can occur in all age-groups and can vary from mildly symptomatic states with slight fever and chills to convulsions and coma (Young, 1976).

Proof of the centuries of influence that malaria has had on sub-Saharan populations is seen in the high prevalence of the sickle hemoglobin gene. Despite the high rates of mortality and morbidity associated with the homozygous expression of the gene (sickle cell disease), the gene has become widespread because of the protective properties provided against malaria by the heterozygote state (Livingston, 1967). Other aspects of the association between malaria and sickle hemoglobin will be discussed later in this chapter.

Unfortunately, attempts to eradicate malaria in Africa have produced less spectacular results than were originally envisioned (Basch, 1978). Efforts at eradication have now been generally abandoned in favor of attempts to control the disease. Some technological developments have actually led to increases in malaria prevalence. Irrigation programs have increased mosquito breeding grounds, and spraying with insecticides have produced resistant strains of the mosquito (Hughes and Hunter, 1970).

Trypanosomiasis is more prevalent in Africa than in any other continent. The African form of the disease (sleeping sickness) is endemic in various foci throughout the entire geographic area bounded by 15°N and 20°S (Hawking, 1976). The distribution of the disease depends on the availability of a suitable habitat for its vector, the tsetse fly. In western and central Africa where the vectors are the riverine flies *G. palpalis* and *G. tachinoides,* the disease is confined to peoples dependent on rivers and streams for washing, drinking, and fishing. In East Africa where the vectors are the woodland flies *G. palidipes* and *G. morsitans,* the persons affected live in game-inhabited dry savannas and woodlands (Cahill, 1975; Benenson, 1975).

Trypanosomiasis has had a much greater impact on sub-Saharan African populations than just its effect on human morbidity and mortality. The disease also can attack cattle and other domestic animals, resulting in the nonuse of large domestic animals for food, labor, or transportation in most parts of sub-Saharan Africa (Gourou, 1966; Basch, 1978). The total impact of this loss must be immense. For example, the lack of these animals can be linked to malnutrition. Kwashiorkor exists in many areas because of a lack of protein that might have been provided in part by beef and milk products (Basch, 1978). Other forms of protein energy malnutrition abound because of the shortage of foods produced through laborious and nonproductive hand agricultural methods that do not utilize animal labor.

Unfortunately, the necessary means to control trypanosomiasis are still too elaborate and technical for much of Africa. The control methods consist primarily of destruction of the tsetse fly population and early diagnosis and treatment of human and animal cases (Benenson, 1975). The infrastructure needed to carry out these actions on a continuing basis frequently does not exist. Although chemoprophylactic agents of varying effectiveness do exist, their use has not been well received by the local populations (Hawking, 1976). Therefore, trypanosomiasis will probably remain a major problem in Africa until economic and technological development has reached a level where control of the disease becomes feasible.

A large number of other arthropod-borne diseases are found in sub-Saharan Africa. Examples include: viral diseases including the hemorrhagic fevers such as yellow fever, and viral fevers such as West Nile Virus, Bwamba, and Bunyamwera; filarial diseases such as onchocerchiasis; bacterial diseases such as silvatic plague and tick-borne relapsing fever; and diseases resulting from human infestation of insects such as scabies and pediculosis (Benenson, 1975). These diseases, have had a major impact on development in Black Africa.

B. Sewerage and Water Treatment

Another group of important infectious diseases is composed of those that primarily infect the gastrointestinal tract. Almost all of these are transmitted by the dissemination of fecal material containing the responsible microorganisms. Frequently it is food, water, and milk that are contaminated. The diseases, therefore, are spread through populations usually by means of a fecal–oral cycle that may necessitate or permit intermediate vectors and hosts. The microorganisms must be swallowed and infect the bowel of one person, thus making his feces a source of contamination for others. Some diseases have a closely related life cycle in which the microorganisms instead of being swallowed, enter the body by penetrating the skin of susceptible persons. The mature worms eventually lodge in the lumen or wall of the bowel.

The types of microorganisms that can cause clinical disease through the oral–

fecal route are varied. They include bacteria which cause typhoid and paratyphoid fevers, cholera, bacillary dysentery (shigellosis), food poisoning, and milder diarrheas; viruses now recognized for their role in severe diarrheas of infancy and childhood and for other specific disease entities such as hepatitis A and poliomyelitis; and larger parasites varying from protozoa that can cause amebiasis and giardiasis to well-adapted and highly prevalent intestinal helminths such as *Ascaris* (roundworm) and *Trichuris* (whipworm) and *Ancylostoma* or *Necator* (hookworm). In all cases, control of these diseases depends on interrupting the oral–fecal or skin–fecal cycles. Control measures include proper sewage disposal, water treatment, pasteurization and proper storage of milk, appropriate food handling and storage procedures, personal hygiene and cleanliness, prevention of the use of contaminated bodies of water for swimming and wading, and control of flies and other potential mechanical vectors (Burnet and White, 1972).

Because of the degree of economic development and health education needed to control these diseases, such procedures have not been easily introduced throughout sub-Saharan Africa. The infectious enteric diseases are highly prevalent and responsible for large amounts of morbidity and mortality. Three of these diseases, cholera, the weanling diarrheas, and schistosomiasis (which also has nonenteric forms), will be discussed in more detail to demonstrate some of the problems that have arisen in attempts to control them.

C. Cholera

Cholera, caused by ingestion of *Vibrio cholerae,* in contaminated food or water is transmitted through a fecal–oral cycle in which man is the only host. Following an incubation period ranging from a few hours to a few days, the disease begins with a sudden onset of profuse watery stools and vomiting. The amount of diarrhea can reach several liters per day, which may produce dehydration and lead to hypovolemic shock and death within hours after onset, especially in children. Mortality can be as high as 60%, but with only basic educational campaigns and fluid replacement centers, mortality should approach zero (Carpenter *et al.,* 1978; Benenson, 1975).

Sub-Saharan Africa remained virtually free of cholera until 1970. In August of that year an epidemic began in West Africa which ultimately involved 150,000 cases and 20,000 deaths. The epidemic began in Guinea and spread regularly and consistently from west to east along the West African coast, skipping no areas and rarely penetrating inland. In each new area there was approximately a 2-month cycle beginning with a slow rise to epidemic proportions, a prolonged regression, and usually a subsequent endemic focus. The major direction for the spread of the disease was along waterways and rarely by inland routes. Those habitations built in close association with slow-moving waters, such as lagoons or pools, were particularly at risk. Particularly problematic in this epidemic was the fact that the involved organism was biotype El Tor, known for its high infection-to-case ratio, which is estimated to range from 36:1 to as high as 100:1. The overall mortality for clinically apparent cases was high, averaging 10–15% (Goodgame and Greenough, 1975).

The popular reaction to such a lethal disease in a extremely primitive environment might have been predictable. In Mali the general belief was that the disease was caused by God because Moslems had not been fastidious enough in their religious practices (Imperato, 1974). People also believed that the vaccine was the most effective preventive measure and would travel great distances to obtain it. This popular reaction probably developed from previous experiences with the smallpox and measles vaccines. Unfortunately, the vaccine is of very limited effectiveness and is not generally recommended for use during epidemics. There were health education messages encouraging people to boil their water and seek treatment. Urban dwellers generally responded, but in rural areas, where 90% of the population lived, the messages were largely ignored (Imperato, 1974).

D. Weanling Diarrhea

Weanling diarrhea is the name given to diarrheal diseases occurring during and after the weaning period (Morley, 1973). During this period the child is first exposed to foods other than breast milk, which has previously comprised his entire diet. Some of these foods may be contaminated because of poor preparation facilities or lack of knowledge of how to correctly prepare weaning foods. In addition, as breast feeding decreases, the resultant loss of nutritive elements, especially protein, can lead to malnutrition and an accompanying decrease in immunologic competence of the child. The result is frequent bouts of diarrhea with potentially high case-fatality rates. Each episode also contributes to increasing degrees of malnutrition (Morley, 1973).

The microorganisms involved in weanling diarrhea are usually various bacteria and viruses. No matter what organism is present, it is the diarrhea and subsequent dehydration that causes the mortality. The treatment is rehydration, replacement of the deficient electrolytes, and provision of an energy source such as glucose (Pierce and Hirschhorn, 1977).

Although common to most developing countries, the problems of controlling weanling diarrhea represent some of the most basic barriers to health in Black Africa. Mothers frequently react more to the nuisance of diarrhea than to the more serious unrecognized threat of dehydration to the child's general health. Some degree of forced starvation is usually an essential part of the management (Morley, 1973). Even when mothers understand the necessity for rehydration, the availability of medical care with intravenous rehydration is lacking, especially in rural areas. For these reasons there has been a growing interest in the developing programs of oral rehydration therapy that will allow mothers to treat their infants themselves in their own villages (Diarrhea Dialogue, 1980). The permanent solutions to weanling diarrhea probably lie in socioeconomic development and elimination of the sources of contamination, but oral rehydration offers an attractive approach to adapting treatment to the primitive conditions that exist.

E. Schistosomiasis

Schistosomiasis (*Bilharzia*) represents a water-borne disease transmitted by a fecal-skin or urine-skin cycle rather than by the fecal-oral cycle characteristic of cholera and weanling diarrhea. In this cycle, the parasite is deposited via feces or urine in water, where it hatches and penetrates a snail host. After several generations it emerges from the snail ready to penetrate the skin of humans who come in contact with the water. With the exception of *S. haematobium*, which lodges in the wall of the bladder, all major species ultimately lodge in the wall of the intestines (Hunter *et al.*, 1976).

Two of the four major species of schistosomes are found throughout sub-Saharan Africa and a third is found in isolated focal areas (Hunter *et al.*, 1976). It has been estimated that in 14 selected African countries, 34,000,000 of the total 100,000,000 population are infected. In some countries the infection rate is over 50% (Hughes and Hunter, 1970). Most infected persons are initially asymptomatic; however, more severe cases lead to hepatosplenic, pulmonary, and urinary tract complications, and sometimes death due to fibrosis secondary to the parasite ova laid in the involved tissues (Hunter *et al.*, 1976).

The available forms of medical treatment for schistosomiasis are highly toxic and difficult to administer to whole populations through public health programs. Current attempts to control the disease therefore are limited to preventive public health measures. These include sanitary control of feces and urine, molluscocides, and other attempts to kill the snail host, and education of the population to discourage fecal and urine contamination of water sources (Benenson, 1975).

The problems associated with maintaining sewage control and water treatment have already been emphasized. In view of the water shortage in many parts of Africa, it is not surprising that most populations simply use the available water and expose themselves to infection rather than worry about the long-term consequences of this chronic disease.

Certain water project development efforts in Africa are also associated with the spread of schistosomiasis. Many agricultural improvement schemes include the construction of dams and irrigation systems. Unfortunately these new water sources often act as transmission networks for the diffusion of the snail host (Hughes and Hunter, 1970).

F. Immunizations

Diseases that have had a major impact on Black African populations have been reduced to relatively minor importance in more developed parts of the world through the use of immunizations. Any examination of morbidity and mortality in pediatric age-groups in both urban and rural areas of sub-Saharan Africa indicates that immunizable diseases are still highly prevalent and often fatal (Morley, 1973; Williams and Jelliffe, 1972). Diseases of major importance include pertussis, measles, tetanus, diphtheria, poliomyelitis, and in endemic areas, yellow fever and typhoid, among others.

Two diseases that illustrate some of the differences in impact of these diseases in Africa and in developed nations are tetanus and measles. Tetanus, although globally distributed, rarely causes death in the United States (mortality about 1/100,000) because of widespread primary immunizations and frequent boosters for people with contaminated wounds. In Africa, however, the death rates can be as high as 26.5/100,000. These high rates appear to be due to a combination of several factors including the inaccessibility of medical care, increased prevalence of the organism in rural areas, and certain unhygienic practices, particularly those involving the cutting of the umbilical cord at birth (Cruickshank, 1976).

Neonatal tetanus occurs secondary to infection of the umbilical stump and has been estimated to be 80–90% fatal and responsible for about 80% of all tetanus deaths in developing countries (Cruickshank, 1976). With the lack of prenatal health care and the frequent use of traditional midwives in much of Africa, these opportunities to protect the infant against neonatal tetanus are often lacking.

Even before the development of the measles vaccine, the case fatality rate for measles in the United States had dropped to 1/10,000 with an encephalitis rate of 1/1000 (Basch, 1978). In parts of West Africa, however, case fatality rates are estimated as being 3–5% and up to 20–40% for hospitalized patients (Morley, 1973). The differences are largely attributed to the interaction between measles infection and malnutrition. In the malnourished child, measles is much more severe. "In no other common disease is there so much difference in the course and outcome of the disease . . ." (Morley, 1976). Measles also makes the malnutrition worse. A longitudinal study in Africa demonstrated that nearly one-fourth of the children with measles lost 10% of their weight. The fact that measles frequently leads to marasmus or kwashiorkor in children is well recognized (Morley, 1976).

VI. DISEASES ASSOCIATED WITH BIOLOGICAL COMPOSITION

Prevalence of diseases associated with the biological composition of black Africans demonstrates a variety of patterns in comparison with other populations.

Some diseases, such as certain hemoglobinopathies, are related to specific changes in DNA, which have been well delineated. In others, such as certain skin diseases, their high prevalence is well established and believed to be related to physical characteristics. However, the exact genetic mechanisms involved remain open to conjecture. In still other cases, such as hypertension, the diathesis is believed to be genetic but the course of the disease can be modified through interaction with the environment.

In contrast to diseases related to the environment that are discussed in the previous section, diseases associated with the biological composition of black Africans are responsible for much less morbidity and mortality. This section will discuss a limited number of these diseases and explore their various mechanisms of expression and their interrelationship with environmental and cultural factors.

A. Hemoglobinopathies

Perhaps the most widely studied group of diseases associated with the biological composition of sub-Saharan Africans is that composed of the hemoglobinopathies and associated erythrocyte abnormalities. Although a large number of these abnormal hemoglobin and erythrocyte disorders have been identified, the number that have been shown to produce overt disease is much lower. The most widely studied hemoglobins that produce disease states are hemoglobins S and C and thalassemia; enzyme disorder most studied is G6PD deficiency.

Sickle cell hemoglobin or hemoglobin S (HbS) is produced by a substitution of valine for glutamic acid in position six of the N terminal of the β chain. Erythrocytes of persons homozygous for the HbS gene form a sickle shape under appropriate conditions, such as deoxygenation (Bullock and Pongrac, 1975).

The clinical picture of persons homozygous for HbS is characterized by a chronic hemolytic anemia with painful crises and infarctions secondary to vascular obstruction by the abnormal erythrocytes. The disease begins in early childhood with a high mortality in Africa. Persons who are heterozygous for the gene (sickle cell trait) are generally asymptomatic (Lehman *et al.*, 1977).

The HbS gene is distributed widely throughout sub-Saharan Africa in an equatorial belt that stretches across the continent from the Sahara in the north to the Zambesi River in the south. The average frequency of the gene is 20%, with variation from 0 up to 40% (Wintrobe *et al.*, 1974).

Originally, there was much speculation as to why a deleterious gene for hemoglobin should be maintained at such high frequencies. Subsequently, HbS was shown to provide protection against malaria. Although persons homozygous for HbS were found to be at high risk for mortality from sickle cell disease, those heterozygous for HbS were found to have a protective advantage against malaria. There is also some evidence for increased fertility for those with sickle cell trait

(Livingstone, 1971). Therefore, the high frequency of HbS in malarious regions can be viewed as a gradual genetic adaptation to a particularly harsh selective agent in the environment, malaria.

Other diseases of red blood cells in black Africans have also been associated with malaria. Erythrocytes with G6PD deficiency have been found to be much less frequently parasitized by *Falciparum* malaria in hemizygous males and homozygous and heterozygous females. Nevertheless, the locus of the G6PD gene and the higher frequencies of the defect in areas less malarious than Africa prevent drawing a conclusive association between G6PD deficiency and malaria (Livingstone, 1971). Similarly, HbC is suspected of having an association with malaria but none has yet been proven (Livingstone, 1971). Like the S gene, it is autosomal and in its homozygous expression is associated with a reduced erythrocyte life span, chronic hemolytic anemia, and splenomegaly. In parts of West Africa, particularly Ghana, the gene is present in 17–28% of the population (Lehman *et al.*, 1977).

Both α- and β-thalassemias are found in sub-Saharan African populations. β-Thalassemia is found throughout West Africa and especially in parts of Liberia, where it reaches a frequency of 10% (Livingstone, 1976; Weatherall, 1977). There are also varying frequencies of hemoglobin Bart's in umbilical cord blood of various black African populations, which probably indicate the presence of α-thalassemia. The frequencies vary from 2% to a high of 18% in certain equatorial groups in Zaire (Piliszek, 1979).

Livingstone proposes that the high frequencies of the three β-hemoglobin chain abnormalities, HbS, HbC and β-thalassemia in West Africa represent a genetic replacement phenomenon. He hypothesizes that before the introduction of yam cultivation in about 2500–1500 BC, the human population was neither dense enough nor the endemicity of malaria high enough for these abnormal hemoglobins to be of selective advantage against malaria. Following the increase in population density, the selective advantage became important. After about 100 generations, the gene reached its current level in the population (Livingstone, 1976). Assuming HbS and HbC are each single point mutations spread from a single population, the areas of their highest density probably reflect their starting places. Therefore, HbS would have begun east of West Africa and HbC would have started in Ghana. Simulation studies indicate that both HbS and HbC are probably replacing β-thalassemia as they advance through West Africa. However, it is not as clear which of the hemoglobin variants HbS or HbC is replacing the other (Livingstone, 1976).

In addition to the hemoglobinopathies discussed above, a number of others occur in sub-Saharan African populations but either are not causes of clinical disease or are prevalent in frequencies too low to be discussed individually. These include, among others, hemoglobin K, Stanleyville-1 and -2, and HbS in combination with other hemoglobin abnormalities (Bullock and Pongrac, 1975).

There are also nonhemoglobin variations in erythrocytes found in certain populations. One is the Duffy-negative phenotype present in many African populations. There is now evidence that it is associated with innate resistance to infection with *P. vivax* (Welch *et al.*, 1977).

B. Skin Disorders

Because black Africans represent an extreme in the spectrum of skin colors found in human populations of the world, not surprisingly they also differ in the incidence, prevalence, and clinical course of certain dermatologic diseases. One of these differences is manifest in the higher prevalence of keloids among blacks than among lighter complexioned peoples (Domonokos, 1971).

No keloid surveys of unselected Negro or African populations have been made (Oluwasanmi, 1974); however, the increased prevalence of keloids in black African populations as opposed to other populations has been reported in the literature since the 1950s. Interestingly, keloids have not been documented in African albinos, accentuating the fact that their prevalence seems dependent on dark skin color more than on other physical characteristics (Oluwasanmi, 1974).

Oluwasanmi studied keloids through a survey in rural Nigeria and found the prevalence to be about the same for both sexes (5.4% male and 6.2% female), in contrast to the condition depicted in much of the literature based on hospital records. He hypothesized that women demand treatment more frequently than do men. The factors most frequently found to predispose to keloid formation were nonspecific trauma followed by vaccinations and tattooing. Prevalence was found to be low in the first decade of life, high in the second and third decades of life, and to slowly diminish after that (Oluwasanmi, 1974). Pseudofolliculitis, a syndrome that results from ingrown hairs following shaving and that leads to multiple formation of small keloids, illustrates the daily problems that keloids can present even in more developed urban areas (McDonald and Kelly, 1975).

Albinism represents a genetic state that occurs in all world populations but which has a particularly devastating clinical course in Africans (McDonald and Kelly, 1975). Undoubtedly, a great deal of the problem is rooted in the daily social activities and cultural practices that are well adapted to the usual presence of strong sunlight. Preventive health behavior must be especially difficult for albinos, whose well-being directly depends on avoiding the sun.

The dangers of increased incidence of cancerous and precancerous lesions of the skin in albinos are well known (McDonald and Kelly, 1975). While these lesions are more a nuisance than a threat to life in more developed countries, the situation is different in Africa. In a study of 1000 Nigerian albinos, Okoro (1975) found evidence that less of the albino population reached ages greater than 30 years than the nonalbino population. His interpretation is that the increased mortality among albinos is due to advanced skin cancers.

There appears to be a great variation in the rates of many skin diseases in blacks versus other groups. For example, *dermatosa papulosa nigra* occurs almost solely in blacks and various of the nevi occur with greater frequency in blacks, whereas seborrheic keratoses and xanthomatosis occur less frequently than in whites. The prevalence of psoriasis almost matches the 2.5% level in white people in East Africa, but is less than 0.1% in West Africans (McDonald and Kelly, 1975). Most skin cancers and precancerous lesions have a much lower incidence in blacks than in other groups. Perhaps the difference may be due to protection against sunlight afforded by the increased melanin in black skin (Murray, 1975).

C. Cancer

An important exception to the apparent reduction of the incidence of skin cancers in blacks is Kaposi's sarcoma. First reported by Kaposi in 1872, this malignancy has become known as Kaposi's sarcoma or multiple idiopathic hemorrhagic sarcoma (D'Oliveira and Oliveira Torres, 1972). The disease has been found to be more prevalent in parts of Africa than elsewhere. Studies examining the relative frequency of reported cases as a percentage of all reported cancers show Kaposi's sarcoma to be the most frequent cancer in northeast Zaire, Rwanda, and Burundi; its frequency diminishes radially from that focus (Taylor *et al.*, 1972). According to reports from this region, Kaposi's sarcoma comprises 9.9% of all tumors and 17.2% of all tumors in males (D'Oliveira and Oliveira Torres, 1972).

Other parts of sub-Saharan Africa also have reported higher incidence of Kaposi's sarcoma in blacks than in whites. In South Africa, the Bantu population has been found to have the disease with a frequency that is ten times higher than that among whites (Oettle, 1962). A study in Uganda found a greater frequency of reported disease among the Bantu than among the Nilotic tribes, but lower rates than among the Sudanic tribes. Kaposi's sarcoma shows a steady increase in frequency with age (Taylor *et al.*, 1972) and a predilection for males varying from a reported rate of 33:1 in Uganda to 2:1 in the Bantu of Durban (D'Oliveira and Oliveira Torres, 1972). Evidence regarding the cause of Kaposi's sarcoma is still unclear.

In addition to the skin cancers mentioned earlier, several neoplasms appear to have a relatively high prevalence in certain black African populations. Geographically, Burkitt's lymphoma has been shown to occur most commonly in a "lymphoma belt" across moist tropical and subtropical Africa between the latitudes of about 15°N and 15°S (Burkitt, 1970a). The tumor usually presents clinically with swelling of the jaw and primarily affects children under 15 years of age (Lythcott *et al.*, 1975). Strong evidence now suggests that development of this neoplasm depends on previous infection with Epstein-Barr virus (de-Thé *et al.*, 1978). The actual clinical expression of the disease, however, may be dependent on other factors such as the presence of severe malaria (Biggar and Nkrumah, 1979).

Nasopharyngeal cancer has also been shown to occur with high incidence in some parts of sub-Saharan Africa. In a study in Uganda, these tumors were found to occur at a young age, with 25% of them occurring in persons under the age of 20 years. Variation in incidence was found among tribal groups. Nilotic and Para-Nilotic peoples showed a higher incidence at an earlier age than Bantu or Sudanic peoples. The specific causative agents remain unknown (Schmauz and Templeton, 1972). A study in Kenya tended to implicate endocrinologic factors associated with the much higher incidence in males (Bulbrook *et al.*, 1968).

Surveys of all types of cancers in black Africans point to a wide spectrum of possible causative agents. High levels of genitourinary cancers tend to occur in areas where schistosomiasis is prevalent. Penile cancers are sometimes associated with lack of circumcision and poor hygiene of the prepuce. The association between dietary habits and certain cancers such as cancers of the liver and esophagus will be discussed later. Predisposing factors have not yet been found for several cancers of high incidence, such as antral cancers of the respiratory tract (Keen, 1975).

D. Hypertension

Another disease associated with the biological composition of black Africans is hypertension. Various studies have documented the high prevalence of hypertension among black Africans (Akinkugbe, 1972; Stamler *et al.*, 1967; Vaughn, 1977), including both essential and renal hypertension (Vaughn, 1977). Essential hypertension is believed to be related to a genetic predisposition, but inheritance must be polygenic. The ultimate effect of this genetic predisposition appears to be closely associated with certain environmental factors. Salt intake, urbanization, stress, and other factors have all been implicated (Robbins and Cotran, 1979; Dollery, 1979). The association of hypertension with certain cultural phenomena will be treated in the next section.

VII. DISEASES ASSOCIATED WITH CULTURAL PATTERNS

The existence of a relationship between culture and disease patterns has long been acknowledged in the Western medical tradition, although the significance of particular aspects of culture continue to be controversial. In a wider perspective, entire medical systems have been analyzed within their cultural contexts to understand the relationship between patient and practitioner, to uncover the function of syndromes that are linked to specific ethnic groups, and to determine the principles on which either local or cosmopolitan systems of healing are based. According to Press (1980), there are links between a group's medical system and its social structure and world view. Glick (1967) stated that the aspects of social structure reflected in the medical system are the sources of power (religious, economic, and political) that are capable of causing or treating illness within the group. In discussing the relationship between medical systems and world view, Press cites Ackerknecht's (1942) earlier declaration that a medical system and its practices reflect cultural patterns and are consistent with ideas and behavior of everyday life.

A. Traditional Categories and Classifications of Disease

Investigations of the relationship between social structure and world view and traditional African medical systems have revealed that these systems diverge in numerous ways from the one that is usually labeled as Western or scientific. According to contemporary anthropologists, these divergences are perhaps most clearly seen in the categories or classifications of disease on which the different systems are built. Western researchers' attempts to describe such categories have produced various schemes, conflicting interpretations of the same information, and a wide range of complexity.

Bryant's (1966) study of the Zulu considers the disease categories of the local population to be of secondary importance, as evidenced in the organization of his work, which provides descriptions of health problems using Western categories with which Zulu diseases, when they were cited, are made to correspond. When multiple Zulu lexemes are grouped under one Western disease, no information is provided to indicate their degree of synonymy.

In one section of Bryant's work, a discussion of local medicinal agents provides some clue to categories in the Zulu medical system. A limited idea of disease categories emerged from this classification of traditional medicines:

ama Khuhale: medicine for self-fortification against evil
imi Khando: medicine for destroying power in others
im Bhulelo: medicine laid on an enemy's path to cause fatal disease
izin Telez: medicine sprinkled in the Kraal to ward off lightning
izim Pundu: medicine for causing confusion
izin Ggunda: medicine to "take the edge off" when an act is completed
imi Thi emayama: black medicine—the first used on a patient for the expulsion of the afflicting evil
imi Thi emblopha: white medicine—to follow black medicine as a kind of sedative
ama Khambhi: green medicine—fresh herbs and roots which form the largest class of medicines

A totally different approach to the Zulu medical system is found in Conco's (1973) study, which divides traditional diseases in a dualistic fashion, into naturally caused and supernaturally caused afflictions. Diseases of natural causation may be further labeled as "specific" or "nonspecific," according to the specificity of the signs and symptoms associated with them. Illnesses that have identifiable signs and symptoms (e.g., asthma, measles, and worms) are "specific." On the other hand, "nonspecific" illnesses (e.g., colds, mild infectious fevers, and gastroenteritis) generally show the same symptomatology and signs. The Zulu term for common sickness, *mKhuhlane,* can be used specifically or nonspecifically. Nonspecific use of *mKhuhlane* indicates a naturally caused disease that is neither serious nor fatal but is incapacitating and endemic. A specific use of the term , for example *mKhuhlane—cough*—refers to a disease with these same features, but in which the specific term (coughing in this example) is the main symptom. The Zulu diseases of supernatural causation are extraordinary, generally nonspecific, and develop through a combination of magical and spiritual forces. These illnesses are known as *uKufa Kwabanto* or diseases of the people. As such, they are understood only by Africans and have to be treated in a traditional fashion (Ngubane, 1976).

The interpretation offered by Evans-Pritchard (1937) of the Azande concept of illness is the most often cited example of a system in which all sicknesses, especially serious conditions, tend to be attributed to either witchcraft or sorcery. Disease causation, however, has a dual course. That is, any affliction generally has a magical or mystical cause that is remote and invisible, and a natural cause that is proximate. Effective treatment involves the patient's action on both supernatural and natural levels. The only serious illnesses not attributed to magic and sorcery are two diseases of infants, *Kazo amadi* and *ngorombe,* which are present in high frequency and for which the mortality is considerable, and incurable conditions such as smallpox and sleeping sickness, which are attributed to a supreme god.

The relationship of this classification of disease causation to other aspects of social structure is demonstrated by Evans-Pritchard to be associated with the tendency of the Azande to blame fellow tribesmen rather than spirits or ancestors for their misfortunes. The result is that almost everyone in the society is open to accusations of witchcraft or sorcery and thus becomes a possible agent of disease.

As in the Azande system, the Ndembu system is one in which calamities and adversities of all kinds appear to be caused by mystical forces that are tied in some fashion to conscious agents (Turner, 1964).

Similarly, Price-Williams' (1962) study of the Tiv of central Nigeria shows that the principal feature of illness among this group is its framing of interpretations of disease causation in terms of the functioning of witchcraft and malevolent forces. A person who becomes ill can assume that his fate is due to these factors or to his having offended an *akombo*, or supernatural agency. Nevertheless, although disease is a recognizable entity, it is not isolated by the Tiv as a category that is distinct from other misfortunes that can affect one's compound, farm, or kin relationships. Rather, it is merely one of several *akombo* that include separate agents for illness, birth, hunting, rendering arrows efficacious, fertility of crops, good luck, and obtaining wives.

Ayoade (1979), in his study of the Yoruba, uses a similar scheme. He states that among the Yoruba, illnesses are attributed to a supernatural cause when no known visible acts have led to the condition and to a nonsupernatural cause when the affliction is known to be the consequence of a cause-and-effect relationship. The supernatural causation may take the form of sorcery, witchcraft, and spirit possession. A third category of disease consists of ailments caused by a god. Those diseases are identifiable by their persistence, resistance to the usual medication, and ultimate incurableness. In Ayoade's analysis, natural and supernatural causations of illness are not presented as absolutely distinct categories, but as different points on a continuum. For example, the same illness can be seen as being supernaturally caused in one person and naturally caused in another. In addition, a condition that is initially interpreted as a supernatural affliction can later be interpreted as an ailment of natural cause.

Bisilliat's (1976) classification of diseases among the Songhai is also based on this division into natural and supernatural forms of causation. She, however, uses the terms village disease and bush disease to indicate this difference and to construct a typology. Village diseases are of natural causation and are analyzed according to traditional principles of physiology and anatomy. These principles involve movement of the blood (not equivalent to circulation), movement of heat and cold within the body, and movement of the disease itself via routes or pathways that link the various organs and parts of the body. An excess of blood around a particular organ, a reversal in its flow, or a cooling of the blood may be given as causes or as consequences of illness. Bush diseases are of supernatural causation and are linked to bush-residing spirits that enter a person's body to produce illness.

Although Bisilliat attempts to analyze the two categories as separate entities as in Ayoade's analysis of the Yoruba system, she acknowledges that in a complete description of a disease, bush and village are not in opposition but are complementary. The complexity of the traditional healer's task is evident. He must classify the disease within one of the two categories, but treatment involves the recognition of their unity.

Harley (1970) in his study of the Mano of Liberia, as Bryant in his study of the Zulu, does not use traditional categories in his discussion of disease. Rather, he presents an analysis organized on the basis of Western terminology. Because his major interest is the treatment process, he indicates the preferred medicine for each condition. Harley does, however, present a classification of diseases among the Mano in terms of causative factors, and in each case indicates whether the treatment is rational, magical, or mixed: (1) natural causes—rational treatment, (2) witchcraft and poisoning—mixed treatment, (3) broken taboo—mixed treatment, (4) fetish power—magical or mixed treatment, and (5) were-animals—rational treatment.

Gillies' (1976) classification of disease among the Akoko of Ogori in Nigeria focuses on distinctions based on the type of medical specialist and medicines. At one's disposal are both curers and diagnosticians, and herbal and magical medicines. For natural diseases, divination is not needed and treatment does not entail the use of magical remedies. Diseases of natural causation include afflictions such as malaria, which is believed to be a type of sunstroke; gonorrhea, which is known to be sexually transmitted; guinea worm, which is seen as related to impure drinking water; and other conditions including hepatitis and yellow fever. The diseases that need the help of a diviner are often cases in which the chance of recovery is slight or death is believed to be the outcome.

According to Gillies, the system is coherent and the classification of illness is part of the culture's total semantic arrangement of reality. This classification is based on a series of dichotomies that include diviner/medicine man; good magical medicine/bad magical medicine; and private misfortune/public calamity.

In an attempt to compare views of disease causation in cross-cultural fashion, Weisz (1972) collected data that point to similarities and differences among twelve East African tribal groups. The causes of illness that she examines are (1) ancestor spirits, (2) broken rules, (3) contagion, (4) evil eye, (5) evil spirits, (6) God, (7) heredity, (8) natural causes, (9) vague evil forces, and (10) witchcraft. Her results indicated that the most commonly held beliefs about disease causation implicate witchcraft in eleven groups and ancestral spirits and broken rules in each of ten groups. The least commonly held beliefs about disease causation are those implicating evil eye and vague evil forces, each of which is found in four groups. All the tribes reported more than one theory of disease causation. The most complex patterns are those of the Sebei, which are listed as having seven of the causes, followed by the Nyamwezi Sukum, Toro and Digo, each with six causes.

The importance of native categories and concepts of health and illness has been pointed out by several authors. Among the Digo of East Africa, ricketts, kwashiorkor, and the loss of strength in children are placed under one heading, *Chirwa,* which is caused by the sexual transgression of parents. This belief led to the group's strong resistance to claims of Westerners that improved diets could change these conditions. In cases such as these, a health team's knowledge of such native categories can be essential information in the design of programs to improve a group's health status.

Last (1976) points out, however, that among the Maguzawa, non-Muslim Hausa, the infusion of new health information does not always change ideas that already exist. The government introduced the term *Sank'arau* to indicate cere-brospinal meningitis. But the Maguzawa used *Sank'arau* to indicate a type of neck ailment rather than meningitis, a condition that they already recognized but for which they had no name. In effect, as Last indicates, the government created a new disease.

Another new disease among Maguzawa women is *gishiri*, which unlike *Sank'arau* has evolved from within the group. Last suggested that this affliction of the vagina, which is considered to be passed between women from cooking stool to cooking stool, may relate to women's general health anxiety and specifi-cally a concern regarding their reproductive ability. He suggests that because symptoms for new diseases such as *gishiri* are so vague, they are "caught in conversation."

The conclusion reached by Warren (1979) in his study of the Bono of Ghana has perhaps the most far-reaching implications in this matter. After an extensive study of the Bono medical system, he challenges the conclusion of researchers who stressed supernatural, sorcery, or witchcraft theories in African disease classification. In a prior study of the Bono conducted by Field (1960), this approach to illness did receive emphasis, and because her work influenced the attitudes of local health workers and was used to help structure health programs to alter these beliefs, Warren claimed that a considerable amount of human and economic resources were needlessly wasted.

According to Warren, the analysis provided by Field misses the larger portion of Bono disease classification, which deals with naturally caused affliction. His own work focused on 1266 recorded disease lexemes, of which 742 were primary terms and 524 were synonyms. Through an arrangement of these data in contrast-ing sets related through vertical class inclusion, it appears to Warren that most Bono disease names and causes of illness have nothing to do with supernatural causation. He does admit, however, that many of the lexemes that indicate a natural cause referred to minor illnesses, whereas those that indicate a super-natural cause refer to serious conditions. Additionally, some lexemes fit into either category, depending on the content within which the affliction develops.

The significance of classification and language generally was indicated in a study by Conco (1973), who challenges another currently held assumption. From his research among the Zulu, Conco believes that the assertion that the diseases of Western civilization were a rarity in rural Africans is unjustified. In his own practice in such rural areas, he claims to have seen over one-half of the condi-tions that Burkitt (1970b) and Gelfand (1957) listed as rare, including heart disease.

In a test of translation of medical terms from English to Zulu, measuring loose and exact translation, Conco finds terms concerning the cardiovascular system to have a communication potential of 6%, based on exact translation. It is difficult or impossible to find equivalences for such notions as failing heart and blood pressure. In comparison, terms referring to obstetrics show a higher (43%) exact communication potential. In a comparison of disease terminology a high correspondence exists between the English and the Zulu for conventional diseases, such as coughs, asthma, worms, and dizziness. Here no communication problem exists. The infectious fevers, such as infectious hepatitis, shigella infections, and filariasis are all categorized in Zulu under *mKhuhlane*. In dealing with these disorders, the communication problem was significant. Similarly, the Zulu designations for traditional diseases such as "trail disease," "dreaded men's disease," and "mental disease made by Africans" have no English equivalents. Here a communication problem is significant also. Conco concludes that the apparent rarity of certain diseases may be due, in part, to a communication problem.

In any discussion of disease or health problems in Africa, it becomes clear that language in general, and classification within the domain of illness terminology specifically, become critical matters. When there is little correspondence between traditional and Western classificatory systems, the signs and symptoms, so important for Western medicine, may be ignored, be combined to form different syndromes, or be more inclusive or exclusive than what might be expected by individuals oriented to the Western system. In essence, the physical body, and in this case its afflictions, become an expression of culture.

B. Patterns of Disease in Traditional Cultures

With increasing contact between the Western countries and traditional tribal groupings in Africa, two views of the health status of these regions emerged, as Polunin (1977) pointed out. On the one hand were those who believed that pre-contact peoples had lived in a state of perpetual good health and that illness was essentially a consequence of conquest and colonization. On the other hand were those who believed that the "primitive" world was disease-ridden and that one of the tasks of modernization was to provide proper medical care. As Polunin states, there is an amount of truth in both positions.

As the experience of Western-trained health teams increased in Africa, it became clear that some traditional cultural patterns not only interfered with the introduction of new ideas about health, but also appeared to be linked to particular patterns of disease. Although carefully collected epidemiological data are not generally available, some patterns of the relationship between traditional culture and illness have emerged.

The cultural context of high infant mortality has become one of the main areas of concern of health workers, and efforts to identify practices associated with this phenomenon often have been undertaken. In one study, Jelliffe and Bennett (1960) described two customs that appear to have endangered the lives of newborns. In many parts of the continent, after the cutting of the umbilical cord, a paste substance has often been placed on the stump. They pointed out that the danger to the infant of contracting tetanus is considerable due to the nature of this mixture. In Nigeria, an herbal infusion, *agbo omo*, is given after birth to expel meconium. In other parts of the continent, enemas are similarly used on young children. These irritants, sometimes made of pepper water, may cause severe diarrhea, proctitis, or anal fissures.

The practice of circumcision of both males and females, which served as a rite of passage to adulthood, was widespread in traditional African cultures. Roles (1966) describes these rituals as they existed in nineteenth century East Africa, and Harley (1970) outlined these rites as part of the Poro and Sande initiation schools among the Mano of Liberia. Although details of the rite of circumcision are not available, the sorts of stone and metal instruments used in the operation coupled with a lack of sanitation would have made a certain amount of sepsis inevitable (Roles, 1966; Hughes, 1959).

The insertion of ear and lip plugs, and chipping of teeth, and scarification have also been used over a widespread area of the continent as a means of tribal identification, initiation, and adornment. According to Hughes (1959) the former practice of the Thonga of filing the front teeth apparently resulted in faster decay. Harley (1970) maintains that scarification in the Poro initiation could result in hermorrhage and infection, and Hughes (1959) pointed out that the effects of extensive keloid formation that results from this practice are not known.

A study of the Kikuyu by Wilkinson (1957) indicates that intestinal anthrax and tapeworm were more commonly found in males than females due to a group custom that limited eating meat to males. For ceremonial uncleanness to be avoided, the consumption of two sources of animal protein, game birds and fish, was forbidden and thereby reduced the amount of protein available for human consumption. Traditional house construction of the Kikuyu, consisting of mud over a wattle framework and grass thatch roof, also posed threats to health. The custom of surfacing the structure's walls with a layer of cow manure left exposed spores of *Clostridium tetani*. Dirt floors attracted insects, thatched roofs were nests for rats and snakes, and the dampness of the hut was common, not only during the rainy season but often through the dry season as well.

The classification of African plant life, the use for herbs in traditional healing, and the value of these for modern pharmacology have received considerable attention. Nevertheless, McKhobo (1976) points out that among the plants widely used in medication, as food preparations, or ingested directly are some that apparently are linked to illness. Species of *Senecio* in Lesotho have been classified as principal sources of hepatotoxic alkaloids and may play a role in the development of herbal hepatitis, cirrhosis, and hepatoma, as well as disorders of other organs.

Several studies have shown that liver cell cancers are highly prevalent in sub-Saharan Africa. Although the variations among countries is wide, the prevalence generally tends to decrease as one proceeds northward (Linsell and Higgins, 1976). Males tend to develop it twice as frequently as females. The younger age-groups show an even greater difference between the sexes (Linsell and Higgins, 1976). Various possible causative and predisposing factors have been hypothesized, most of which relate to the environment and culture. Alcoholism, hepatitis B infection, malnutrition, iron overload (sometimes related to the consumption of alcoholic beverages), parasitosis (especially schistosomiasis), and aflatoxins (involved in food contamination) have been implicated in the high prevalence of liver cell cancer in sub-Saharan Africa (Anthony, 1976).

Incidence of cancer of the esophagus has been shown to be high in certain black African populations as well. In particular, the Transkei and Ciskei of South Africa have a much higher rate of neoplasm than the neighboring Basuto or Zulu, with the difference being of fairly recent origin. Possible causative agents include nitrosamines in food, specific plant foods, and toxins produced by molds that contaminate grains, among others (Rose, 1967). Central African studies of esophageal cancer suggested as possible causative agents the carcinogens in pots used to make beer, cigarette smoking, and nitrosamines (Wapnick *et al.*, 1972).

In addition to the studies that have uncovered linkages between traditional behavior and identifiable Western disease entities, there have been studies that examined the relationship of behavior patterns to those disorders labeled as culture-bound syndromes. Such afflictions include attacks of the evil eye among the Amhara of Ethiopia. Reminick's (1974) analysis of this disorder emphasizes that the dominant theme of the Amhara belief centers on the fear that members of a high status group have of being envied by a member of a lower status group, and the interpretation of certain misfortunes as the consequence of this envy. Persons at high risk of attack are those who show signs of fear, worry, or anxiety. Symptoms of the disorder may have immediate onset or be delayed and result in either illness or death.

A syndrome known as *Pobough Lang* among the Serer of Senegal is characterized by compulsive geophagia, pallor, weakness, edema, depression, anxiety, and social isolation. According to recent studies (Beiser *et al.*, 1974), the dirt-eating feature of the disorder is possibly linked to dietary deficiency of iron and other nutrients. In addition, the feature is speculated to be a possible famine-related behavioral response. Other aspects of this syndrome are thought to be related to a cultural belief in which geophagia is disapproved and conflicts with Moslem food taboos.

C. Patterns of Disease and Modernization

Although traditional cultural patterns can be linked with a variety of illnesses, modernization and the changes it entails also have adverse health consequences. In a general fashion, Lightman (1977) characterizes the acculturation of tribal groups into contemporary civilization as a process that results in poor nutrition, overcrowding, and an increase in droplet and fecal–oral contamination, new chronic and epidemic diseases, and the introduction of new patterns of stress and stress-related disorders. As a result of a search for a specific marker that might serve as an early manifestation of imminent Western disease patterns, Kloppens and Fehrsen (1977) suggest the use of phleboliths, end products of veinal thrombosis that appear as shadows on pelvic radiographs. According to their findings, phleboliths are seldom seen in radiographs of black Africans who live in traditional groupings, but are commonly seen in whites in South Africa, as well as in other Westerners, and may be increasing in younger, more acculturated blacks.

In a review of development projects in Africa, Hughes and Hunter (1970) point out numerous examples in which the acculturation process was one that resulted in both intended and unintended consequences. Programs that are not carefully planned before execution have resulted in the construction of model villages and dams in the Nargedi area of northern Ghana where onchocerciasis was endemic. New dams and irrigation systems have spread bilharzia throughout Africa. In addition, new roads designed to transport people have become new links for disease as well. Migrant laborers moving along these roads on the west coast from north to south in past years have been unintentionally provided with access to areas within the tsetse belt. Here they contracted sleeping sickness only to move on and reinfect zones where the disease had previously been eliminated.

The effects of urbanization on health has become a matter of increasing concern in all parts of Africa. Patterson (1979), however, indicates that this is by no means a recent phenomenon. In Accra, major changes between 1908 and 1940 to develop the city's water supply, improve sewerage, expand housing, and increase mosquito control have not provided the maximum hoped-for benefits. Piped water was considered a vitally necessary replacement for the old system of wells and became the major contribution of the colonial government to the city's health. A pure-water system was needed to reduce the incidence of conditions such as amebic and bacillary dysentery, diarrhea, typhoid fever, and guinea worm. In terms of improved personal hygiene, it was designed to help control yaws and louse-borne relapsing fever. Patterson points out, however, that pure water at neighborhood taps does not insure pure water at the time of use. It might be collected in dirty vessels or become contaminated either during transport through dusty streets, or in home storage.

Similar problems resulted from other city health projects during that time. Intestinal diseases were spread because of an inadequate system of pan collection and cleaning of the city's new latrines. The implementation of rubbish collection posed threats as a result of infrequent collection and improperly discarded garbage. Although certain diseases, such as smallpox, yaws, and guinea worm were considerably reduced during these years, infant mortality remained high because of infantile diarrhea, worms, and postweaning protein deprivation. Patterson maintains that public health projects in the early 1970s, including sewage disposal, rubbish collection, and improvements in housing, have continued to pose problems.

According to Seftel (1977), there are both similarities and differences in the health of urban and rural blacks in southern Africa. The similarities include high rates of tuberculosis, infantile gastroenteritis, venereal disease, malnutrition, rheumatic heart disease, and idiopathic congestive cardiomyopathy. Disorders that are more common in rural areas than in cities include goiter in certain regions and esophageal and hepatic cancer. For example, Zaire does have well-defined geographic areas known as "goiter belts" where goiter is prevalent (Delange, 1974). Urban blacks tend to have more obesity, hypertension, lung cancer, and other diseases that are associated with Westernization. Donaldson (1971) found that in Central Africa acculturation of traditional groups is characterized by a decrease in parasitic diseases, such as bilharzia, hand-to-mouth nematode disease, and scabies. Nutritional deficiency disorders such as avitaminosis, kwashiorkor, and anemia decrease, but disorders associated with nutritional excess, such as obesity and dental caries, tend to increase. Infectious diseases are less severe and are treated earlier, while stress-related conditions, such as hypertension and emotional disorders, increase.

In addition there is a large group of diseases in sub-Saharan Africa that appears to be associated with a combination of crowded, unhygienic living conditions and unavailability of adequate medical care. Although infectious in nature, these diseases follow chronic clinical courses and maintain an endemic level that is much higher than that seen in more developed countries. Examples of such diseases include leprosy, tuberculosis, syphilis, and gonorrhea. World prevalence studies by the World Health Organization (WHO) indicate that leprosy has the highest rates by far in sub-Saharan Africa. Rates between 3 and 4% are not uncommon and several countries report rates greater than 4%. No other continent approaches this high level of endemicity (Bechelli and Martinez Dominguez, 1966). The prevalence of leprosy in sub-Saharan Africa in part results from the inadequate availability of treatment and case follow-up capabilities.

Another endemic disease is gonorrhea. Belsey of WHO reports that infertility in sub-Saharan Africa is common and can affect up to 40% of the women. He hypothesizes that the major underlying etiology is gonorrhea (Belsey, 1976). The spread of gonorrhea can be tied to certain cultural practices. For example, studies in rural Uganda show that the polygamous marriage structure is intimately connected with its spread (Arya *et al.*, 1973). Any successful control program would have to examine and take into account the specific cultural practices of the society for which it is designed.

Malnutrition is currently of major importance throughout sub-Saharan Africa and is closely linked to the culture in terms of both cause and consequence. Any discussion of diseases inherent to sub-Saharan Africa must be framed by the chronic problem of famine which, as this discussion is written, is again raging throughout the eastern part of the continent. According to World Bank statistics, most African nations are found among those countries with the world's lowest average index of food production per capita (World Bank, 1980). During the 1970s, on a per capita basis, food production has declined 1% each year. Although this decline has been primarily due to a high population growth rate, averaging 2.9% per year, it characterizes a region with significant problems relating to the most basic element of health maintenance.

In addition to protein–energy malnutrition, specific conditions caused by lack of vitamins and minerals, such as scurvy, goiter, xerophthalmia, and iron deficiency anemias, are found unevenly distributed throughout the subcontinent. The exact prevalence of each depends on availability of certain food types in each area and cultural factors determining food utilization. For example, Zaire has a relatively high level of protein-energy malnutrition, yet xerophthalmia is virtually nonexistent, even during the famine conditions, due to the generous use of palm oil, which is rich in vitamin A (Kabamba *et al.*, 1978; R. R. Franklin, unpublished data).

Interest in blood pressure of Africans has become considerable. Scotch (1963) shows in a comparison between rural and urban Zulu that readings are similar to those of United States whites. The blood pressure of the rural Zulu is lower than that of urban Zulu. Scotch attributes this difference to stress factors. Persons who are less well adapted to urban life have higher blood pressure than those who are better adapted. Among urban Zulu women, those with higher blood pressure more than those with normal blood pressure tend to maintain more traditional cultural patterns, such as living in extended families, having many children and believing in sorcery. Among women with normal blood pressure, modern behavioral patterns prevailed, such as church membership and use of medical clinics. The relative absence of hypertension and the indication of no increase in blood pressure with advancing age among the Masai (Mann *et al.*, 1964), the Pygmies (Mann *et al.*, 1962), and the San (Truswell and Hansen, 1976), all of whom live in traditional rural areas, provide support for linkages between hypertension and factors of modernization, including stress.

Although many people assume that the introduction of the Western medical system into traditional African culture has resulted in an unambiguous achievement, a number of critics indicate that this assumption may not be the case. Harrison (1979a) points out that although health care was a high priority of the Nigerian government, the level of health services throughout the country was generally poor. This paradox arose because of three factors: first, the country had inherited from its colonial past a two-tiered health system of curative and preventive medicine in which the curative is given priority; second, the construction of health care facilities overshadowed the importance of public health measures;

and third, the low ratio of doctors to population was worsened by the poor distribution of these health care resources. Given the social, political, and economic obstacles that presently impede a resolution of these problems to allow for the successful implementation of a Western health care delivery system, Harrison questions the very need of developing such a system in nations such as Nigeria.

Serious consideration in a number of African countries is currently being given to using traditional healers to fill a part of the void in present health care modernization efforts. In a discussion of indigenous healers, Dunlop (1975) indicates that governments have three policy options in this matter: legalization of traditional medicine, recognition of its existence through cooperative efforts, or denial of any legal status or protection. Although the second option presently appears to be the most favored, steps toward legalization have been taken in Botswana and areas of Nigeria are pressing for this type of recognition.

Confidence in the values of indigenous healers is a matter of considerable debate. According to Asuni (1979), the preference of Africans for traditional medicine has resulted in high rates of morbidity and mortality in the face of epidemics of smallpox and cholera in rural areas. Dunlop (1975) points out that it is society that must bear the costs when traditional medicine fails because of inappropriate therapy leading to complications (e.g., unsterile equipment producing secondary infections and unsanitary practices in childbirth resulting in tetanus).

On the other hand, Harrison (1979b) indicates that there are numerous similarities between Western physicians and traditional healers in terms of social role, status, preparation, and general perspective of multiple causation within the respective systems. In addition, Asuni (1979) claims that where the two complement each other, as in circumstances where Western medicine functions in a curative fashion with respect to the physical organism, and traditional medicine searches for causes within the supernatural order or social structure, there is no problem. Janzen (1979) shows that in Zaire, herbalists, magicians, kinship therapists, prophets, and physicians are all engaged in healing and often treat the same person. As stated earlier, most traditional Africans regard illness within the larger context of misfortune and a concern for "wholeness," interpreted as an individual's well-being, health, and harmony with others. It is here that modern medicine fails to satisfy and gives tradition a reason for persisting (Swartz, 1979).

This concern for the use of traditional healers has prompted the World Health Organization to re-examine its role as a defender of the Western model of medicine. According to Bibeau (1979), the equating of health care with medical technology and Western-trained specialists in the past made indigenous healers unpopular. Their use in certain functions, however, may possibly produce a new model of care and improve the health status of populations in all parts of the continent.

VIII. CONCLUSIONS

From the preceding discussion of the spectrum and severity of diseases with high prevalence or incidence in black African populations, it is apparent that to understand the pathogeneses of these diseases, one cannot consider them to be caused by a single agent. Rather, the sub-Saharan African environment, the biological makeup of the black Africans, and the existing cultural attitudes toward disease and responses to disease all interact to modify the expression of these diseases in the populations. Of these three interacting influences, the environment is currently probably the most dominant factor. The high prevalence and incidence of infectious diseases in sub-Saharan Africa take such a high toll in morbidity and mortality that the other factors affecting health status seem dwarfed by comparison. This situation need not always exist. As the epidemic and endemic infectious diseases are gradually brought under control, the culturally and biologically unique aspects of black African populations will come to play increasingly important roles as determinants of health status.

REFERENCES

Ackerknecht, E. H. (1942). Primitive medicine and culture pattern. *Bull. Hist. Med.* **12,** 545–574.

Akinkugbe, O. O. (1972). "High Blood Pressure in the African." Churchill-Livingstone, Edinburgh.

Alland, A. (1973). Human biological diversity in Africa. *In* "Peoples and Cultures in Africa" (E. Skinner, ed.), pp. 59–70. Doubleday, Garden City, New York.

Anthony, P. P. (1976). The background to liver cell cancer. *In* "Liver Cell Cancer" (H. M. Cameron, D. A. Linsell, and G. P. Warwick, eds.), pp. 93–130. Elsevier, Amsterdam.

Arya, O. P., Nsanzumuhite, H., and Taber, S. R. (1973). Clinical, cultural, and demographic aspects of gonorrhea in a rural community in Uganda. *Bull. W. H. O.* **49,** 587–595.

Asuni, T. (1979). Modern medicine and traditional medicine. *In* "African Therapeutic Systems" (Z. A. Ademuwagun, J. A. A. Ayoade, I. E. Harrison, and D. M. Warren, eds.), pp. 176–181. Crossroads Press, New York.

Ayoade, J. A. (1979). The concept of inner essence in Yoruba traditional medicine. *In* "African Therapeutic Systems" (Z. A. Ademuwagun, J. A. A. Ayoade, I. E. Harrison, and D. M. Warren, eds.). pp. 49–55. Crossroads Press, New York.

Basch, P. F. (1978). "International Health." Oxford Univ. Press, London and New York.

Bechelli, L. M., and Martinez Dominguez, V. (1966). The leprosy problem. *Bull. W. H. O.* **34,** 811–826.

Beiser, M., Burr, W. A., Collomb, H., and Ravel, J. L. (1974). *Pobough Lang* in Senegal. *Soc. Psychiatry* **9,** 123–129.

Belsey, M. A. (1976). The epidemiology of infertility: A review with particular reference to sub-Saharan Africa. *Bull. W. H. O.* **54,** 319–341.

Benenson, A. S., ed. (1975). "Control of Communicable Diseases in Man," 12th ed. Am. Public Health Assoc., Washington, D.C.

Bibeau, G. (1979). The World Health Organization in encounter with African traditional medicine: Theoretical conceptions and practical strategies. *In* "African Therapeutic Systems" (Z. A.

Ademuwagun, J. A. A. Ayoade, I. E. Harrison, and D. M. Warren, eds.), pp. 182–186. Crossroads Press, New York.

Biggar, R. J., and Nkrumah, R. K. (1979). Burkitt's lymphoma in Ghana: Urban–rural distribution, time–space clustering and seasonality. *Int. J. Cancer* **23**, 330–336.

Bisilliat, J. (1976). Village diseases and Bush diseases in Songhay: An essay in description and classification with a view to a typology. *In* "Social Anthropology and Medicine" (J. B. Loudon, ed.), pp. 553–593. Academic Press, New York.

Bohannan, P., and Curtin, P. (1971). "Africa and Africans." Doubleday, Garden City, New York.

Bryant, A. T. (1966). "Zulu Medicine and Medicine Men." Struik, Cape Town.

Bulbrook, R. D., Wang, D. Y., and Clifford, P. (1968). Endocrine aspects of cancer of the nasopharynx. *In* "Cancer in Africa" (P. Clifford, D. A. Linsell, and G. P. Warwick, eds.), pp. 299–314. East Afr. Publ. House, Nairobi.

Bullock, W. J., and Pongrac, N. J. (1975). Hematology. *In* "Textbook of Black-related Diseases" (R. A. Williams, ed.), pp. 199–316. McGraw-Hill, New York.

Burkitt, D. P. (1970a). Geographical distribution. *In* "Burkitt's Lymphoma" (D. P. Burkitt and D. H. Wright, eds.), pp. 186–197. Livingstone, London.

Burkitt, D. P. (1970b). Relationship as a clue to causation. *Lancet* **ii**, 1237–1240.

Burnet, M., and White, D. O. (1972). "Natural History of Infectious Diseases," 4th ed. Cambridge Univ. Press, London and New York.

Cahill, K. M. (1975). "Tropical Diseases, A Handbook for Practitioners." Octopus Books, London.

Carlson, L. (1973). African landscapes. *In* "Peoples and Cultures in Africa" (E. Skinner, ed.), pp. 7–33. Doubleday, Garden City, New York.

Carpenter, C. C. J., Mahmoud, A. A. F., and Warren, K. S. (1978). Cholera. *In* "Geographic Medicine for the Practitioner. Algorithms in the Diagnosis of and Management of Exotic Diseases" (K. S. Warren and A. A. F. Mahmoud, eds.), pp. 17–20. Univ. of Chicago Press, Chicago, Illinois.

Cavalli-Sforza, E. (1977). Biological research on African Pygmies in population structure. *In* "Human Variation" (G. A. Harrison, ed.), pp. 273–284. Cambridge Univ. Press, London and New York.

Conco, W. Z. (1973). Diseases in the Tropics: A confrontation in an African medical practice. *Br. Med. J.* **iii**, 331–333.

Coon, C. S. (1965). "The Living Races of Man." Knopf, New York.

Cruickshank, R. (1976). Tetanus and diphtheria. *In* "Epidemiology and Community Health in Warm Climate Countries" (R. Cruickshank, K. L. Standard, and H. B. L. Russell, eds.), pp. 77–82. Churchill-Livingstone, Edinburgh.

de Blij, H. J. (1964). "A Geography of Sub-Saharan Africa." Rand McNally, Chicago, Illinois.

Delange, F. (1974). "Endemic Goitre and Thyroid Function in Central Africa," Monographs in Pediatrics, Vol. 2. Karger, Basel.

de-Thé, G., Geser, A., Day, N. E., Tukei, P. M., Williams, E. H., Beri, D. P., Smith, P. G., Deon, A. G., Bronkamm, G. W., Feroni, P., and Henle, W. (1978). Epidemiological evidence for causal relationship between Epstein–Barr virus and Burkitt's lymphoma from Ugandan prospective study. *Nature (London)* **274**, 756–7.

Diarrhea Dialogue (1980). No. 1, May.

D'Oliveira, J. J., and Oliveira Torres, F. (1972). Kaposi's sarcoma in the Bantu of Mozambique. *Cancer (Philadelphia)* **30**, 553–561.

Dollery, C. T. (1979). Arterial hypertension. *In* "Cecil Textbook of Medicine" (P. B. Beeson, ed.), 15th ed., Vol. 1, pp. 1199–1218. Saunders, Philadelphia, Pennsylvania.

Domonokos, A. N. (1971). "Andrew's Diseases of the Skin: Clinical Dermatology." Saunders, Philadelphia, Pennsylvania.

Donaldson, J. F. (1971). Changes in African disease patterns with western acculturation. *Cent. Afr. J. Med.* **17,** 51-54.

Dunlop, D. W. (1975). Alternatives to modern health delivery systems in Africa: Public policy issues of traditional health systems. *Soc. Sci. Med.* **9,** 581-586.

Du Toit, B. M., ed. (1978). Introduction. *In* "Ethnicity in Modern Africa," pp. 1-16. Westview Press, Boulder, Colorado.

Evans-Pritchard, E. E. (1937). "Witchcraft, Oracles and Magic Among the Azande." Oxford Univ. Press, London and New York.

Field, M. J. (1960). "Search for Security: An Ethnopsychiatric Study of Rural Ghana." Faber & Faber, London.

Fordham, P. (1972). "The Geography of World Affairs," 3rd ed. Penguin Books, London.

Fortes, M., and Evans-Pritchard, E. E. (1940). "African Political Systems." Oxford Univ. Press, London and New York.

Frankenberg, R., and Leeson, J. (1976). Disease, illness and sickness: Social aspects of the choice of healer in a Lusaka suburb. *In* "Social Anthropology and Medicine" (J. B. Loudon, ed.), pp. 223-258. Academic Press, New York.

Frierman, S. (1979). Change in African therapeutic systems. *Soc. Sci. Med.* **13B,** 277-284.

Gann, L. H., and Duignar, P. (1972). "Africa and the World: An Introduction to the History of Sub-Saharan Africa from Antiquity to 1840." Chandler, San Francisco, California.

Gelfand, M. (1957). "The Sick African: A Clinical Study." Juta, Johannesburg.

Gillies, E. (1976). Causal criteria in African classifications of disease. *In* "Social Anthropology and Medicine" (J. B. Loudon, ed.), pp. 358-395. Academic Press, New York.

Glick, L. (1967). Medicine as an ethnographic category: The Gimi of the New Guinea highlands. *Ethnology* **6,** 31-56.

Goodgame, R. W., and Greenough, W. B. (1975). Cholera in Africa: A message for the West. *Ann. Intern. Med.* **82,** 101-106.

Gourou, P. (1966). "The Tropical World: Its Social and Economic Conditions and its Future Status" (S. H. Beaner and E. D. Laborde, transl.). Longman, New York.

Greenberg, J. H. (1966). "The Languages of Africa." Indiana Univ. Press, Bloomington.

Harley, G. W. (1970). "Native African Medicine." Frank Cuss, London.

Harrison, I. E. (1979a). Traditional healers: A neglected source of health manpower. *In* "African Therapeutic Systems" (Z. A. Ademuwagun, J. A. A. Ayoade, I. E. Harrison, and D. M. Warren, eds.), pp. 197-201. Crossroads Press, New York.

Harrison, I. E. (1979b). Traditional healers as a source of traditional and contemporary powers. *In* "African Therapeutic Systems" (Z. A. Ademuwagun, J. A. A. Ayoade, I. E. Harrison, and D. M. Warren, eds.), pp. 95-97. Crossroads Press, New York.

Hartwig, G. W., and Patterson, K. D., eds. (1978). "Disease in African History: An Introductory Survey and Case Studies." Duke Univ. Press, Durham, North Carolina.

Hawking, F. (1976). African trypanosomiasis. *In* "Tropical Medicine" (G. W. Hunter, J. C. Swartzwelder, and D. F. Clyde, eds.), pp. 430-439. Saunders, Philadelphia, Pennsylvania.

Herskovits, M. J. (1962). "The Human Factor in Changing Africa." Knopf, New York.

Hiernaux, J. (1966). The peoples of Africa from 22°N to the equator: Current knowledge and suggestions for future research. *In* "The Biology of Human Adaptability" (P. T. Baker and J. S. Weiner, eds.), pp. 91-110. Oxford Univ. Press (Clarendon), London and New York.

Hiernaux, J. (1975). "The People of Africa." Scribner's, New York.

Hiernaux, J. (1977). Long-term biological effects of human migration from the African savanna to the equatorial forest: A case study of human adaptation to a hot and wet climate. *In* "Human Variation" (G. A. Harrison, ed.), pp. 187-218. Cambridge Univ. Press, London and New York.

Hughes, C. C. (1959). Public health in non-literate societies. *In* "Man's Image in Medicine and Anthropology" (I. Gladston, ed.), pp. 157–236. Interantional Univ. Press, New York.

Hughes, C. C., and Hunter, J. M. (1970). Disease and development in Africa. *Soc. Sci. Med.* **3**, 443–493.

Hunter, G. W., Swartzwelder, J. C., and Clyde, D. F. (1976). The schistosomes. *In* "Tropical Medicine" (G. W. Hunter, J. C. Swartzwelder, and D. F. Clyde, eds.), pp. 543–568. Saunders, Philadelphia, Pennsylvania.

Imperato, P. J. (1974). Cholera in Mali and popular reactions to its first appearance. *J. Trop. Med. Hyg.* **77**, 290–296.

Janzen, J. M. (1979). Pluralistic legitimation of therapy systems in contemporary Zaire. *In* "African Therapeutic Systems" (Z. A. Ademuwagun, J. A. A. Ayoade, I. E. Harrison, and D. M. Warren, eds.), pp. 208–216. Crossroads Press, New York.

Jelliffe, D. B., and Bennett, F. J. (1960). Indigenous medical systems and child health. *J. Pediatr.* **57**, 248–261.

Kabamba, N., Makwala, M. B., Franklin, R. R., Rico-Velasco, J., Carter, J., and Bertrand, W. (1978). "Department of Health Investigation of Nutritional Consequences of the Drought in Bas-Zaire," Rep. No. VIII. Zaire Nutr. Plann. Cent.

Keen, P. (1975). The epidemiology of cancer in Africans in southern Africa. *S. Afr. J. Surg.* **13**, 105–114.

Kloppens, P. J., and Fehrsen, G. S. (1977). Western diseases in developing peoples: In search of a marker. *S. Afr. Med. J.* **51**, 745–746.

Last, M. (1976). The presentation of sickness in a community of non-Muslim Hausa. *In* "Social Anthropology and Medicine" (J. B. Loudon, ed.), pp. 104–149. Academic Press, New York.

Lehman, H., Huntsman, R. G., Casey, R., Lang, A., and Lorkin, P. A. (1977). Sickle cell disease and related disorders. *In* "Hematology" (J. W. Williams, E. Beutler, A. J. Erslev, and R. W. Rudles, eds.), 2nd ed., pp. 495–523. McGraw-Hill, New York.

Lightman, S. (1977). The responsibilities of intervention in isolated societies. *In* "Health and Disease in Tribal Societies," Ciba Foundation Symposium, No. 49, pp. 303–313. Elsevier, Amsterdam.

Linsell, D. A., and Higgins, J. (1976). The geographic pathology of liver cell cancer. *In* "Liver Cell Cancer" (H. M. Cameron, D. A. Linsell, and G. P. Warwick, eds.), pp. 1–16. Elsevier, Amsterdam.

Little, K. (1957). The role of voluntary associations in West African urbanization. *Am. Anthropol.* **59**, 579–596.

Livingstone, F. B. (1958). Anthropological implications of the sickle cell gene distribution in Africa. *Am. Anthropol.* **60**, 553–557.

Livingstone, F. B.(1967). "Abnormal Hemoglobins in Human Populations: A Summary and Interpretation." Aldine, Chicago, Illinois.

Livingstone, F. B. (1971). Malaria and human polymorphisms. *Annu. Rev. Genet.* **5**, 33–64.

Livingstone, F. B. (1976). Hemoglobin history in West Africa. *Hum. Biol.* **48**, 487–500.

Lythcott, G. I., Sinnette, C. H., and Hopkins, D. R. (1975). Pediatrics. *In* "Textbook of Black-Related Diseases" (R. A. Williams, ed.), pp. 129–298. McGraw-Hill, New York.

McDonald, J. C., and Kelly, A. P. (1975). Dermatology and venereology. *In* "Textbook of Black-Related Diseases" (R. A. Williams, ed.), pp. 513–592. McGraw-Hill, New York.

McKhobo, K. P. (1976). Herb use and necrodegenerative hepatitis. *S. Afr. Med. J.* **50**, 1096–109.

Mann, G. V., Roels, O. A., Price, D. L., and Merrill, J. M. (1962). Cardiovascular disease in African Pygmies. *J. Chronic Dis.* **15**, 341–371.

Mann, G. V., Shaffer, R. D., Anderson, R. S., and Sanstead, H. H. (1964). Cardiovascular disease in the Masai. *J. Atheroscler. Res.* **4**, 289–342.

Maquet, J. (1972). "Africanity: The Cultural Unity of Black Africa" (J. R. Rayfield, transl.). Oxford Univ. Press, London and New York.

Montagu, M. F. A. (1960). "An Introduction to Physical Anthropology." Thomas, Springfield, Illinois.

Morley, D. (1973). "Paediatric Priorities in the Developing World." Butterworth, London.

Morley, D. (1976). Measles and whooping cough. In "Epidemiology and Community Health in Warm Climate Countries" (R. Cruickshank, K. L. Standard, and H. B. L. Russell, eds.), pp. 63–76. Churchill-Livingstone, Edinburgh.

Morris, D. M. (1979). "Measuring the Condition of the World's Poor," Pergamon Policy Studies. Pergamon, New York.

Mourant, A. E., Kopec, A. C., and Domaniewski-Sabezak, K. (1976). "The Distribution of the Human Blood Groups and Other Polymorphisms," 2nd ed. Oxford Univ. Press, London and New York.

Murdock, G. P. (1959). "Africa: Its People and Their Culture History." McGraw-Hill, New York.

Murray, R. F. (1975). Medical genetics and black-related diseases. In "Textbook of Black-Related Diseases" (R. A. Williams, ed.), pp. 31–98. McGraw-Hill, New York.

Ngubane, H. (1976). Some aspects of treatment among the Zulu. In "Social Anthropology and Medicine" (J. B. Loudon, ed.), pp. 318–357. Academic Press, New York.

Oettle, A. G. (1962). Geographical and racial differences in the frequency of Kaposi's sarcoma as evidence of environmental or genetic causes. Acta Unio Int. Contra Cancrum 18, 330–363.

Okoro, A. N. (1975). Albinism in Nigeria: A clinical and social study. Br. J. Dermatol. 92, 485–492.

Oluwasanmi, J. O. (1974). Keloids in the African. Clin. Plast. Surg. 1, 179–195.

Owusu, M. (1978). Ethnography of Africa: The usefulness of the useless. Am. Anthropol. 80, 310–334.

Patterson, K. D. (1979). Health in urban Ghana: The case of Acra. Soc. Sci. Med. 13B, 251–268.

Pierce, N. R., and Hirschhorn (1977). Oral-fluid—A simple weapon against dehydration in diarrhea. WHO Chron. 31, 87–93.

Piliszek, T. S. (1979). Hb Bart's and its significance in the South African Negro. Acta Haematol. 60, 33–38.

Polunin, I. V. (1977). Some characteristics of tribal peoples. In "Health and Disease in Tribal Societies," Ciba Foundation Symposium, No. 49, pp. 5–19. Elsevier, Amsterdam.

Press, I. (1980). Problems in the definition and classification of medical systems. Soc. Sci. Med. 14B, 45–57.

Price-Williams, D. R. (1962). A case study of ideas concerning disease among the Tiv. Africa 32, 123–131.

Reminick, R. A. (1974). The evil eye belief among the Amhara of Ethiopa. Ethnology 13, 279–291.

Robbins, S. L., and Cotran, R. S. (1979). "Pathologic Basis of Disease," 2nd ed. Saunders, Philadelphia, Pennsylvania.

Roles, N. C. (1966). Tribal surgery in East Africa during the XIX century, Part I, Ritual operations. East Afr. Med. J. 43, 577–594.

Rose, E. F. (1967). A study of esophageal cancer of the Transkei. In "Symposium on Tumors of the Alimentary Tract in Africans" (J. F. Murray, ed.), Monogr. No. 25, pp. 83–96. Natl. Cancer Inst., Bethesda, Maryland.

Schmauz, R., and Templeton, A. C. (1972). Nasopharyngeal carcinoma in Uganda. Cancer (Philadelphia) 29, 610–621.

Scotch, N. (1963). Sociocultural factors in the epidemiology of Zulu hypertension. Am. J. Public Health 53, 1205–1213.

Seftel, H. C. (1977). Diseases in urban and rural black populations. S. Afr. Med. J. 51, 121–123.

Seligman, C. G. (1966). "Races of Africa." Oxford Univ. Press, London and New York.

Ssebabi, E. C. T. (1975). Characteristics of African blood. *CRC Crit. Rev. Clin. Lab. Sci.* **6,** 19–45.

Stamler, J., Stamler, R., and Pullman, T. N., eds. (1967). "The Epidemiology of Hypertension." Grune & Stratton, New York.

Swartz, M. L. (1979). Community and healing among the Zarano in Tanzania. *Soc. Sci. Med.* **13B,** 169–173.

Taylor, J. F., Smith, P. G., Bull, D., and Pike, M. C. (1972). Kaposi's sarcoma in Uganda: Geographical and ethnic distribution. *Br. J. Cancer* **26,** 483–497.

Tobias, P. (1966). The peoples of Africa south of the Sahara. *In* "The Biology of Human Adaptability" (P. Baker and J. S. Weiner, eds.), pp. 111–200. Oxford Univ. Press (Clarendon), London and New York.

Truswell, A. S., and Hansen, J. D. L. (1976). Medical research among the !Kung. *In* "Kalahari Hunter–Gatherers" (R. B. Lee and I. Devore, eds.), pp. 166–194. Harvard Univ. Press, Cambridge, Massachusetts.

Turnbull, C. M. (1977). "Man in Africa." Anchor/Doubleday, Garden City, New York.

Turner, V. (1964). An Ndembu doctor in practice. *In* "Magic, Faith, and Healing" (A. Kiev, ed.), pp. 230–263. Free Press, New York.

Vaughn, J. P. (1977). A brief review of cardiovascular disease in Africa. *Trans. R. Soc. Trop. Med. Hyg.* **71,** 226–231.

Wapnick, S., Zanamwe, L. N. D., Chitigo, M., and Mynors, J. M. (1972). Cancer in the esophagus in Central Africa. *Chest* **61,** 649–654.

Warren, D. M. (1979). The role of emic analysis in medical anthropology. *In* "African Therapeutic Systems" (Z. A. Ademuwagun, J. A. A. Ayoade, I. E. Harrison, and D. M. Warren, eds.), pp. 36–42. Crossroads Press, New York.

Weatherall, D. M. (1977). The thalassemias. *In* "Hematology" (J. W. Williams, E. Beutler, A. J. Erslev, and R. W. Rudles, eds.), 2nd ed., pp. 291–412. McGraw-Hill, New York.

Weisz, J. R. (1972). East African medical systems. *Soc. Sci. Med.* **6,** 323–333.

Welch, S. G., McGregor, I. A., and Williams, K. (1977). The Duffy Blood Group and malaria prevalence in Gambian West Africa. *Trans. R. Soc. Trop. Med. Hyg.* **71,** 295–296.

Wilkinson, J. (1957). The influence of heredity and environment upon disease amongst the Kikuyu people. *East Afr. Med. J.* **34,** 627–642.

Williams, C. D., and Jelliffe, D. B. (1972). "Mother and Child Health, Delivering the Services." Oxford Univ. Press, London and New York.

Wilson, H. S. (1977). "The Imperial Experience in Sub-Saharan Africa Since 1870." Univ. of Minnesota Press, Minneapolis.

Wintrobe, M. M., Lee, G. R., Boggs, D. R., Bithell, T. C., Athens, J. W., and Foerester, J. (1974). "Clinical Hematology." Lea & Febiger, Philadelphia, Pennsylvania.

World Bank (1980). "Annex. World Development Indicators." World Bank, Washington, D.C.

World Health Organization (1977). "World Health Statistics Annual, Vol. II, Infectious Diseases: Cases and Deaths." WHO, Geneva.

World Health Organization (1979). "World Health Statistics Annual, Infectious Diseases: Cases." WHO, Geneva.

Young, M. D. (1976). Malaria. *In* "Tropical Medicine" (G. W. Hunter, J. C. Swartzwelder, and D. F. Clyde, eds.), 5th ed., pp. 353–393. Saunders, Philadelphia, Pennsylvania.

16
Diseases of the Jews

HENRY ROTHSCHILD

I. ORIGINS

The history of the Jewish people dates back over 3500 years (Sachar, 1964). Out of a cluster of small nomadic tribes of hunters and farmers who had become a nation settling in Canaan, they subsequently dispersed over the entire globe. In modern times some Jews have been assimilated into the indigenous cultures and societies of many countries, others have maintained loose and informal associations within their nationality, some have remained in tightly knit groups, and still others have created a new Jewish culture in Israel. Although no longer a specific designator, the Jewish religion, a system of monotheistic worship, accompanied by a moral code or guide for ethical living that is an integral part of the faith, historically determined who was a "Jew." Now the spectrum of that religion's acceptance ranges from orthodox to reformed. The Jewish people are as physically, mentally, and emotionally diverse as any other people on earth; most Jews would be classified as Caucasian, but some are Negroid or Oriental. Con-

BIOCULTURAL ASPECTS OF DISEASE
Copyright © 1981 by Academic Press, Inc.

sequently, today confusion and diversity of opinion exist as to whether the approximately 14 million Jews should be recognized as a race, as an ethnic group, or even as more than one group of people.

A brief description of their origins may help to explain their classification into primarily three distinct major subgroups, the Ashkenazic, the Sephardic, and the Oriental Jews (Darlington, 1969), and the association of certain diseases with these subgroups.

According to biblical legend, the twelve tribes of Israel represent the descendants of the twelve sons of Jacob. The tribes, which had been united under David and Solomon, separated after the latter's death into the kingdoms of Judea (the tribes of Judah and Benjamin) and Israel (the other ten tribes). After the conquest of the kingdoms of Judea in 721 BC and Israel in 586 BC, a large number of inhabitants were deported to Assyria and Babylon. This event marked the beginning of the Diaspora, or Dispersion, of the Jewish people. The two kingdoms remained separated, and probably did not mix, at least not intentionally, until 538 BC when Cyrus, king of the Medes and Persians, after having conquered Assyria and Babylon, permitted the Jews to return to Palestine.

Not all Jews returned to their homeland, however, and the Jewish communities of Asia Minor, Iraq, Turkey, and Iran are generally believed to include descendants of the exile. Today, their descendants and those who remained in India and Yemen form one of the three major subgroups of Judaism and are often referred to as "Oriental" Jews. Iraq, having the largest Oriental Jewish community, dating back about 2500 years, provided the scholastic center of Judaism until about 1000 AD. The Oriental Jews appear to have a distinctive genetic constitution with disease problems that differ not only from those of the main body of world Jewry, but also among themselves. Unlike the other two major subgroups, they do not have a distinct language, their primary languages having been Persian, Arabic, and Judeo-Arabic.

In pre-Islamic times Jews often dominated the political and cultural life of Arabian principalities such as the kingdom of Yemen, which was mainly under Jewish rule from 200 to 460 AD (Mourant et al., 1978). Apparently the whole of the Jewish communities of Yemen and Habban of the Arabian Peninsula have emigrated to Israel; the former now constitutes one of the largest ethnic communities in Israel, whereas the latter constitutes only about 350 persons. An interesting feature of the Oriental Jews is their high rate of consanguinity. The "Black Jews" of Cochin, India, numbering about 2000, have a rate of consanguinity estimated at about 40% (Cohen and Bloch, 1963).

During the period of the Second Temple in Jerusalem (516 BC), groups of Jews emigrated to cultural centers around the Mediterranean, such as Alexandria and Rome. The beginning of the final Dispersion followed the destruction of Jerusalem and the Second Temple by Titus' Roman soldiers in 70 AD. After the revolt of Bar Kochba from 132 to 135 AD, the Jews were dispersed to various parts of the Roman Empire.

Although they first developed into a distinct subgroup in medieval Poland and Lithuania, the Jews who descended from the tribes of Judah and Benjamin and initially settled Western Europe formed the second major subgroup of modern Judaism, the Ashkenazim—the Hebrew word for German. In the early decades of the third century, Jewish tradesman followed Roman legions and settled in towns along the Rhine Valley. Charlemagne, who ruled France, Germany, and northern Italy at the end of the eighth century, promoted the Dispersion by encouraging the settlement of Jews in France and the Rhineland.

By the time of the Crusades (1096 AD) and the intensified discrimination against Jews of that period, from 100,000 to 250,000 Jews (Neel, 1979) had settled in communities all over western and central Europe. By the middle of the fourteenth century the migration to eastern Europe had begun.

The history of the Ashkenazim has been one of large-scale migrations, re-peated expulsions, and decimations. For example, the Jewish population of Poland was decimated from more than 500,000 to fewer than 100,000 in the seventeenth century, primarily because of the Cossack massacres of 1648.

During the nineteenth century, this subgroup flourished both numerically and culturally, especially in an area of eastern Europe known as the Pale, an area that extended from the Austro-Hungarian border to the western parts of Russia. This area became the largest Jewish community during the first half of the twentieth century.

From the Medieval period until after the French Revolution, the Ashkenazic Jews existed as a distinct ethnic group, despite their lack of a homeland. Often they were recognized as an *imperium in imperio,* a state within a state, and were granted a significant degree of autonomy, many times as a form of apartheid. A vestige of this status still exists in the Soviet Union, which recognizes Jews as one of its constituent nationalities, although at the same time practicing an-tisemitism as a state policy in the guise of anti-Zionism.

Apart from the religion itself, a common language, Yiddish, unwritten until the beginning of the nineteenth century, was the main unifying feature of the Ashkenazic Jews. It is low German from the Rhineland, with touches of Old French, Italian, and several Slovic tongues, and spiced with Hebrew-Aramaic.

Descendants of the Ashkenazim have emigrated to North, Central, and South America, South Africa, Australia, and Israel. Whereas eastern Europe and Ger-many were originally the hub of Ashkenazim, the United States and Israel be-came the centers of this subgroup after the holocaust of World War II. There are now about 11.5 million Ashkenazim, half of whom live in the United States. About 2.5 million remain in the Soviet Union, 1.1 million in the rest of Europe, and 1.4 million in Israel (Adam, 1973).

Other Jews whose ancestors lived in the countries around the Mediterranean constitute the third major subgroup of modern Jewry, the Sephardim, a term derived from the Hebrew word for sunset or Spain. Their history dates back more than 2000 years, their ancestors having lived in the coastal plains of Palestine and in Galilee in the late biblical and early Christian era. After the fifth century, when the Roman Empire collapsed and was unable to defend the region against attacks by nomadic raiders, the ancestors of this group migrated to Asia Minor and along the Mediterranean, where they found refuge with and support from Jews who had previously settled there. They probably moved to Spain after its conquest by the Arabs (740 AD). Most of the descendants remained for centuries around the Mediterranean, where they prospered, especially as administrators and physicians, until the Christians recaptured Spain. Toward the end of the fifteenth century, a considerable number who were driven out of Spain and Portugal by the Inquisition settled in Turkey, the Balkans, North Africa (including Morocco and Libya), Italy, Holland, and England. More than half of the present-day Sephardim, who number about 1.5 million, live in Israel, whereas the majority of Ashkenazim live elsewhere. About 200,000 Sephardim reside in the United States. They share a common language, Ladino, a form of ancient Castillian Spanish written in Hebrew characters.

Several minor subgroups that are not included in the three major subgroups contribute to the population that may be considered the Jewish people. The Karaites, a sect that accepts only the Old Testament as the source of religious authority, but rejects the later interpretative literature and traditions accepted by most other Jewish communities, was founded in the eighth century in Babylon and later spread to Egypt, Morocco, Spain, Israel, and even the Soviet Union. They number about 10,000 (Goldschmidt *et al.*, 1976).

The Samaritans, the only biblical group that has continuously remained *in situ*, now divide into two subgroups living in the same general geographic area, Jordan and Israel. The Samaritan tradition, an offshoot of the Jewish religion, split from the mainstream of Judaism in 500 BC over the question of the location of the temple and other conflicts. From a nation consisting initially of several hundred thousands, the Samaritans gradually became a small sect, decreasing to a minimum of 150 at the end of the nineteenth century and now numbering about 300 persons. Despite this reduction in numbers, from a few centuries BC to present they remained strictly endogamous.

Many other Jewish splinter groups exist in Africa, the Balkans, and other places, although their biological relationship to the biblical Jews is tenuous.

The recent demographics of the Jewish populations of Israel are reviewed by Bonne-Tamir *et al.* (1979).

II. GENETIC POLYMORPHISMS

Populations may be described by their gene pools, i.e., the total number of alleles distributed among the members of an interbreeding group and differentiated in allele frequencies at single structural loci. Originally, physical anthropological structures and simple genetic traits were used as genetic markers to provide data about the drift, selection, and gene flow within and across the ethnic boundaries. Now, polymorphic blood groups, serum and cell proteins, enzyme variants that have altered catalytic activity, kinetic properties, stability, or electrophoretic mobility are used.

Genes that are selectively neutral, e.g., haptoglobin, probably give evidence of remote history and a common heritage of the bearers, whereas those that are subject to selective pressure give evidence of recent history. This subject has been reviewed in an excellent book by Mourant *et al.* (1978), from which I have drawn extensively.

Genetic differentiation among the Jewish subgroups is reflected in the gene frequencies at many loci governing the genetic polymorphisms. Gene frequencies for many polymorphic systems have been established in the Jews as a group, and the findings in the subgroups have been compared.

Because of the uncertainties concerning the original gene frequencies, computing genetic flow is difficult. Today, probably no Jewish group's gene frequencies, except possibly those of the Samaritans, even approximate the original frequencies among the ancient Jews. Because of their small number, the Samaritans must have been considerably affected by drift and thus do not provide the base for a valid estimate of gene flow.

Although historically relatively few converts were accepted into the Jewish fold, there have been exceptions. Koestler (1976) theorized that the Ashkenazim are genetically derived almost entirely from the Khazars, a Turkish tribe in the lower Volga region that converted almost en masse in 740 AD. Subsequent blood group data, however, do not support that theory (Mourant *et al.*, 1978), although the Karaites and Krimchaks (Orthodox Jews of the Crimea) may be descendants of the Khazars.

Another deterrent to gene flow was religious precepts. Among the tenets of Judaism is a strong stricture against intermarriage. The migrating groups of Jews, even those in the United States, tended to remain reproductively isolated from the rest of the population, at least in the first generation after immigration.

Some gene flow, however, is probably always present, even among groups that try to remain isolated. A notable exception to this generalization was the Jewish ghetto in Rome. Between 1554 and 1870, Jews were virtually sealed off from the rest of Italy and probably maintained a high degree of endogamy with little if any gene flow occurring into or out of that ghetto. As a result of that isolation, the blood group frequencies of present-day Roman Jews differ from those of the other populations of Italy. For instance, the frequency of the B allele among them is 27%, whereas in no other group on the Italian mainland does it rise above 11%.

In general, although Jews may have not only cultural but also some physical differences from their neighbors, and although some genetic uniformity exists among the major Jewish subgroups, gene frequencies in Jewish populations tend to be similar to those among the non-Jews inhabiting the same geographic region. The frequencies of the ABO, MN blood group genes in Jews of any given area are similar to those of non-Jews of that area, whereas Jews from other areas differ in their ABO and MN frequencies (Patai Wing, 1974). Yemenite Jews, unlike other "Oriental" Jews, are low in A and B, and high in O blood groups, as are Yemenite Arabs, whereas Cochin Jews are reasonably high in A and B, as are the Cochin Hindus. The Kurdish Jews of Iran show a scatter of gene frequencies but are similar to non-Jewish Kurds. The Jews whose ancestors lived in Russia, Poland, France, and Germany for perhaps as long as 2000 years show some effect of local population on their genetic-marker frequencies (Mourant *et al.*, 1978); that suggests gene flow or an environmentally caused equilibrium polymorphism that both Jews and non-Jews have reached at each location.

Patai and Patai Wing (1975) concluded that interbreeding and conversion had a considerable impact on the Jewish gene pool. Whereas Karlin *et al.* (1979) concluded that the flow has been largely from Jewish to non-Jewish, Szeinberg (1979) concluded that the contribution of non-Jews to the Jewish gene pool has been small.

Differing gene frequencies demonstrate the high degree of genetic variability among the various Jewish subgroups. For example, the frequency of the glucose-6-phosphate dehydrogenase (G6PD) deficiency varies among the Israelis of different geographic origins. Szeinberg (1963) found the frequency of G6PD deficiency in Ashkenazim to be extremely rare (0.4%), a frequency similar to that of other European populations who have not lived in malarial environments. The frequency in Sephardic Jews was about 2%, whereas among Iraqi Jews it was 25%, and among Kurdish Jews, 60%.

Although the gene frequencies of Jews from different parts of the world vary widely, some frequencies may indicate the persistence of a common heritage. In the Rh system, Ashkenazic and Sephardic Jews have a relatively high frequency of the cDe compared with that of non-Jews of the same region (Mourant, 1959). The higher frequency of the typically African rhesus genotype was presumably acquired by the Jews through admixture during their prolonged sojourn in Egypt. Also, adenylate kinase, acid phosphatase, haptoglobulin, and some of the HLA haplotype frequencies have suggested a common ancestry for the Jewish people. Perhaps these polymorphisms have been subject to less selective pressure and thus better reflect the history of the Jews.

III. DISEASES PREVALENT AMONG JEWS

Since biblical times, many diseases have been considered unique to the Jews. Physicians began to write about the increased prevalence of certain diseases among Ashkenazim as early as the eighteenth century (Friedenwald, 1967).

A. Altered Frequency Attributable to Custom

The increased or decreased prevalence of several diseases may be attributable to religious practices and customs. Public health measures may have been incorporated into the formal religion, accounting for some of the increased or decreased prevalence. Biblical and Talmudic precepts (the authoritative collection of Jewish oral tradition), including sanitation, personal hygiene, dietary laws, and social relations, may still play a role in disease prevention among Jews, especially in underdeveloped countries.

Alcoholism has been reported to be less frequent in several ethnic groups including Jews, but alcoholism appears to be on the rise in acculturated Jews (Snyder, 1979). The lesser frequency of alcoholism has been postulated as possibly due to genetic factors (Schuckit et al., 1972). Although this possibility cannot be eliminated completely, the most probable explanation is sociocultural.

The religious custom of circumcision appears to play a role in cancer prevention. Representing the fulfillment of the covenant between God and Israel, circumcision has such profound religious significance that Jews refused to relinquish the rite even under the threat of death during the conquest by the Greeks and later by the Romans. When Antiochus tried to prevent the practice, mothers allowed themselves to be put to death rather than to give up circumcision of their sons. This religious ritual is thought by many to be the reason for the low incidence of not only cancer of the glans penis among Jewish men, but also cancer of the cervix among Jewish women. This viewpoint is supported by a ten-city survey of the incidence of cancer of the cervix—the reported 1977 rate in American white women being 32.2/100,000, in American nonwhite women, 51.2/100,000 and among Israeli and American Jewish women in the United States, 2.2/100,000 (Sharon et al., 1977). Although cancer of the cervix is not uncommon among some circumcised groups, in India genital cancer is much more frequent among the Hindus than among the Moslems, who practice circumcision as a ritual of puberty. Furthermore, nuns and virginal women also have a decreased incidence of cervical cancer.

An example of local custom affecting disease prevalence is Creutzfeldt–Jakob disease. A progressive, dementia-producing central nervous system disease of middle life, it has an unusually high incidence among Jews of Libyan origin in Israel. Although the disease has a worldwide distribution, its incidence varies widely among Jews of different origin living in Israel. Jews from western and central Europe and native-born Israelis have an incidence of only 1.0/million, an incidence similar to that worldwide. In contrast, Libyan Jews have a remarkably high incidence (31.3/million) (Kahana et al., 1974).

The prevalence of the disease may be related to the custom among Bedouin and Moroccan Arabs of eating sheep's eyeballs and brains, considered gastronomic delicacies (Alter, 1978). This custom, shared by Libyan Jews, may play a role in causing the high incidence of Creutzfeldt–Jakob disease in these ethnic groups.

Thus, the ingestion of brains or eyes from animals such as sheep infected with scrapie virus may lead to the zoonotic transmission of the suspected causative agent to humans (Gajdusek, 1978).

B. Genetic Diseases

Although the genetic diseases of most other ethnic groups have been studied only limitedly, the genetic diseases affecting various subgroups of Jews, especially those of the Ashkenazim, have been studied and written about extensively. The literature of the genetic diseases among the Jews has been reviewed comprehensively in numerous articles and in three recent books (Mourant *et al.*, 1978; Goodman, 1979; Goodman and Motulsky, 1979). These excellent works have been major sources for the brief reviews of the diseases discussed in this section.

Most genetic diseases that preponderantly affect Jews are transmitted as autosomal recessive genes. One contributing factor appears to be consanguineous marriages. Religious law forbids certain types of marriages, such as intermarriage with all other groups. Other laws and customs have encouraged marriage between certain relatives. Jewish law decrees, for example, that if a man dies childless, his brother, if unwed, must marry the widow. Custom extended this injunction to the nearest kinsman no matter how distantly related. A meritorious marriage among Ashkenazim was between an uncle and niece. Some of these customs are still practiced among certain groups in Israel and may account also for the high incidence of congenital malformations, which is the third leading cause of infant death in Israel.

Several hypotheses have been postulated to explain why some of the rarer genetic diseases are more frequent in Jewish subgroups than in the other subgroups or other ethnic groups. Some have postulated that certain alleles are more common in a Jewish population due to selective advantage. Others have postulated a founder effect with subsequent genetic drift. The unique history and mating patterns of the Jews may have allowed some mutations to be expressed more frequently in these ethnic subgroups than in others. Many factors, including selection, gene flow, mutation, size, and breeding patterns may also account for genetic diversity in various Jewish subgroups.

A few diseases occur in more than one of the subgroups, but most are limited to one. Lactase deficiency has been reported in all three major Jewish subgroups. Brachydactyly type D, or stub thumb, a disorder determined by an autosomal dominant gene, has been reported to have a high frequency in both Ashkenazic and Sephardic Jews.

C. Genetic Diseases of Ashkenazic Jews

Of the genetic diseases shown to have an unusually high incidence among Ashkenazim, all but the Gilles de la Tourette syndrome are recessively inherited diseases. The following list is far from complete.

1. Abetalipoproteinemia

The clinical features of abetalipoproteinemia, also referred to as Bassen–Kornzweig syndrome, include steatorrhea, pigmentary degeneration of the retina, and a peculiar "burr-cell" malformation of red blood cells called acanthocytosis (Bassen and Kornzweig, 1950). Defective intestinal absorption of lipids resulting in steatorrhea and abdominal distention begins in infancy. Neurological manifestations are characterized by ataxia, dysarthria, muscle weakness, abnormal reflexes, and sensory deficits, but no cerebral abnormalities.

Autopsy and biopsy of the intestinal mucosa show the cytoplasm of the cells to be foamy and vacuolated. The peripheral nerves, posterior columns, spinocerebellar tracts, and the cerebellum show extensive demyelination. Serum cholesterol levels are low and serum chylomicrons and β-lipoproteins (low-density lipoproteins) are absent. The basic defect is unknown, and whether all the patients examined have the same biochemical defect has not been established. Lees (1967) demonstrated that the lipid-free apoprotein of β-lipoprotein is present in abetalipoproteinemia, suggesting a defect in the formation of the complete macromolecule. Gotto *et al.* (1971), however, later showed that both low-density lipoprotein and its principal protein component, apo LP-Ser, were absent in a patient with abetalipoproteinemia.

Of the fewer than 50 cases described, about 25% have been in Ashkenazic Jews, but the disease has also been reported in several other ethnic groups. Consanguinity is common in the non-Jewish parents.

2. Bloom's Syndrome

First described by Bloom (1954), this syndrome is characterized by dwarfism, typical thin facies with a relatively large nose, dolichocephaly, spotty hypopigmentation and hyperpigmentation, telangiectatic lesions of the face, and clinodactyly. Intelligence appears to be normal. Exposure to sunlight exacerbates the skin lesions and may also affect other exposed parts of the body. The disease occurs more commonly in males. Decreased immunoglobulins result in frequent infections. The life span is shortened; the mean life expectancy among affected persons is about 16 years. Chromosomal breakage and rearrangement, often with abnormal nuclear morphology and sister chromatid exchanges, are unusually frequent. The cytogenetic abnormalities may be a useful cytologic marker for the diagnosis, including the prenatal diagnosis of the syndrome. The frequency of sister-chromatid exchanges is not abnormal in heterozygotes (German *et al.*, 1977). A predisposition to leukemia and, to a lesser extent, to other cancers has been reported. The basic biochemical defect is unknown; no deficiency in a DNA repair enzyme has been found, although an enzyme required for DNA synthesis and for the repair of ultraviolet-induced damage has been suggested by Giannelli *et al.* (1977).

Although fewer than 100 cases have been reported, about half of those cases affected Jews who had originated from southeastern Poland and southwestern Ukraine (German *et al.*, 1979). It has also been observed in other ethnic groups such as Japanese, blacks, and Turks. Consanguinity is low in Jewish families and high in affected non-Jewish families. The incidence in Ashkenazic Jews has been estimated to be about 1:161,000, with a carrier rate of about 1 in 120.

3. Dysautonomia

First described by Riley *et al.* (1949), dysautonomia is also known as Riley–Day syndrome. It is characterized by autonomic instability and impaired perception of pain, temperature, and taste. Patients have characteristic facies with wide mouth, difficulty in feeding and swallowing during infancy, absence of overflow tears, skin blotching, excessive perspiration, breath-holding attacks, emotional lability, episodic vomiting, hyporeflexia, and motor incoordination. Symptoms often include postural hypotension and scoliosis. Affected persons have diminished or absent tendon reflexes, ataxia, pathognomonic lack of fungiform papillae on the tongue and taste buds, and loss of histamine flare response (Axelrod *et al.*, 1974). There appears to be no intellectual impairment (Welton *et al.*, 1979). About 50% of those affected die by the age of 20 years, most of them of pulmonary infection. Pathological characteristics are demyelination of the medulla, pontine reticular formation, and dorso-longitudinal tracts, and degeneration, pigmentation, and loss of cells in autonomic ganglia.

Weinshilboum and Axelrod (1971) reported a decreased level of dopamine-β-hydroxylase, the enzyme that converts dopamine to norepinephrine, resulting in a decreased excretion of vanilylmandelic acid and its precursors and an increased excretion of homovanillic acid, a urinary metabolite of dopamine.

Siggers *et al.* (1976) reported finding a lack of large-calibre myelinated axons, no myelinated axons of the sural nerve, and a threefold increase in serum nerve-growth factor. Levi-Montalcini (1976) described an elevation in the β fraction of nerve growth factor in patients with this disease.

Although rare cases have been reported in non-Jews, most cases have been found among persons of Ashkenazic descent, especially among those originating from southeastern Central Europe around Galicia. The clustering of ancestors similar to that of Tay–Sachs disease suggested a founder effect to Brunt and McKusick (1970). The incidence is between 1 in 10,000 and 1 in 20,000 Ashkenazim live births, with an estimated gene frequency of 1:100 to 1:140.

4. Dystonia Musculorum Deformans

Also known as torsion dystonia, dystonia musculorum deformans comprises a group of genetically heterogeneous disorders of the central nervous system characterized by irregular sustained grotesque twisting movements of the trunk and extremities. In the form of the disease found in Jews, symptoms begin between the ages of 4 and 16 years, usually in the hand or foot on the dominant side, preceded by a period of normal neurological and intellectual development. It may quickly progress to involve all limbs and to a lesser degree the axial musculature. The progression of symptoms may slow down or the symptoms may actually improve after adolescence. The degree of involvement varies in affected persons. Similar involuntary movements can be produced by administration of dopamine receptor blocking agents. Abnormal asymmetrical postures result in great distortion of the ankles, hands, and spine. The disorder is not accompanied by dementia or other organ system disease but may be accompanied by superior intelligence and emotional stability (Eldridge, 1970).

Grossman and Kelly (1976) found evidence of atrophy of the basal ganglia. However, no distinctive histopathological or biochemical abnormalities have been identified.

Autosomal dominant, autosomal recessive, and X-linked forms of the disease have been described, as have some nongenetic cases due to such primary causes as vascular diseases or neoplasms. Only the autosomal recessive form, which differs from the autosomal dominant form in earlier onset and greater severity, has a higher incidence in Ashkenazim, but it also occurs in Sephardic and Oriental Jews (Alter *et al.,* 1976). Both Oppenheim (1911) and Mendel (1919), in the early decades of this century, called attention to the frequent Russian–Jewish ancestry of patients with this disease. Half of the reported cases occurred in non-Jews. Consanguinity appears to be important in the non-Jewish cases (Eldridge and Koerber, 1979). Eldridge and Gottlieb (1976) estimated that the incidence is about 1:17,000 in Ashkenazim and that about 1 in every 65 Ashkenazim carries the gene.

5. Glycosphingolipidoses

Three autosomal recessive metabolic defects due to lysosomal hydrolases have been reported to have an increased frequency in Ashkenazic Jews. The degradation of sphingolipids, which are a major lipid class in the central nervous system, where they form an essential part of the membranes, is a defect in several diseases that affect Ashkenazic Jews. The absence of a substrate-specific hydrolytic lysosomal enzyme results in accumulation of sphingolipid in the brain, nerve-ending membranes, and most extraneural tissues such as muscle, liver, and mammary glands. The fact that three biochemically related diseases occur at a relatively high frequency in one ethnic group has suggested a common selective factor to some investigators. Tuberculosis has been suggested as the selective factor for at least one of these diseases, Tay-Sachs disease (Perla and Marmorston, 1941).

a. Gaucher's Disease. About 100 years ago, Gaucher (1882) described a syndrome characterized by chronic progressive hepatosplenomegaly and other organ involvement. Subsequently, at least three forms of Gaucher's disease have been distinguished on the basis of clinical manifestations and age of onset. All three types have hepatosplenomegaly, "Gaucher cells" (20–100 μm in size, with an eccentric nucleus) in the bone marrow, and increased serum acid phosphatase activity. A rare, acute, infantile form (type 2) is characterized by development of neurological abnormalities during the first year of life, and the patient dies after a short course. With juvenile or subacute (type 3) Gaucher's disease, neurological symptoms appear later and the patients usually survive beyond 2 years. The chronic nonneuropathic or adult Gaucher's disease (type 1), the most common form of the disorder, is characterized by pingueculae, anemia, thrombocytopenia with accompanying bleeding tendency, low white blood cell count, frequent infections, bone pain and fractures (especially of the weight-bearing joints), and a peculiar pattern of yellow pigmentation on exposed skin surfaces, but usually no central nervous system involvement. X-ray findings may suggest erosion of the cortices of the long bones. This form of the disease has a wide range of clinical severity; some patients have symptoms as early as the third decade, whereas others may have symptom-free lives for seven or eight decades. Histopathologically, the presence of Gaucher cells is characteristic.

Little is known about the biochemical or genetic basis for the clinical variation among the forms of Gaucher's disease. The basic metabolic defect in all forms appears to be the same. Accumulation of glucocerebroside, primarily in lysosomes of reticuloendothelial cells, occurs probably as a result of a structural defect of the lysosomal enzyme hydrolase glucocerebrosidase (β-glucosidase), which catalyses the hydrolytic cleavage of glucocerebroside into ceramide and glucose. That enzyme also has glucosidase activity. The degree of enzyme deficiency is not related to the extent of pathology or organ involvement in the various forms of the disease. Some investigators suggested that the biochemical basis for the differential neurological involvement and rapidity of progression in the three forms of the disease result from attenuation of glucocerebrosidase activity or multiple glycosidase deficiencies (Chiao *et al.*, 1978).

Both homozygote and heterozygote can be identified by chemical analysis of fibroblasts and by thin-layer chromatography separation and gas–liquid chromatography quantitation, of the urine. Because cultured amniotic cells have glucocerebrosidase activity, they have been used to monitor the fetus at risk, and the disease has been diagnosed prenatally.

Infantile and juvenile forms and their variants appear to occur with equal frequency among various ethnic groups, but the adult form is about 30 times more common among Ashkenazic Jews (Meals, 1971) than among other populations. It is rare among Sephardic and Oriental Jews and non-Jews. The crude prevalence for the Ashkenazim is about 1:3000 to 1:6000. Estimates of the carrier frequency in Ashkenazic Jews range from 1:100 to as high as 1:20.

b. Niemann–Pick Disease. First described by Niemann (1914), a German pediatrician, Niemann–Pick disease comprises degenerative disorders involving storage of sphingomyelin. Because of the variability of manifestations, Niemann–Pick disease has been subdivided into five categories (Crocker, 1961). Type A, the acute classical form, accounts for most reported cases and is more common in Ashkenazic Jews. Visceral organs and the central nervous system are affected early in infancy, and the disease has a rapidly fatal course. It is characterized by hepatosplenomegaly, poor state of nutrition, yellow–brown discoloration and thickening of the skin, gastrointestinal bleeding, lymphadenopathy, jaundice, a cherry-red spot on the retina in about half of the patients, mental retardation, and moderate anemia. Death usually occurs by the fourth year because of neurological deterioration. Foamy histiocytes due to the ganglioside sphingomyelin accumulate in the reticuloedothelial system. The cells are scattered throughout the spleen, bone marrow, liver, lungs, and lymph nodes and may be distinguished from "Gaucher cells" by phase contrast or electron microscopy. The defect is caused by deficiency of sphingomyelinase, an enzyme that cleaves sphingomyelin to phosphorylcholine and ceramide. This deficiency can be diagnosed *in utero* as well as in the carrier (Wenger *et al.*, 1978).

Type B, a chronic form with severe visceral involvement, does not involve the central nervous system; type C, a subacute form, involves both visceral organs and the nervous system; type D, a Nova Scotia variant, has clinical manifestations similar to those of type C and an atypical protracted course; and type E is an adult, nonneuropathic form with mild visceral involvement.

The disorder is panethnic, but most patients, especially those with the type-A form, have been Ashkenazic Jews, especially those whose heritage was Lithuanian (Meals, 1971). The proportion of Jewish to non-Jewish infants affected is about 3:1. The gene frequency has been estimated to be greater than 1:100,000 among Ashkenazic Jews, with a carrier rate of 1:100 to 1:140.

c. Tay–Sachs Disease. Of all diseases that affect Jews, Tay–Sachs disease (GM2 gangliosidosis type I), or infantile amaurotic idiocy, has received most attention in recent years. The disease was first described by Tay (1881), a British ophthalmologist. It is characterized by onset in infancy of developmental retardation, cherry-red spot in the macula, blindness, mental retardation, apathy, and a flaccid paralysis followed by spastic convulsions, with death occurring by the second to fifth year of life. A ganglioside glycosphingolipid containing sialic acid in its oligosaccharide chain (GM2) is deposited in central nervous system cells. Okada and O'Brien (1969) showed a deficiency of β-hexosaminidase A (hex A) activity with artificial substrates in these patients. Tissues from patients with Tay–Sachs disease were also shown to be incapable of degrading GM2 ganglioside *in vitro*. The hex A locus has been assigned to chromosome 15 (McKusick and Ruddle, 1977).

Heterozygous carriers of the affected gene are clinically normal, but may be distinguished by reduced levels of the enzyme. The diagnosis in an affected fetus has been made from cultured amniotic cells. All attempts at therapy, including intrathecal injections of purified enzyme, have been unsuccessful.

Striking deficiency of the hex A activity with the synthetic substrate has been reported in a few healthy adults (Navon *et al.*, 1976). Parents with the enzyme deficiency produced offspring with variants of Tay–Sachs disease.

Several other types of GM2 ganglioside storage diseases affect a variety of ethnic groups. The clinical and pathological manifestations of these storage diseases are similar to those of Tay–Sachs disease. One of these, Sandhoff's disease, lacks both hexosaminidase A and B.

Many observers have noted that the disease is particularly common in Jews of Eastern European origins. The gene frequency is ten times higher and the birth incidence of affected children a hundred times greater among the Ashkenazim than among any other ethnic group. The incidence among Ashkenazim has been estimated to be 1:6000 to 1:3600 and the heterozygote frequency, based on more than 60,000 serum enzyme screenings in the United States, at about 0.03 in Ashkenazim and about 0.003 in non-Jewish populations (Kaback *et al.*, 1977). The incidence among Sephardim is about intermediate between Ashkenazim and non-Jews (Kolodny, 1979). Today, 30–50 children with Tay–Sachs disease are conceived each year in the United States. Parental consanguinity is frequent in non-Jewish cases and relatively infrequent in Jewish cases.

Controversy persists on why the Tay–Sachs disease gene, despite its mass elimination through homozygotes, is found in such high frequency among a restricted population. Myrianthopoulos and Aronson (1966) found that most of the ancestors of children with Tay–Sachs disease in the United States originated principally from provinces neighboring on the Baltic Sea, Grodno, Kovno, and Suwalki, with fewer originating from the Ukrainian and Moldavian regions and even less from the western Balkan areas of Germany. They noted a moderate increase in fitness in the siblings of the affected and that the Ashkenazic Jews had survived the high tuberculosis attack rate of the crowded ghettos for many generations. Perla and Marmorston (1941) had shown that, although the rate of tuberculosis infection as determined by skin testing was similar in Jews and non-Jews, tuberculosis mortality was significantly less in Jews. They suggested tuberculosis as a possible selective factor imparting advantage to carriers. That suggestion does not explain why non-Jews, living in the same environment, do not have a similar increase in Tay–Sachs gene frequency.

Chase and McKusick (1972) favored the founder effect. This hypothesis proposes a disproportionate contribution from a founder with manifestation of the phenotype later in history. Wagener *et al.* (1978) concluded that the elevated frequency of Tay–Sachs disease among Ashkenazim is due to drift, and Chakravarti and Chakraborty (1978) asserted that heterozygote selective advantage together with random genetic drift is responsible.

The combination of heterozygote detection and prenatal differentiation among normal, carrier, and affected fetuses has allowed the first large-scale prospective prevention program of a genetic disease because Tay–Sachs disease meets the following prerequisites: (1) the disease occurs preponderantly in a defined population; (2) heterozygotyes can be identified simply, accurately, and inexpensively; and (3) the disease can be detected *in utero* early in pregnancy. By 1979, there were more than 100 worldwide Tay–Sachs screening centers. More than 250,000 persons have been tested, with more than 10,000 carriers detected and more than 200 couples at risk identified M. M. Kaback, personal communication). Of more than 600 pregnancies with possibly affected fetuses, 148 fetuses were found to have the disease.

6. Mucolipidosis Type IV

This disorder, first reported by Berman *et al.* (1974), is characterized by bilateral congenital corneal opacities and slow psychomotor development resulting in inability to speak and to respond to verbal commands, hypotonia, and hyperactive deep-tendon reflexes. The retinas of affected children may degenerate, as shown on the electroretinogram. In conjunctival biopsies, inclusions in the lysosomes of epithelial cells are particularly striking. Electron microscopic examination of conjunctival biopsies and aborted fetuses have shown two types of abnormal fibroblast lipidlike material: (1) single-membrane-limited cytoplasmic vacuoles containing both fibrillogranular material and membranous lamellae and (2) lamellar and concentric bodies resembling those of Tay–Sachs disease. The basic biochemical defect is not known. Abnormal distribution of GM3 and GD3 gangliosides have been reported in several patients (Bach *et al.*, 1975). These gangliosides and acid mucopolysaccharides, mainly hyaluronic acid, accumulate and are abnormally distributed in cultured skin fibroblasts. Patients do no excrete elevated amounts of mucopolysaccharides. Berman *et al.* (1974) postulated that the basic defect may be due to a sialidase deficiency because both GM3 and GD3 gangliosides serve as substrates for this enzyme.

Most of the cases reported to date have Ashkenazic heritage; and the family origins can be traced to southern Poland. Consanguinity has not been reported in these families. The incidence is not known.

7. Pentosuria

First described in 1892 by Salkowski and Jastrowitz (1892), essential or idiopathic pentosuria is a benign defect in glucouronic metabolism that should not really be classified as a disease because it results in no discomfort or disability to the patient and has no life-shortening effect. The only difficulty encountered is the likelihood of a mistaken diagnosis of diabetes mellitus. Transient pentosuria may appear in normal persons after ingestion of large amounts of fruit. Patients with the defect excrete L-xylulose, a five-carbon sugar, in the urine, the amount being fairly constant for a particular patient but varying from one patient to the next. The excretion rate appears to be independent of diet, although certain L-xylulose-like drugs (e.g., aminopyrine) may alter the rate, since they are probably excreted in a similar chemical form—as glucuronates.

Wang and Van Eys (1970) demonstrated that the basic defect is in NADP-linked xylitol dehydrogenase in erythrocytes. Heterozygotes can be identified by an intermediate level of the enzyme.

About 3000 cases of idiopathic pentosuria have been reported. All but rare cases, including several in Lebanese Arab families, have involved Ashkenazic Jews, who have an estimated prevalence of about 1 in 2000–2500 births. Lasker (1955) estimated one in 50 Jews in the United States are heterozygous for this condition. She found a wide distribution of origin of these cases from Riga on the Baltic to Odessa on the Black Sea, and from Holland to Hungary. No one city or area was the site of origin for all the cases. Lasker estimates that this mutation may have occurred from about 1000–2000 years ago if all cases of this condition were derived from a single mutation.

8. Plasma Thromboplastin Antecedent, Factor XI Deficiency

Hemophilia, both the classical X-linked factor VIII (hemophilia A) and other bleeding disorders, is mentioned in the Bible. Jewish law concerning circumcision even made exceptions for affected persons.

Hemophilia due to factor XI (plasma thromboplastin antecedent) deficiency, first described by Rosenthal *et al.* (1953), is characterized by minor bleeding episodes, occasional severely protracted bleeding after surgical procedures, abnormal prothrombin consumption, prolonged partial thromboplastin and recalcification times, and abnormal factor XI assay. Factor XI is a glycoprotein that participates in the activation of factor IX in the intrinsic clotting system.

Inheritance is autosomal recessive, and heterozygotes may have a mild bleeding tendency.

Almost all reported affected persons have been Ashkenazim (Seligsohn, 1979). Muir and Ratnoff (1974) estimated the prevalence of 1:12,000 and a carrier rate of 1:56 in Ashkenazim.

9. Spongy Degeneration of the Central Nervous System

This rare disease is characterized by onset at early infancy of atonia of the neck muscles, flexion of the arms, and hyperextension of the legs, blindness, mental retardation, and megalocephaly, with death by 2 years of age. Histopathologically, there is widespread vacuolation and disintegration of the cortical and subcortical white matter. The biochemical abnormality has not been identified. More than half of the reported cases have been among Ashkenazic Jews originating in Eastern Europe, with a male to female ratio of about 2:1. In the affected non-Jewish families, consanguinity was more common and the sex ratio was reversed (Banker and Victor, 1979).

Gilles de la Tourette Syndrome. This neurological disorder, first reported by Gilles de la Tourette (1885), is characterized by both motor and behavioral abnormalities, a distinctive combination of multifocal involuntary vocalizations and movements (Golden, 1979). The age of onset is usually between 2 and 14 years. The initial symptom is usually involuntary tic-like movements; progressive echolalia, grunting, and coprolalia may develop. In about half of the patients, self-mutilation is a symptom.

No consistent histopathological finding has been reported in this disease. Van Woert *et al.* (1977) reported normal hypoxanthine guanine phosphoribosyltransferase (HGPRT) and adenine phosphoribosyltransferase (APRT) activities of red blood cell lysates, but unstable red blood cell HGPRT and abnormal enzyme peaks have been detected by isoelectric focusing. The self-mutilation and biochemical findings prompted a trial of L-5-hydroxytryptophan, the precursor of serotonin, which had been reported to relieve self-mutilation in patients with the Lesch-Nyhan syndrome. Van Woert *et al.* (1977) described a 15-year-old boy who was much improved while taking the medication and who returned to aggressive behavior, tics, biting, and facial punching while taking a placebo. Haloperidol and phenothiazines, which block postsynaptic dopaminergic activity, have been reported to ameliorate symptoms. Cohen *et al.* (1979) found that clonidine, an α-adrenergic agonist, improves the condition in some children who are unresponsive to haloperidol. Drugs (such as amphetamines) that release catecholamines exacerbate the symptoms, suggesting that the disorder is caused by a relative excess of catecholaminergic activity.

About three-fourths of patients with Gilles de la Tourette syndrome are male. The mode of genetic transmission is still in dispute, but the most likely form found in Jews is autosomal dominant (Eldridge *et al.*, 1979). This form of disease has been reported in many ethnic groups, including Mexicans, American Indians, and blacks, but it has been reported most frequently in Ashkenazic Jews.

10. Others

X-linked red–green color blindness and several other genetic diseases (some rare) have been reported to occur with relatively high frequency in Ashkenazic Jews.

D. Genetic Diseases of Sephardic Jews

Until recently the genetic diseases of the Sephardic Jews have not been as extensively studied as those of the Ashkenazic Jews.

1. Familial Mediterranean Fever

Also known as recurrent polyserositis, familial Mediterranean fever (FMF) is an autosomal recessive disorder marked by recurrent sporadic acute attacks of fever, an erysipelas-like erythema, accompanied by polyserositis manifested by pain in the chest, abdomen, and joints, and with a normal white blood cell count (Sohar *et al.*, 1967). Although symptoms may begin in infancy, in most patients they begin between the ages of 5 and 15 years and recur at regular intervals. Death occurs usually between 10 and 30 years of age due to renal failure, usually secondary to amyloidosis, which often is associated with renal vein thrombosis.

Amyloidosis, which occurs in about one-fourth of the patients, is manifested by renal involvement of the perireticular type. Amyloidosis has been found in kinships who never had clinical attacks. Sohar *et al.* (1967) divided FMF into two types. In phenotype I, the more common type, the attacks appear first; in phenotye II, amyloidosis is the first manifestation.

Pathologically, it is characterized by hyperemia and nonbacterial inflammation of the serous membranes. The biochemical defect, however, has not been identified.

Colchicine, when taken chronically, appears to be effective in preventing attacks in most patients, and when taken intermittently it can, in many patients, abort a developing attack (Wolff, 1978). The attacks of fever and abdominal pains may be suppressed by hemodialysis (Rubinger *et al.*, 1979).

The disease is prevalent in Arabs, Turks, Italians, and Greeks, but especially in Armenians and in Sephardic Jews (Schwabe and Peters, 1974). Originally, it was thought to affect only Sephardic Jews, but, as is now clear, Ashkenazim are also affected sporadically. One in about 600 Libyan Jews is affected, compared with about 1:4000 among other Sephardic Jews and 1:80,000 among Ashkenazim. Amyloidosis is frequent in Sephardim but rare in Armenians.

2. Others

The prevalence of other genetic diseases that affect Sephardim at higher frequencies than they do other ethnic groups has not been studied as extensively. Cystinosis and congenital adrenal hyperplasia, mainly due to 21-OH deficiency, have been reported in high frequency in this subgroup.

Ataxia-telangiectasia, a disorder characterized by immunological defects, thymic abnormalities, chromosomal instability, and a predisposition to lymphoma and acute lymphocytic leukemia, has been reported to have high frequencies in Moroccan Jews. Autosomal recessive deafness and glycogen storage disease type III, or Cori–Forbes disease (debrancher enzyme deficiency), is a disease of childhood—characterized by liver dysfunction with hepatomegaly, fasting hypoglycemia, and seizures, signs and symptoms that regress at puberty—which has also been reported to be high in this group of Sephardic Jews.

Autosomal recessive cystinuria, types II and III, resulting in renal calculi and crystalluria has been noted to be more common in Libyan Jews.

Selective vitamin B_{12} malabsorption with proteinuria and the infantile form of cystinosis resulting in a renal tubular defect are common among Sephardic Jews of Tunisian origin.

E. Genetic Diseases of Oriental Jews

The incidence of inbreeding of Ashkenazic and Sephardic Jews has been lower than among most of the Oriental groups. Fewer recessive diseases, however, have been reported in this group, probably because they have not had the medical scrutiny of the former two subgroups.

Yemenite Jews have a high incidence of α-thalassemia, autosomal dominant benign familial neutropenia, autosomal recessive phenylketonuria, and deficiency of peroxidase and phospholipid in the eosinophils of the blood. They and the Maori of New Zealand have a high incidence of autosomal recessive cystic disease of the lung.

Selective hypoaldosteronism, an autosomal recessive syndrome characterized by salt wastage, hyponatremia, hyperkalemia, high level of plasma renin activity, and inappropriately low levels of aldosterone has been described in Iranian Jews mainly from Isfahan. This population isolate also has one of the highest frequencies in the world of the benign Dubin–Johnson syndrome, which consists of chronic, mainly conjugated hyperbilirubinemia of unknown cause, and a grossly black liver. The incidence in Iranian Jews is about 1:1300. Increased frequency of G6PD deficiency has been described in this population as well as in Iraqi and Kurdish Jews.

A recessive syndrome consisting of nerve deafness and infantile tubular acidosis has been described in Kurdish Jews. As noted earlier, Kurdish Jews also have a high incidence of β-thalassemia and G6PD deficiency.

Jews of Iraqi origin have been found to have a high incidence of X-linked ichthyosis, benign familial hematuria, and Glanzmann thrombasthenia, a severe bleeding disorder due to a platelet aggregation abnormality.

Autosomal dominant ichthyosis and β-thalassemia have been observed frequently in Jews from India.

Oriental Jews from Habban, South Arabia, have been reported to have a high rate of metachromatic leukodystrophy.

Many other rare genetic syndromes have been described in the Jewish populations. Because they have been extensively catalogued in Goodman's (1979) excellent book, they will not be discussed further here.

F. Complex Diseases

Several complex diseases whose genetic bases are tenuous are reported to be more or less frequent among Jews than among non-Jewish populations. Diabetes mellitus, idiopathic hypercholesterolemia, ischemic heart disease, Kaposi's idiopathic sarcoma dermatosis, polycythemia vera, and ulcerative colitis have been reported to be more frequent among the Ashkenazic Jewish population than among most other ethnic groups. Nevertheless, because these diseases are not uncommon among non-Jewish populations, because they have been extensively described, and because they have not been definitely established as occurring more commonly among Jews, they will not be discussed further.

Regional enteritis and pemphigus vulgaris have also been reported to be more frequent among Jews. All 14 of the original patients with regional enteritis whom Crohn *et al.* (1932) described were Jewish. Later, however, Crohn and Janowitz (1954) stated, "no ethnic group predominates." Nevertheless, many, though not all, of the reported series of cases, even those from non-Jewish institutions, have shown a disproportionate number affecting Ashkenazic Jews. Of a series of 600 cases reported from the Mayo Clinic, 153 affected patients were Jewish (Van Patter *et al.*, 1954). Several other studies, including one by Acheson (1960) of all the Veterans Administration hospitals in the United States, showed a disproportionately large number of Jewish veterans admitted for regional enteritis.

Pemphigus vulgaris, which may have been mentioned in the Bible (Exodus 9:9), is an adult-onset illness characterized by scanty or numerous giant bullae involving the skin and mucous membranes. Familial clustering has been described but no genetic basis for the disease has been established. A number of reports suggested that the disease was more common in Ashkenazic Jews than in other groups but might also occur more frequently in other Jewish subgroups than in non-Jews (Ziprkowski and Schewach-Millet, 1964). Park *et al.* (1979) found an association of HLA-A10 and HLA-DRw4 with the disease among Jewish patients but less of an association in non-Jewish patients. HLA-A10 also has an excess frequency in pemphigus patients in Japan.

As mentioned above, cancer of the cervix and glans penis, alcoholism, pyloric stenosis, and tuberculosis appear to be less frequent in Jews.

G. Spurious Associations

Differences in disease frequencies observed among Jewish populations compared with those of non-Jews are not necessarily real but may be the result of an ascertainment bias. Buerger's disease, or thromboangiitis obliterans, for example, was at first thought to be more frequent among Jews. The inflammatory and occlusive changes in arteries and veins of legs were first described by Buerger (1908) at Beth Israel Hospital in Boston, where a high percentage of patients were Jewish. He reported that it occurred frequently in Polish or Russian Jews. For a time after that, Jews were believed to be particularly prone to the disease. Evans and Dumas (1933–1934) later reported that, of 52 patients with Buerger's disease at the Veterans Administration Hospital in Minneapolis, 14 were Jewish.

Gradually, however, observations accumulated showing that other groups were probably just as liable to be affected as were Jews. Subsequently, Wessler *et al.* (1960) showed that the percentage of Jews diagnosed with the disease was not larger than the percentage of Jews listed on general hospital admissions.

More thorough reporting among the Jews may account for the reported increased frequency of some diseases. The initially apparent increased incidence of such diseases as angiitis obliterans may only mean that the Jews obtained better medical care or congregated in cities and used academic medical institutions to a disproportionate degree. Physicians in such institutions are more likely to recognize and report unusual disorders than would those in smaller, less specialized hospitals.

IV. CONCLUSIONS

Thus, the high frequency of rare diseases in Jewish populations is probably real in some cases and spurious in others. In those instances where it is real it may be due not only to social and religious customs but also to Jewish history.

The history of all Jewish subgroups is replete with pogroms and imposed social and economic restrictions and periods of population expansion. Their relative small number, often living in small communities, allowed opportunities for genetic drift and a second founder effect. Moreover, their religious customs may be responsible for certain diseases manifesting in lesser or greater frequency in the subgroups.

Although there are no "Jewish diseases" as such, unquestionably some diseases and alleles have a higher frequency in the various Jewish subgroups or subpopulations of these subgroups. There are three separate subgroups, not a monolithic group that shares a common gene pool, or even a common culture or religion. Nonetheless, many still consider Jews to be a distinctive ethnic group. Most significant is their historical continuity and their self perception as an ethnic group, maintained and nurtured by adversity throughout their history.

REFERENCES

Acheson, E. D. (1960). The distribution of ulcerative colitis and regional enteritis in the United States veterans with particular reference to the Jewish religion. *Gut* 1, 291–293.

Adam, A. (1973) Genetic diseases among Jews. *Isr. J. Med. Sci.* 9, 1383–1392.

Alter, M. (1978). Creutzfeldt–Jakob disease: Hypothesis for high incidence in Libyan Jews in Israel. *Science* 186, 848.

Alter, M., Kahana, E., and Feldman, S. (1976). Differences in torsion dystonia among Israeli ethnic groups. *In* "Advances in Neurology" (R. Eldridge and S. Fahn, eds.), Vol. 14, pp. 115–120. Raven, New York.

Axelrod, F. B., Nachtigal, R., and Dancis, J. (1974). Familial dysautonomia: diagnosis, pathogenesis and management. *Adv. Pediatr.* **21,** 75–96.

Bach, G., Cohen, M. M., and Kohn, G. (1975). Abnormal ganglioside accumulation in cultured fibroblasts from patients with mucolipidosis IV. *Biochem. Biophys. Res. Commun.* **66,** 1483–1490.

Banker, B. Q., and Victor, M. (1979). Spongy degeneration of infancy. In ``Genetic Diseases Among Ashkenazi Jews'' (R. M. Goodman and A. G. Motulsky, eds.), pp. 201–216. Raven, New York.

Bassen, F. A., and Kornzweig, A. L. (1950). Malformation of the erythrocytes in a case of atypical retinitis pigmentosa. *Blood* **5,** 381–387.

Berman, E. R., Livni, N., Shapira, E., Merin, S., and Levij, I. S. (1974). Congenital corneal clouding with abnormal systemic storage bodies: a new variant of mucolipidosis. *J. Pediatr.* **84,** 519–526.

Bloom, D. (1954). Congenital telangiectatic erythemia resembling lupus erythematosus in dwarfs. *Am. J. Dis. Child.* **88,** 754–758.

Bonne-Tamir, B., Karlin, S., and Kenett, R. (1979). Analysis of genetic data on Jewish populations: I. Historical background, demographic features, and genetic markers. *Am. J. Hum. Genet.* **31,** 324–340.

Brunt, P. W., and McKusick, V. A. (1970). Familial dysautonomia. A report of genetic and clinical studies with a review of the literature. *Medicine (Baltimore)* **49,** 343–349.

Buerger, L. (1908). Thrombo-angiitis obliterans: A study of the vascular lesions leading to presenile gangrene. *Am. J. Med. Sci.* **136,** 567–580.

Chakravarti, A., and Chakraborty, R. (1978). Elevated frequency of Tay–Sachs disease among Ashkenazic Jews unlikely by genetic drift alone. *Am. J. Hum. Genet.* **30,** 256–261.

Chase, G. A., and McKusick, V. A. (1972). Founder effect in Tay–Sachs disease. *Am. J. Hum. Genet.* **24,** 339–340.

Chiao, Y.-B., Hoyson, G. M., Peters, S. P., Lee, R. E., Diven, W., Murphy J. V., and Glew, R. H. (1978). Multiple glycosidase deficiencies in a case of juvenile (type 3) Gaucher disease. *Proc. Natl. Acad. Sci. U.S.A.* **75,** 2448–2452.

Cohen, D. J., Nathanson, J. A., Young, J. G., and Shaywitz, B. A. (1979). Clonidine in Tourette's syndrome. *Lancet* **ii,** 551–553.

Cohen, T., and Bloch, N. (1963). Immigrant Jews from Cochin. In ``The Genetics of Migrant and Isolate Populations'' (E. Goldschmidt ed.), p. 352. Williams & Wilkins, Baltimore, Maryland.

Crocker, A. C. (1961). The cerebral defect in Tay–Sachs disease and Niemann–Pick disease. *J. Neurochem.* **7,** 69–80.

Crohn, B. B., Ginzburg, L., and Oppenheimer, G. D. (1932). Regional ileitis: pathological and clinical entity. *J. Am. Med. Assoc.,* **99,** 1323–1329.

Crohn, B. B., and Janowitz, H. D. (1954). Reflections on regional ileitis twenty years later. *J. Am. Med. Assoc.* **156,** 1221–1225.

Darlington, C. D. (1969). ``The Evolution of Man and Society.'' Simon & Schuster, New York.

Eldridge, R. (1970). The torsion dystonias: Literature review and genetic and clinical studies. *Neurology* **20,** Suppl., Part 2, 1–78.

Eldridge, R., and Gottlieb, R. (1976). The primary hereditary dystonias: Genetic classification of 768 families and revised estimate of gene frequency, autosomal recessive form and selected bibliography. In ``Advances in Neurology'' (R. Eldridge and S. Fahn eds.), Vol. 14, pp. 457–474. Raven, New York.

Eldridge, R., and Koerber, T. (1979). Torsion dystonia: autosomal recessive form. In ``Genetic Diseases Among Ashkenazi Jews'' (R. M. Goodman and A. G. Motulsky, eds), pp. 231–252. Raven, New York.

Eldridge R., Wassman, E. R., Nee, L., and Koerber, T. (1979). Gilles de la Tourette syndrome. *In* "Genetic Diseases among Ashkenazic Jews" (R. M. Goodman and A. G. Motulsky, eds), pp. 231–252. Raven, New York.

Evans, E. T., and Dumas, A. G. (1933–1934). Thromboangiitis obliterans: report of fifty-two cases. *Med. Bull. Vet. Adm.* **10**, 99–109.

Friedenwald, H. (1967). "The Jews and Medicine." Ktav, New York.

Gajdusek, D. C. (1978). Unconventional viruses. *In* "Human Diseases Caused by Viruses" (H. Rothschild, F. Allison, Jr., and C. Howe, eds), pp. 231–258. Oxford Univ. Press, London and New York.

Gaucher, P. C. E. (1882). De l'épitheliome primitif de la rate, hypertrophic idiopathique de la rate sans leucémie. Theses de Paris, pp. 4–31.

German, J., Schonberg, S., Louie, E., and Chaganti, R. S. K. (1977). Bloom's syndrome: IV: Sister-chromatid exhanges in lymphocytes. *Am. J. Hum. Genet.* **29**, 248–255.

German, J., Bloom, D., and Passarge, E. (1979). Bloom's syndrome: VII. Progress report for 1978. *Clin. Genet.* **15**, 361–367.

Giannelli, F., Benson, P. F., Pawsey, S. A., and Polani, P. E. (1977). Ultraviolet light sensitivity and delayed DNA-chain maturation in Bloom's syndrome fibroblasts. *Nature (London),* **265**, 466–469.

Gilles de la Tourette, G. (1885). Étude sur une affection nerveuse caractérisée par l'incordination motrice accompagnée d'écholalie et de coprolalie. *Arch. Neurol. (Paris)* **9**, 19–42; 158–200.

Golden, G. S. (1979). Tics and Tourette syndrome. *Hosp. Pract.* **14**, 91–100.

Goldschmidt, E., Fried, K., Steinberg, A. G., and Cohen, T. (1976). The Karaite community of Iraq in Israel: a genetic study. *Am. J. Hum. Genet.* **28**, 243–252.

Goodman, R. M. (1979). "Genetic Disorders Among the Jewish People." Johns Hopkins Press, Baltimore, Maryland.

Goodman, R. M., and Motulsky, A. G., eds. (1979). "Genetic Diseases Among Ashkenazi Jews." Raven, New York.

Gotto, A. M., Levy, R. I., John, K., and Frederickson, D. S. (1971). On the protein defect in abetalipoproteinemia. *N. Engl. J. Med.* **284**, 813–818.

Grossman, R. G., and Kelly, P. J. (1976). Physiology of the basal ganglia in relation dystonia. *In* "Advances in Neurology" (R. Eldridge and S. Fahn, eds.), Vol. 14, pp. 49–57, Raven, New York.

Kaback, M. M., Nathan, T. J., and Greenwald, S. (1977). Tay–Sachs disease: Heterozygote screening and prenatal diagnosis—U.S. experience and world perspective. *In* "Tay–Sachs Disease: Screening and Prevention" (M. M. Kaback, ed.), pp. 13–36. Alan R. Liss, New York.

Kahana, E., Alter, M., Jackson, B., and Sofer, D. (1974). Creutzfeldt–Jakob disease: focus among Libyan Jews in Israel. *Science* **183**, 90–91.

Karlin, S., Kenett, R., and Bonne-Tamir, B. (1979). Analysis of biochemical genetic data on Jewish populations: II. Results and interpretations of heterogeneity indices and distance measures with respect to standards. *Am. J. Hum. Genet.* **31**, 341–365.

Koestler, A. (1976). "The Thirteenth Tribe." Random House, New York.

Kolodny, E. H. (1979). Current status of Tay–Sachs disease. *In* "Genetic Diseases in Ashkenazi Jews" (R. M. Goodman and A. G. Motulsky, eds.), pp. 285–300. Raven, New York.

Lasker, M. (1955). Mortality of person with xyloketosuria: a follow-up study of a rare metabolic anomaly. *Hum. Biol.* **27**, 294–300.

Lees, R. S. (1967). Immunological evidence for the presence of beta protein (apoprotein of beta-lipoprotein) in normal and abetalipoproteinemia plasma. *J. Lipid Res.* **8**, 396–405.

Levi-Montalcini, R. (1976). Nerve-growth factor in familial dysautonomia. *N. Engl. J. Med.* **295**, 671–673.

McKusick, V. A., and Ruddle, F. H. (1977). The status of the gene map of the human chromosomes. *Science* **196**, 390–405.

Meals, R. A. (1971). Paradoxical frequencies of recessive disorders in Ashkenazic Jews. *J. Chronic. Dis.* **23**, 547–554.

Mendel, K. (1919). Torsion dystonie. (Dystonia musculorum deformans, Torsions spasms.) *Monatsscher. Psychiatr. Neurol.* **46**, 309–361.

Mourant, A. E. (1959). The blood groups of the Jews. *Jew. J. Sociol.* **1**, 155–176.

Mourant, A. E., Kopec, A. C., and Domaniewska-Sobczak, K. (1978). "The Genetics of Jews." Oxford Univ. Press, London and New York.

Muir, W. A., and Ratnoff, O. D. (1974). The prevalence of plasma thromboplastin antecedent (PTA Factor XI) deficiency. *Blood* **44**, 569–570.

Myrianthopoulos, N. C., and Aronson, S. M. (1966). Population dynamics of Tay–Sachs disease. I. Reproductive fitness and selection. *Am. J. Hum. Genet.* **18**, 313–327.

Navon, R., Geiger, B., Ben Yoseph, Y., and Rattazzi, M. C. (1976). Low levels of beta hexosaminidase A in healthy individuals with apparent deficiency of this enzyme. *Am. J. Hum. Genet.* **28**, 339–349.

Neel, J. V. (1979). History and the Tay–Sachs allele. *In* "Genetic Diseases Among Ashkenazi Jews" (R. M. Goodman and A. G. Motulsky, eds.), pp. 285–300. Raven, New York.

Niemann, A. (1914). Ein unbekanntes Krankheitsbild. *Jahrb. Kinderheildkd.* **79**, 1–10.

Okada, S., and O'Brien, J. S. (1969). Tay–Sachs disease: generalized absence of a beta-D-N-acetylhexosaminidase component. *Science* **165**, 698–700.

Oppenheim, H. (1911). Verber eire eigerartige Krampfkrankheit des kindlichen and jugendlicken Alters (Dysbasia lordotica progressiva, Dystonia musculorum deformans). *Neurol. Centralbl.* **30**, 1090–1107.

Park, M. S., Ahmed, A. R., Terasaki, P. I., and Tiwari, J. L. (1979). HLA-DRw4 in 91% of Jewish pemphigus vulgaris patients. *Lancet* **ii**, 441–442.

Patai, R., and Patai Wing, J. (1975). "The Myth of the Jewish Race." Scribner's, New York.

Patai Wing, J. (1974). Blood protein polymorphisms in Jewish populations. *Hum. Hered.* **24**, 323–344.

Perla, D., and Marmorston, J. (1941). "Natural Resistance and Clinical Medicine." Little, Brown, Boston, Massachusetts.

Riley, C. M., Day, R. L., Greely, D. McL., and Langford, W. S. (1949). Central autonomic dysfunction with defective lacrimation: report of five cases. *Pediatrics* **3**, 468–470.

Rosenthal, R. L., Dreskin, O. A., and Rosenthal, N. (1953). New hemophilia-like disease caused by deficiency of a third plasma thromboplastin factor. *Proc. Soc. Exp. Biol. Med.* **82**, 171–174.

Rubinger, D., Friedlaender, M. M., and Popovtzer, M. M. (1979). Amelioration of familial Mediterranean fever during hemodialysis. *N. Engl. J. Med.* **301**, 142–144.

Sachar, A. L. (1964). "A History of the Jews." Knopf, New York.

Salkowski, E., and Jastrowitz, M. (1892). Ueber eine bisher nicht beobachtete Zuckerart im Harn. *Zentralbl. Med. Wissenschaften* **30**, 337–339.

Schuckit, M. A., Goodwin, D. A., and Winokur, G. (1972). A study of alcoholism in half siblings. *Am. J. Psychiatry* **128**, 1132–1136.

Schwabe, A. D., and Peters, R. S. (1974). Familial Mediterranean fever in Armenians: analysis of 100 cases. *Medicine (Baltimore)* **53**, 453–562.

Seligsohn, U. (1979). Factor XI (PTA) deficiency. *In* "Genetic Diseases Among Ashkenazi Jews" (R. M. Goodman and A. G. Motulsky, eds.), pp. 141–148. Raven, New York.

Sharon, Z., Shani, M., and Modan, B. (1977). Clinicoepidemiologic study of uterine cancer, comparative aspects of the endometrial and cervical sites. *Obstet. Gynecol.* **50**, 536–540.

Siggers, D. C., Rogers, J. G., Boyer, S. H., Margolet, L., Dorkin, H., Shailesh, P. B., and Shooter,

E. M. (1976). Increased nerve-growth-factor beta chain cross reacting material in familial dysautonomia. *N. Engl. J. Med.* **295**, 629–634.

Snyder, C. R. (1979). Alcoholism: its rarity among Jews. *In* "Genetic Diseases Among Ashkenazi Jews" (R. M. Goodman and A. G. Motulsky, eds.), pp. 353–362. Raven, New York.

Sohar, E., Gafni, J., Pras, M., and Heller, H. (1967). Familial Mediterranean fever: a survey of 470 cases and review of the literature. *Am. J. Med.* **43**, 227–253.

Szeinberg, A. (1963). G6PD deficiency among Jews: genetical and anthropological considerations. *In* "The Genetics of Migrant and Isolate Populations" (E. Goldschmidt, ed.), pp. 69–72. Williams & Wilkins, Baltimore, Maryland.

Szeinberg, A. (1979). Polymorpic evidence for a Mediterranean origin of the Ashkenazi Jewish community. *In* "Genetic Diseases Among Ashkenazi Jews" (R. M. Goodman and A. G. Motulsky, eds.), pp. 77–91. Raven, New York.

Tay, W. (1881). Symmetrical changes in the region of the yellow spot in each eye of an infant. *Trans. Ophthal. Soc. U. K.* **1**, 155.

Van Patter, W., Bargen, J., Dockerty, M. B., Feldman, W. H., Mayo, C. W., and Waugh, J. M. (1954). Regional enteritis. *Gastroenterology* **26**, 347–450.

Van Woert, M. H., Yip, L. C., and Bayles, M. E. (1977). Purine phosphoribosyltransferase in Gilles de la Tourette syndrome. *N. Engl. J. Med.* **296**, 210–212.

Wagener, D., Cavalli-Sforza, L. L., and Barakat, R. (1978). Ethnic variation of genetic disease: roles of drift for recessive lethal genes. *Am. J. Hum. Genet.* **30**, 262–270.

Wang, Y. M., and Van Eys, J. (1970). The enzymatic defect in essential pentosuria. *N. Engl. J. Med.* **282**, 892–896.

Weinshilboum, R. M., and Axelrod, J. (1971). Reduced plasma dopamine-beta-hydroxylase activity in familial dysautonomia. *N. Engl. J. Med.* **285**, 938–942.

Welton, W., Clayson, D., Axelrod, F. B., and Levine, D. B. (1979). Intellectual development and familial dysautonomia. *Pediatrics* **63**, 708–712.

Wenger, D. A., Wharton, C., Sattler, M., and Clark, C. (1978). Niemann–Pick disease: prenatal diagnoses and studies of sphingomyelinase activities. *Am. J. Med. Genet.* **2**, 345–356.

Wessler, S., Ming, S. C., Gurewich, V., and Freiman, D. G. (1960). A critical evaluation of thromboangiitis obliterans: the case against Buerger's disease. *N. Engl. J. Med.* **262**, 1149–1160.

Wolff, S. M. (1978). Familial Mediterranean fever: a status report. *Hosp. Pract.* **13**, 113–123.

Ziprkowski, L., and Schewach-Millet, M. (1964). A long term study of pemphigus. *Proc. Tel-Hashomer Hosp.* **3**, 46–53.

17

Disease Patterns of Isolated Groups

RALPH M. GARRUTO

I. INTRODUCTION

Human population isolation, generally considered synonymous with geographic isolation, is usually explained in terms of genetic isolation. There are, in fact, many types of human population isolates with a variety of distinguishing characteristics. Populations may be socially isolated (e.g., religious, economic, political, linguistic, ethnic, traditional) as well as geographically isolated, by

BIOCULTURAL ASPECTS OF DISEASE
ISBN 0-12-598720-X

choice or nonchoice situations; they may be large or small, technologically simple or technically advanced, mating or nonmating, and represent either closed or semiclosed systems of mating behavior. The more classical isolated groups are often small, living as hunter–gathers, as fisherfolk or primitive hoe-and-digging-stick agriculturalists, or, with varying degrees of isolation, as migratory herders or peasants, and they present medical problems that are often unique or unusual.

The variation among isolated groups from the Arctic tundra to tropical rain forests, from small island atolls to central continental plains and mountain ranges, and from rural to urban population centers probably exceeds that of genetically open, technologically advanced societies. Isolates are characterized by a geographically or culturally restricted territory and the lack of travel outside it, a "simplified" ecology and fixed habitat, a close association with the flora and fauna, a high degree of inbreeding (in mating groups), and unique social and behavioral patterns that are often inextricably tied to a particular disease expression or strange epidemiologic pattern. The importance of such isolates to medicine in elucidating the etiology, pathogenesis, ecology, and epidemiology of disease is inordinately high.

Field and laboratory studies in such areas as epidemiology, genetics and associated molecular biology, immunology, virology, endocrinology, biochemistry, nutrition, fertility and reproduction, growth and development, maturation and aging, differential genetic susceptibility to disease, and human biological adaptation to diverse and extreme environmental conditions have been directed toward solving problems that may be more appropriately studied in isolates than in large Western societies. In large genetically open cosmopolitan communities, numerous cultural and environmental variables may complicate the analysis of major medical problems and inquiries. The opportunistic study of "natural experiments" in isolated populations has already resulted in major biomedical discoveries of importance far beyond their application to the isolated communities themselves. Yet the value of these findings to the people who usually suffer considerably from the disorders studied is obvious.

In considering the diseases of isolated groups, attention will be focused on the natural history of disease and on the factors affecting disease in isolated communities. Concepts of optimal and critical levels are important in understanding disease states and in assessing the degree to which isolates are in equilibrium with their environment. For example, small shifts in availability of iodine in the presence of already severe, yet asymptomatic, iodine deficiency may "drive" a population into severe clinical disease. Thus, isolated populations living in marginal ecological settings may be precariously adapted to their natural environments. Examples of natural disease phenomena will be presented, including infectious disease, nutritional, toxic or deficiency disease, genetic disease and culturally specific psychoses. The "myths" of increased susceptibility and increased resistance of isolates to disease will also be discussed.

The interaction of biology and behavior in a natural setting is nowhere more obvious than among isolated communities. Therefore, consideration will be given to specific behavioral patterns of isolates associated with unusual patterns of disease and, to the converse, specific disease patterns resulting in changes in sociocultural phenomena.

With isolated groups rapidly vanishing and peasant populations undergoing severe cultural change through contact with and assimilation into cosmopolitan communities, investigating such populations in unaltered natural settings may soon be impossible. Nevertheless, studying changing patterns of disease in acculturating groups continues to be important, and the factors associated with such patterns in groups exposed to the effects of increased contact and westernization will be discussed.

Finally, the neurobiology of population isolates in the Western Pacific and the implications of "natural experimental models" for solving etiological and epidemiological problems will be specifically considered.

Isolated communities offer unparalleled opportunities for studying disease as agents of natural selection, as factors influencing population stability and size, and as natural experimental models for solving etiological and epidemiological problems of widespread medical significance. One must, therefore, not attempt to arrive at some parochial scheme of research with regard to isolate studies but, rather, to capitalize on the unique features of each isolate to answer the particular problems for which it is most suited. Consequently, the study of disease patterns in isolated groups should be holistic, integrative, and necessarily opportunistic.

II. NATURAL HISTORY OF DISEASE IN ISOLATED GROUPS

The natural history of disease in isolated groups represents a system of dynamic interaction. The associated factors affecting the expression of disease among isolates are:

1. Degree of isolation and contact
2. Demographic characteristics of the population including size, density, and age and sex distribution
3. Group mobility
4. Ecosystem stability
5. Uniformity of food sources
6. Physical environmental stress

7. Close physical proximity during work and play
8. Similar housing
9. Culturally specific hygienic practices
10. Degree of natural resistance and differential genetic susceptibility.

The specific characteristics of the disease agent must also be considered, including virulence, persistence, and potential reactivation. Certainly the above list is not all-inclusive nor the categories clearly definitive. The examples of disease patterns of isolates that follow have been selected to reflect the interaction of several of the above factors.

A. Infectious Diseases

Most infections do not lead to overt disease but only to subclinical infections that also confer immunity. Burnet and White (1972) offer three general considerations on the spread of infections, which can be summarized as identification of the reservoir and mode of liberation of the infectious agent from it; transmission from infected host to new susceptibles; and mode of entry into the tissues. Specific factors such as route of inoculation, number of organisms needed to produce clinical symptoms, number of persons shedding microorganisms, duration of disease, resistance and virulence of the agent, and probability of contact with new susceptibles are also important in determining the epidemiological characteristics of infectious disease.

Infectious diseases affecting isolates can be divided into two categories: (1) Those that persist in a population over a long period of time, maintaining themselves in either human or nonhuman hosts, are referred to as endemic or endogenous infections. They are characterized by high incidence and low morbidity, frequently due to the large number of subclinical infections that confer natural immunity. Such infections tend to survive well in small isolated populations as they do not normally kill their hosts. (2) Those infections that produce only acute symptomatic disease and generally have no reservoir other than man are referred to as epidemic or exogenous diseases. In isolated groups they tend to have a high incidence, high morbidity, and high mortality. Such diseases generally ''burn-out'' quickly after introduction, because a large population is needed to supply new groups of susceptibles as those previously affected either die or become immune.

1. Endemic Diseases

The examples of endemic infections selected are those that have long persistence, usually as latent infections that may sometimes be reactivated to produce late or recurrent disease.

The nonvenereal treponemal infections of yaws, pinta, and bejel are evolutionarily very old and today almost exclusively associated with isolated population groups. Unlike venereal syphilis, these infections elicit a natural immunity.

Pinta, characterized by areas of white depigmented mottled skin in late-stage lesions, typically affects adolescents and young adults and now appears limited to river basins in tropical Central and South America, particularly the upper reaches of the Amazon Basin. Transmission generally necessitates a break in the skin and close contact with an infected person. Demis (1977) reported that the Pura-pura Indians of the Amazon Basin have a tribal ritual in which affected adults and noninfected youths are alternately whipped in order to transmit the disease, presumably because of their preference for mottled skin. Biting insects may also play a direct role in the transmission of pinta, but such insect involvement has not been proved.

Bejel, also called endemic syphilis, is rapidly disappearing. Found mostly among prepubertal children in Africa and several eastern Mediterranean countries, the disease is spread by contact with infected lesions of the mouth or through common drinking vessels. The disease is known among Bedouins, among tribal populations of Iran and Afghanistan, and among Yugoslavs, where it is sometimes referred to as "drinking spout disease." It spreads easily within a household or in groups where communal drinking vessels are used.

Yaws, the most important and widespread nonvenereal treponemal infection of man, is found in almost all hot and humid tropical environments. Rarely fatal, it can be debilitating, affecting the skin and bone through destructive late-stage lesions. Infection results from close contact in early childhood, and the early-stage lesions can remain infectious for 4 or 5 years. An asymptomatic latent stage then develops for 3 or more years until final-stage destructive lesions appear (Fig. 1). Unlike bejel, yaws spreads through close contact with susceptible children from other households as older sibs within the same household have probably already passed into the latent noninfectious stage.

Because of its long infectious stage, yaws may persist in small isolated tropical populations, where it remains endemic, affecting a few newly susceptible children each year. Yaws and venereal syphilis do not normally occur simultaneously, leading to the generally accepted conclusion that yaws provides strong, if not total, protection from venereal syphilis. Thus yaws, free of the cardiovascular and neurological sequelae of syphilis, limits the debilitating disease load on these groups.

The second example of endemic diseases is illustrated by several of the herpesviruses, which maintain themselves endemically in isolated groups by their persistent infections, are ubiquitous, and are acquired at a very early age. Cytomegalovirus (CMV) and Epstein–Barr virus (EBV), two members of this group, have been studied extensively in cosmopolitan and in isolated communities throughout the world. They often present as inapparent subclinical infections, although both agents have been implicated in overt disease, CMV

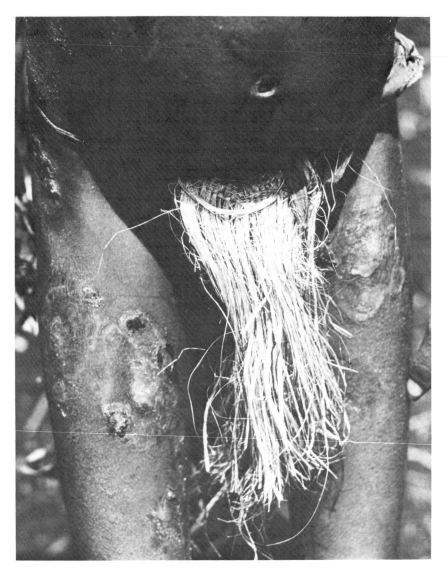

Fig. 1.   Yaws lesions of the lower extremities of a Mamusi girl from the central highlands of New Britain (DCG 56 M 69).

mainly in congenital infections and EBV in infectious mononucleosis, Burkitt's lymphoma, and nasopharyngeal carcinoma. In a survey of isolated communities in the Solomon Islands, New Hebrides, and New Guinea, virtually all persons were found to have acquired infections with both CMV and EBV at a very early age (Lang *et al.*, 1977). These studies suggest that the spread of CMV and EBV is probably determined by the pattern of interpersonal contact, the prevalence of virus shedders, and the amount of virus shed. In such groups infection is most likely through contamination with saliva, urine, feces, breast milk, semen, or cervical excretions. Direct mouth-to-mouth food sharing, especially with infants, is a widespread practice; many different individuals premasticate food for an infant or pass food from their mouths to an infant or toddler. In all three populations, babies are seldom out of the arms of children or adults during the daylight hours, and the number of different close and distant relatives who hold and carry the infant, often kissing or playing with the baby in the act of nose rubbing and mouth-to-mouth contact, may exceed a dozen every day. This intensity of interpersonal contact with many different infant handlers clearly differentiates the opportunity for acquiring herpesvirus infections in infancy in these cultures, rather than with a few restricted individuals as in closed Western nuclear families.

Under certain circumstances, exposure to CMV and EBV at an early age and the establishment of persistent inapparent infections may be advantageous to the host. Although significant fetal dissemination and damage may follow primary maternal CMV infection, previous maternal experience with any CMV serotype seems to protect the fetus against significant virus-induced injury. Among people who acquire CMV infections universally during early childhood, congenital infection associated with fetal injury should, therefore, occur rarely, or not at all. Additionally, early exposure to EBV provides protection against later onset of infectious mononucleosis or other EBV-associated diseases (Epstein and Achong, 1979).

Finally, we can consider the diseases of chickenpox (*varicella*) and shingles (*Herpes zoster*), two different disease expressions caused by the same infectious agent, varicella–zoster virus (V–Z virus), a third member of the herpesvirus group. Although the agent can be either endemic or epidemic in natural populations, the endemic model is presented because of the fascinating evolutionary adaptation of the V–Z virus to the human host through its reactivation abilities.

Chickenpox, a highly contagious disease spread by the respiratory route through droplet infections, is primarily a childhood disease that confers natural immunity on recovery.

Shingles, on the other hand, is a sporadic reactivation of the V–Z virus in already partially immune older persons who have had chickenpox. The mechanism responsible for reactivation is not known, although it is widely supposed that the V–Z virus enters the sensory nerve system during the initial chickenpox infection and establishes a chronic latent infection in the dorsal-root ganglia (Hope-Simpson, 1965). The virus particles are contained by the host's circulating antibodies until resistance falls below a critical level. The reactivated virus, no longer contained, then multiplies and passes down the sensory nerve to the skin.

Shingles, although mildly debilitating and often painful, only rarely leads to serious central nervous system complications. The epidemiological importance of this disease lies in the fact that from a single case of sporadic shingles, new susceptibles in the population can contract chickenpox. Thus, the agent maintains and perpetuates itself in humans, its only known natural host. The reverse situation, chickenpox causing shingles or secondary infections with shingles, is rare or nonexistent. In isolated populations, therefore, the natural situation allows for "epidemics" of chickenpox with an endemic agent. Because of its latent abilities even small populations with a critical size of less than 1000 persons are affected, because the V–Z virus may remain latent for many years until reactivation during adulthood, allowing the accumulation of new susceptibles (Hope-Simpson, 1965).

2. Epidemic Diseases

Epidemic diseases of isolated groups are best exemplified by measles and influenza, infections commonly introduced into such groups and causing high morbidity and mortality.

Measles represents the classical example of a severe epidemic in previously isolated communities having no previous immunological experience with the disease. Such outbreaks are called "virgin-soil" epidemics. However, measles epidemics can also occur cyclically in moderately isolated groups with intervals as long as one, two, or three decades before reintroduction of the agent. Because few groups live in absolute isolation, the cyclic occurrence of measles is the more usual situation, with the oldest members of the group having already experienced at least one measles epidemic. Reports of such epidemics representing diverse geographic areas come from isolated communities in New Guinea, Micronesia, Australia, the Amazon Basin, Greenland, and the Canadian Arctic (Adels and Gajdusek, 1963; Black *et al.*, 1977; Christensen *et al.*, 1953; Peart and Nagler, 1954).

Black (1966) suggested that measles needs a population base of 200,000 to 500,000, depending on the population density, for the virus to persist endemically without reintroduction from the outside. Such a critical community size is dictated by several factors. First, measles virus has no reservoir other than man capable of causing human epidemics. Second, lifelong immunity follows infection and thus a sizeable continuous supply of new susceptibles must be born each year. Third, the disease has an infectious acute stage of only several days.

Finally, measles virus, unlike chickenpox virus, is not latent and able to be reactivated except in rare cases of delayed and chronic measles encephalitis (subacute sclerosing panencephalitis) wherein patients release no infectious virus and thus cannot infect other susceptibles. It therefore seems likely that measles virus is evolutionarily a new organism, with the disease probably not antedating the great civilizations of 5000 or 6000 years ago (Black, 1966, 1975).

Measles epidemics in isolated groups are often severe, with attack rates of nearly 100% and case mortalities of almost 30% (Black et al., 1977). Such a high mortality is probably due to secondary bacterial infections and inadequate medical care (Adels and Gajdusek, 1963; Polunin, 1967; Black et al., 1977). Such epidemics result in complete collapse of village life with virtually everyone becoming sick at once. Mothers are unable to nurse their infants, food supplies wane, and hygiene deteriorates. Fear and depression often ensue and social continuity within the group diminishes (Polunin, 1967; Brown and Gajdusek, 1970; Neel, 1970; Dubos, 1965). It is perhaps this phenomenon that has implicated unusual racial susceptibility as an explanation for greater severity of introduced diseases in such groups.

Influenza represents a second example of an introduced disease with widespread medical significance for isolated populations. Like measles, influenza causes high morbidity and mortality in these communities, with a short contagious period. Animal reservoirs of influenza viruses are known, but none is a cause of human epidemics. Yet primary infections from animals to man have occurred, and the 1976 outbreak of swine influenza in about 500 Fort Dix army recruits suggests that secondary man-to-man transmission of infections acquired from animals may occasionally occur (Kilbourne, 1978). Many reports of influenza epidemics in isolated communities have appeared since 1933, when it became possible to certify the cause of the disease by isolation of the agent (summarized in Brown et al., 1966). However, the 1969–1970 Hong Kong influenza epidemic in New Guinea, with its unusual progression and shifting clinical severity, gave new insights into the behavior of the virus in isolated island-like communities (Garruto and Gajdusek, 1975; Gajdusek, 1971). Hong Kong flu was late in reaching many isolated New Guinea villages allowing the determination of antibody levels to the virus in many persons before the epidemic arrived. On arrival, it behaved erratically: in some communities nearly 100% of the inhabitants contracted influenza in less than a month. In other communities the epidemic lasted many months, with prevalence never exceeding 10%. Influenza passed through some schools affecting only a few students, to return many months later to infect those missed during the first passage. Virus isolation confirmed that both waves were caused by the same strain of influenza. Influenza-associated mortality was from 1 to 10% in some communities whereas in others, both large and small, no cases were fatal. In the New Guinea Highlands the main cause of death was pneumonia—usually secondary bacterial pneumonia, with the pneumococcus the prime offender. Secondary gastroenteritis in some villages and meningitis in others also contributed to mortality.

Carrier rates of meningococcus, pneumococcus, *H. influenzae*, and streptococcus in the community were important in determining the incidence and nature of secondary complications of influenza. The impact of the influenza epidemic on a community appeared to depend on how much crowded indoor living was necessitated by inclement weather and on the immune status of the population. The possibility that some patients were particularly active and intense spreaders of infection may also have been important.

Like measles, fatal outcome of influenza may result from lack of prompt medical care, as noted in studies of isolated Eskimo communities, of South American Indian tribal populations, and, most distinctly, among Micronesians from the Outer Islands of the Yap district (Pettit *et al.*, 1936; Black *et al.*, 1977; Brown *et al.*, 1966). In the Micronesian epidemic, the best medical care was provided on Ulithi with some care on Woleai and the least on the smallest and most isolated of the three islands, Ifaluk. The mortality rates were 1, 3, and 6.5%, respectively.

Finally, although active immunity from an influenza attack persists for many years, the protection afforded is specific to the subtype variant of the virus involved. With the virus's unusually high ability to mutate, the disease not only reaches epidemic proportions but can and does become pandemic as well.

B. Nutritional, Toxic, or Deficiency Disease

Perhaps no single factor influences the patterns of disease as much as the nutritional practices of the world's populations. Nutrition is also one of the most difficult factors to evaluate, particularly at a secondary level of association with disease. Nutrition is affected by the degree of a population's isolation and by its demographic characteristics, group mobility, uniformity of food sources, specific cultural practices, and ecosystem stability. Many populations, for instance, clearly are precariously adapted to their environment. Concepts of optimal and critical levels of nutrition are important in assessing the degree to which people are in nutritional balance with their environment. Among the !Kung Bushman, hunter–gatherers who live in the harsh environment of Botswana with limited and seasonal variation in food sources, no qualitative deficiencies of specific nutrients were found (Truswell, 1977). There was no obesity, coronary heart disease, high blood pressure, elevated blood lipid levels, or dental caries. Accidents and infectious diseases were the major causes of morbidity and mortality. The generally poor nutrition of some isolated horticulturalists is associated with protein deficiency, as in the Ekari (Kapauku) of the Central Highlands of West New Guinea (Couvée, 1962). Birth weights and infantile growth rates among the

Mulia Dani, their eastern neighbors, are among the lowest reported for New Guineans and are in part associated with the severely protein-deficient diet of pregnant mothers in the Mulia Valley (Gajdusek *et al.*, 1974). Populations living on small Pacific islands and atolls characteristically have low-fat, high-carbohydrate, and high-protein (fish and shellfish) diets. Although a limited land mass exists, the ocean provides plentiful foodstuffs rich in vitamins, protein, and other nutrients. However, such nutrition may be periodically interrupted by typhoons that devastate natural food supplies, forcing whole populations to move to other islands or suffer severe nutritional stress.

Among less-isolated aboriginal populations, including native American Indians, Eskimo, and certain Melanesians, Micronesians, and Polynesians, the prevalence and clinical manifestations of diabetes have been extensively documented (West, 1974). However, the extent to which diet, degree of adiposity, genetic predisposition, population variability, peculiarities of glucose metabolism, insulin secretion, and social, cultural, and economic factors are involved in the patterns of diabetes and hyperglycemia observed in these groups remains unclear.

Hyperuricemia and chronic debilitating gout are highly prevalent in the Pacific Basin, with high levels reported for Micronesians, including Chamorros and Carolineans (Reed *et al.*, 1972; Burch *et al.*, 1966); Polynesians, including New Zealand Maori, Cook Islanders, and Samoans (Prior and Rose, 1966; Healy and Jones, 1970); Filipinos (Healy *et al.*, 1966; Decker *et al.*, 1962); and Indonesian Malayans (Duff *et al.*, 1968). Obesity, high caloric and fat intake, diabetes, and alcohol use are often associated with the disease. Diet as a causative factor in high uric acid levels is difficult to evaluate; Reed and co-workers (1972) found no association with sociocultural factors or degree of acculturation and suggested that the disease may be genetically influenced among Micronesians.

Isolated groups frequently use highly toxic plants and animals as foodstuffs or as traditional healing remedies including known poisonous or occasionally poisonous fish, goiterogenic agents, tapioca root, toxic mushrooms, species of wild lima beans, and cycad nuts. Some are rendered harmless by extraction of the toxin, others are tolerated after several prior ingestions of small amounts, and still others result in uncalculated violent deaths. With the close association of a population to its indigenous flora and fauna, people in all isolates are cognizant of the toxic substances in their environment that cause acute disease or poisoning. On Guam for example, cycad, the highly toxic nut of *Cycas circinalis*, has been an important carbohydrate food source (Whiting, 1964; Kurland, 1972) and is still used today, although on a more restricted basis. The nut contains water-soluble substances that are highly carcinogenic and hepatotoxic. It may also contain neurotoxic substances previously postulated as extrinsic factors associated with amyotrophic lateral sclerosis and parkinsonism-dementia, chronic degenerative neurological diseases common among Guamanian Chamorros.

The nuts are opened, sliced, washed for several days with frequent water changes to elute the toxin, dried, and ground into flour. However, nuts more highly toxic than normal or washing that is improper and inadequate can result in ingestion of small amounts of toxin that may remain after such treatment. In addition, traditional healers, called *suruhanos,* have on occasion prepared the unwashed cycad as a poultice in the treatment of skin ailments (Kurland, 1978).

Dental caries appear to be associated with degree of isolation and increased consequences of westernization. Among most traditional isolates, little if any oral hygiene is practiced. Yet the prevalence of caries among these groups is frequently much lower than would be expected in cosmopolitan westernized populations (Pedersen, 1938; Schamschula *et al.,* 1977; Liu, 1977; Masi, 1973). The consequences of decreased isolation and increased westernization with increased dietary intake of refined fermentable carbohydrates seem clear. In contrast, attrition of occlusion surfaces results from a traditional diet high in abrasives, as evidenced by widespread chewing of coca leaves among Andean Indians of South America and betel nut in Pacific populations (Polunin, 1953–1954).

Finally, deficiency diseases other than protein–calorie malnutrition include vitamin, calcium, iron, and iodine deficiencies. Less than a decade ago endemic goiter and cretinism posed a major medical problem in many inland mountainous regions of the world, but with the advent of iodized oil injections and iodized salt the problem has been brought under control (Figs. 2–4). One of the largest foci of hyperendemic goiter and cretinism, often associated with a high level of congenital deaf-mutism, was discovered in the Central Highlands of Western New Guinea. The two conditions presented a crippling load of defect on the isolated Dani population of the Mulia Valley, wherein 50% of the female adults from most villages suffered from goiter (Gajdusek, 1962; Gajdusek and Garruto, 1975). Among the Dani children, there is a wide spectrum of cretinoid defects with severe dwarfism occurring in only a few children and occasionally in those who are neither deaf-mutes nor severely mentally defective (Gajdusek, 1962). Clearly, iodine deficiency is the cause of endemic goiter and cretinism in these inland populations, and endemic cretinism results from fetal damage *in utero* due to iodine deficiency in the mother during pregnancy; this form is distinguished from the sporadic hypothyroid cretinism usually associated with severe dwarfism.

These studies demonstrate that within a single cultural and linguistic group the incidence of goiter may be extremely high in one region and extremely low in an adjacent region without any change in diet, other cultural factors, language, or genetic origin. Additionally, populations in some regions with low-incidence goiter may have no higher serum protein-bound iodine (PBI) levels than do severely affected populations with goitrous patients having only slightly lower PBIs than normal nongoitrous persons (Garruto *et al.,* 1974). In areas where such extremely low levels of iodine exist, populations may be "pregoitrous" and adapted to low "critical" levels of intake; even a slight decrease in iodine intake,

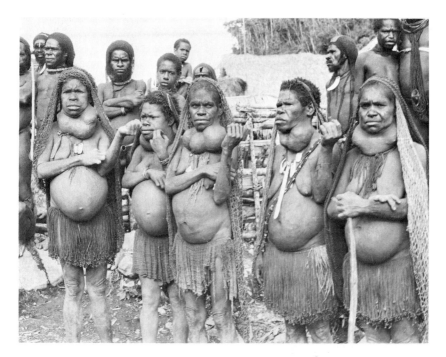

Fig. 2. Five western Dani women and two men from Mulia, Central Highlands, West New Guinea, with large goiters. The photograph was taken in 1959 a few minutes after blood specimens were collected for iodine determinations. One goitrous man stands between the first and second women and another between the fourth and fifth women from the left (DCG 59 DNG II).

for example after ingestion of a mild goiterogenic substance like that postulated for iron-binding sweet potato leaves, may be critical in provoking marginal-risk persons into "full-blown" disease (Gajdusek, 1962). This situation may have occurred in the Jimi River area of Papua New Guinea, where the introduction of uniodized salt for barter rapidly replaced use of salt from traditional mineral springs that had been a source of at least some iodine in the already iodine-deficient "pregoitrous" population.

C. Genetic Disorders and Congenital Anomalies

Specific genetic disorders and congenital anomalies may attain unusually high frequencies in highly inbred, isolated communities. The example just presented of endemic cretinism and the spectrum of damage it causes to fetuses of severely iodine-deficient mothers is a case in point. Certainly the genetic load of defect on any isolate is determined by numerous factors, including size, mating patterns and structure, socioeconomic circumstances, gene flow, selection, and drift (Fig.

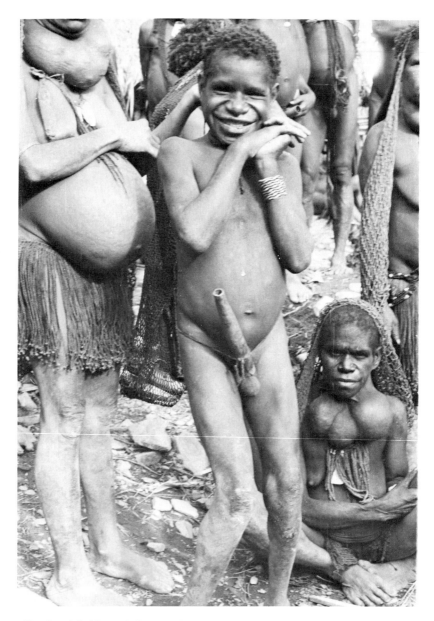

Fig. 3. A feeble-minded cretinoid adolescent boy from Mulia in hyperlordotic stance between two women with huge goiters. Partially deaf and severely mentally retarded, he nevertheless took an active part in the social life and work of the community (DCG 59 DNG II).

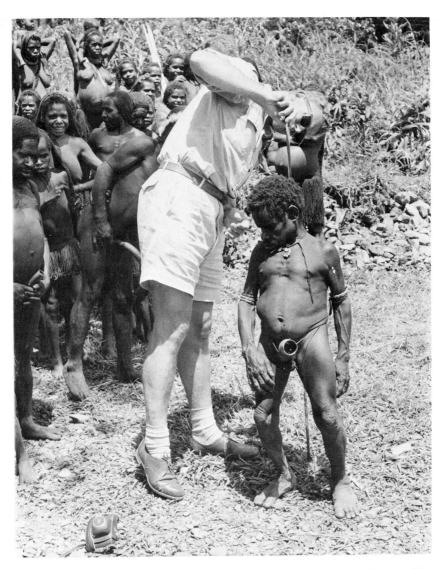

Fig. 4. An intelligent adult male cretin dwarf from the Guderi Valley of western Dani people. He understood gestures and cooperated well with Dr. J. ten Brink. Severe dwarfism is not always a feature of the cretinoid syndrome in this focus of endemic goiter (DCG 61 WP II).

5). For some isolates, infanticide is a well-known method for removing recognized congenitally defective children from the population (Neel, 1970, 1977; Glasse, 1963). Thus, the load of defect may be higher in isolates without similar practices.

Isolated communities often have a wide spectrum of genetic disorders and congenital defects that sometimes occur in foci within larger populations. Thus, albinism may be sporadic or attain high frequencies within a single endogamous group like the Zuni Indians of the American southwest, where the condition is 100 times more prevalent than in the general population (Mohindra and Nagaraj, 1977) (Fig. 6). In some communities albinos are socially accepted whereas in others they are rejected and even destroyed (Gajdusek, 1964a).

A focus of male pseudohermaphroditism among the Simbari Anga in the Papua New Guinea highlands has recently been fully described (Gajdusek, 1964b, 1977a). The people recognize the defect as congenital yet accept those with malformed genitalia as members of the community (Figs. 7a and b). In a society that practices extreme sex segregation with complicated age-grade initiations, those malformed members are not killed but are allowed to function as males in the culture, having abandoned in such cases the awkward and inappropriate male initiation ceremonies which are instead verbally explained.

There is a high incidence of lactase deficiency in American Indians and Australian Aborigines, autosomal recessive dwarfism among the Amish, autosomal recessive muscular dystrophy among the Hutterites of Canada, familial Mediterranean fever among Sephardic Jews, and Tay-Sachs disease among Ashkenazic Jews. Sporadic hypothyroid cretinism, generally caused by the absence of a structural or transport protein of a metabolic enzyme, occurs in families on the isolated islands of Rennell and Bellona in the Solomon Islands (D. C. Gajdusek and R. M. Garruto, unpublished data).

Congenital achromatopsia, total color blindness (rod monochromatism), is an autosomal recessive disease found in high incidence among Pingelapese, a genetic isolate in the Eastern Caroline Islands of Micronesia (Brody et al., 1970; Carr et al., 1971; Hussels and Morton, 1972). The disease, also characterized by aversion to bright light and poor visual acuity, occurs much less commonly in the general population than forms of X-linked color blindness. This disorder exemplifies the effects of historical accident and closed breeding systems on small populations. In the late eighteenth century, the tiny atoll of Pingelap was struck by a severe typhoon that devastated the population of 500 inhabitants, leaving about 20 survivors; their descendents repopulated the island to numbers of several hundred by the early twentieth century. During the German administration of the islands, a portion of the Pingelapese population was moved to the island of Ponape, where they set up a community with endogamous marriage practices. Thus, the number of persons with achromatopsia on the atoll as well as on Ponape reached about 5%, with more than one-third of the popula-

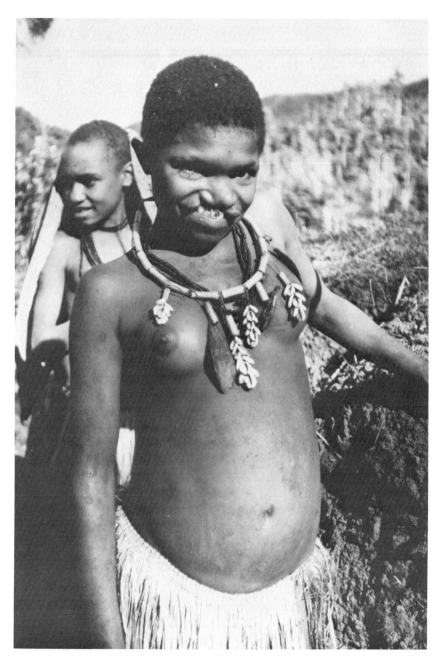

Fig. 5. A Simbari Anga girl with harelip from the Dunkwi group in the Eastern Highlands province of Papua New Guinea who had been followed since infancy in our study. She was the only living patient with harelip among the Simbari (DCG 72 NG 30).

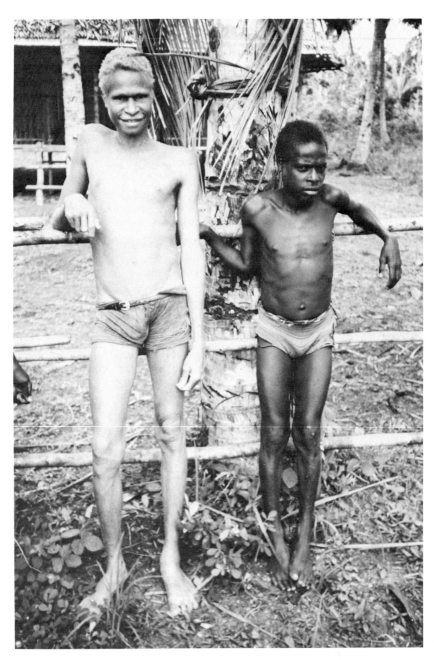

Fig. 6.   An albino male of the Khogi linguistic group from the southeastern coastal plain of West New Guinea (DCG 74 WNG 49).

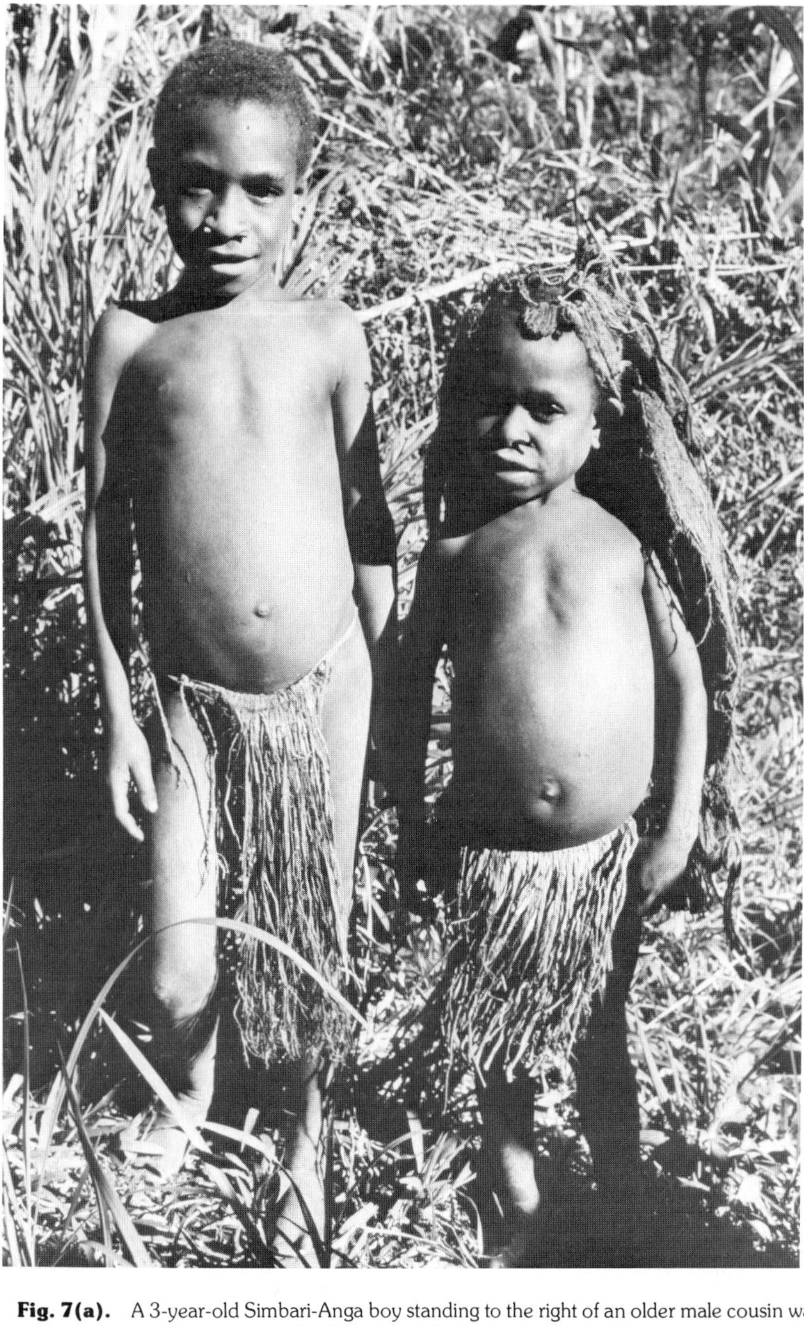

Fig. 7(a). A 3-year-old Simbari-Anga boy standing to the right of an older male cousin was recognized as a pseudohermaphrodite (*kwalatmala*) shortly after birth. He wears the attire of a small girl with a girl's grass skirt and bark cape covering the buttocks to avert having visitors mock him as a "girl" in boy's attire (DCG 76 PNG 25).

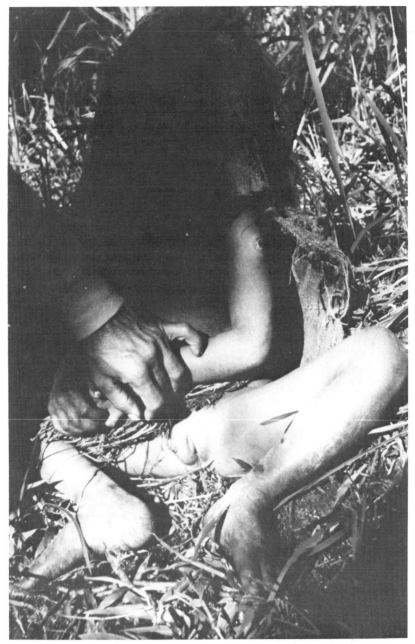

Fig. 7(b).   The same boy showing the external genetalia (DCG 76 PNG 27).

tion being carriers of the recessive gene (Carr *et al.*, 1971; Hussels and Morton, 1972). Such historic accidents in small isolated groups with closed or semiclosed mating systems are claimed not to have been unique, and thus founder effects and drift may have dramatically influenced the genetics of small isolates during the course of human evolution (Gajdusek, 1964a).

The recent discovery that autosomal recessive inheritance correlates with susceptibility to *tinea imbricata* (Tokelau ringworm), a fungal infection of isolates in Papua New Guinea (Schofield *et al.*, 1963; Serjeantson and Lawrence, 1977) and Southeast Asia (Polunin, 1952), represents an important genetic model of an infectious disease (Fig. 8). The disease is a superficial skin infection with non-localized, itching, patchy concentric rings affecting most group members by 2 years of age. The occurrence of the disease (8–30%) is promoted by a hot, wet tropical environment, close contact between infected relatives and uninfected infants, and the nutritional status of the person (Schofield *et al.*, 1963). The failure of infants to gain weight, or weight loss in adults as a result of illness and pregnancy, was a consistent pattern associated with the disease.

The disease is not serious clinically but has profound social implications because it reduces the overall crude fertility rate of the community while selectively fixing gene frequencies. Infected women tend to marry much later than unaffected women and are frequently only a second or third choice mate in polygamous unions (Schofield *et al.*, 1963). Although in 1963 direct evidence for a genetic factor had not been found, children of nonaffected parents or with one affected parent had lower incidences than if both parents were commonly affected, with frequencies of 16, 40, and 63%, respectively. More substantial evidence for genetic susceptibility became available in 1977, when Serjeantson and Lawrence (1977) demonstrated in an untreated New Guinea population that the disease was compatible with an autosomal recessive mode of inheritance. With continued studies to further substantiate the genetic implications, *tinea imbricata* should become an important genetic model of an infectious disease. The exact conditions for expression of the disease remain undefined, however, and thus the relative contribution of genetic susceptibility to the expression of the disease remains unknown.

D. Culturally Specific Psychoses

Unusual culture- or group-specific psychological disorders or "exotic syndromes" range from mild possession states and beliefs to severe psychopathic reactions with homicidal tendencies. Such culture-bound syndromes are surprisingly common. *Susto*, found among Andean Quechua Indians, is a possession syndrome characterized by anxiety and depression following fright or shock, and *amok*, a well-known reactive psychosis, is associated with suicidal and homicidal tendencies in Malaya. Other culturally related conditions have been reported:

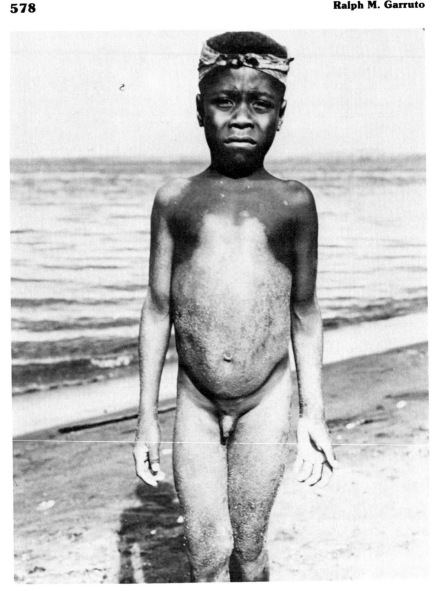

Fig. 8. A prepubertal boy from Rapuri Village, West Nakanai, New Britain, with *tinea imbricata*, called *grile* in Pidgin. The fungal infection is nonlocalized and covers much of his body with characteristic patchy concentric rings (DCG 56 WN 202).

epidemics of laughter in the Lake Victoria area of East Africa; fear of penile shrinkage and retraction associated with acute anxiety and intense panic, known as *koro* among Southeast Asians; dissociation syndromes of *piblokto*, a form of Arctic hysteria, among Eskimos; and *windigo*, a possession syndrome among Canadian Indians. Other culture-specific psychoses include *latah* in Malaya or *mali-mali* in the Philippines and *lulu* and "wildman" (*long-long*) behavior in New Guinea.

The conditions cited are not all-inclusive but represent a spectrum of culturally specific psychoses that are sometimes viewed within the group as abnormal but at times may be culturally sanctioned to various degrees. The specific causes associated with such syndromes can be obscure but are thought to be associated with psychological shock, fear, stress, depression, and hysteria. Yap (1968, 1969) believed that such "reactive" psychoses are affected by sociocultural factors, including value systems, shared beliefs, and influences during the socialization process. Evidence associating certain of these syndromes to physiological, metabolic, or dietary deficiencies remains unclear (Foulks and Katz, 1975).

E. Myths of Increased Susceptibility and Increased Resistance to Disease among Isolated Populations

The "myth" of increased susceptibility of certain isolated racial and ethnic groups to acute infections comes from accounts of great epidemics among previously isolated groups. Generally such an outbreak can be attributed to the immunologically virgin status of a group relative to a particular disease agent and by the concomitant sociocultural collapse from diseases of high morbidity and mortality. Additionally, observed differences in infectious disease between populations (as with dengue hemorrhagic fever in Southeast Asia in the 1960s) may arise from their differing previous exposures to a similar or antigenetically related agent (Halstead *et al.*, 1969; Gajdusek, 1977a; Fazekas de St. Groth and Webster, 1966).

The "converse myth" of increased resistance to disease in isolated groups results from impressions of early Pacific explorers who saw the islanders as healthy, happy, and well adapted to their environment. Several factors contribute to that picture:

(1) In most traditionally isolated groups infanticide is often practiced when congenital malformations and defects are recognized at birth.

(2) Cultural patterns, hygienic practices, and intimate contact with the natural environment result in inapparent infections from endemic agents during infancy

and childhood with early acquisition of immunity against potentially more severe
late-onset infections.

(3) Immunoglobulin levels are elevated, with high maternal antibody transfer
probably occurring during pregnancy (Couvée, 1962; Neel, 1977).

(4) Long-term breast-feeding results in reasonably good nutrition and lowered
completed fertility.

(5) Major infectious diseases such as influenza, measles, smallpox, cholera,
plague, and typhoid are not endemic as a consequence of small group size.

(6) There is a low incidence of overt chronic diseases associated with increased
westernization and of diseases associated with old age (Dunn, 1968). The latter is
due to a shortened life span, probably as a result of accidents, homicides,
suicides, group conflict, and early death from acute bacterial infections among
chronically ill persons.

Differential genetic susceptibility to disease is extremely difficult to verify or
evaluate (Neel, 1977). Its existence in animals is well documented (Allison, 1975;
Schull, 1963). In man, however, the evidence is limited. The well-known associations between hemoglobin S and resistance to *falciparum* malaria, the
resistance of Duffy-negative blood groups to *vivax* malaria (Miller *et al.*, 1975;
1976), and the demonstration of autosomal recessive inheritance in susceptibility
to the fungal infection *tinea imbricata* (Serjeantson and Lawrence, 1977) provide good evidence for genetic susceptibility in man. However, most associations are unclear, and the clarity has not been improved by the voluminous
literature on histocompatibility antigens (HLA) and disease.

III. INTERACTION OF BIOLOGY AND BEHAVIOR IN THE NATURAL ENVIRONMENT

A. Specific Behavioral Patterns of Isolates Resulting in Unusual Patterns of Disease

Some isolates present unusual patterns of disease as a direct consequence of
their behavioral or cultural practices. Patterns of leprosy and pulmonary tuberculosis described by Schofield (1970) in separate communities of Ethiopian
hermit monks illustrate the point. In one community more than one-third of those
examined had leprosy (Fig. 9). Affected and unaffected persons were not segregated nor were leprous monks excluded from joining the community. All monks
refused treatment, believing that the more maimed they were with leprous lesions, the purer their souls became. In the second community, much the same
philosophy existed. Monks with pulmonary tuberculosis refused treatment and
unaffected monks understood that they were at high risk of becoming infected.

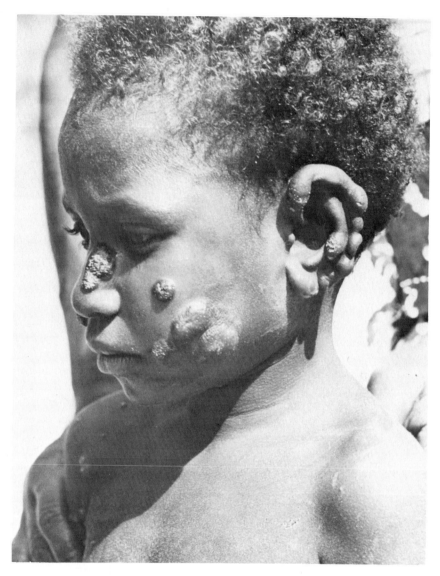

Fig. 9. A young boy on the Papuan coast of Papua New Guinea, showing the characteristic deforming leprous lesions of the face, nose, and ear.

Perhaps one of the most unusual patterns of disease expression results from the practice of endocannibalism among the Fore people and neighboring residents in the Eastern Highlands of Papua New Guinea. Kuru, a chronic degenerative infectious disease of the central nervous system, was first described medically by Gajdusek and Zigas (1957). They soon associated the spread of the disease with ritualistic cannibalism of dead relatives practiced mainly by women and children. The route of inoculation is not necessarily through ingestion, but more importantly through contamination of peripheral routes that include the conjunctiva, nasal passage, auditory canal, and skin abrasions in the act of body dismemberment and handling of infectious tissue. The Australian administration and missionaries pursued a vigorous campaign among Eastern Highland populations in the 1940s and 1950s to eliminate the practice of eating dead relatives. Cannibalism ceased, and kuru is now rapidly disappearing. No one born after the practice was discontinued has ever developed the disease, and the youngest patients are now more than 20 years of age (Gajdusek, 1977b).

In the Wissel Lakes area of West New Guinea, the Ekari people are currently suffering from cysticercus epilepsy as a result of the recent introduction of pigs infected with *Taenia solium*, the pork tapeworm (Gajdusek, 1977a; 1978) (Figs. 10 and 11). Through close interaction between highland New Guinea man and his pigs, the parasite soon spread from the recently introduced infected pigs to the Ekari population. Ingestion of the cysticercus cysts in pig flesh ("measley pork") resulted in an intestinal infection with *T. solium* in a population previously free of the tapeworm. Soon thereafter, secondary infections in man acquired from contamination with human feces containing *T. solium* ova caused, not intestinal taeniasis with the pig tapeworm, but cysticercosis in man with the penetration of the larval form to *T. solium* into muscle, subcutaneous tissues, viscera, and central nervous system (CNS) tissue. In many of those affected, the larvae formed encapsulated cysts in the brain causing epileptic seizures. In the particular cultural setting of the Wissel Lakes area, where the highland population sleeps huddled close to house fires during the cold nights, cysticercosis resulted in a unique epidemic of severe burns, many fatal and others requiring amputations, as patients with cysticercus epilepsy often rolled into their house fires during grand mal seizures.

B. Specific Disease Patterns of Isolates Resulting in Changes in Sociocultural Practices

Also well documented is the fact that specific disease patterns result in changes in sociocultural phenomena. *Tinea imbricata,* already mentioned, results in mating segregation by socially restricting the choice of a partner, with uninfected persons preferring uninfected partners (Schofield *et al.,* 1963). Similarly, strict mating segregation associated with endemic leprosy also occurs in the Ethiopian

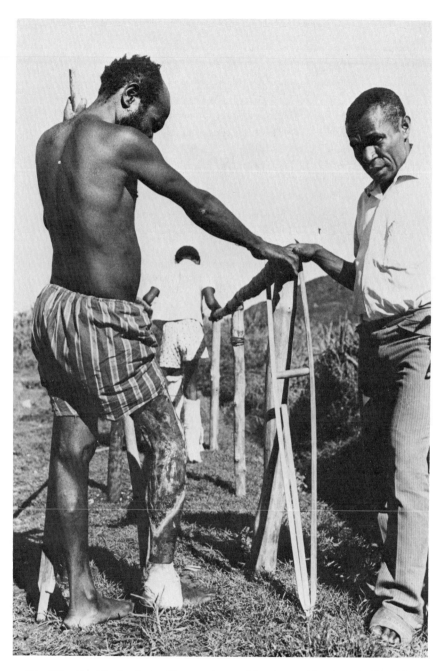

Fig. 10. Two Ekari patients with severe burns of their legs and feet from the Wissel Lakes area of West New Guinea. Both had cysticercosis epilepsy resulting from the recent introduction of the tapeworm into the area. While sleeping close to their house fires on cold nights both developed grand mal seizures, rolled into the fire, and, being unconscious, were unable to withdraw (Donkers 621–624).

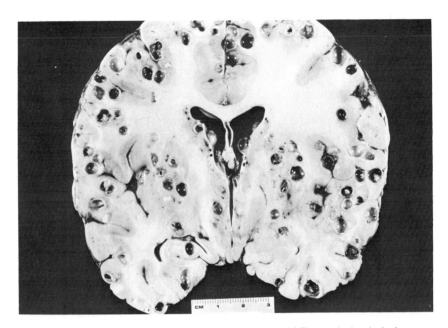

Fig. 11. This coronal section of brain from a 13-year-old Ekari girl who died of cysticercosis shows the multiple cysts that invaded the tissue. The estimated total number of cysts in the entire brain would exceed 2000. Microscopic examinations showed the cysts contained *Taenia solium* larvae (AFIP 76 7706).

highlands, although no physical isolation takes place because the disease is not considered infectious (Schofield, 1970).

The effects of kuru, with deaths preponderant in young adult women, resulted in a male to female sex ratio of 2:1 in many Fore communities and in other hamlets a ratio greater than 3:1 among those who had reached marriageable age. The polygamous Fore society, therefore, accumulated a large number of unmarried men and motherless nuclear families. In such families, men performed activities previously ascribed to women, including gardening and caring for infants (Glasse, 1962). Kuru has also led to many reprisal murders of suspected sorcerers who the Fore believed were responsible for these deaths (Lindenbaum, 1979).

In East Africa, a central core of 51 tribal groups extract or mutilate incisor teeth, a practice postulated as a response to high-incidence tetanus (Garruto and Willey, 1967 and unpublished data). Evidence of tooth evulsion has been found in skeletal remains as far back as the upper paleolithic era in northwest Africa (Wells, 1964) and is described in the Ebers Papyrus from eighteenth dynasty Egypt (Lefebvre, 1956). Upper and/or lower incisors are generally removed before infection allowing a tube to be introduced into the patient's mouth during the lockjaw stage of tetanus to prevent suffocation and provide a means for liquid feeding (Lefebvre, 1956). Native explanations of the custom range from extracting incisors to protect against tetanus to filing of teeth for reasons of beauty. Although an association between tetanus and the cultural practice of tooth evulsion exists, the extent to which this practice affects the course of the disease remains uncertain.

Extreme depopulation as a direct consequence of disease has had a major impact on the demographic and sociocultural patterns of many isolates (Scragg, 1954; Kooijman *et al.*, 1953–1954; Simmons *et al.*, 1967; Simmons and Gajdusek, 1966; Baruzzi *et al.*, 1977). Among the Marind-Anim and Yei-Anim people of coastal West New Guinea, the population had declined from an estimated 12,000 persons at the time of major European contact in 1902 to about 7000 by 1915. Around 1905, granuloma venereum was observed and its eventual spread linked to promiscuous ritual sexuality, an aspect of the traditional culture. The population soon became acutely ill, with the disease attaining frequencies as high as 25%. Considerable infertility followed, although granuloma venereum was not thought solely responsible for the population decline (Simmons *et al.*, 1967). Likewise, before and during World War II, gonorrhea had been implicated in the altered demographic structure of postwar Rennell Island in the New Hebrides, where a 1951 government census indicated an absence of children between the ages of 5 and 16 years (Simmons and Gajdusek, 1966).

IV. CHANGING PATTERNS OF DISEASE IN ACCULTURATING GROUPS

Traditional isolates are rapidly changing because of increased westernization and contact. The complex alteration of disease patterns in such groups is associated with a number of interacting and interrelated factors, including:

1. Decreased isolation
2. Decreased group mobility
3. Altered group size, increased in some and decreased in others
4. Major disturbances in the ecology
5. Dietary changes
6. Deteriorating sanitary and housing conditions
7. Decreased physical activity
8. Development of agricultural systems and cash economies
9. Increased exposure to toxic substances in air and water
10. Cultural and social disruption resulting in new forms of cultural stress

Major epidemic diseases including measles, smallpox, influenza, pertussis, and venereal disease are constantly reintroduced with shorter time intervals between epidemics as isolation continues to decrease. Intestinal parasitic infections increase, and epidemics of bacterial dysentery, including typhoid and cholera, appear, often as a consequence of crowding, decreased group mobility, and deteriorating sanitary and housing conditions. Development of tropical urban centers, the use of slash and burn agriculture, and the building of dams and reservoirs increases the occurrence of arbovirus infections such as "urban malaria" while decreasing the incidence of "jungle malaria" and yellow fever. In such groups endemic yaws is rapidly eliminated through easy and effective treatment, but venereal syphilis, lymphogranuloma, and gonorrhea are more severe replacements.

Breast feeding, normally of long duration (2 or 3 years) with resultant population control, is often shortened or abandoned in favor of bottle-feeding with cow's milk. Thus, previously good infant nutrition and immunological benefits from maternal milk are lost, and with the absence of high sanitation standards and refrigeration, bottle-feeding leads to severe diarrheas. Increased use of refined foods such as fermenting carbohydrates leads to the rapid appearance of dental caries in previously caries-free populations. Deficiencies in the diet, such as iodine, which result in huge goiters with associated congenital cretinism in inland mountain regions, readily disappear in isolated groups through the use of iodized-oil injections and dietary supplements of iodine.

Chronic and degenerative diseases are more noticeable as a consequence of increased westernization and include high frequencies of diabetes, obesity, hypertension, and cardiovascular disease, and some malignant neoplasms. Such chronic and degenerative diseases may result directly from increased use and mismanagement of processed foods, with increased consumption of sugar and fats and a decline in bulk fiber consumption, from radical changes in the local ecology with the introduction of chemical carcinogens such as sulfur, hydrocarbons, and insecticides or from the toxicity of soil, water, and air with heavy-metal pollutants.

Accidents—especially those involving moving vehicles—homicides, poisonings, and other violent forms of death are often leading causes of mortality in many acculturating communities (Reed, 1977). Alcoholism and some forms of drug abuse, as a direct consequence of increased contact and associated cultural impoverishment, are major widespread problems affecting many previously isolated groups, including Amerindians, Micronesians, Melanesians, and Australian Aborigines.

Finally, the cultural and social disruption incurred by the acculturating groups results in new forms of culture stress. Psychological stress and the anxiety of life in such "unsettled" societies result from new life-styles, imposed cultural mores, ideals, and similar circumstances.

As the process of acculturation and decreased isolation continues, new patterns of disease emerge and old ones disappear. Some changes are beneficial, others are surely detrimental, but the altered patterns of disease morbidity and mortality and the altered age structure of the population that follows loss of isolation result in far-reaching social changes for the entire community.

V. IMPLICATIONS OF NATURAL EXPERIMENTAL MODELS FOR SOLVING ETIOLOGICAL AND EPIDEMIOLOGICAL PROBLEMS OF WIDESPREAD MEDICAL SIGNIFICANCE

Foci of disease in isolated groups frequently offer a unique opportunity to increase our understanding of medical problems having worldwide as well as local significance. Recognition of the importance of such studies as other than just exotic phenomena was no doubt recently fostered by the awarding of the 1976 Nobel prize in physiology or medicine jointly to D. Carleton Gajdusek and Baruch S. Blumberg for their respective investigations of biomedical and anthropological phenomena in isolated human communities. The examples that follow have been specifically selected from studies of CNS diseases in high incidence among isolated groups in the western Pacific and represent disorders that have wider significance than the serious local problem they present.

A. Kuru: The Model and Its Implications

Kuru, a chronic progressive degenerative disease of the central nervous system caused by a transmissible virus with many unconventional properties, is found among the Fore and neighboring peoples in the eastern highlands of Papua New Guinea (Gajdusek, 1973) (Figs. 12 and 13). This uniformly fatal disease of slow neuronal destruction thought to be transmitted through the practice of ritualistic cannibalism is now rapidly disappearing. However, the "natural model" of a slowly progressive infection of man with long incubation periods and absence of an inflammatory response has led to the discovery of the transmissibility of another degenerative neurological disorder, Creutzfeldt–Jakob disease, having considerable similarities to kuru but found in worldwide distribution. Thus the investigation of kuru not only led to the discovery of new mechanisms for the origin and dissemination of infectious diseases and the recognition of a new group of microorganisms with atypical, unconventional physical and chemical properties but also led to the discovery of a "slow virus etiology" in a number of chronic diseases of man, such as delayed and chronic measles encephalopathy (SSPE), progressive multifocal leukoencephalopathy (PML), some forms of chronic epilepsy, and transmissible virus dementias. Furthermore, these investigations gave new impetus to the idea that similar slow unconventional virus infections may be involved in the chronic degenerative diseases of multiple

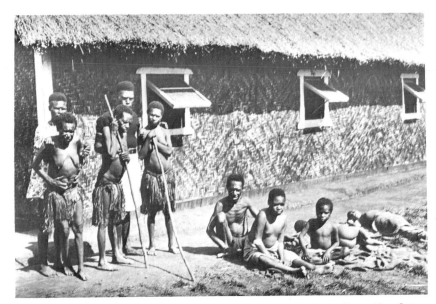

Fig. 12. Seven kuru patients at the Kuru Research Hospital in Okapa, Papua New Guinea, in 1957. The four children at the right are in stage two of the disease. The three adult women at the left are still ambulatory, but characteristically already require sticks to hold and maintain their balance (DCG 57 PNG 1090).

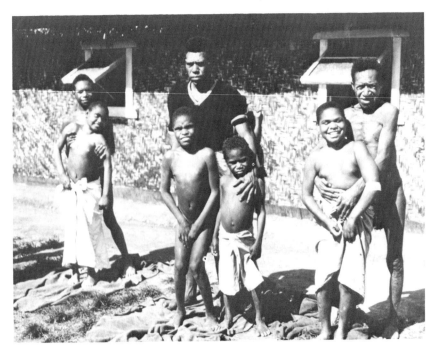

Fig. 13. Five Fore kuru children, including two boys in the center and a girl on each side, at the Kuru Research Hospital. The adolescent boy supporting the girl on the left is himself a kuru victim but in an earlier stage of the disease (DCG 57 PNG 1087).

sclerosis, amyotrophic lateral sclerosis, Parkinson disease, parkinsonism-dementia, and Alzheimer disease.

B. Foci of Motor Neuron Disease in the Western Pacific

Almost simultaneously with the discovery and initial medical descriptions of kuru, an extraordinary concentration of amyotrophic lateral sclerosis (ALS), another chronic progressive uniformly fatal disease, was found afflicting the Chamorro people of Guam and Rota in the southern Mariana Islands. Unlike kuru, ALS is found sporadically throughout the world, although certain clinical and pathological features of the disease led to the suggestion of a "Guam form" of ALS. Locally known as *lytico*, ALS is a disease of the motor neurons of the brain and spinal cord characterized by progressive atrophy of skeletal muscles. It appeared in the Chamorro population at a prevalence rate nearly 100 times that of the continental United States (Kurland and Mulder, 1954; Brody and Chen, 1969; Reed and Brody, 1975). No satisfactory explanation exists as yet for the high frequency of ALS on Guam (Fig. 14). The major contribution toward understanding the disease has been negative findings, which have excluded simple genetic, toxic, deficiency, or infectious etiologies. Studies on Guam have delineated a second uniformly fatal neurological disease, parkinsonism-dementia (PD), which occurs in association with ALS, the two disease patterns occurring simultaneously within the same sibship and even within a single patient more often than chance association would predict. In contrast to ALS, PD (locally referred to as *bodig*) is characterized by profound mental deterioration combined with slowness of voluntary motor activity, muscular rigidity, tremor and blank facial masking. Both disorders are late onset and together account for one in five Guamanian deaths in persons over 25 years of age (Brody and Kurland, 1973).

The Chamorro people of Saipan and Tinian in the more northern Mariana Islands do not have an unusually high incidence of ALS or PD, whereas the population of Rota shares the phenomenon of a high incidence of both diseases with the Guamanians. On Guam itself, the large non-Chamorro Caucasian population of predominantly transient American military personnel and their dependents has failed to show an unusual incidence of either disease. However, recent studies have demonstrated an increasing number of cases of ALS and PD in long-term Filipino migrants to Guam and in long-term Chamorro migrants to the United States (Garruto *et al.*, 1979, 1980, 1981). These observations suggest that toxic, infectious, metabolic, or deficiency factors on Guam, with or without genetic interaction, may be a cause of either disease.

Recent epidemiological data on ALS, like that on kuru, indicates a progressive decrease in incidence. Although the disease now appears relatively stable in women, it continues to decrease in men from a sex ratio of 2.5:1 three decades

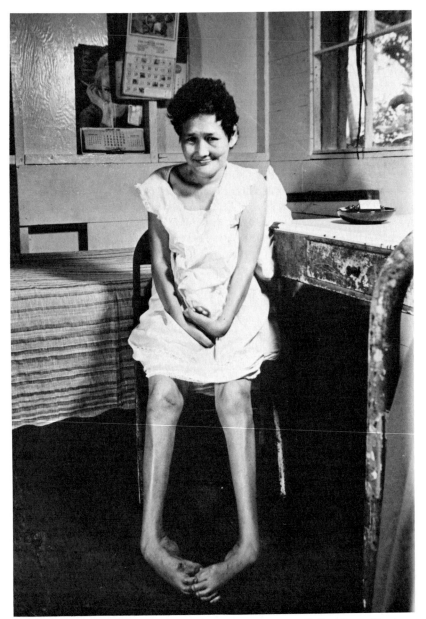

Fig. 14. A Chamorro patient with amyotrophic lateral sclerosis (ALS) of Guam. She shows the characteristic muscle atrophy of the limbs as a result of motor dysfunction and associated joint deformity. Onset of her ALS occurred at age 39 with a rather long-term duration of 14 years. (Courtesy of Dr. Kwang-Ming Chen.)

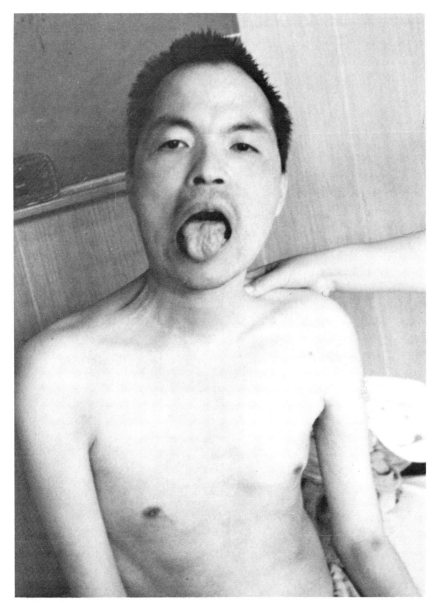

Fig. 15. A 36-year-old male ALS patient from the Kii peninsula focus in Japan. He had dysarthric speech and characteristic tongue atrophy. (Courtesy of Dr. Yoshiro Yase.)

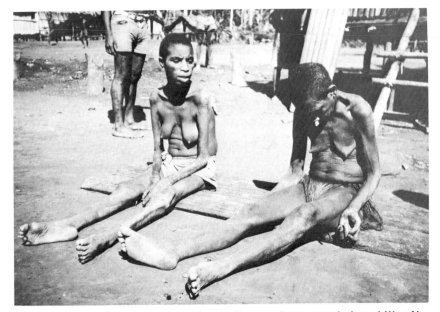

Fig. 16. Two Auyu women from Siyen village, southwest coastal plain of West New Guinea, with advanced ALS; both lived in the same household. Neither could walk without extensive support. The woman on the right with head drop, as a result of muscle atrophy in the neck, could not maintain a sitting posture. The duration of their illnesses was 4 and 4½ years, respectively (DCG 74 WNG 74).

ago to a ratio of 1:1 today (Garruto *et al.*, 1981b). No clear epidemiological trends for PD, however, are evident.

Two additional foci of high-incidence ALS and associated PD-like complex have been discovered among isolated groups living in the Kii Peninsula of Japan (Kimura *et al.*, 1963; Yase *et al.*, 1968) and among the Auyu and Jakai peoples in the southern lowlands of West New Guinea (Gajdusek, 1977a; 1979) (Figs. 15 and 16). In the latter isolate the prevalence rate has been estimated to be at least 500 times more than the rates for the United States and western Europe. The three foci of ALS with associated PD in these isolates represent a great medical riddle, the solution of which ultimately may have worldwide significance.

VI. OVERVIEW

The natural history of disease in isolated groups has been illustrated through many sometimes exotic examples that have focused attention on (1) the associated interaction of biology and behavior in the natural environment; (2) the effects of acculturation and decreased isolation of disease patterns in such groups; (3) the importance of "natural experimental models" represented by isolates that assist in the understanding of the mechanisms for the origin and dissemination of disease; and (4) the impact such discoveries have on modern medicine and the community of man. Many isolated groups are now rapidly vanishing as a result of culture change and assimilation into more cosmopolitan communities. Continued monitoring and accumulation of information on disease patterns in such groups facilitates the understanding of biomedical phenomena in these isolates as they undergo their current rapid process of change.

ACKNOWLEDGMENTS

I wish to thank Dr. D. Carleton Gajdusek and Dr. David Asher for their comments and critical review of this chapter. I am thankful for the many still photographs that have been generously supplied by Dr. Gajdusek, Dr. Kwang-Ming Chen, and Dr. Yoshiro Yase. The extensive assistance by Judith D. Garruto during the preparation of this chapter is also gratefully acknowledged.

REFERENCES

Adels, B. R., and Gajdusek, D. C. (1963). Survey of measles patterns in New Guinea, Micronesia and Australia. With a report of new virgin soil epidemics and the demonstration of susceptible primitive populations by serology. *Am. J. Hyg.* **77**, 317–343.

Allison, A. C. (1975). Interactions of genetic predisposition, acquired immunity and environmental factors in susceptibility to disease. *In* "Man-Made Lakes and Human Health" (N. F. Stanley and M. P. Alpers, eds), pp. 401–426. Academic Press, New York.

Baruzzi, R. G., Marcopito, L. F., Serra, M. L., Souza, F. A., and Stabile, C. (1977). The Keren-Akorore: a recently contacted indigenous tribe. *In* "Health and Disease in Tribal Societies," Ciba Foundation Symposium, No. 49, pp. 179–200. Elsevier, Amsterdam.

Black, F. L. (1966). Measles endemicity in insular populations: critical community size and its evolutionary implication. *J. Theor. Biol.* **11**, 207–211.

Black, F. L. (1975). Infectious diseases in primitive societies. *Science* **187**, 515–518.

Black, F. L., Pinheiro, F. De P., Hierholzer, W. J., and Lee, R. V. (1977). Epidemiology of infectious disease: the example of measles. *In* "Health and Disease in Tribal Societies," Ciba Foundation Symposium, No. 49, pp. 115–130, Elsevier, Amsterdam.

Brody, J. A., and Chen, K.-M. (1969). Changing epidemiologic patterns of amyotrophic lateral sclerosis and parkinsonism-dementia on Guam. *In* "Motor Neuron Diseases: Research on Amyotrophic Lateral Sclerosis and Related Disorders" (F. H. Norris, Jr. and L. T. Kurland, eds.), Vol. 2, pp. 61–79. Grune & Stratton, New York.

Brody, J. A., and Kurland, L. T. (1973). Amyotrophic lateral sclerosis and parkinsonism-dementia in Guam. *In* "Tropical Neurology" (J. D. Spillane, ed.), pp. 355–375. Oxford Univ. Press, London and New York.

Brody, J. A., Hussels, I., Brink, E., and Torres, J. (1970). Hereditary blindness among Pingelapese people of Eastern Caroline Islands. *Lancet* **1**, 1253–1257.

Brown, P. W., and Gajdusek, D. C. (1970). IX Disease patterns and vaccine response studies in isolated Micronesian populations. *Am. J. Trop. Med. Hyg.* **19**, 170–175.

Brown, P. W., Gajdusek, D. C., and Morris, J. A. (1966). Epidemic A2 influenza in isolated Pacific Island populations without pre-epidemic antibody to influenza virus types A and B, and the discovery of other still unexposed populations. *Am. J. Epidemiol.* **83**, 339–344.

Burch, T. A., O'Brien, W. M., Need, R., and Kurland, L. T. (1966). Hyperuricaemia and gout in the Mariana Islands. *Ann. Rheum. Dis.* **25**, 114–116.

Burnet, F. M., and White, D. O. (1972). "Natural History of Infectious Disease," 4th ed. Cambridge Univ. Press, London and New York.

Carr, R. E., Morton, N. E., and Siegel, I. M. (1971). Achromatopsia in Pingelap islanders. Study of a genetic isolate. *Am. J. Ophthalmol.* **72**, 746–756.

Christensen, P. E., Schmidt, H., Bang, H. O., Andersen, V., Jordal, B., and Jensen, O. (1953). An epidemic of measles in Southern Greenland, 1951. Measles in virgin soil II. The epidemic proper. *Acta Med. Scand.* **144**, 430–449.

Couvée, L. M. J. (1962). The nutritional condition of the Kapauku in the central Highlands of West New Guinea II. Clinical and hematological data. *Trop. Geogogr. Med.* **14**, 314–324.

Decker, J. L., Lane, J. J., and Reynolds, W. E. (1962). Hyperuricemia in a male Filipino population. *Arthritis Rheum.* **5**, 144–155.

Demis, D. J. (1977). Nonsyphilitic treponematoses. In "Infectious Diseases" (P. D. Hoeprich, ed.), 2nd ed., pp. 823–835. Harper, New York.

Dubos, R. (1965). "Man Adapting." Yale Univ. Press, New Haven, Connecticut.

Duff, I. F., Mikkelson, W. M., Dodge, H. J., and Himes, D. S. (1968). Comparison of uric acid levels in some Oriental and Caucasian groups unselected as to gout or hyperuricemia. *Arthritis Rheum.* **11**, 184–190.

Dunn, F. L. (1968). Epidemiological factors: health and disease of hunter–gatherers. In "Man the Hunter" (I. De Vore, ed.), pp. 221–228. Aldine, Chicago, Illinois.

Epstein, M. A., and Achong, B. G. (1979). "The Epstein–Barr Virus." Springer-Verlag, Berlin and New York.

Fazekas de St. Groth, S., and Webster, R. G. (1966). Disquisitions on original antigenic sin. I. Evidence in man. *J. Exp. Med.* **124**, 331–341.

Foulks, E. F., and Katz, S. H. (1975). Biobehavioral adaptation in the Arctic. In "Biosocial Interrelations in Population Adaptation" (E. Watts, F. E. Johnston, and G. W. Lasker, eds.), pp. 183–193. Mouton, The Hague.

Gajdusek, D. C. (1962). Congenital defects of the central nervous system associated with hyperendemic goiter and cretinism in a neolithic highland society of Netherlands New Guinea. I. Epidemiology. *Pediatrics* **29**, 345–363.

Gajdusek, D. C. (1964a). Factors governing the genetics of primitive human populations. *Cold Spring Harbor Symp. Quant. Biol.* **29**, 121–135.

Gajdusek, D. C. (1964b). Congenital absence of the penis in Muniri and Simbari Kukukuku people of New Guinea. *Program Abstr. Annu. Meet. Am. Pediatr. Soc., 74th* Abstr. No. 128, p. 138.

Gajdusek, D. C. (1971). "Journal of Expeditions to the Soviet Union, Africa, the Islands of Madagascar, la Reunion and Mauritius, Indonesia and to East and West New Guinea, Australia and Guam to Study Kuru and Other Neurological Diseases, Epidemic Influenza, Endemic Goitrous Cretinism and Child Growth and Development with Explorations on The Great Papuan Plateau and on the Lakes Plain and Inland Southern Lowlands of West New Guinea, June 1, 1969 to March 3, 1970." Natl. Inst. Neurol. Dis. Stroke, Natl. Inst. Health, Bethesda, Maryland.

Gajdusek, D. C. (1973). Kuru in the New Guinea highlands. In "Tropical Neurology" (J. D. Spillane, ed.), pp. 376–383, plates pp. 29–31. Oxford Univ. Press, London and New York.

Gajdusek, D. C. (1977a). Urgent opportunistic observations: the study of changing, transient and disappearing phenomena of medical interest in disrupted primitive human communities. In

"Health and Disease in Tribal Societies," Ciba Foundation Symposium, No. 49, pp. 69-102. Elsevier, Amsterdam.

Gajdusek, D. C. (1977b). Unconventional viruses and the origin and disappearance of kuru. *In* "Les Prix Nobel en 1976," Nobel Foundation, pp. 167-216. P. A. Norstedt and Söner, Stockholm.

Gajdusek, D. C. (1978). Introduction of *Taenia solium* into West New Guinea with a note on an epidemic of burns from cysticercus epilepsy in the Ekari people of the Wissel Lakes area. *P. N. G. Med. J.* **21**, 329-342.

Gajdusek, D. C. (1979). A focus of high incidence amyotrophic lateral sclerosis and parkinsonism and dementia syndromes in a small population of Auyu and Jakai people of South West New Guinea. *In* "Amyotrophic Lateral Sclerosis" (T. Tsubaki and Y. Toyokura, eds.), pp. 287-305. Japan Medical Research Foundation, Publ. No. 8. Univ. of Tokyo Press, Tokyo.

Gajdusek, D. C., and Garruto, R. M. (1975). The focus of hyperendemic goiter, cretinism and associated deaf-mutism in Western New Guinea. *In* "Biosocial Interrelations in Population Adaptation" (E. Watts, F. E. Johnston, and G. W. Lasker, eds.), pp. 267-285. Mouton, The Hague.

Gajdusek, D. C., and Zigas, V. (1957). Degenerative disease of the central nervous system in New Guinea. The endemic occurrence of "kuru" in the native population. *N. Engl. J. Med.* **257**, 974-978.

Gajdusek, D. C., Garruto, R. M., and Dedecker, R. (1974). Congenital defects of the central nervous system associated with hyperendemic goiter in a Neolithic Highland society of Western New Guinea. V. A note on birth weights and infantile growth rates in the Mulia population. *Hum. Biol.* **46**, 339-344.

Garruto, R. M., and Gajdusek, D. C. (1975). Unusual progression and shifting clinical severity, morbidity and mortality in the 1969 Hong Kong (A/New Guinea/1/69 H_3N_2) influenza epidemic in New Guinea. *Am. J. Phys. Anthropol.* **42**, 302-303. (Abstr.)

Garruto, R. M., and Willey, L. M. (1967). A biocultural study of tetanus and tooth extraction in East Africa. *Annu. Meet. Northeast. Anthropol. Assoc., 7th, Montreal, Abstr. Commun.*, p. 3.

Garruto, R. M., Gajdusek, D. C., and ten Brink, J. (1974). Congenital defects of the central nervous system associated with hyperendemic goiter in a Neolithic Highland society of Western New Guinea: III. Serum and urinary iodine levels in goitrous and adjacent non-goitrous populations. *Hum. Biol.* **46**, 311-329.

Garruto, R. M., Gajdusek, D. C., Chen, K.-M., and Plato, C. C. (1979). Amyotrophic lateral sclerosis in parkinsonism-dementia in long-term Filipino migrants to Guam. *Asian Oceanian Congr. Neurol., 5th, Manila* Abstr. 90, Excerpta Medica/Asia Pacific Congress Series No. 1, p. 43.

Garruto, R. M., Gajdusek, D. C., and Chen, K.-M. (1980). Amyotrophic lateral sclerosis among Chamorro migrants from Guam. *Ann. Neurol.*, **8**, 612-619.

Garruto, R. M., Gajdusek, D. C., and Chen, K.-M. (1981a). Amyotrophic lateral sclerosis and parkinsonism-dementia among Filipino migrants to Guam. *Ann. Neurol.* (in press).

Garruto, R. M., Gajdusek, D. C., Chen, K.-M., and Gibbs, C. J., Jr. (1981b). Changing epidemiological and clinical characteristics of amyotrophic lateral sclerosis and parkinsonism-dementia in the Mariana Islands. 12th World Congress of Neurology, Kyoto, Sept. 20-25. Abstract (in press).

Glasse, R. M. (1963). "Cannibalism in the Kuru Region," Mime. Dep. Public Health, Territ. Papua New Guinea.

Glasse, S. (1962). "The Social Effects of Kuru," Mimeo. Dep. Public Health, Territ. Papua New Guinea.

Halstead, S. B., Scanlon, J. E., Umpaivit, P., and Udomsakdi, S. (1969). Dengue and chickungunya virus infection in man in Thailand, 1962-1964: IV. Epidemiologic studies in the Bangkok metropolitan area. *Am. J. Trop. Med. Hyg.* **18**, 977-1021.

Healey, L. A., and Jones, K. W. (1970). The epidemiology of hyperuricemia. *Bull. Rheum. Dis.* **20,** 600–603.

Healy, L. A., Caner, J. E., and Decker, J. L. (1966). Ethnic variation in serum uric acid: I. Filipino hyperuricemia in a controlled environment. *Arthritis Rheum.* **9,** 288–294.

Hope-Simpson, R. E. (1965). The nature of herpes-zoster: a long term study and a new hypothesis. *Proc. R. Soc. Med.* **58,** 9–20.

Hussels, I. E., and Morton, N. E. (1972). Pingelap and Mokil atolls: achromatopsia. *Am. J. Hum. Genet.* **24,** 304–309.

Kilbourne, E. D. (1978). Influenza. In "Human Diseases Caused by Viruses" (H. Rothschild, F. Allison, and C. Howe, eds.), pp. 79–98. Oxford Univ. Press, London and New York.

Kimura, K., Yase, Y., Higashi, Y., Uno, S., Yamamoto, K., Iwasaki, M., Tsumato, I., Sugiura, M., Yoshimura, S., Namikawa, K., Kumura, J., Iwamoto, W., Yamamoto, I., Handa, Y., Yata, M., and Yata, Y. (1963). Epidemiological and geomedical studies on amyotrophic lateral sclerosis. *Dis. Nerv. Syst.* **24,** 155–159.

Kooijman, S., Borren, M., Veeger, L., Verschueren, J., and Luyken, R. (1953–1954). "Report of the Investigation into the Problem of Depopulation Among the Marind-Anim of Netherlands New Guinea," South Pac. Comm. Popul. Stud., S. 18. Noumea, New Caledonia.

Kurland, L. T. (1972). An appraisal of the neurotoxicity of cycad and the etiology of amyotrophic lateral sclerosis on Guam. *Fed. Proc., Fed. Am. Soc. Exp. Biol.* **31,** 1540–1542.

Kurland, L. T. (1978). Geographic isolates: their role in neuroepidemiology. In "Neurological Epidemiology: Principles and Clinical Applications" (B. S. Schoenberg, ed.), Advances in Neurology, Vol. 19, pp. 69–82. Raven, New York.

Kurland, L. T., and Mulder, D. W. (1954). Epidemiologic investigations of amyotrophic lateral sclerosis. 1. Preliminary report on geographic distribution, with special reference to the Mariana Islands, including clinical and pathologic observations. *Neurology* **4,** 355–448.

Lang, D. J., Garruto, R. M., and Gajdusek, D. C. (1977). Early acquisition of cytomegalovirus and Epstein–Barr virus antibody in several isolated Melanesian populations. *Am. J. Epidemiol.* **105,** 480–487.

Lefèbvre, G. (1956). "Essai sur la Médecine Egyptienne de l'époque Pharaonique." Presses Univ. de France, Paris.

Lindenbaum, S. (1979). "Kuru Sorcery, Disease and Danger in the New Guinea Highlands." Mayfield Publ. Co., Palo Alto, California.

Liu, K. L. (1977). Dental condition of two tribes of Taiwan aborigines-Ami and Atayal. *J. Dent. Res.* **56,** 117–127.

Masi, M. B. (1973). The pattern of dental disease in the South Pacific area of the Pacific basin. *Int. Dent. J.* **23,** 573–578.

Miller, L. H., Mason, S. J., Dvorak, J. A., McGinniss, M. H., and Rothman, I. K. (1975). Erythrocyte receptors for (*Plasmodium knowlesi*) malaria: Duffy Blood Group determinants. *Science* **189,** 561–563.

Miller, L. H., Mason, S. J., Clyde, D. F., and McGinniss, M. H. (1976). The resistance factor to *Plasmodium vivax* in blacks. The Duffy blood group genotype, FyFy. *N. Engl. J. Med.* **295,** 302–304.

Mohindra, I., and Nagaraj, S. (1977). Astigmatism in Zuni and Navajo Indians. *Am. J. Optom. Physiol. Opt.* **54,** 121–124.

Neel, J. V. (1970). Lessons from a "primitive" people. *Science* **170,** 815–822.

Neel, J. V. (1977). Health and disease in unacculturated Amerindian populations. In "Health and Disease in Tribal Societies," Ciba Foundation Symposium, No. 49, pp. 155–177. Elsevier, Amsterdam.

Peart, A. F. W., and Nagler, F. P. (1954). Measles in the Canadian Arctic, 1952. *Can. J. Public Health* **44,** 146–156.

Pedersen, P. O. (1938). Investigations into dental conditions of about 3000 ancient and modern Greenlanders. *Dent. Rec.* **58,** 191-198.

Pettit, H., Mudd, S., and Pepper, D. S. (1936). The Philadelphia and Alaska strains of influenza virus: epidemic influenza in Alaska, 1935. *J. Am. Med. Assoc.* **106,** 890-892.

Polunin, I. V. (1952). Tinea imbricata in Malaya. *Br. J. Dermatol.* **64,** 378.

Polunin, I. V. (1953-1954). The medical natural history of Malay Aborigines. *Med. J. Malaya* **8,** 55-174.

Polunin, I. V. (1967). Health and disease in contemporary primitive societies. *In* "Diseases in Antiquity" (D. Brothwell and A. T. Sandison, eds.), pp. 67-97. Thomas, Springfield, Illinois.

Prior, I. A. M., and Rose, B. S. (1966). Uric acid, gout and public health in the South Pacific. *N.Z. Med. J.* **65,** 295-300.

Reed, D. M. (1977). Current health problems in the South and Central Pacific. *N. Z. Med. J.* **85,** 326-329.

Reed, D. M., and Brody, J. A. (1975). Amyotrophic lateral sclerosis and parkinsonism-dementia on Guam, 1945-1972: I. Descriptive epidemiology. *Am. J. Epidemiol.* **101,** 287-301.

Reed, D. M., Labarthe, D., and Stallones, R. (1972). Epidemiologic studies of serum uric acid levels among Micronesians. *Arthritis Rheum.* **15,** 381-390.

Schamschula, R. G., Adkins, B. L., Barmes, D. E., Charlton, G., and Davey, B. G. (1977). Caries experience and the mineral content of plaque in a primitive population in New Guinea. *J. Dent. Res.* **56,** Spec. Issue C, C62-C70.

Schofield, F. D. (1970). VIII. Some relations between social isolation and specific communicable diseases. *Am. J. Trop. Med. Hyg.* **19,** 167-169.

Schofield, F. D., Parkinson, A. D., and Jeffrey, D. (1963). Observations on the epidemiology, effects and treatment of tinea imbricata. *Trans. R. Soc. Trop. Med. Hyg.* **57,** 214-227.

Schull, W. J., ed. (1963). Selection. *Proc. Macy Conf. Genet., 3rd.,* 1961. Univ. of Michigan Press, Ann Arbor,

Scragg, R. F. R. (1954). Depopulation of New Ireland: a study of demography and fertility. Administration of Papua and New Guinea. M. D. Thesis, Univ. of Adelaide, Southern Australia.

Serjeantson, S., and Lawrence, G. (1977). Autosomal recessive inheritance of susceptibility to tinea imbricata. *Lancet* **1,** 13-15.

Simmons, R. T., and Gajdusek, D. C. (1966). A blood group genetic survey of children of Bellona and Rennell Islands (B. S. I. P.) and certain northern New Hebridean Islands. *Arch. Phys. Anthropol. Oceania* **1,** 155-174.

Simmons, R. T., Gajdusek, D. C., and Nicholson, M. K. (1967). Blood group genetic variations in inhabitants of West New Guinea, with a map of the villages and linguistic groups of South West New Guinea. *Am. J. Phys. Anthropol.* **27,** 277-298.

Truswell, A. S. (1977). Diet and nutrition of hunter-gatherers. *In* "Health and Disease in Tribal Societies," Ciba Foundation Symposium, No. 49, pp. 213-226.

Wells, C. (1964). "Bones, Bodies and Disease." Praeger, New York.

West, K. M. (1974). Diabetes in American Indians and other native populations of the New World. *Diabetes* **23,** 841-855.

Whiting, M. G. (1964). Food practices in amyotrophic lateral sclerosis foci in Japan, the Marianas and New Guinea. *Fed. Proc., Fed. Am. Soc. Exp. Biol.* **23,** 1343-1344.

Yap, P. M. (1968). Classification of the culture-bound reactive syndromes. *Aust. N. Z. J. Psychiatry* **1,** 172-179.

Yap, P. M. (1969). The culture-bound reactive syndromes. *In* "Mental Health Research in Asia and the Pacific" (W. Caudill and T. Y. Lin, eds.), pp. 33-53. East-West Center Press, Honolulu.

Yase, Y., Matsumoto, N., Yoskimasu, F., Handa, Y., and Kumamoto, T. (1968). Motor neuron disease in the Kii Peninsula, Japan. *Proc. Aust. Assoc. Neurol.* **5,** 335-339.

18

Genetic Disparities of Senescence

LEONARD HAYFLICK

Of all the conflicting views on the causes of biologic aging, few gerontologists disagree with the axiom that, after reaching sexual maturity, individual members of a species accumulate physiologic decrements that lead to an increase in their likelihood of dying. In fact, for man the actuarial data, first analyzed by the English actuary Gompertz in 1825, reveal that the force of mortality doubles

599

BIOCULTURAL ASPECTS OF DISEASE
ISBN 0-12-598720-X

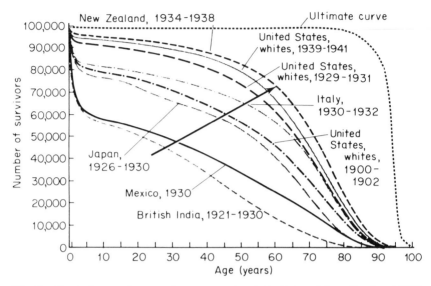

Fig. 1. Survival curves for several countries and periods. (Adapted from Comfort, 1979.)

every 7 years beyond the age of 30—i. e., after maturity, the rate and probability of dying are exponential with increasing age. A variety of human physiologic functions, although subject to some individual variation, show a slow, nearly linear decline from 30 years of age. The rate constants for this linear loss seem to occur at about 0.8–0.9% loss per year of the functional capacity present at the age of 30 years (Strehler and Mildvan, 1960).

The common impression that the triumphs of modern medicine have lengthened the human life span is not supported by either vital statistics or biologic evidence. The fact is that the prevention and treatment of the ills of early years have improved and, therefore, more people are reaching what appears to be an immutable, upper age limit. Thus, life expectancy has increased, but the human life span has remained virtually unchanged since recorded history. Medical achievements have simply allowed more persons to reach the limit of what appears to be a fixed life span. Deaths in the early years are becoming increasingly less frequent, resulting in life tables that are simply becoming more rectangular, as indicated by the direction of the arrow in Fig. 1. In many privileged countries, one now can expect to become reasonably old, which is a relatively new phenomenon.

I. EFFECTS OF DISEASE RESOLUTION

If the two leading causes of death in this country—heart disease and stroke— are successfully eliminated, approximately 12 years of additional life can be expected (Table I). If the third greatest cause of death—cancer—is eliminated, about 2 years of additional life expectancy will result. The net increase at birth in life expectancy achieved in the United States from 1900 to 1950 was almost 20 years. This increase resulted from the decrease in the large number of deaths that occurred before the age of 65 years. The gain in life expectancy at 65 and 75 years of age from 1900 to 1969 was, respectively, only 2.9 and 2.2 years.

What would be the effect on human longevity and the human life span in a world in which all causes of death resulting from disease and accidents were totally eliminated (Table I)? The effect on human longevity would be to realize the ultimate rectangular curve (Fig. 1) in which citizens would live out their lives, free of the fear of premature death, but with the certain fate that their physiologic decrements would result in death on about their 100th birthdays.

These concepts have forced gerontologists to the conclusion that the disease-oriented approach to medical research might increase life expectancy but will have little impact on increasing the human life span. If such an increase is desirable (and there is considerable doubt that it is), one must first separate the disease-related causes of death from the age-dependent physiologic decrements that give rise to the manifestations of old age. The diseases of old age are simply superimposed on these normal physiologic decrements but must be separately

TABLE I

Gain in Life Expectancy at Birth and at Age 65 That Would Result from Elimination of Various Causes of Death, 1969–1971

Cause of death	Gain (years) in life expectancy if death cause eliminated	
	At birth	At age of 65
Major cardiovascular–renal diseases	11.8	11.4
Diseases of the heart	5.9	5.1
Cerebrovascular diseases	1.2	1.2
Malignant neoplasms[a]	2.5	1.4
Motor vehicle accidents	0.7	0.1
All accidents excluding motor vehicles	0.6	0.1
Influenza and pneumonia	0.5	0.2
Diabetes mellitus	0.2	0.2
Infectious and parasitic diseases	0.2	0.1
Tuberculosis	Less than 0.05	

[a] Including neoplasms of lymphatic and hematopoietic tissues. From U.S. Public Health Service, National Center for Health Statistics, "U.S. Life Tables by Causes of Death: 1969–71," by T. N. E. Greville; *ibid*. "U.S. Decennial Life Tables for 1969–71," Vol. 1, No. 5, 1976.

regarded if one is rationally to consider increasing the human life span. Although age-associated physiologic decrements surely increase vulnerability to disease, the fundamental causes of death are not diseases but the physiologic decrements that make their occurrence more likely.

Biomedical research has trained its heavy artillery almost exclusively on the disease-associated causes of death. Scant attention has been paid to the underlying causes of biological aging that are not disease-associated but which, in clocklike fashion, dictate for each species a specific maximum life span. To be sure, the physiological decrements that occur in advancing years increase vulnerability to disease, but unless more attention is paid to the fundamental nondisease-related biologic causes of aging, the fate of each person will be death on or about his or her 100th birthday.

II. PROSPECTS FOR INCREASING HUMAN LONGEVITY

As stated, there are two ways in which the efforts of biomedical research can be expected to extend human longevity in the next 25 years. The first is to reduce or eliminate the major causes of death, in particular cardiovascular diseases and cancer. The results of reducing the effects of minor diseases will be minimal. For example, if tuberculosis were completely eliminated, the gain in life expectancy at birth would be less than a 0.05 year (Table I). Thus, it could be argued that if an increase in life expectation becomes the main goal of biomedical research, all such research should be directed toward the elimination of the two major causes of death. This position, although less than humane, and not likely to attract many adherents, is nonetheless the most logical conclusion to be derived from life-table studies and the projections dealt with in Table I.

The second way in which biomedical research can deal with human longevity is to address itself specifically to the underlying nondisease-related fundamental biological causes of age changes. These are not diseases but are the basic biological changes that result in those physiological decrements characteristic of aging and on which are superimposed an increasing vulnerability to disease. That statement, in fact, defines the science of gerontology. Such an approach, then, does not directly concern itself with efforts to increase human life expectancy but rather to extend what appears to be a fixed life span that differs in its length for man and all other animal species.

As a measure of the current effort put forth toward these two approaches, funds spent on cardiovascular disease and cancer research are about 20 times greater than the funds spent in gerontology. It is also probable that the number of researchers, and consequently the amount of effort, in both these areas also differs by 20-fold. Consequently, the likelihood that any significant increase in human longevity will occur in the next 25 years depends on (1) significantly better cure rates for cardiovascular disease and/or cancer and/or (2) significant advances in our understanding and ability to manipulate the biological clocks that set for each species a mean maximum life span.

If potential success in either of these endeavors can be measured by the current attitudes and priorities of the biomedical research establishment, then clearly the search for cardiovascular disease and cancer cures are more likely to effect human longevity than is gerontological research. The further conclusion is that by curing these two diseases a maximum of 14 years of additional life expectancy could be attained, but with successful efforts to increase the life span itself no fixed end point is ruled out. Furthermore the resolution of the two leading killers will in no way reverse or halt the decline in physiological decrements characteristic of age changes, whereas efforts to increase the life span could lead to such a reversal. Clearly, research in cardiovascular diseases and cancer should not be stopped, but if our goal is to maximize opportunities to effectively increase human longevity, then our current priorities are seriously out of balance. If this imbalance continues unchanged, the likelihood is extremely small indeed.

III. DEMOGRAPHIC PROJECTIONS

That the proportion of persons in our society over the age of 65 has been steadily increasing is well known. In the last 100 years, their proportions of the total population have increased from 3 to 10% (Fig. 2), and the aged have become a larger proportion of the nonworking component of the population, which includes the nonworking youth. This nonworking population component is largely supported by the work force itself, and, if current population trends continue, the elderly will command increasingly more support.

Within 50 years those over 65 are expected to number nearly 40 million (Fig. 3). This prediction does not take into account any major resolution within 50 years of the two leading causes of death—cardiovascular disease and cancer. If some significant cure rate were to occur, however, we might have as many persons over 65 as under 15 years of age in the year 2025.

If zero population growth were achieved and maintained, the family size of old persons would obviously be reduced, and along with that reduction would be a diminuation in the economic, social, and psychological benefits that now accrue from adult children. The inevitable consequence would be a further acceleration of current trends, in which the government would provide more health care, food, housing, recreation, and income to the elderly. Because one could safely assume that the proportion of those in government over 65 years would also increase, the closest thing to a gerontocracy could prevail in 2025.

Since zero population growth might be achieved by 2025, it is interesting to speculate on the consequences of another extreme condition—a population in

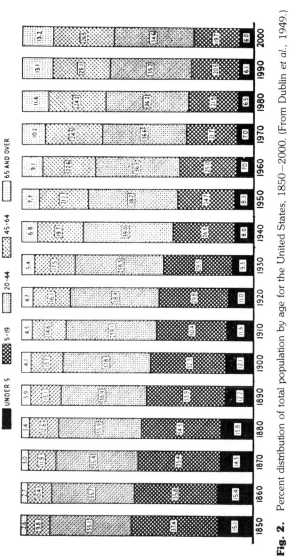

Fig. 2. Percent distribution of total population by age for the United States, 1850–2000. (From Dublin et al., 1949.)

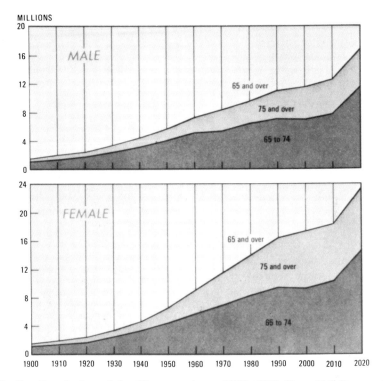

Fig. 3. Growth of population 65 years and over, 1900–2020. (From U. S. Bureau of the Census, 1973.)

which no one dies at all. The immediate effect on the growth rate of the total population would be significant, since the growth rate would be increased by the amount of the current death rate. In the long run, however, the increase would not be dramatic (Siegel, 1976). The increase in growth rate would be somewhat less than one-half million persons per year in a U.S. population of 250 million—that is, over and above the number of births now being added to the population each year. (In 1974, the number of U.S. births was approximately 3 million. With no mortality, the number of births would be an additional one-half million, based on the projection that those females who now die in childhood would survive and would bear children.)

Consequently, even the stupendous achievement of attaining biological immortality would not greatly increase the total population—that is, if those achieving biological immortality did not concomitantly gain fecundity. However, even a steady-state annual increase of one-half million persons greater than the present annual increase of three million in the United States would have a significant impact after several years.

After the initial large impact of a shift to zero mortality, the rate of increase of the elderly would change slowly. Because with the current life expectancy of 70 years any large reductions in death rates would be limited to persons over 60, the elimination of all deaths would increase the proportion of older people. If the birthrate were to decline to zero—the most unlikely event of all—then obviously the population would eventually consist entirely of centenarians and then of supercentenarians.

IV. AGING, RUSSIAN STYLE

No discussion of genetic disparities of human longevity would be complete without considering the claims of superlongevity attributed to three geographically disparate peoples. Were these claims true, one could reasonably conclude that genetic or environmental factors might exist that lead to increased human longevity and, more importantly, that if these factors were known, they could be manipulated to apply equally to other persons as well.

Of the three groups, one is found in the Andean village of Vilcabamba in Ecuador, the second is found in Hunza in the Karakoram Range of the Pakistani region of Kashmir, and the third is found predominantly in the Abkhazia and Osetia regions in the Caucasus of the Georgian Republic of the Soviet Union.

To appreciate the magnitude of the claims made by these groups, one must realize that in other parts of the world the number of centenarians in the population is normally about two or three per 100,000. Only one person in a million reaches the age of 105, and only one in 40 million will live to be 110. Yet in the three regions mentioned, not only are higher proportions of centenarians claimed, but many individuals claim ages of 120, 130, and even 150 and 160 years.

In addition to the Georgian Republic, the whole Caucasus area, with a population of 21,290,400 (in 1959), was reported to have 8890 centenarians (45 per 100,000) and about 500 persons claiming to be between 120 and 170 years of age. In certain areas of Azerbaijan, claims of 300–400 centenarians per 100,000 have been made! In the census of 1971, the village of Vilcabamba in Ecuador, which had a population of 819, claimed nine centenarians among whom one person was purportedly 123 years of age. This extrapolates to an incredible rate of 1100 centenarians per 100,000 persons.

Unhappily, however, none of these claims, which have enjoyed widespread popularity in the news media, can be authenticated.

In Hunza, few statistical data are available, and the Hunzukuts, who have no written language, cannot even point to falsified birth records. The Vilcabambans are isolated and their birth records are either nonexistent or totally unreliable. One gerontologist who returned from his second trip to this village after a lapse of 5 years was told by several supercentenarians that during his absence their ages had increased by 7–10 years!

In the three areas of Hunza, Vilcabamba, and Soviet Georgia, some as yet unidentified common geographical, climatological, dietary, genetic, or lifestyle situation has long been suspected as accounting for the claims. More important, however, is that the claims of superlongevity themselves cannot be substantiated in any of these regions. The best studied situation is that found in the Soviet Union, where the evidence is a curious admixture of social mores, pseudoscience, and politics, sadly reminiscent of the Lysenko affair.

First and foremost is the complete lack of valid documentation for these claims, as all census information is based on verbal replies unsubstantiated by documentation. Curiously, census data in the Soviet Union reveal that the number of centenarians outside of the Caucasus area dropped from 1926 to 1970 but increased within this area. Zhores Medvedev, the Russian gerontologist, now a London resident, speculates that this imbalance is most probably connected with an improvement in the cultural and educational levels outside of the Caucasus and where, therefore, the likelihood of collecting spurious information is reduced (Medvedev, 1974). (Medvedev draws an analogy with similar claims for large numbers of centenarians among black Americans, and he suggests that the claims are attributable to the same cause.)

As for birth records, internal identity cards only came into use in the Soviet Union in 1932 for urban areas only, and dates of birth were recorded only from oral information. Furthermore, in the Moslem areas of the Caucasus, where the centenarian claims are most exaggerated, births are not registered at all. It has been suggested that the Moslem year, which spans a 10-month period, caused some misunderstandings when census takers arrived. In Christian areas birth records were kept before 1917 in special church registers, but because 90% of all churches were destroyed between 1922 and 1940, these records are almost completely lost. Not one of 500 supercentenarians questioned in the Caucasus could produce a valid document in support of his claim.

General census statistics in the Soviet Union clearly show that, for the age-group 90 to 99 years, the ratio of women to men, was 3:1, yet in the group of Georgian centenarians the ratio after the age of 100 clearly favors the men. Are centenarian men more likely than women to exaggerate their ages? A further curiosity is that tendencies to exaggerate age in most industrialized countries occur more frequently in the very young and very old age-groups. Persons in their middle years are more likely to reduce their real ages.

Medvedev, in further investigations on the superlongevous persons of the Georgian Republic, offers some interesting notions on why these claims persist. Extremely old persons in those regions enjoy the highest levels of social authority, and the older a person is, the more respect and honor he receives. "The most elderly people are almost regarded as saints." These traditions create a stimulus for age exaggeration, especially when documentation does not exist and when no living witnesses can contradict the claims. Furthermore, the national and international publicity surrounding the superlongevous, such as images on postage stamps, frequent news media photographs and stories, and establishment of centenarian bands, chorales, and dance groups, have made these areas profitable tourist attractions. The Novosti Press Agency itself derives income from the sale of stories and photographs of the supercentenarians to the gullible Western news media.

The villages compete to have the oldest resident in the Soviet Union, where the competition is fueled by a circus atmosphere and longevity records are pushed upward annually. Associated with these claims, and providing further impetus to the exaggerations, is the political propaganda that refers to these people unabashedly as a special social achievement of the Soviet Union. Articles in central newspapers and magazines with such titles as "The U.S.S.R.—State of Longevity" promote the legend. Medvedev cites statements such as the following, appearing in what are purported to be scholarly academic publications: "The Soviet Union is the country with the record longevity of human beings. The number of centenarians is increasing, parallel with our approach to the creation of a Communist Society."

The fact that Joseph Stalin was a Georgian must also be taken into account in the legend of the Soviet centenarians. Stalin himself was much interested in the phenomenon, and because of that interest, local Georgian authorities were anxious to provide more and more cases of longevous people. But perhaps the most reasonable explanation for the appearance of this phenomenon in the Soviet Union is the likelihood that hundreds of thousands of known deserters and draft dodgers of World War I and the Russian Revolution (most of whom were from the Caucasus) used their fathers' documents to falsify their ages. To maintain the fiction, they have had to continue the masquerade, and have exaggerated it even further when the several benefits cited here were likely to accrue.

V. THE GENETIC BASIS FOR SENESCENCE

Most gerontologists believe that a cell's genetic apparatus is the major arena for the primary events that lead to the decrements associated with biological aging.

The principal evidence that aging is, at least in part, genetically determined is based on the following kinds of observations.

A. Species-Specific Life Spans

Gerontologists generally agree that all animal species age and that each species has a characteristic life span. Consequently, and regardless of the kind and degree of trauma suffered by individual animals during their lifetimes, genetically determined factors exist that operate independent of the environment. Differences in life spans of members of various animal groups argue strongly in favor of a species-specific genetic basis for longevity. The eagle owl (*Bubo bubo*) has a maximum recorded longevity of 68 years, whereas the crowned pigeon (*Goura cristata*) lives a maximum of 16 years (Comfort, 1979). Marions tortoise (*Testudo sumeiri*) has survived at least 152 years, whereas the loggerhead turtle (*Caretta caretta*) lives only 33 years (Comfort, 1979). In mammals, the longest-lived species is man (about 115 years) and the shortest-lived species are small rodents, where, for example, the golden hamster (*Cricetus auratus*) lives between 2 and 3 years (Comfort, 1979).

B. Hybrid Vigor

The effect of genetic constitution on longevity is perhaps best exemplified by those experiments in which "hybrid vigor" or heterosis has been demonstrated. Pearl *et al.* (1923) found that the F_1 hybrid of two *Drosophila melanogaster* strains had a greater longevity than either parental strain. Clarke and Maynard Smith (1955) and Maynard Smith (1959) obtained even more striking results when they crossed two geographically isolated strains of *Drosophila subobscura* and found that the hybrid lived longer and had a less variable life span than did its inbred parents. Most explanations of heterosis suggest that recessive, harmful, but nonlethal mutations are produced by inbreeding; hence, hybrid vigor results from the reciprocal dominance between wild-type alleles of one strain and the recessive, suboptimal genes of the other parental strain. Nevertheless, worth considering is that the increased longevity seen in heterosis has not been shown to exceed the life span characteristic of wild strains that had been lost by inbreeding.

C. Sex and Longevity

Sex differences in longevity are well-established facts. In the human population, the penalty for maleness is that almost every disease has a higher incidence in males than in females. This difference in vulnerability is also expressed in life span, where a white female born in the United States in 1974 can expect to outlive her male counterpart by 7.7 years (Siegel, 1976). If genes carried on the sex chromosomes dictate life span, then factors on the X chromosome may decrease vulnerability to degenerative diseases. Contrariwise, genes on the Y chromosome may exert life-shortening effects that are incidental to their main function. Although the male sex is the shorter-lived in most animal species, some mouse and rat strains show the opposite state of affairs (Oliff, 1953; Woolley, 1946; Hamilton, 1948), as do pigeons (Levy, 1957). Regardless of which sex might be favored, the fact that one is, strongly suggests a fundamental genetic basis for the difference exists.

D. Influence of Parental Age

Actuarial data for man lead to the conclusion that genetic factors play a principal role in determining individual longevity. Figure 4 graphically shows that life expectation for persons with older parents is greater than for persons whose parents died earlier. Figure 5 shows that fathers of long-lived sons lived longer than fathers of short-lived sons. Conversely, sons of long-lived fathers live longer than sons of short-lived fathers. Pearl and Pearl (1934) found that the summed ages at death of the six immediate ancestors of centenarians and nonagenarians were significantly greater than those of persons in a control series. Long-lived persons (older than 70 years) had at least one long-lived parent. Of nonagenarians, 48.5% had two such parents, and of centenarians, 53.4% had two long-lived parents. All these figures are significantly higher than those found in control groups. Kallman and Sander (1948, 1949) found that in 1062 pairs of twins, the mean difference in longevity between dizygotic twin persons was twice that found in monozygotics.

These principal lines of evidence, although by no means complete, constitute a reasonable basis for the notion that genetic factors play an important role in those events that lead to the aging and death of individual members of a species. It should be stressed, nevertheless, that nongenetic factors must also play a role in those decrements that lead to manifestations of aging. Changes that occur in molecular structures and biochemical reactions over time are certainly not all governed by genetic events. The cross-linking of collagen may be one good example of the kind of change that occurs over time and that is probably not directly influenced by a genetic program, yet one that might contribute to senescent changes. Thus, at the level of macromolecules, a "program" could be the stability of the macromolecule itself, which does not require any genetic basis. The accumulation of lipofuscin and the denaturation of organelles and enzyme molecules having regular turnover rates may represent other examples of molecular changes occurring over time that do not necessarily require instructions from information-containing molecules. Other extrinsic aging mechanisms are endocrine and neural factors that apparently regulate age changes in target cells (Finch, 1976). However, a clear demonstration that these factors are not under the control of gene expression has not been achieved.

If genetic factors do play a role in longevity, the next question to be answered is: What is the mechanism? Current thought on this question has led to speculation within four general categories:

1. Unprogrammed Senescence
    i. Instability of the genome. This is unprogrammed senescence resulting from the random acquisition of genetic damage.

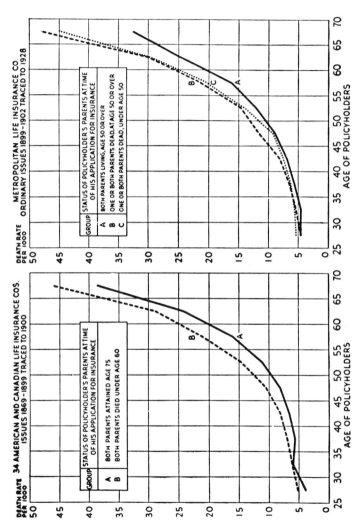

Fig. 4. Inheritance of longevity. Death rates at successive ages among white male policyholders classified according to longevity of parents. (From Dublin *et al.*, 1949.)

612   Leonard Hayflick

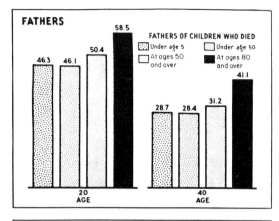

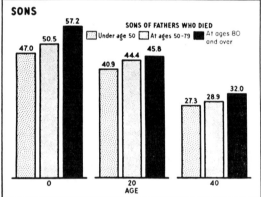

Fig. 5. Expectation of life of (top) fathers according to longevity of their children and (bottom) sons according to longevity of their fathers. (From Dublin *et al.*, 1949.)

ii. Slow accumulation of nongenetic damage, which has a minor influence on a person's survival before reproductive maturity. These events would not cause evolutionary selection of compensating genetic properties.

2. Programmed Senescence

i. The presence of "aging genes," that is, genes that slow down or shut down vital processes. This would be an active process where genes are selected through evolution because they confer a direct advantage to survival of the species but at the expense of individual death.

ii. Programmed senescence where the degenerative processes of aging are accidentally incurred as a passive by-product of the genetic selection of advantageous properties.

A detailed description of several theories applicable to some of the above mechanisms has been published (Hayflick, 1975).

In any consideration of the role of genetics or any other possible root cause of aging, one must come to terms with at least two important biological principles. The first principle is that death from old age is almost certainly confined to man and those animals that he chooses to protect, that is, his domestic or zoo animals. Animals in the wild are generally killed by predators or struck down by disease or accidents well before they show physiological decrements analogous to those expressed in elderly humans. The prolongation of the life span beyond reproductive maturation, therefore, has no survival value for the species. In cold biological terms, persons more than, say, age 40 do not contribute to the biological survival of the species. Says Bidder (1925): "If primitive man begat a son, the species had no more need of him by 37, when his son could hunt for the food for the grandchildren." Aging, in its most profound expressions in man, simply does not occur in wild animals. One must cope with the thought that man's success in dealing with his environment, to the extent that his life expectation is now well beyond the period of reproductive maturity and child-rearing, has simply revealed a Pandora's Box of vicissitudes that were never intended for him to see in the first place.

The second principle that impacts on any consideration of the role of genetics, or any other root cause of aging, is to account for those biological systems that have seemingly escaped from aging's inevitability. These are the continuity of their germ plasm and continuously reproducing abnormal or cancer-cell populations. Why these systems are immortal remains speculation.

VI. MUTATIONS AND AGING

Brown (1979) has reviewed the possible role of mutations in human aging. He considered whether longevity genes exist and whether their mutations effect aging. Sacher and Staffeldt (1974), Sacher (1975, 1976), and Cutler (1975, 1976a, 1979) have discussed the role of genetic changes in the evolution of human longevity. Seemingly, the human life span has doubled in the last 2 million to 3 million years. This estimate is based on the increased ratio of brain weight to body weight, which ratio is thought to correlate well with vertebrate life spans.

Cutler estimates that between 40 and 250 genes could have undergone mutation, which resulted in an adaptive amino acid substitution during the last 2 million to 3 million years. This estimate is based on known rates of amino acid substitutions in several species and the known nucleotide differences found between man and lower primates. The estimate permits a notably small number of structural gene mutations, many of which probably had no important effect on longevity. Alternatively, King and Wilson (1975) suggest that the rapid evolution of increased longevity in primates is due to regulatory changes in levels of certain key enzymes that profoundly affect morphological development and increase brain size.

Brown (1979) points out that indirect evidence from studies on enzyme concentrations, suggests that regulatory mutations may play an important role in the adaptive evolution of higher animals. The concentration of many enzymes in a variety of tissues in homotherms varies by more than an order of magnitude. This variation suggests that regulatory gene mutations govern enzyme levels (Wilson *et al.*, 1977). In the cow, for example, ribonuclease is present in 1200-fold greater concentration per gram of pancreas than in humans. This difference may have resulted from the evolutionary requirement by the cow's digestive system for higher levels of this enzyme to digest RNA from cellulose-metabolizing microorganisms. Regulatory gene mutations may contribute to animal evolution and, in particular, to longevity. The observations of Hart *et al.* (1979) may support this concept, as he finds a good correlation between ultraviolet-induced DNA repair capacity and life span in a broad range of animals. Differences in repair capacity may be due to regulatory variations in the level of common DNA repair enzymes rather than differences in specific enzyme activity (Brown, 1979). No clear evidence exists for the presence of regulatory genes in eukaryotic cells, although such genes have been suggested by Hart to play a role in β-thalassemias. Thus, the contribution of regulatory genes to the evolution of human longevity is, at present, a speculative notion.

VII. GENETIC DISEASES AND HUMAN AGING

Brown (1979) has also discussed the role of genetic factors in the rate of aging in humans. The studies of Jarvik *et al.* (1960) on twins older than 60 years of age are particularly revealing. The mean difference in life span for monozygotic twins was found to be consistently less than that for dizygotic twins. As the twins aged, however, the differences decreased, due perhaps to the approaching maximum life span. Jarvik *et al.* (1960) concluded that dizygotic twins show more variation in their ages at death than do monozygotic twins. The difference was significant only in younger-aged females. Thus, individual genetic factors may tend to shorten life expectation rather than increase it.

About 20% of the human population is thought to suffer from genetic anomalies that contribute to reduced life expectation. These would include familial hyperlipidemias, adult-onset diabetes, juvenile diabetes, α-1 antitrypsin deficiency, and cystic fibrosis. Childs (1975) estimates that 40% of infant mortality is traceable to genetically determined conditions.

Brown (1979) suggests that the abundance of human genetic variations may allow certain mutations to effect longevity genes. Glueck *et al.* (1976) report that the rare autosomal dominant conditions of hypo-β- and hypo-α-lipoproteinemia appear to increase life expectation (not life span) by reducing deaths from myocardial infarction. No single mutation is known to increase human life span, but several mutations reduce it. It is unclear whether life-shortening mutations occur in specific longevity genes or whether the anomalies that they produce only incidentally shorten life.

Martin (1979) has examined McKusick's (1975) catalog of 2336 human autosomal recessive, autosomal dominant, and sex-linked recessive loci. About 7% appear to be involved with the pathobiology of aging. If man has a maximum of 100,000 genetic loci, 7000 loci are probably involved. However, many loci overlap, and Martin concluded that no more than 70 of these 7000 loci are involved in the pathobiology of aging. Apparently, no single gene mutation is involved in longevity, so that aging is most likely polygenic. The kind of genes involved are probably regulator, not structural, genes. That regulator genes may be involved is compatible with the probable role of this kind of gene in the evolution of longevity, as discussed previously (Wilson *et al.*, 1977).

The mechanism by which regulator genes modulate aging is, of course, highly speculative. Martin (1979) suggests that they could enhance rates of enzyme synthesis and maintain the stability of DNA and its associated information-containing molecules.

Burnet (1974) refers to this as the "intrinsic mutagenesis" theory of aging. The basis for this theory is that the genetic loci that account for most of the 40- to 50-fold variation in maximum mammalian life spans are those responsible for quantitative differences in somatic mutation rates. The best candidates for these loci are genes coding for various DNA polymerases, which would be expected to replicate DNA with varying degrees of fidelity, and those genes coding for the several DNA repair systems. As indicated previously, Hart and Setlow (1974) showed a striking positive correlation between the efficiency of excision repair enzyme activity induced by ultraviolet light damage and maximum life span in mammals.

Martin (1979) points out that other loci relevant to the intrinsic mutagenesis hypothesis may be those that participate in the metabolism of premutagens and mutagens, either of endogenous or exogenous origin. Thus, the loci for mixed function oxidases or aryl hydrocarbon hydroxylases would be important because they code for the synthesis of enzymes that convert potential mutagens to proximal mutagens. Schwartz (1975) showed that the ability of cultured cells from several mammalian species to metabolize dimethylbenzanthracene into proximal mutagens does not occur in cells of long-lived species, such as humans or elephants, but does occur in several lower animals in proportion to life span. Perhaps the gene loci associated with excision repair capacity and metabolism of carcinogens influence rates of synthesis through position effects (Martin, 1979).

616

VIII. HUMAN DISEASES WITH ACCELERATED AGING PHENOTYPES

A. Progeria (Hutchinson-Gilford Syndrome)

This rare genetic disease is characterized by acceleration of the aging process. Patients by 1 year of age show growth retardation, balding, and loss of eyebrows and eyelashes. Subcutaneous tissue loss occurs and superficial veins in the scalp become prominent. Ths skin becomes thin with pigmented spots and sclerodermatous changes. Patients are short and the weight-to-height ratio stays low. Complete sexual maturation does not ordinarily occur, and the voice is thin and high-pitched. Features include prominent eyes, beaked nose, cranial-facial disproportionality, small jaw, crowded teeth, large cranium, and remodeling of sutures. The bones show distinctive changes with (1) clavicle resorption and replacement by fibrous tissue, (2) resorption of the terminal phalanges, (3) stiffening of finger joints, and (4) coxa valga, a characteristic "horse riding" stance. Patients have normal or above-average intelligence. The median age of death is 12 years, with more than 80% of deaths attributable to heart disease. Widespread atherosclerosis and interstitial fibrosis of the heart is apparent at autopsy. Some features associated with aging are not found, such as diabetes, increased frequency of tumors, cataracts, and osteoporosis.

Because progeria is rare, the genetics are unclear. The incidence is about one in 8 million live births. Five families have had more than one case each, one involving identical twins (Mostafa and Gabr, 1954; Erecinski *et al.*, 1960; Rava, 1967; Franklin, 1976; Rautenstrauch *et al.*, 1977; Viegus *et al.*, 1974). In two of the five families consanguinity occurred, which is consistent with autosomal recessive inheritance. However, in the remaining 80 cases described, consanguinity occurred in only 6% (Franklin, 1976).

We found that the ability of normal human fibroblasts to replicate in cell cultures was finite (Hayflick and Moorhead, 1961; Hayflick, 1965) and that the number of population doublings was inversely related to donor age (Hayflick, 1976, 1977).

A reduced *in vitro* life span has been reported for cultured fibroblasts derived from patients with progeria (Goldstein, 1969; Danes, 1971; Martin *et al.*, 1970; DeBusk, 1972), but this finding often varies (Brown *et al.*, 1976; Martin *et al.*, 1970; Little *et al.*, 1975; Goldstein and Moerman, 1975). Epstein *et al.* (1974) found diminished DNA repair capacity in X-irradiated progeric cells, and Brown *et al.* (1976, 1977) made similar findings in cells at mid-passage. Rainbow and Howes (1977) also found decreased repair capacity in γ-ray-damaged DNA of cultured progeric cells.

B. Cockayne's Syndrome

This syndrome is a rare autosomal recessive disease with features of premature age (Cockayne, 1936; Schmickel et al., 1977). By 2–4 years of age, growth retardation occurs and the skin shows severe photosensitivity. Additional characteristics include microcephaly, sunken eyes, prominent ears, loss of subcutaneous fat, long arms, big hands, progressive joint deformities, hypogonadism, retinal hyperpigmentation, optic atrophy, deafness, progressive ataxia, intracranial calcification, and frequent neurological deterioration. Death usually occurs in late childhood or early adolescence. Schmickel et al. (1977) report that Cockayne fibroblast cultures show increased sensitivity to ultraviolet irradiation, with normal dimer excision. An enzymatic defect in DNA repair capacity may be present and correlates with the known relationship of DNA repair capacity and species life span. An ultraviolet DNA repair defect may produce an accelerated aging phenotype.

C. Werner's Syndrome

This syndrome is also a rare autosomal recessive disease. It is characterized by growth retardation, short stature, premature graying and loss of hair, cataracts, thin skin, thick subcutaneous tissue, leg ulcers, loss of teeth, osteoporosis, adult-onset diabetes mellitus, and generalized atherosclerosis (Epstein et al., 1966). Some patients develop sarcomas, and the mean age of survival is 47 years. Cultured fibroblasts from these patients have a greatly reduced life span (Martin et al., 1970) and are reported to have an increased level of thermolabile proteins (Goldstein and Moerman, 1975). Normal levels of ultraviolet and X-irradiation damage repair capacity were reported by Fujiwara et al. (1977).

D. Down's Syndrome

Down's syndrome (trisomy 21) patients also show evidence of premature aging. These characteristics include premature graying and loss of hair, increased lipofuscin concentration, neoplasms and leukemia, adipose tissue variations, amyloidosis, increased autoimmune diseases, hypogonadism, degenerative vascular system diseases, cataracts, and senile dementia indistinguishable from Alzheimer's disease in all patients more than age 40 years (Viegus et al., 1974; Smith and Berg, 1976). Only 8% of Down's syndrome patients reach 40 years, and at age 10 years life expectation is 26 years (Smith and Berg, 1976). The etiology of the disease is probably attributable to quantitative differences in gene expression located on chromosome 21 and, perhaps, affecting other genes. This expression differs from the specific qualitative gene defects that may underlie the autosomal diseases of progeria, Cockayne's and Werner's syndromes. The trisomy 21 condition may permit life only because this chromosome is one of the smallest and is thought to have the least number of active genes of any of the autosomes (Martin and Hoehn, 1974).

Cultured Down's syndrome cells also show a diminished capacity to replicate (Schneider and Epstein, 1973). Cultures from other genetic anomalies have also been assessed for replicative capacity compared with that of normal controls. Boué *et al.* (1975) have reported a mean limit of from 20 to 28 population doublings for cells derived from aneuploid human abortuses showing monosomy X, trisomy C, D, G, and triploidy. Normal controls had a mean of 41 population doublings. Although there is considerable scatter in data of this kind, the *in vitro* expression of a reduced population doubling capacity may soon be shown to have useful predictive value in assessing the longevity of anomalous genetic conditions. Variations in gene dosage may lead to accelerated *in vitro* senescence and may also affect mechanisms that regulate the quantitative levels of important enzymes (Brown, 1979). Variations in enzyme levels may produce a phenotype resembling premature aging.

Analyses of human mutations that appear to accelerate age changes may provide important insights into the mechanism that leads to normal age changes.

IX. ANEUPLOIDY AND HUMAN AGING

Jacobs *et al.* (1961) first described a substantial increase in aneuploidy in chromosome studies on human blood lymphocytes. Later, a sex difference in the development of this aneuploidy was reported (Jacobs *et al.*, 1963). A greater proportion of hypodiploid cells was found in females than males, and, instead of showing a linear increase, the data for females fitted a quadratic curve, with a steeper rate of increase of hypodiploidy between the ages of 45 and 64 years than at other times. The chromosome loss apparently is not random, because a disproportionate number of female hypodiploid cells lacked a C-group chromosome. The loss of a Y chromosome from the cells of older males was common, and it was, therefore, proposed that the chromosome lost frequently from the female cells might be an X chromosome (Jacobs *et al.*, 1963). The increase in hyperdiploidy also involved a large number of cells with an extra C-group chromosome. A number of subsequent studies have confirmed and extended these observations (Jacobs *et al.*, 1964; Hamerton *et al.*, 1965; Sandberg *et al.*, 1967; Goodman *et al.*, 1969; Jarvik and Kato, 1970; Jarvik *et al.*, 1974, 1976; Mattevi and Salzano, 1975). Some discrepancies are reported, but there is general agreement that proportions of hypodiploid cells increase with age and that this is more pronounced in females than in males. The study of a Japanese population by Bloom *et al.* (1967) is at variance with these reports, because no significant age-associated change in aneuploidy was found. All of these reports used conventional staining techniques that did not permit the identification of each chromosome pair. Galloway and Buckton (1978) examined a random sample of the general population using the newer banding techniques to identify each chromosome lost, gained, or involved in rearrangements. This study confirmed that the incidence of hypodiploid blood lymphocytes increased with age in males and females. In females, hyperdiploid levels also rise, although such cells were much less common than were hypodiploid cells. The cells reported in previous studies as having lost or gained a C-group chromosome are, in fact, 45 X and 47 XXX cells.

Galloway and Buckton (1978) also showed that the total number of cells missing chromosomes of groups other than the C group also rises significantly with age. In females, the occurrence of a "fragment" of an X chromosome also correlated with increasing age, and this "fragment" appears to be an X chromosome that has divided prematurely at the centromere.

As is often the case in studies of this kind, it is uncertain whether these chromosome changes are a cause or an effect of the aging process. The timing of the aneuploid change in females correlates with hormonal changes that occur at menopause (Jacobs et al., 1963), in thyroid autoimmunity (Fialkow, 1970), and, possibly, in high blood pressure (Pero et al., 1976). These chromosome studies show large individual variations in proportions of abnormal karyotypes, and Galloway and Buckton (1978) suggest that the observed aneuploidy may reflect (1) nondisjunction due to a mutation in the normal mitotic control mechanism; (2) changes in membrane fragility; (3) somatic mutation; or (4) an accumulation of errors in translation and transcription.

X. CURRENT THEORIES OF BIOLOGICAL AGING

Probably no other area of biological inquiry is underpinned by so many theories as is the science of gerontology. This abundance of theories is due not only to the lack of sufficient fundamental data in the field, but also to the manifestations of biological changes that with time affect almost all biological systems from the molecular level to the whole organism.

Because biological aging is thought to emanate from changes commencing at the molecular level, and thence up to the level of the whole animal, theories based on changes occurring at each increasingly greater level of complexity have been advanced. If the modern notions of biological development are rooted in signals originating from information-containing molecules, attributing fundamental causes of aging to similar molecular events would seem reasonable. Although many age changes, like developmental processes, occur at complexities greater than those at the genetic or epigenetic level, the root causes of senescence seemingly should have a genetic basis also. Or, at the least, they must be the result of fundamental changes that occur in information-containing molecules. If this supposition is to be believed, then those classes of theories of biological aging that are based on observations made at the supramolecular level (for example, organelle, cell, tissue, and organ changes) are not likely to yield information on those fundamental molecular events that are presumed to be the essential variables leading to manifestations of aging at all higher organizational levels.

For this reason I have chosen to restrict this discussion to those theories of aging that depend on molecular changes at the genetic or epigenetic level.

A. Error Theories

In 1963, Orgel proposed a model for biological aging that was based on a decrease in the fidelity of protein synthesis. This notion was first postulated by Medvedev (1961). Protein synthesis involves two steps in which discrimination between related molecules occurs. A unique amino acid must be selected by each activating enzyme, and it must be attached to the appropriate tRNA. A codon of messenger RNA must then pair with the anticodon of an appropriate tRNA. These processes are probably prone to a small degree of error. The fidelity of protein synthesis could also be decreased by errors in RNA synthesis (Orgel, 1963, 1973). A repetition of events such as these, in which errors in proteins occur, could result in a convergence to a stable value of errors or it would diverge. If the former were the case, aging would not occur. In the latter case, the error frequency would eventually become great enough to impair cell function. Although Orgel originally supported the latter possibility, he has now abandoned that position for this reason: a protein-synthesizing system containing a small number of errors might be capable of synthesizing a new protein-synthesizing system containing fewer errors. That such is the case is more plausible in view of evidence for the existence of enzymes capable of scavenging error-containing proteins (Goldberg, 1972). In *Neurospora,* one case of direct evidence exists for protein error frequencies increasing to the point where cell death ensues (Printz and Gross, 1967). This "error-catastrophe" hypothesis is also supported by evidence obtained by Lewis and Holliday (1970), who showed that the accuracy of protein synthesis in Leu-5 in *Neurospora* falls when the mutant is shifted from 25° to 35°C and then remains virtually constant. After about 70 hours, cell aging occurs rapidly with a simultaneous increase in the thermostability of glutamic dehydrogenase and a concomitant dramatic drop in the specific activity of this enzyme. Another conjecture is that distinguishing contributions to cellular aging caused by errors in protein synthesis from those due to an accumulation of somatic mutations may not be possible. Inaccurate protein synthesis may be indistinguishable from inaccurate DNA synthesis, and in that sense they may be coupled phenomena (Orgel, 1973). The accuracy of one process may depend completely on the fidelity of the other. Orgel now subscribes to this more general notion, in which positive feedback occurs whereby "the greater the number of errors that have accumulated in the macromolecular constituents of the cell, the faster the accumulation of further errors" (Orgel, 1973). It is also envisioned that extracellular and intracellular mechanisms of aging are coupled, because inaccurate protein synthesis must affect extracellular events.

B. Redundant Message Theory

Medvedev is the chief proponent of a notion that has considerable merit as a fundamental theory of biological aging. He proposes that the selective repetitions of some definite genes, cistrons, operons, and other linear structures on the DNA molecule, the bulk of which are repressed, behave as redundant messages to be called into action when active genome messages become faulty (Medvedev, 1972). He argues that the total genome of mammals is composed of not fewer than 10^5 structural genes or cistrons, but that in each cell hardly more than 0.2–0.4% of those genes are expressed during biological development and maturity. If 1/500 of all genes are active and 499/500 are specifically repressed, and if mutagenic factors act equally on the repressed and active cistrons, the mutation rate of repressed genes must yield more mutations than those occurring in active genes. Medvedev asserts that the life spans of different species may be a function of the degree of repeated sequences. Long-lived species should then have more redundant message than short-lived species. As errors accumulate in functioning genes, reserve sequences containing the same information take over until the redundancy in the system is exhausted, resulting in biological age changes. The differences in species' life spans is then thought to be a manifestation of the degree of gene repetition (Medvedev, 1972). That gene repetition may be a universal mechanism for phylogenetic evolution in eukaryotes has, of course, been suggested (Britten and Kohne, 1968a,b, 1969).

Thus, the phenomenon of linear repetition of some genes can have not only evolutionary, but also gerontological, implications where a protective role of gene repetition against random molecular accidents occurs. Conceptually this phenomenon has merit not only as an explanation for the wide differences found in the life span of species but also for the less variable life span of individual members within a species. A repeated nucleotide sequence simply has a greater chance of preserving intact the final gene product during evolution or during a long life span than does any unique sequence. It follows, therefore, that if errors accumulate in unique genes then age changes may result from this kind of event. Certainly not all unique genes could be expected to have equal value for cell function or maintenance of cell life. The vital unique sequences are likely to be restricted to some universally important genes of general metabolism. They may represent the essential group of genes whose failure ultimately results in manifestations of biological aging. Medvedev prefers the view that the derepression of unique genes during postembryonal or adult stages in development are the real initiators of age changes. This derepression would be a manifestation of the deterioration with time of nonrepeated nucleotide sequences.

The theory that aging is due to the accumulation of gene mutations and chromosome anomalies has many supporters (Burnet, 1973, 1974; Curtis, 1966; Szilard, 1959). Despite this support, the failure of this theory to explain the quantitative aspects of normal and radiation-induced aging has been repeatedly observed (Alexander, 1966; Clark, 1964; Strehler, 1959).

C. Control of Age Changes by Transcriptional Events

This thesis, championed by von Hahn (1970), suggests that the control of cellular aging is functional at the level of the transcription of genetic information from DNA into the intermediary messenger RNA. This notion maintains that (1) with increasing age, deleterious changes occur in the metabolism of differentiated postmitotic cells; (2) the alterations are the result of primary events occurring within the nuclear chromatin; (3) in the nuclear chromatin complex exists a control mechanism responsible for the appearance and the sequence of the primary aging events; and (4) this control mechanism involves the regulation of transcription, although other regulated events may occur.

Von Hahn notes that several *a priori* assumptions are involved in this hypothesis, the most important being that a universal physiological aging process exists, one that is deleterious to the cell, due to intrinsic causes, and progressively acting with increasing chronological age. These are the essential criteria characterizing biological aging that have been proposed by Strehler (1977) and appear to be generally valid.

The central event of aging, at whatever level of biological complexity, seems to be the progressive diminution in adaptation to stress and in the system's capacity to maintain the homeostatic equilibrium characteristic of the adult animal at maturity (Comfort, 1968).

Von Hahn suggests that two types of primary events, previously referred to here in another context, can interfere with transcription. One is genetically controlled and is based on a genetic program, and the other is random, involving stochastic processes similar to those discussed in the "error hypothesis."

Von Hahn offers data suggesting that an age-related increase in the stability of the DNA double helix depends on the presence and degree of binding of certain proteins. In old nucleoprotein, a particular protein fraction is bound to DNA in such a way as to increase the energy required for the separation of the two strands in the helix. Because strand separation is an essential step in transcription, blocking the process will block transcription, leading to a loss of genetic information within the cell.

D. Proliferating and Nonproliferating Cells

Most gerontologists agree that there is probably no single cause of aging. A phenomenon that probably comes close to a unifying theory relates to those concepts based on genetic instability as a cause of aging. Also, the genetic contribution to the aging process seems foremost in determining a life span that is characteristic of each species. This is so because the range of variation in the maximum life span among different species is obviously much greater than the range of individual life spans within the species. One fundamental problem in relating genetic processes to aging is to attempt to separate the genetic basis of differentiation from a possible genetic basis for aging. I believe that a distinction should be drawn, at least operationally, between processes of development and of aging—or the concept of "first we ripen, and then we rot."

In metazoan aging, we are concerned essentially with three types of cell populations. The first are fixed postmitotics, represented by neurons and muscle cells that are essentially unable to divide. A second category includes slowly dividing cells, for example, those found in the liver. The third group would be intermitotic cells, those that divide at a faster rate, that is, fibroblasts and blast cells generally.

To illustrate the processes by which these last two categories of dividing cells replicate, one can use essentially three types of proliferative cell populations. The first would be a population whose numbers increase with time, for example, embryonic tissue or tumor tissue, the latter case exemplifying antisocial behavior. The second type of proliferation would be a steady-state renewal system, where the rate of cell death equals the rate of cell birth, for example, the hair follicles in the skin. Finally, one population might decrease in numbers, perhaps programmed as a part of differentiation, for example, the cells massively destroyed during vertebrate embryogenesis (Saunders, 1966) or in the thymus.

Genetic instability as a process can be further subdivided. One category is the progressive functional deterioration of these fixed postmitotic cells. The second is the progressive accumulation of faulty copying in dividing cells, or the accumulation of errors. These errors can be categorized as previously described. A third class consists of cross-linking effects in information-carrying molecules postulated by von Hahn (1970), which is relevant not only with respect to DNA but to RNA as well. Cross-linkages occurring between proteins and DNA are known, and this concept of permanent gene repression may be responsible for the manifestations of aging, where repressors are irreversibly bound to structural genes.

The progressive accumulation of errors in function of either fixed postmitotics or actively dividing cells could act as a clock. This process would initiate secondary types of mischief that would ultimately be manifest as biological aging as we know it. Thus, aging could be a special case of morphogenesis. Cells may be programmed simply to run out of program.

E. Functional and Mitotic Failure

We may call the lapse of time during which these results become manifest as the "mean time to failure." The concept of mean time to failure has a precise relevance to the deterioration of mechanical as well as biological systems, and it can be simply illustrated by considering the mean times to failure of, for example, automobiles. The mean time to failure may be 5–6 years, which may be extended or decreased by the competence of repair processes. Barring total replacement of all vital elements, deterioration is inevitable. Similarly, the progressive decrease in the adequacy of the cellular transcription mechanism may ultimately result in a catastrophe of errors in which cell function or cell division is impaired or wrongly directed.

By virtue of the fact that biological activities (and repair mechanisms) are imperfect, we are led to conclude that the ultimate death of a cell, or loss or misdirection of its functionality, is a programmed event having a mean time to failure. Just as mechanical systems of different purpose have different mean times to failure, I have proposed that such differences have their counterpart in informational molecules. Consequently, the mean time to failure may ultimately be applicable to a single cell, clone, tissue, organ, or the intact animal itself. It is proposed that the genetic mechanism simply runs out of accurate program, which results in a mean time to failure of all the dependent biological systems.

The different average life spans for each animal species and among the cells, tissues, and organs of different animals may be the manifestation of the evolution of more perfect repair mechanisms in those biological systems having greater longevity.

In what way can we fit this concept to account for those biological systems that, seemingly, have escaped from the inevitability of aging? Specifically, one must consider the continuity of the germ plasm and continuously propagable or transplantable tumor cell populations. Cancer cells can replicate indefinitely *in vitro* and *in vivo*. Is it possible that cancer cells, unlike normal cells, can exchange genetic information, thereby ensuring their apparent immortality? Gametes do not have an unlimited propensity to multiply unless they unite to form a zygote. Thus, the exchange of genetic material may serve to program or to reset a more perfect biological clock. By this mechanisms, species' survival is guaranteed but the individual animal is ultimately programmed to failure.

ACKNOWLEDGMENTS

This work was supported in part by the Glenn Foundation for Medical Research, Manhasset, New York, and by Grant 1 RO1 AG 00850 from the National Institute on Aging, National Institutes of Health.

REFERENCES

Alexander, P. (1966). Is there a relationship between aging, the shortening of life-span by radiation and the induction of somatic mutations? *In* "Perspectives in Experimental Gerontology" (N. W. Shock, ed.), pp. 266–279. Thomas, Springfield, Illinois.

Bidder, G. P. (1925). The mortality of plaice. *Nature (London)* **115**, 495.

Bloom, A. D., Archer, P. G., and Awa, A. A. (1967). Variation in the human chromosome number. *Nature (London)* **216**, 487–489.

Boué, A., Boué, J., Cure, S., Deluchat, C., and Perraudin, N. (1975). *In vitro* cultivation of cells from aneuploid human embryos: inhibition of cell lines and longevity of the cultures. *In Vitro* **11**, 409–415.

Britten, R. J., and Kohne, D. E. (1968a). Repeated nucleotide sequences. *Year Book—Carnegie Inst. Washington* **66**, 73–88.

Britten, R. J., and Kohen, D. E. (1968b). Repeated sequences in DNA. *Science* **161**, 529–540.

Britten, R. J., and Kohne, D. E. (1969). Repetition of nucleotide sequences in chromosomal DNA: implications of repeated nucleotide sequences. *In* "Handbook of Molecular Cytology" (A. Lima-de-Faria, ed.), pp. 21–51. North-Holland Publ., Amsterdam.

Brown, W. T. (1979). Human mutations affecting aging—a review. *Mech. Ageing Dev.* **9**, 325–336.

Brown, W. T., Epstein, J., and Little, J. B. (1976). Progeria cells are stimulated to repair DNA by co-cultivation with normal cells. *Exp. Cell Res.* **97**, 291–296.

Brown, W. T., Little, J. B., Epstein, J., and Williams, J. R. (1977). DNA repair defect in progeria cells. *Birth Defects, Orig. Artic. Ser.* **13**.

Burnet, M. J. (1973). A genetic interpretation of aging. *Lancet* **ii**, 480–483.

Burnet, M. J. (1974). "Intrinsic Mutagenesis: A Genetic Approach to Aging." Wiley, New York.

Childs, B. (1975). Prospects for genetic screening. *J. Pediatr.* **87**, 1125–1132.

Clark, A. M. (1964). Genetic factors associated with aging. *In* "Advances in Gerontological Research" (B. L. Strehler, ed.), pp. 207–255. Academic Press, New York.

Clarke, J. M., and Maynard Smith, J. (1955). The genetics and cytology of *Drosophila subobscura*, XI. Hybrid vigor and longevity. *J. Genet.* **53**, 172.

Cockayne, E. A. (1936). Dwarfism with retinal atrophy and deafness. *Arch. Dis. Child.* **11**, 1–5.

Comfort, A. (1968). Physiology, homeostasis and ageing. *Gerontologia* **14**, 224–234.

Comfort, A. (1979). "The Biology of Senescence," 3rd ed. Elsevier/North Holland, New York.

Curtis, H. J. (1966). The possibility of increased longevity by the control of mutations. *In* "Perspectives in Experimental Gerontology" (N. W. Shock, ed.), pp. 257–265. Thomas, Springfield, Illinois.

Cutler, R. G. (1975). Evolution of human longevity and the genetic complexity governing aging rate. *Proc. Natl. Acad. Sci. U.S.A.* **72**, 4664–4668.

Cutler, R. G. (1976a). Evolution of longevity in primates. *J. Hum. Evol.* **5**, 169–202.

Cutler, R. G. (1976b). Nature of aging and life maintenance processes. *In* "Interdisciplinary Topics of Gerontology" (R. G. Cutler, ed.), Vol. 9, pp. 83–133. Karger, Basel.

Cutler, R. G. (1979). Evolution of human longevity: a critical overview. *Mech. Ageing Dev.* **9**, 337–354.

Danes, B. S. (1971). Progeria: a cell culture study on aging. *J. Clin. Invest.* **50**, 2000–2003.

DeBusk, F. L. (1972). The Hutchinson–Gilford progeria syndrome. *J. Pediatr.* **80**, 697–724.

Dublin, L. I., Lotka, A. J., and Spiegelman, M. (1949). "Length of Life." Ronald Press, New York.

Epstein, C. J., Martin, G. M., Schultz, A. L., and Motulsky, A. G. (1966). Werner's syndrome: a review of its symptomatology, natural history, pathologic features, genetics and relationship to the natural aging process. *Medicine (Baltimore)* **45**, 177–221.

Epstein, J., Williams, J. R., and Little, J. B. (1974). Rate of DNA repair in progeria and normal fibroblasts. *Biochem. Biophys. Res. Commun.* **59**, 850–857.

Erecinski, K., Bittel-Dobrzynska, N., and Mostowiec, S. (1960). Zespol progeril u dwoch braci. *Pol. Tyg. Lek.* **16**, 806.

Fialkow, P. J. (1970). Thyroid autoimmunity and Down's syndrome. *Ann. N.Y. Acad. Sci.* **171**, 500–511.

Finch, C. E. (1976). The regulation of physiological changes during mammalian aging. *Q. Rev. Biol.* **51**, 49–83.

Franklin, P. P. (1976). Progeria in siblings. *Clin. Radiol.* **27**, 327–333.

Fujiwara, Y., Higashikawa, T., and Tatsum, M. (1977). A retarded rate of DNA replication and normal level of DNA repair in Werner's syndrome fibroblasts in culture. *J. Cell. Physiol.* **92**, 365–374.

Galloway, S. M., and Buckton, K. E. (1978). Aneuploidy and ageing: chromosome studies on a random sample of the population using G-banding. *Cytogenet. Cell Genet.* **20**, 78–95.

Glueck, C. J., Gartside, P., Fallat, R. W., Sieski, J., and Steiner, P. M. (1976). Longevity syndromes: familial hypobeta and familial hyperalpha lipoproteinemia. *J. Lab. Clin. Med.* **88**, 941–957.

Goldberg, A. J. (1972). Degradation of abnormal proteins in Escherichia coli. *Proc. Natl. Acad. Sci. U.S.A.* **69**, 422–426.

Goldstein, S. (1969). Life-span of cultured cells in progeria. *Lancet* **i**, 424.

Goldstein, S., and Moerman, E. (1975). Heat-labile enzymes in skin fibroblasts from subjects with progeria. *N. Engl. J. Med.* **292**, 1305–1309.

Gompertz, B. (1825). On the nature of the function expressive of the law of human mortality and on a new mode of determining life contingencies. *Philos. Trans. R. Soc. London, Ser. A* **115**, 513–585.

Goodman, R., Fechheimer, N., Miller, F., Miller, R., and Zartman, O. (1969). Chromosomal alterations in three age groups of human females. *Am. J. Med. Sci.* **258**, 26–33.

Hamerton, J. L., Taylor, A. I., Angell, R., and McGuire, V. M. (1965). Chromosome investigations of a small isolated human population: chromosome abnormalities and distribution of chromosome counts according to age and sex among the population of Tristan da Cunha. *Nature (London)* **206**, 1232–1234.

Hamilton, J. B. (1948). The role of testicular secretions as indicated by the effects of castration in man and by studies of pathological conditions and the short lifespan associated with maleness. *Recent Prog. Horm. Res.* **3**, 257–322.

Hart, R. W., and Setlow, R. B. (1974). Correlation between deoxyribonucleic acid excision-repair and life-span in a number of mammalian species. *Proc. Natl. Acad. Sci. U.S.A.* **71**, 2169–2173.

Hart, R. W., D'Ambrosio, S. M., and Ng, K. J. (1979). Longevity, stability and DNA repair. *Mech. Ageing Dev.* **9**, 203–223.

Hayflick, L. (1965). The limited *in vitro* lifetime of human diploid cell strains. *Exp. Cell Res.* **37**, 614–636.

Hayflick, L. (1975). Current theories of biological aging. *Fed. Proc., Fed. Am. Soc. Exp. Biol.* **34**, 9-13.

Hayflick, L. (1976). The cell biology of human aging. *N. Engl. J. Med.* **295**, 1302-1308.

Hayflick, L. (1977). The cellular basis for biological aging. *In* "Handbook of the Biology of Aging" (C. Finch and L. Hayflick, eds.), pp. 159-186. Van Nostrand-Reinhold, New York.

Hayflick, L., and Moorhead, P. S. (1961). The serial cultivation of human diploid cell strains. *Exp. Cell Res.* **25**, 585-621.

Jacobs, P. A., Court Brown, W. M., and Doll, R. (1961). Distribution of human chromosome counts in relation to age. *Nature (London)* **191**, 1178-1180.

Jacobs, P. A., Brunton, M., Court Brown, W. M., and Doll, R. (1963). Change of human chromosome count distribution with age: evidence for a sex difference. *Nature (London)* **197**, 1080-1081.

Jacobs, P. A., Brunton, M., and Court Brown, W. M. (1964). Cytogenetic studies in leucocytes on the general population: subjects aged 65 years or more. *Ann. Hum. Genet.* **27**, 353-365.

Jarvik, L. F., and Kato, T. (1970). Chromosome examinations in aged twins. *Am. J. Hum. Genet.* **22**, 563-573.

Jarvik, L. F., Falek, A., Kallmann, F. J., and Lorge, I. (1960). Survival trends in a senescent twin population. *Am. J. Hum. Genet.* **12**, 170-179.

Jarvik, L. F., Yen, F. S., and Moralishvili, E. (1974). Chromosome examinations in ageing institutionalized women. *J. Gerontol.* **29**, 269-276.

Jarvik, L. F., Yen, F., Fu, T., and Matsuyama, S. S. (1976). Chromosomes in old age: a six year longitudinal study. *Hum. Genet.* **33**, 17-22.

Kallman, F. J., and Sander, G. (1948). Twins studies on aging and longevity. *J. Hered.* **39**, 349.

Kallman, F. J., and Sander, G. (1949). Twin studies in senescence. *Am. J. Psychiatry* **106**, 29.

King, M. C., and Wilson, A. C. (1975). Evolution at two levels in humans and chimpanzees. *Science* **188**, 107-116.

Levy, W. H. (1957). "The Pigeon." Sumter, South Carolina.

Lewis, C. M., and Holliday, R. (1970). Mistranslation and ageing in Neurospora. *Nature (London)* **228**, 877-880.

Little, J. B., Epstein, J., and Williams, J. R. (1975). Repair of DNA strand breaks in progeria fibroblasts and aging human diploid cells. *In* "Mechanisms for the Repair of DNA" (R. B. Setlow, ed.), pp. 793-799. Plenum, New York.

McKusick, V. A. (1975). "Mendelian Inheritance in Man," 4th ed. Johns Hopkins Press, Baltimore, Maryland.

Martin, G. M. (1979). Genetic and evolutionary aspects of aging. *Fed. Proc., Fed. Am. Soc. Exp. Biol.* **38**, 1962-1967.

Martin, G. M., and Hoehn, H. (1974). Genetics and human disease. *Hum. Pathol.* **6**, 387-405.

Martin, G. M., Sprague, C. A., and Epstein, C. J. (1970). Replicative life-span of cultivated human cells: effects of donor's age, tissue, and genotype. *Lab. Invest.* **23**, 86-92.

Mattevi, M. S., and Salzano, F. M. (1975). Senescence and human chromosome changes. *Humangenetik* **27**, 1-8.

Maynard Smith, J. (1959). Rate of ageing in Drosophila subobscura. *Ciba Found. Colloq. Aging* **5**, 269-281.

Medvedev, Z. A. (1961). Aging of the body on the molecular level. *Usp. Sovrem. Biol.* **51**, 299-316.

Medvedev, Z. A. (1972). Repetition of molecular-genetic information as a possible factor in evolutionary changes of life-span. *Exp. Gerontol.* **7**, 227-238.

Medvedev, Z. A. (1974). Caucasus and Altay longevity: a biological or social problem? *Gerontologist* **14**, 381-387.

Mostafa, A. H., and Gabr, M. (1954). Hereditary progeria with follow-up of two affected sisters. *Arch. Pediatr.* **71**, 163–172.

Oliff, W. D. (1953). The mortality, fecundity and intrinsic rate of natural increase of the multimammate mouse *Rattus (Mastomys) natelensis* Smith in the laboratory. *J. Anim. Ecol.* **22**, 217.

Orgel, L. E. (1963). The maintenance of the accuracy of protein synthesis and its relevance to aging. *Proc. Natl. Acad. Sci. U.S.A.* **49**, 517–521.

Orgel, L. E. (1973). Aging of clones of mammalian cells. *Nature (London)* **243**, 441–445.

Pearl, R., and Pearl, R. de W. (1934). "The Ancestry of the Long-Lived." H. Milford, London.

Pearl, R., Parker, S. L., and Gonzales, B. M. (1923). Experimental studies on the duration of life VII. The mendalian inheritance of duration of life in crosses of wild type and quintuple stocks of *Drosophila melanogaster*. *Am. Nat.* **57**, 153–192.

Pero, R. W., Bryngelsson, C., Mittelman, F., Thulin, T., and Norden, A. (1976). High blood pressure related to carcinogen induced unscheduled DNA synthesis, DNA carcinogen binding, and chromosomal aberrations in human lymphocytes. *Proc. Natl. Acad. Sci. U.S.A.* **73**, 2496–2500.

Printz, D. B., and Gross, S. R. (1967). An apparent relationship between mistranslation and an altered leucyl-tRNA synthetase in a conditional lethal mutant of *Neurospora crassa*. *Genetics* **55**, 451–467.

Rainbow, A. J., and Howes, M. (1977). Decreased repair of gamma ray damaged DNA in progeria. *Biochem. Biophys. Res. Commun.* **74**, 714–719.

Rautenstrauch, T., Shigula, F., Kreig, T., Gay, S., and Muller, P. V. (1977). Progeria: a cell culture study and clinical report of familial incidence. *Eur. J. Pediatr.* **124**, 101–111.

Rava, G. (1967). Su un nucleo familiare de progeria. *Minerva Med.* **58**, 1502–1509.

Sacher, G. A. (1975). Maturation and longevity and relation to the cranial capacity in hominid evolution. *In* "Antecedents of Man and After. I. Primates: Functional Morphology and Evolution" (R. Tuttle, ed.), pp. 417–441. Montox, The Hague.

Sacher, G. A. (1976). Evaluation of the ectrophy and information terms governing mammalian longevity. *In* "Interdisciplinary Topics of Gerontology," (R. G. Cutler, ed.), Vol. 9, pp. 69–82. Karger, Basel.

Sacher, G. A., and Staffeldt, E. F. (1974). Relationship of gestation time to brain weight for placental mammals: implications for the theory of vertebrate growth. *Am. Nat.* **108**, 593–615.

Sandberg, A. A., Cohen, M. M., Rimm, A. A., and Levin, M. L. (1967). Aneuploidy and age in a population survey. *Am. J. Hum. Genet.* **19**, 633–643.

Saunders, J. W. (1966). Cell death in embryos: Accelerated senescence? *In* "Topics in the Biology of Aging" (P. L. Krohn, ed.), pp. 159–169. Wiley (Interscience), New York.

Schmickel, R. D., Chu, E. H. Y., Trosko, J. E., and Chang, C. C. (1977). Cockayne syndrome: a cellular sensitivity to ultraviolet light. *Pediatrics* **60**, 135–139.

Schneider, E. L., and Epstein, C. J. (1973). Replication rate and life-span of cultured fibroblasts in Down's syndrome. *Proc. Soc. Exp. Biol. Med.* **141**, 1092–1094.

Schwartz, A. G. (1975). Correlation between species life-span and capacity to activate 7, 12-dimethylbenz(a)anthracene to a form mutagenic to a mammalian cell. *Exp. Cell Res.* **94**, 445–447, 1975.

Siegel, J. S. (1976). "Demographic Aspects of Aging and the Older Population in the United States," Current Population Reports, Special Studies, Series P-23, No. 59. U.S. Gov. Print. Off., Washington, D.C.

Smith, G. F., and Berg, J. M. (1976). "Down's Anomaly," pp. 239–245. Churchill-Livingstone, Edinburgh.

Strehler, B. L. (1959). Origin and comparison of the effects of time and high-energy radiations on living systems. *Q. Rev. Biol.* **34**, 117–142.

Strehler, B. L. (1977). "Time, Cells and Aging," 2nd ed. Academic Press, New York.

Strehler, B. L., and Mildvan, A. S. (1960). General theory of mortality and aging. *Science* **132**, 14–21.

Szilard, L. (1959). On the nature of the aging process. *Proc. Natl. Acad. Sci. U.S.A.* **45**, 30–45.

U.S. Bureau of the Census (1973). "Some Demographic Aspects of Aging in the United States," Current Population Reports, Series P-23, No. 43. U.S. Gov. Print. Off., Washington, D.C.

U.S. Public Health Service, National Center for Health Statistics, "U.S. Life Tables by Causes of Death: 1969–71," by T. N. E. Greville; *ibid*. "U.S. Decennial Life Tables for 1969–71," Vol. 1, No. 5, 1976.

Viegus, J., Souza, P. L. R., and Salzanio, F. M. (1974). Progeria in twins, *J. Med. Genet.* **11**, 384–386.

von Hahn, H. P. (1970). The regulation of protein synthesis in the aging cell. *Exp. Gerontol.* **5**, 323–334.

Wilson, A. C., Carlson, S. S., and White, T. J. (1977). Biochemical evolution. *Annu. Rev. Biochem.* **46**, 573–639.

Woolley, G. (1946). *In* Hamilton, J. B. (1948). *Recent Prog. Horm. Res.* **3**, 257.

Index

A

Aarskog syndrome, in Scandinavia, 391
Abetalipoproteinemia, among Jews, 539
ABO blood group system, *see* Blood groups
Acatalasemia, in Japan, 313–314
Accidents
    acculturation and, 586
    in Eastern Europe, 465
    in Western Europe, 419
    rural, 441
Acculturation, of isolates, changing disease patterns and, 585–587
Acheiropodia, in Latin America, 284
Achlorhydria, among Amerinds, 212
Achondroplasia, in Western Europe, 450
Achromatopsia, *see* Color blindness
Acrodermatitis enteropathica, in Scandinavia, 391
Acropigmentatio reticularis, in Japan, 318–319
Acute intermittent porphyria (AIP), in Finland, 385
Acute myocardial infarction (AMI), among Amerinds, 209, 210–211
Adaptation, 14–15
    disease concept and, 70
Adrenal hyperplasias
    congenital
        human leukocyte antigens and, 115
        in Finland, 385
        among Jews, 548
    in Western Europe, 450
Adrenogenital syndrome, in Western Europe, 451
Africa, colonization of, disease and, 163–166
Africans, *see* Black Africans

Age
    causes of death in Western Europe and, 419–423
    Kaposi's sarcoma and, 511
    parental, senescence and, 610–613
    oral contraception and, in Western Europe, 444, 445
Agglutination
    ABO blood group system and, 97
    immunoglobulin allotypes and, 110
Aging, 599–600
    accelerated, diseases associated with, 616–618
    aneuploidy and, 618–619
    current theories of, 619–620
        error theories, 620–621
        functional and mitotic failure, 624
        proliferating and nonproliferating cells, 623–624
        redundant message theory, 621–622
        transcriptional events, 622–623
    demographic projections and, 603–606
    in Eastern Europe, 465–466
    effects of disease resolution on, 600–602
    genetic basis for, 608
        hybrid vigor and, 609
        parental age and, 610–613
        sex and, 609–610
        species-specific life spans and, 608–609
    genetic diseases and, 614–615
    mutations and, 613–614
    in Russia, 606–608
Agriculture, disease patterns and, 259–260, 264–265
AGU, *see* Aspartylglucosaminuria
Akoko, disease concept of, 516